DENTAL MANAGEMENT OF THE MEDICALLY COMPROMISED PATIENT

DENTAL MANAGEMENT OF THE MEDICALLY COMPROMISED PATIENT

JAMES W. LITTLE, D.M.D., M.S.

Professor of Oral Diagnosis and Radiology
University of Minnesota School of Dentistry
Minneapolis, Minnesota

DONALD A. FALACE, D.M.D.

Section Leader, Oral Diagnosis
Department of Oral Health Science
The University of Kentucky College of Dentistry
Lexington, Kentucky

FOURTH EDITION

*With **234** illustrations*

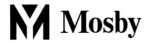

St. Louis Baltimore Boston Chicago London Philadelphia Sydney Toronto

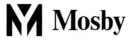

Publisher: George Stamathis
Editor-in-Chief: Don Ladig
Executive Editor: Linda L. Duncan
Assistant Editor: Melba Steube
Project Manager: John Rogers
Production Editor: George B. Stericker, Jr.
Designer: Gail Morey Hudson
Manufacturing Supervisor: Theresa Fuchs

FOURTH EDITION

Printed in the United States of America

Mosby–Year Book, Inc.
11830 Westline Industrial Drive St. Louis, Missouri 63146

Library of Congress Cataloging in Publication Data

Little, James W., 1934–
    Dental management of the medically compromised patient / James W.
  Little, Donald A. Falace.—4th ed.
      p.   cm.
    Includes bibliographical references and index.
    ISBN 0-8016-6837-9
    1. Sick—Dental care.   2. Chronically ill—Dental care.   3. Oral
  manifestations of general diseases.   I. Falace, Donald A., 1945–
    II. Title.
    [DNLM: 1. Dental Care.   2. Diseases.   3. Oral Manifestations.   WU
29 L778d]
  RK55.S53l57   1993
  617.6–dc20
  DNLM/DLC   92-48217
  for Library of Congress   CIP

93 94 95 96 97 GW/DC 9 8 7 6 5 4 3 2 1

Dedicated to the memory
of
my teacher, friend, and dad,

James A. Little

Foreword

The dental management of medically compromised patients continues to assume increased importance in oral health care delivery. There are many reasons for this, but foremost is the expanding senior citizen group, with those over 65 accounting for about 13% of America's population, which is expected to grow to 20% slightly beyond the year 2000. With extended longevity, there is an inevitable increase in diseases and disabilities, which will demand larger responsiblilities from and lay greater burdens on health care delivery. Extended longevity will be accompanied by an increase in the use of medicines. In turn, there will be a continual growth in the number of individuals both seeking and in need of oral health care, which will lead to a concomitant expansion of patients with a variety of health risks that influence dental-oral diseases and treatment.

Some examples of diseases that will affect dental care in the years ahead are cancer, blood dyscrasias, diabetes, transplants and implants, atherosclerosis, and cardiomyopathy. Regarding the last two, although they remain the leading cause of mortality in the United States, the number of deaths from atherosclerotic heart disease is decreasing, which indicates that more Americans are living in this somewhat compromised state and stresses the need for knowledge in this area in order to deliver optimal care and minimize problems related to dental health and treatment. The most dramatic example of medical-dental interaction relates to infectious disease epidemics that strike both the young and the elderly. Therefore, knowledge and understanding of the human immunodeficiency and hepatitis-B viruses are critical to managing a dental facility and delivering oral health services.

Since the majority of medically compromised patients either elect or are required to have dental care for optimal health and function, knowledge of the multitude of compromised states is essential for dental professionals. This knowledge will support the high standards for oral health care delivery, which include recognizing and diagnosing conditions that reflect compromised states, preventing adverse side effects of procedures and drugs utilized in dentistry, and formulating treatment plans that are consistent with a patient's medical status.

It is obvious that the compromised patient forms a complex part of dentistry. Such individuals will require from their dentist, in addition to sound dental skills, all of the following: a knowledge of many medical diseases and conditions, a background in oral manifestations and detection of systemic diseases, insight into testing procedures, familiarity with the implications of pharmacotherapeutics, and an ability to assess the significance of history data, signs, and symptoms before, during, and after dental procedures. Therefore the usefulness of this text as a reference at all levels of dentistry, for the student as well as the practitioner, is evident.

Although care of the medically compromised patient is a complex problem requiring specialists in the field, its occurrence is so common that practitioners and students must be acquainted with these conditions in order to have the competence necessary to recognize and prevent problems associated with dental management and to utilize consultations and referrals appropriately. The text supplies this type of information in the form of practical organization, summary tables, and overviews of diagnosis and management; and yet it contains sufficient information that allows some insight into most of these conditions. This is accomplished by comprehensively covering, in 27 well-organized chapters, most conditions that lead to compromised states affecting a patient's well-being. It is bolstered by summary tables for easy access, adequate figures, and appendices that further allow the reader to identify disease states rapidly, recognize important features, be aware of potential complications, and select an approach to drug management in a prescription format. Explanations and rationale are presented for additional understanding. Although the main focus is on the management of compromised patients during dental procedures, the text very effectively includes causation, medical management, pathophysiology, and prognosis. In its present format, it serves as both a quick reference and a well-referenced resource for this critical interface of medicine and dentistry. It will help ensure high standards of care and reduce the occurrence of adverse reactions, for which compromised patients are at risk, by improving knowledge and encouraging judgment in the management of these patients.

Sol Silverman

Preface

The need for a fourth edition of *Dental Management of the Medically Compromised Patient* became apparent because of the ever increasing flow of new knowledge and changing concepts in medicine and dentistry.

The purpose of the book remains to provide the dental practitioner with an up-to-date, concise, factual reference work describing the dental management of patients with selected medical problems. The more common medical disorders that may be encountered in a dental practice continue to be the focus. This book is not a comprehensive medical reference, but rather a book that contains only enough core information about each of the medical conditions covered to enable the reader to recognize the basis for various dental management recommendations. Where appropriate, medical problems are organized to provide a brief overview of the basic disease process, pathophysiology, signs and symptoms, laboratory findings, and currently accepted medical therapy of each disorder. This is followed by a detailed explanation and recommendations for specific dental management.

We have found that those who may benefit from reading this book include practicing dentists, practicing dental hygienists, dental graduate students in specialty or general practice programs and dental and dental hygiene students.

Several major changes have been made in this fourth edition. New chapters on organ transplantation (26) and infection of prosthetic devices (27) have been added. The material on infection control has been updated and moved to Appendix A for easier access. The American Heart Association's newest recommendations for prevention of endocarditis have been incorporated into the appropriate chapters. Chapter 14, on AIDS, has been rewritten to reflect the rapid changes that are taking place in this most important area. New recommendations have been made on adrenal insufficiency (Chapter 11). Major updating and reorganization have been done to the chapters on hypertension (6), hepatitis (12), arthritis (15), diabetes mellitus (17), allergy (21), bleeding disorders (22), blood dyscrasias (23), oral cancer (24), and psychiatric disorders (25). The remaining chapters have been updated where necessary.

Even more emphasis has been placed on the medications used to treat the medical conditions covered in this fourth edition. Dosages, side effects, and drug interactions with agents used in dentistry — including those used during pregnancy — are discussed in greater detail than in the third edition. Tables have been added, and all tables have been made to stand out and be easier to read. Illustrative material has been added to better describe certain concepts and clinical findings.

Our sincere thanks and appreciation are extended to those many individuals who have contributed their time and expertise to the writing and revision of this text. Particular thanks is extended to Anne Langley, Rebecca Turpin, and Joyce Wallace for their typing and editing of the drafts of new chapters and revisions of the old.

James W. Little
Donald A. Falace

Contents

Dental Management of the Medically Compromised Patient

DENTAL MANAGEMENT
A SUMMARY

This table, *Dental Management: A Summary,* presents the more important factors to be considered in the dental management of medically compromised patients. Each medical problem is outlined according to the potential problems related to dental treatment, the prevention of these complications, the effect of the complications on dental treatment planning, oral changes that may be associated with the medical condition, and modifications indicated when rendering emergency dental care for patients with the condition.

The information contained in this table will be more easily understood if the text has been read first. The table has been designed for use by dentists, dental students, graduate students, dental hygienists, and dental assistants as a convenient reference work for the dental management of patients who have the medical diseases covered in this book.

Dental Management: A Summary

Medical problem	Potential problem related to dental care	Prevention of complications
Murmurs *(p 134)*	1. No problem if murmur is functional in nature 2. If murmur is organic (pathologic), infective endocarditis must be prevented	1. Medical consultation or referral to confirm nature of murmur 2. If organic murmur, management same as for patient with rheumatic heart disease

Rheumatic fever and rheumatic heart disease *(pp 123-134)*	If rheumatic heart disease is present, patient is susceptible to infective endocarditis following dental procedures that may cause transient bacteremias	1. Medical consultation to confirm presence or absence of rheumatic heart disease
		2. Medical referral to evaluate patient for presence or absence of rheumatic heart disease
		  a. Electrocardiogram
		  b. Chest x-ray
		  c. Physical examination of chest including auscultation for murmurs
		  d. Echocardiogram
		3. Patients with rheumatic heart disease require prophylactic antibiotic coverage for all dental procedures (including certain examination procedures)
		  a. In patients not allergic to penicillin, 3 g amoxicillin, orally, at least 1 hour before dental procedure followed 6 hours later by 1.5 g orally
		  b. In patients allergic to penicillin, clindamycin 300 mg, orally 1 hour before procedure, then 150 mg orally 6 hours after initial dose; or erythromycin ethylsuccinate 800 mg or erythromycin stearate 1 g orally 2 hours before procedure, then ½ dose 6 hours after initial dose
		  c. In patients taking low daily oral dose of penicillin or monthly injections of penicillin to prevent recurrent attacks of rheumatic fever
		    (1) Continue medication
		    (2) Then add clindamycin 300 mg, orally, 1 hour before procedure and then 150 mg, orally, 6 hours after initial dose; or one of erythromycin regimens shown above
		  d. See Tables 2-17 and 2-18 for children's dose of above agents
		  e. Use of chlorhexidine mouth rinse and sulcular irrigation before extractions and periodontal therapy can be considered

Treatment plan modifications	Oral complications	Emergency care
1. Patients with functional murmur would be treated as normal patient 2. Patients with organic murmur would be managed same as patient with rheumatic heart disease or congenital heart disease	Usually none	1. Patients with history of murmur during childhood or pregnancy that since has disappeared do not require prophylactic coverage unless history is not clear 2. Other patients with murmur who require emergency dental care should be protected from infective endocarditis with prophylactic antibiotics; medical consultation by phone can be used in attempt to determine nature of murmur

1. No dental procedures are contraindicated for asymptomatic patient with rheumatic heart disease
2. Management plan should include
  a. Carry out as much treatment as possible during 2 to 3 hours following waiting period after loading dose (1 to 2 hours)
  b. Allow at least 1 week to elapse before starting new coverage period to allow penicillin-resistant organisms to disappear from oral flora
  c. If multiple coverage periods are needed, antibiotics used can be alternated, first penicillin and then clindamycin or erythromycin; at least 1 week must elapse between coverage periods
3. Length of coverage period may be extended to 5 to 7 days under certain special conditions
  a. Surgical procedures with sutures or surgical areas that are slow to heal
  b. Clindamycin or erythromycin can be used for last 2 to 3 days of an extended coverage period to avoid possibility of bacteria developing resistance to amoxicillin
	Usually none	1. Patients with asymptomatic rheumatic heart disease need prophylactic antibiotic coverage for all emergency dental treatment
		2. Patients with history of rheumatic fever who have not been evaluated for presence or absence of rheumatic heart disease must be considered to have rheumatic heart disease until proven otherwise; give prophylactic antibiotic coverage to prevent infective endocarditis
		3. Patients with history of rheumatic fever who have been told they do not have rheumatic heart disease need no antibiotic coverage once this has been confirmed

Dental Management: A Summary—cont'd

Medical problem	Potential problem related to dental care	Prevention of complications

Congenital heart disease *(pp 136-145)*	1. Infective endocarditis
	2. Infective endarteritis
	3. Prolonged bleeding following scaling or surgical procedures; bleeding problem may be present in patients with right-to-left shunting of blood caused by
	  a. Thrombocytopenia
	  b. Lack of coagulation factor as result of thrombosis in small vessels
	  c. Anticoagulation medication used to prevent thrombosis
	4. Congestive heart failure
	  a. Infection
	  b. Cardiac arrest
	  c. Cardiac dysrhythmias
	  d. Breathing difficulties (caused by pulmonary edema)
		1. Detection by history and examination findings
		2. Referral for medical diagnosis and treatment
		3. Consultation with physician before any dental treatment is performed
		4. Prophylactic antibiotic coverage before and after any dental procedure
		  a. Patients with congenital heart disease—coverage same as for patient with rheumatic heart disease
		  b. Patients who have just had surgery to correct congenital heart defect—coverage same as for patient with rheumatic heart disease unless special regimen is needed; see coverage for patient with artificial heart valve or surgically corrected cardiovascular lesions (below)
		  c. After consultation with physician, many patients with treated defects that have healed will no longer need coverage
		5. Avoidance of dehydration in patients with oral infection
		6. Bleeding time and prothrombin time tested before any surgical procedures; consultation with physician if prolonged

Surgically corrected cardiovascular lesions *(pp 146-159)*	1. Infective endocarditis
	2. Infective endarteritis
	3. Prolonged bleeding following scaling or surgical procedures if anticoagulant medication is being used
		1. Antibiotic prophylaxis up to 6 months postoperatively using AHA standard regimens (confirm by medical consultation)
		  a. Patients not allergic to penicillin—3 g of amoxicillin, orally, 1 hour before dental procedure followed 6 hours later by 1.5 g amoxicillin orally; or if practitioner desires parenteral regimen—1 to 2 g of ampicillin, IM or IV, followed by gentamicin 1.5 mg/kg, IM or IV, ½ hour before dental procedure, followed by 1.5 g amoxicillin, orally, 6 hours after loading dose
		  b. Patients allergic to penicillin—clindamycin 300 mg, orally, 1 hour before procedure, then 150 mg 6 hours after initial dose; or if practitioner desires, parenteral regimen—1 g of vancomycin, IV infusion over the 60 minutes prior to dental procedure
		2. Patients with coronary bypass graft surgery usually are not considered susceptible 1 to 2 weeks after surgery; confirm by consultation and treat as normal patient

Treatment plan modifications	Oral complications	Emergency care

Usually none unless congestive heart failure present (p 232)	1. Cyanosis—blue color
	2. Polycythemia—ruddy color
	3. Thrombocytopenia—small hemorrhages
	4. Leukopenia—infection
		1. Asymptomatic patients—as indicated but protect against infective endocarditis or endarteritis
		2. Symptomatic patients with congestive heart failure and/or polycythemia
		  a. Consultation with physician before any treatment
		  b. Analgesics for pain
		  c. Antibiotics for infection
		  d. Avoidance of dehydration in patient with acute infection
		  e. Patient may have bleeding problem, in which case surgery should be avoided

See sections on rheumatic heart disease (pp 128-135) and artificial heart valves (pp 534-535)	Usually none unless patients receiving anticoagulant medication	1. Patients with coronary bypass graft that has healed do not require antibiotic prophylaxis
		2. Patients for whom it has been at least 6 months since surgery
		  a. Foreign material used to correct defect—coverage may be indicated (standard regimen)
		  b. Defect closed or corrected without use of foreign material—coverage not indicated
		3. Patients with artificial heart valve(s) must have coverage (standard or special regimen)
		4. Surgical procedures should be avoided if possible for patient taking anticoagulant medications

Dental Management: A Summary—cont'd

Medical problem	Potential problem related to dental care	Prevention of complications
Surgically corrected cardiovascular lesions—cont'd		3. Six months after surgery most patients are no longer susceptible unless foreign material was used to correct cardiovascular problem; when synthetic materials such as Dacron were used, patient may be susceptible to infective endocarditis or endarteritis—coverage with AHA standard regimen can be considered, by consultation 4. Patients with artificial heart valves remain very susceptible; coverage with AHA regimens listed above and confirmation by consultation

Ischemic heart disease with history of brief pain (angina pectoris) *(pp 175-195)*	1. Stress and anxiety related to dental visit may precipitate angina attack in dental office
	2. Myocardial infarction may occur when patient is in dental office
	3. Sudden death caused by disruption of cardiac rhythm of cardiac arrest without acute myocardial infarction may occur in dental office
		1. Detection of patient with history of angina pectoris
		2. Referral of patient thought to have untreated angina based on medical history for medical evaluation and treatment
		3. Patient under medical treatment for angina—during dental visit every attempt should be made to reduce stress
		  a. Concern and warm approach by staff and dentist
		  b. Make patient feel free to talk aboout fears
		  c. Morning appointments; however, some evidence supports early afternoon appointments as possibly better
		  d. Short appointments
		  e. Premedication—diazepam (Valium), 5 to 10 mg; prophylactic nitroglycerin, one tablet preoperatively
		  f. Nitrous oxide–oxygen
		  g. Effective local anesthetic—1:100,000 epinephrine can and should be used; aspirate; inject slowly (do not use epinephrine in patients with a serious arrhythmia)
		4. Reinforce importance of risk factors that can be influenced by patient
		5. Terminate appointment if patient becomes fatigued or develops change in pulse rate or rhythm
		6. If patient with stable angina develops chest pain during dental treatment, stop procedure and give nitroglycerin tablet sublingually
		  a. If pain is relieved, let patient rest and then continue with appointment or terminate appointment and reschedule for another day

Treatment plan modifications	Oral complications	Emergency care
1. In patients with stable form of angina, any routine dental care 2. In patients with unstable form of angina, only care needed to deal with or prevent dental pain and/or infection	Usually none; however, on rare occasion patients may have lower jaw pain of cardiac origin (referred pain); history of what initiates the pain and how it is relieved should provide clue to its cardiac origin	1. Patients with stable angina need no restrictions 2. Patients with unstable angina should consult with physician; based on patient status, emergency treatment may be as indicated (or conservative, as is possible for very unstable patients) using antibiotics and infection and analgesics for pain

Dental Management: A Summary—cont'd

Medical problem	Potential problem related to dental care	Prevention of complications
Ischemic heart disease with history of brief pain (angina pectoris)—cont'd		b. If pain continues longer than 2 to 3 minutes, monitor vital signs and give two additional nitroglycerin tablets one at a time during next 10 to 15 minutes; if after three nitroglycerins within 15-minute period pain persists and patient's condition is stable, transport to hospital emergency room and call physician; if patient is unstable, call for medical aid and be prepared to render cardiopulmonary resuscitation 7. If patient with unstable angina or history of MI develops chest pain during dental treatment, stop procedure, give nitroglycerin tablet sublingually, and monitor vital signs 　a. If pain is relieved after first, second, or third nitroglycerin tablet (given within 15 minutes) and patient is stable, terminate appointment and inform patient's physician of what happened 　b. If pain is not relieved following three nitroglycerin tablets and/or patient is unstable, call physician, provide immediate emergency care as needed, arrange for transportation to hospital emergency room; dentist must attend patient until in hands of emergency room personnel or patient's physician 8. Avoid use of vasopressors (except 1:100,000 epinephrine) in local anesthetic; aspirate before injecting; inject slowly; no more than three cartridges 　a. Do not use vasopressors to control local bleeding 　b. Do not use gingival packing material that contains vasopressor
Myocardial infarction *(pp 181-195)*	1. Cardiac arrest 2. Myocardial infarction 3. Angina pectoris 4. Congestive heart failure 5. Bleeding tendency secondary to anticoagulant 6. Infective endocarditis complicating implanted pacemaker (rare) 7. Electrical interference with pacemaker	1. No routine dental care until at least 6 months after infarction because of increased risk of new infarction and arrhythmia 2. Consultation with physician before starting routine dental care to confirm patient's current status 3. Morning appointments; again, some evidence suggests that early afternoon might be better 4. Short appointments 5. Termination of appointment if patient becomes fatigued or short of breath or develops change in pulse rate or rhythm—inform patient's physician; if patient develops chest pain during dental appointment, manage as described for unstable angina patient in above section

Treatment plan modifications	Oral complications	Emergency care
1. In patients 6 months or more after infarction with no complications, any routine dental care can be performed 2. If complications such as congestive heart failure are present, dental treatment should be limited to immediate needs only	Usually none except those related to drugs used to treat patient's medical problem	1. During first 6 months after infarction, emergency dental care only is needed after consultation with patient's physician; dental treatment should be as conservative as possible—drugs for pain control, antibiotics for infection, pulpotomy rather than extraction 2. Patients more than 6 months after infarction a. No complications—can receive any treatment indicated

Dental Management: A Summary—cont'd

Medical problem	Potential problem related to dental care	Prevention of complications
Myocardial infarction—cont'd		6. Use of local anesthetic with epinephrine 1:100,000 (no more than three cartridges); aspirate before injecting; inject slowly; avoid use of vasopressors to control local loss of blood; also avoid use of vasopressors in gingival packing material; do not use epinephrine in local anesthetic for patients with severe arrhythmia 7. Premedication before appointment to reduce stress associated with dental visit—diazepam, 5 to 10 mg 8. Anticoagulant medication—if surgery or scaling procedures are planned, physician should be contacted and dosage of anticoagulant reduced so that prothrombin time will be 2½ times normal or less (will take 3 to 4 days); check to see if desired result was obtained on day of procedure by having another prothrombin time done; prophylactic antibiotics can be considered, to prevent postoperative infection if surgery is planned 9. Digitalis—patient more prone to nausea and vomiting; avoid stimulating gag reflex 10. Antisialagogues—atropine, methantheline; may cause tachycardia; check with patient's physician before using 11. Antiarrhythmic agents—quinidine, procainamide; nausea and vomiting may occur; hypotension may occur; oral ulceration may indicate agranulocytosis 12. Antihypertensive agents (pp 167-169) 13. Avoid use of instruments such as Cavitron or electrocautery in patients with pacemaker

Cardiac arrhythmias *(pp 197-222)*	1. Stress associated with dental treatment or excessive amounts of epinephrine can produce life-threatening arrhythmia in susceptible patient
	2. Patients with existing arrhythmia are at increased risk for serious complications—cardiac arrest, etc
		1. Identify patients susceptible to developing cardiac arrhythmia by medical consultation
		  a. History of significant heart disease
		  b. Thyroid disease
		  c. Chronic pulmonary disease
		  d. Open heart surgery
		2. Identify patients with significant arrhythmia by history and clinical findings
		  a. Those taking medications to control arrhythmia—procainamide, quinidine, disopyramide, or propranolol

Treatment plan modifications	Oral complications	Emergency care
		b. Complications—medical consultation is indicated; treatment should be based on medical complication(s) present (refer to appropriate sections)

1. Reduce anxiety
  a. Premedication
  b. Open and honest communication
  c. Morning or early afternoon appointments
  d. Short appointments
  e. Nitrous oxide–oxygen inhalation
2. Avoid excessive amounts of epinephrine
  a. Use 1:100,000 epinephrine in local anesthetic except for patient with severe arrhythmia
	Agents used to control arrhythmias may have side effects that can cause oral manifestations:
	  a. Ulceration
	  b. Lupus-like syndrome
	  c. Xerostomia
	  d. Petechiae
		1. Consult with physician by phone prior to rendering emergency dental care whenever possible
		2. If patient is stable, most emergency procedures can be rendered; follow guidelines listed under treatment planning modifications
		3. Conservative emergency care only should be provided for unstable patients

Dental Management: A Summary—cont'd

Medical problem	Potential problem related to dental care	Prevention of complications

Cardiac arrhythmias—cont'd	3. Patients with cardiac pacemaker are at risk for possible malfunction of pacemaker because of electromagnetic interference from pulp testers, motorized dental chairs, Cavitrons, etc (see section on prosthetic devices)	b. Those with cardiac pacemaker to control arrhythmias
		c. Those with history of palpitation, dizziness, angina, dyspnea, and/or syncope (refer for medical evaluation)
		d. Those with abnormal physical findings—irregular pulse, very fast pulse, very slow pulse, high blood pressure (refer for medical evaluation)
		3. Medical consultation should occur before starting dental treatment to
		  a. Establish current status
		  b. Determine presence of underlying cardiac problem and need for antibiotic prophylaxis
		  c. Confirm medications patient is taking
		  d. Review dental management plan
		  e. Determine need for antibiotic prophylaxis because of presence of cardiac pacemaker (not recommended by AHA, but some physicians may suggest it)
		  f. Patients with atrial fibrillation may be taking coumarin (Coumadin); must adjust dosage prior to surgery to less than 2½ times normal prothrombin time
		4. Dentist must be prepared to deal with life-threatening arrhythmias
		5. Avoid use of instruments such as Cavitron or electrocautery in patients with pacemaker

Congestive heart failure *(pp 223-234)*	1. If polycythemia is present, bleeding resulting from thrombocytopenia and depletion of fibrinogen secondary to thrombosis in small vessels may occur
	2. Sudden death resulting from cardiac arrest or arrhythmia
	3. Myocardial infarction
	4. Cerebrovascular accident
	5. Infection
	6. Infective endocarditis if heart failure is caused by rheumatic heart disease, congenital heart disease, etc
	7. Shortness of breath
	8. Drug side effects
	  a. Orthostatic hypotension (diuretics, vasodilators)
		1. Detection and referral to physician
		2. No routine dental care until under good medical management
		3. Patients under good medical management—cause of heart failure and any other complications must be dealt with
		  a. Hypertension
		  b. Valvular disease (rheumatic heart disease)
		  c. Congenital heart disease
		  d. Myocardial infarction
		  e. Renal failure
		  f. Thyrotoxicosis
		  g. Chronic obstructive lung disease
		4. Antibiotics to prevent postoperative infection can be considered for patients with signs and symptoms of congestion
		5. Patient should be in upright position during treatment to decrease collection of fluid in lung
		6. Bleeding time and prothrombin time should be obtained before any surgical procedures; if abnormal, consult with physician, also avoid dehydration

Treatment plan modifications	Oral complications	Emergency care
b. Use anesthetic without epinephrine in patients with severe arrythmia (confirm by medical consultation) c. Use no more than three cartridges of anesthetic; aspirate before injection d. Do not use epinephrine in gingival packing e. Do not use epinephrine for control of local bleeding 3. Avoid use of general anesthesia 4. If above precautions are taken, any dental procedure can be performed		4. Prophylactic antibiotics must be used when underlying cardiac problem indicates need—rheumatic heart disease, prosthetic heart valve, congenital heart disease, etc

1. Cause of heart failure, presence of complications, and patient's current status must be considered
2. In some patients only urgent dental needs should be taken care of (by conservative methods)
3. In patients under good medical management with no complications, any indicated dental care can be performed
	1. Infection
	2. Bleeding
	3. Petechiae
	4. Ecchymoses
	5. Drug related
	  a. Xerostomia
	  b. Lichenoid mucosal lesions
		1. Conservative for patients with acute congestive failure—drugs for pain control and antibiotics for infection
		2. As indicated for patients under good medical management; must deal with underlying cause and presence of any complications in dental management

Dental Management: A Summary—cont'd

Medical problem	Potential problem related to dental care	Prevention of complications

Congestive heart failure — cont'd	b. Arrhythmias (digoxin, overdosage)
	c. Nausea, vomiting (digoxin, vasodilators)
	d. Palpitations (vasodilators)
		7. Terminate appointment if patient becomes fatigued, etc
		8. Drug considerations
		  a. Digitalis—patient more prone to nausea and vomiting
		  b. Anticoagulants—dosage should be reduced so that prothrombin time is 2½ times normal value or less (takes 3 to 4 days)
		  c. Antidysrhythmic drugs (see cardiac arrhythmias)
		  d. Antihypertensive agents (see hypertension)
		  e. Use of vasoconstrictors—okay in small amounts (1:100,000) in local anesthetic
		  f. Avoidance of general anesthesia

Antibody positive for HIV (AIDS) but asymptomatic
(pp 289-301)
	1. Transmission of infectious agents to dental personnel and patients
	  a. AIDS virus (HIV)
	  b. Hepatitis B virus (HBV)
	  c. Hepatitis C virus (HCV)
	  d. Epstein-Barr virus (EBV)
	  e. Cytomegalovirus (CMV)
	2. To date one dentist appears to have been HIV infected through occupational exposure and ten other dental health care workers are being investigated for possible occupational exposure to HIV; five patients may have been infected by an HIV infected dentist; thus risk of HIV transmission in dental setting is very low, but potential exists
	3. Individuals who are hepatitis carriers can transmit HBV or HCV infection
		1. Identification of HIV-infected patient is difficult; therefore infectious disease control procedures must be used for *all* patients
		2. Extreme care must be taken to avoid needle stick and instrument wounding
		3. All dental personnel should be vaccinated to be protected from HBV infection
		4. One hundred percent of asymptomatic antibody-positive (HIV) individuals may go on to develop AIDS; however, can take as long as 12 years before diagnosis of AIDS is made

Treatment plan modifications	Oral complications	Emergency care
None indicated	None in early stage; however, increased incidence of certain oral lesions associated with AIDS is found when compared to noninfected individuals	As needed

Dental Management: A Summary—cont'd

Medical problem	Potential problem related to dental care	Prevention of complications

Persistent gener-alized lymph-adenopathy (PGL) and AIDS related complex (ARC) *(pp 289-301)*	1. Transmission of infectious agents to dental personnel and patients
	  a. HIV
	  b. HBV
	  c. HCV
	  d. EBV
	  e. CMV
	2. To date, with the exception of possible transmission by a Florida dentist, HIV has not been found to be transmitted to patients in the dental setting; one dentist was reported to have been infected by oc-cupational exposure, and ten other dental health care workers are being in-vestigated for possible oc-cupational exposure; how-ever, HBV and HCV transmission has been well documented on numerous occasions
	3. Patients with advanced ARC may have significant immune suppression and be at increased risk for in-fection
	4. Patients with ARC may be thrombocytopenic and hence potential bleeders
		1. Use of infectious disease control procedure for *all* patients
		2. Dental personnel should be vaccinated for protec-tion from HBV infection
		3. Identify patients by presence of signs and symp-toms associated with PGL and ARC; refer for medical evaluation, counseling, and management
		4. Establish platelet status and immune status of pa-tients with ARC before performing invasive den-tal procedures (see AIDS below)
		5. Inform patients of various support groups avail-able to help in terms of education and emotional, financial, legal, and other issues

AIDS *(pp 289-315)*	1. Transmission of infectious agents to dental personnel and patients
	  a. HIV
	  b. HBV
	  c. HCV
	  d. EBV
	  e. CMV
	2. To date, HIV has not been found to be transmitted to patient in the dental set-ting (possible exception of five patients who may have been infected by a Florida
		1. Use infectious disease control procedures for *all* patients
		2. Dental personnel should be vaccinated for protec-tion from HBV infection
		3. By medical history and examination findings, identify undiagnosed cases and refer for medical evaluation, counseling, and management
		4. Patients with significant immune suppression usu-ally are *not* given antibiotic prophylaxis for surgi-cal or invasive dental procedures
		5. Platelet count or bleeding time should be ordered before any surgical procedure; if significant thrombocytopenia present, platelet replacement may be needed

Treatment plan modifications	Oral complications	Emergency care
None indicated	1. Oral candidiasis 2. Hairy leukoplakia 3. Lymphadenopathy 4. With the exception of Kaposi's sarcoma and non-Hodgkin's lymphoma, other lesions listed under AIDS can be found with increased frequency	As needed
1. None for cases in "remission"; however, complex restorative procedures usually are not indicated because of poor prognosis (death occurs most often within 2 years following diagnosis) 2. Patients in advanced stages of disease should receive emergency and preventive dental care; elective dental treatment is usually not indicated at this stage	1. Kaposi's sarcoma 2. Non-Hodgkin's lymphoma 3. Oral candidiasis 4. Lymphadenopathy 5. Hairy leukoplakia 6. Xerostomia 7. Salivary gland enlargement 8. Venereal warts 9. HIV-gingivitis 10. HIV-periodontitis 11. Necrotizing stomatitis 12. Herpes zoster	1. Any indicated care, except in advanced cases (when care should be as conservative as possible) 2. Significant immune suppression usually does not require prophylactic antibiotic therapy when surgery must be performed 3. Thrombocytopenia may be present; therefore bleeding time or platelet count should be done before any surgical procedure

Dental Management: A Summary—cont'd

Medical problem	Potential problem related to dental care	Prevention of complications
AIDS—cont'd	dentist); eleven dental health care workers may have become HIV infected through occupational exposure; however, HBV and HCV have been transmitted to patients or dental health care workers on a number of occasions in dental setting 3. Patients with advanced disease have significant suppression of their immune system and can be at risk for infection resulting from invasive dental procedures 4. Patients may be bleeders because of thrombocytopenia	

Diabetes mellitus *(pp 341-360)*	1. In uncontrolled diabetic patients
	  a. Infection
	  b. Poor wound healing
	2. In patients treated with insulin, insulin reaction
	3. In diabetic patients, early onset of complications relating to cardiovascular system, eyes, kidneys, and nervous system (angina, myocardial infarction, cerebrovascular accident, renal failure, peripheral neuropathy blindness, hypertension, congestive heart failure)
		1. Detection by
		  a. History
		  b. Clinical findings
		  c. Screening blood glucose level
		2. Referral for diagnosis and treatment
		3. Patients receiving insulin—prevent insulin reaction
		  a. Advise eating normal meals before appointments
		  b. Schedule appointments in morning or mid-morning
		  c. Advise them to inform you of any symptoms of insulin reaction when they first occur
		  d. Have sugar in some form to give in case of insulin reaction
		4. Diabetic patients being treated with insulin who develop oral infection may require increase in insulin dosage; consult with physician in addition to aggressive local and systemic management of infection (including antibiotic sensitivity testing)
		5. Drug considerations
		  a. Insulin—insulin reaction
		  b. Hypoglycemic agents—on rare occasions aplastic anemia, etc
		  c. In severe diabetics, avoid general anesthesia

Treatment plan modifications	Oral complications	Emergency care
	13. Primary or recurrent herpes simplex lesions 14. Major aphthous lesions 15. Herpetiform aphthous lesions 16. Petechiae, ecchymoses 17. Others (Table 14-7)	
In well-controlled diabetic patients, no alteration of treatment plan is indicated unless complication of diabetes present such as 1. Hypertension (p 173) 2. Congestive heart failure (pp 232-233) 3. Myocardial infarction (p 193) 4. Angina (p 192) 5. Renal failure (p 255)	1. Accelerated periodontal disease 2. Periodontal abscesses 3. Xerostomia 4. Poor healing 5. Infection 6. Oral ulcerations 7. Candidiasis 8. Mucormycosis 9. Numbness, burning, or pain in oral tissues	1. Patients with acute infection—physician should increase insulin dosage; if possible, obtain sample of exudate and have antibiotic sensitivity testing performed; then start penicillin therapy; if clinical response is poor, laboratory data can be used to select more effective antibiotic 2. Patients with diabetes not under medical treatment—referral and consultation are necessary so diabetes can be brought under control 3. In general, other emergency problems can be dealt with as in normal patients

Dental Management: A Summary — cont'd

Medical problem	Potential problem related to dental care	Prevention of complications
Hyperthyroidism (thyrotoxicosis) *(pp 374-378, 380-382)*	1. Thyrotoxic crisis (thyroid storm) may be precipitated in untreated or incompletely treated patients with thyrotoxicosis by a. Infection b. Trauma c. Surgical procedures d. Stress 2. Patients with untreated or incompletely treated thyrotoxicosis may be very sensitive to actions of epinephrine and other pressor amines; thus these agents must not be used; once patient is well managed from medical standpoint, these agents can be resumed 3. Thyrotoxicosis increases risk for hypertension and severe arrhythmias	1. Detection of patients with thyrotoxicosis by history and examination findings 2. Referral for medical evaluation and treatment 3. Avoidance of any dental treatment for patient with thyrotoxicosis until under good medical control; however, any acute oral infection will have to be dealt with by antibiotic therapy and other conservative measures to prevent development of thyrotoxic crisis; suggest consultation with patient's physician during management of acute oral infection 4. Avoidance of epinephrine and other pressor amines in untreated or incompletely treated patient 5. Recognition of early stages of thyrotoxic crisis: a. Severe symptoms of thyrotoxicosis b. Febrile c. Abdominal pain d. Delirious, obtunded, or psychotic 6. Initiate immediate emergency treatment procedures: a. Seek immediate medical aid b. Cool with cold towels c. Hydrocortisone (100 to 300 mg) d. Monitor vital signs e. Start CPR if needed
Hypothyroidism *(pp 378-379, 381-382)*	1. Untreated patients with severe hypothyroidism exposed to stressful situations such as trauma, surgical procedures, or infection may develop hypothyroid coma 2. Untreated hypothyroid patients may be very sensitive to actions of narcotics, barbiturates, and tranquilizers	1. Detection and referral of patients suspected of being hypothyroid for medical evaluation and treatment 2. Avoidance of narcotics, barbiturates, and tranquilizers in untreated hypothyroid patients 3. Recognition of initial stage of myxedema coma a. Hypothermia b. Bradycardia c. Hypotension d. Epileptic seizures 4. Start immediate treatment of myxedema coma a. Seek immediate medical aid b. Hydrocortisone (100 to 300 mg) c. CPR as indicated

Treatment plan modifications	Oral complications	Emergency care
1. Once under good medical management, patient may receive any indicated dental treatment 2. If acute infection occurs, physician should be consulted concerning management	1. Osteoporosis may occur 2. Periodontal disease may be more progressive 3. Dental caries may be more extensive 4. Premature loss of deciduous teeth and early eruption of permanent teeth 5. Early jaw development 6. Tumors found in midline of posterior dorsum of tongue must not be surgically removed until possibility of functional thyroid tissue has been ruled out by ^{131}I uptake tests	1. Thyrotoxic patients—conservative treatment—antibiotics for infection, analgesics for pain, consultation with physician 2. Patients under good medical management—emergency dental care as indicated; however, if problem involves acute infection, consult with patient's physician

1. In hypothyroid patients under good medical management, any indicated dental treatment
2. In patients with congenital form of disease and severe mental retardation, assistance with hygiene procedures may be needed
	1. Increase in tongue size
	2. Delayed eruption of teeth
	3. Malocclusion
		1. Untreated hypothyroid patients
		  a. Control of pain with nonnarcotic analgesics
		  b. Avoid precipitation of hypothyroid coma in patients with severe hypothyroidism; thus avoid surgical procedures and treat acute oral infection by conservative measures
		2. Patients under good medical management—render whatever emergency care is indicated

Dental Management: A Summary—cont'd

Medical problem	Potential problem related to dental care	Prevention of complications

Anaphylaxis *(pp 410-411)*	Severe reaction following administration of agent that patient is allergic to
	a. Drugs
	b. Local anesthetic
		1. Take careful history and identify patients who are allergic to agents used in dentistry and who have history of atopic reactions (asthma, hayfever, urticaria, angioneurotic edema).
		2. Avoid use of agents that patient is allergic to as identified in medical history
		3. Patients with history of atopic reactions—use care when giving drugs and materials with high incidence of allergy such as penicillin; be prepared to deal with severe allergic reaction
		  a. Identify reaction as anaphylactic in nature
		  b. Call for medical help
		  c. Place patient in supine position
		  d. Check for open airway
		  e. Administer oxygen
		  f. Check vital signs—respiration, blood pressure, pulse rate and rhythm
		  g. If vital signs depressed or absent, inject 0.5 ml of epinephrine 1:1000 IM into tongue
		  h. Provide CPR as indicated
		  i. Repeat injection of epinephrine if no response
		4. When prescribing drugs, inform patient regarding signs and symptoms of allergic reactions; advise patient to call you if such reaction occurs, or to report to nearest hospital emergency room

Urticaria (angioneurotic edema) *(p 410)*	1. Nonemergency, edematous swelling of lips, cheek, etc following contact with antigen
	2. Emergency, edematous swelling of tongue, pharynx, and larynx with obstruction of airway
		1. Identify patients who have had allergic reactions by history and what drug or materials caused reaction
		2. Avoid use of antigen in allergic persons
		3. If patients develop allergic reaction to drug or material to which they gave no indication of being allergic
		  a. Nonemergency reaction, no further contact with agent—administer diphenhydramine, 50 mg qid, PO or IM
		  b. Emergency reaction, supine position, patent airway, oxygen, inject 0.5 ml epinephrine 1:1000 IM, support respiration if necessary, check pulse, obtain medical assistance
		4. Local anesthetics
		  a. Most patients who say they are allergic to local anesthetic will describe, on questioning, a fainting episode or toxic reaction
		  b. If allergic reaction occurred, identify kind of anesthetic used and select one from different chemical group

Treatment plan modifications	Oral complications	Emergency care
Usually none	Usually none	1. Avoid agents that patient is allergic to 2. Be prepared to deal with mild or severe allergic reactions 3. Inform patient about signs and symptoms of allergic reactions; advise seeking immediate medical care if these occur after patient has left dental office or has just taken medication you prescribed (e.g., penicillin)
1. Avoidance of drug or material to which patient is allergic 2. In rare patient who is allergic to many local anesthetics, diphenhydramine (Benadryl) can be used as local anesthetic or refer to allergist for provocative dose testing	Soft tissue swelling	As indicated; avoid any agent that patient is allergic to; diphenhydramine can be used as local anesthetic for patients allergic to more than one local anesthetic or who have had allergic reaction to local anesthetic but cannot identify what agent was used

Dental Management: A Summary—cont'd

Medical problem	Potential problem related to dental care	Prevention of complications

Urticaria (angio-neurotic edema)—cont'd		c. Inject 1 drop (aspirate first) of alternate anesthetic; wait 5 minutes; if no reaction, proceed with injection of remaining anesthetic
		d. If anesthetic that patient reacted to cannot be identified
		  (1) Refer to allergist for provocative dose testing, or
		  (2) Use diphenhydramine (Benadryl) with epinephrine 1:100,000 as local anesthetics (1% solution, 1 to 4 ml)
		5. Penicillin
		  a. In allergic individual an alternate choice would be erythromycin
		  b. In nonallergic person, administer by oral route whenever possible—lowest incidence of sensitization
		  c. Do not use in topical form

Bleeding problems as suggested by examination and history findings but no clues as to underlying cause *(pp 432-433)*	Excessive blood loss following surgical procedures, scaling, etc	1. Screen patients with following—if one or more are abnormal, refer for diagnosis and medical treatment
		  a. Prothrombin time
		  b. Partial thromboplastin time
		  c. Thrombin time
		  d. Bleeding time
		  e. Platelet count
		2. Avoid use of aspirin

Thrombocytopenia (primary or secondary) due to chemicals, radiation, or leukemia *(pp 435-436)*	1. Prolonged bleeding
	2. Infection in patients with bone marrow replacement or destruction
	3. In patients being treated with steroids, stress may lead to serious medical emergency
		1. Identification of patients
		  a. History
		  b. Examination findings
		  c. Screening tests—bleeding time, platelet count
		2. Referral and consultation with hematologist
		3. Correction of underlying problem or replacement therapy before surgery
		4. Local measures to control blood loss—splint, thrombosis, etc
		5. Prophylactic antibiotics in surgical cases to prevent postoperative infection can be considered
		6. Additional steroids for patients being treated with steroids if indicated (see section on adrenal insufficiency)
		7. Avoid aspirin, aspirin-containing compounds, and nonsteroidal antiinflammatory drugs (NSAIDs)

Treatment plan modifications	Oral complications	Emergency care
None unless test(s) abnormal, then manage based on nature of underlying problem once diagnosis established by physician	Excessive bleeding following dental procedures	Conservative — antibiotics and analgesics, but avoid use of aspirin or aspirin-containing compounds
No dental procedures unless replacement of platelets is done before procedure or unless underlying problem has been corrected	1. Spontaneous bleeding 2. Prolonged bleeding following certain dental procedures 3. Petechiae 4. Hematomas	Conservative management of infection and pain; avoid aspirin, aspirin-containing compounds, and nonsteroidal antiinflammatory drugs (NSAIDs); acetaminophen (Tylenol) with or without codeine can be used

Dental Management: A Summary—cont'd

Medical problem	Potential problem related to dental care	Prevention of complications
Vascular wall alterations (scurvy, infection, chemical, allergic, autoimmune, other) *(pp 414, 435)*	Prolonged bleeding following surgical procedures or any insult to integrity of oral mucosa	1. Identification of patients 　a. History 　b. Clinical findings 　c. Screening test, bleeding time 2. Consultation with hematologist 3. Splint 4. Local measures to control blood loss 5. Prophylactic antibiotics in surgical cases to avoid postoperative infection can be considered 6. If allergy involved in etiology, and antigen has been identified, it must be avoided
Congenital disorders of coagulation (hemophilia, Christmas disease) *(pp 414, 436-438)*	Excessive bleeding following dental procedures	1. Identification of patients 　a. History—bleeding problems in relatives, excessive bleeding following trauma or surgery 　b. Examination findings 　　(1) Ecchymoses 　　(2) Hemarthrosis 　　(3) Dissecting hematomas 　c. Screening tests—prothrombin time (normal), partial thromboplastin time (prolonged), bleeding time (normal) and thrombin time (normal) 2. Consultation and referral for diagnosis and treatment and for preparation before dental procedures 　a. Antihemophilic factor inhibitors 　b. Steroids, if inducible inhibitors found 　　(1) Surgery very difficult 　　(2) Requires hospitalization 　c. Selection of replacement factor and supportive medication 　　(1) Factor VIII concentrate 　　(2) Cryoprecipitate 　　(3) Fresh frozen plasma 　　(4) 1-desamino-8-darginine vasopressin (DDAVP) 　　(5) Epsilon-aminocaproic acid (EACA) 　　(6) Tranexamic acid (Cyklopron) 　　(7) Nonactivated prothrombin-complex concentrate 　　(8) Activated prothrombin-complex concentrate 3. May be treated on outpatient basis depending on results of consultation (mild to moderate deficiency, no inhibitors) 4. Local measures for control of bleeding—splints, thrombin, microfibrillar collagen, etc

Treatment plan modifications	Oral complications	Emergency care
Surgical procedures must be avoided in these patients unless underlying problem has been corrected or patient has been prepared for surgery by hematologist and dentist is prepared to control excessive loss of blood by local measures (see section on hemophilia)	1. Excessive bleeding following scaling and surgical procedures 2. Petechiae 3. Hematomas	Conservative management of infection and pain
No dental procedures unless patient has been prepared based on consultation with hematologist	1. Spontaneous bleeding 2. Prolonged bleeding following dental procedures that injure soft tissue or bone 3. Petechiae 4. Hematomas 5. Oral lesions associated with HIV infection in patients who receive infected replacement products (most occurred prior to 1985–1986)	1. Conservative management of infection and pain, if possible; otherwise, patient must be prepared for surgery (cryoprecipitate, fresh frozen plasma, desmopressin, epsilon-aminocaproic acid, tranexamic acid, etc) 2. Avoid aspirin, aspirin-containing compounds, and NSAIDs

Dental Management: A Summary—cont'd

Medical problem	Potential problem related to dental care	Prevention of complications
Congenital disorders of coagulation (hemophilia, Christmas disease)—cont'd		5. Prophylactic antibiotics to prevent postoperative infection in surgical cases can be considered 6. Avoid aspirin, aspirin-containing compounds, and NSAIDs

von Willebrand's disease *(pp 425-426, 437-438)*	Excessive bleeding following invasive dental procedures	1. Identification of patients
		  a. History of bleeding problems in relatives and of excessive bleeding following surgery or trauma, etc
		  b. Examination findings
		    (1) Petechiae
		    (2) Hematomas
		  c. Screening laboratory tests—prolonged bleeding time, possible prolonged partial thromboplastin time
		2. Consultation and referral for diagnosis and treatment and preparation before dental procedures
		  a. Fresh frozen plasma
		  b. Cryoprecipitate
		3. May be treated on outpatient basis depending on results of consultation
		4. Local measures for control of bleeding
		  a. Splints
		  b. Gelfoam with thrombin
		  c. Oxycel, Surgicel
		5. Consider prophylactic antibiotics to prevent postoperative infection in surgical cases

Acquired disorders of coagulation (liver disease, broad spectrum antibiotics, malabsorption syndrome, biliary tract obstruction, heparin, coumarin drugs, others) *(pp 429-435, 437-438)*	Excessive bleeding following dental procedures that result in soft tissue or osseous injury	1. Identification of patients with disorder
		  a. History
		  b. Examination findings
		  c. Screening laboratory tests—prothrombin time (prolonged), bleeding time (in liver disease prolonged if hypersplenism present)
		2. Consultation and referral
		3. Preparation before dental procedure
		4. Local measures to control blood loss
		5. Prophylactic antibiotics can be considered
		6. Reduction of anticoagulant so prothrombin time is 2½ normal or less
		7. In patients with liver disease; avoidance of drugs metabolized by the liver or reduction in dosage
		8. Avoid aspirin, aspirin-containing compounds, and NSAIDs

Treatment plan modifications	Oral complications	Emergency care
No invasive dental procedures unless patient has been prepared based on consultation with hematologist	1. Spontaneous bleeding 2. Prolonged bleeding following dental procedures that injure soft tissue or bone 3. Petechiae 4. Hematomas	1. Conservative management of infection and pain, if possible; otherwise patient must be prepared for surgery (fresh frozen plasma or cryoprecipitate) 2. Avoid aspirin, aspirin–containing compounds, and NSAIDs
No dental procedure unless patient prepared based on consultation with hematologist	1. Excessive bleeding 2. Spontaneous bleeding 3. Petechiae 4. Hematomas	1. Conservative 2. Vitamin K injection can be given if surgical procedure is necessary 3. Avoid aspirin, aspirin-containing compounds, and NSAIDs for pain control

Dental Management: A Summary—cont'd

Medical problem	Potential problem related to dental care	Prevention of complications

Disseminated intravascular coagulation (DIC) *(pp 426-427)*	Excessive bleeding following invasive dental procedures; in chronic form of disease widespread thrombosis may occur	1. Identification of patients
		 a. History—excessive bleeding following minor trauma; spontaneous bleeding from nose, gingiva, gastrointestinal tract, or urinary tract; recent infection, burns, shock and acidosis, or autoimmune disease; history of cancer most often associated with chronic form of DIC, in which thrombosis is usually the major clinical problem rather than bleeding
		 b. Examination findings
		  (1) Petechiae
		  (2) Ecchymoses
		  (3) Spontaneous gingival bleeding, bleeding from nose, ears, etc
		 c. Screening laboratory findings
		  (1) Acute DIC—prothrombin time (prolonged), partial thromboplastin time (prolonged), thrombin time (prolonged), bleeding time (prolonged), platelet count (decreased)
		  (2) Chronic DIC—most tests may be normal but fibrin split products present
		2. Referral and consultation with physician if invasive dental procedures must be performed
		 a. Acute DIC—cryoprecipitate, fresh frozen plasma, and/or platelets
		 b. Chronic DIC—anticoagulants such as heparin or vitamin K antagonists
		3. Avoid aspirin, or aspirin-containing products
		4. Local measures to control bleeding
		5. Consider antibiotic therapy to prevent postoperative infection

Disorders of platelet release *(pp 426-427)*	Excessive bleeding following invasive dental procedures	1. Identification of patient a. History—recent use of aspirin, indomethacin, phenylbutazone, ibuprophen, or sulfinpyrazone; presence of other platelet or coagulation disorders b. Examination—often negative unless signs present relating to other platelet or coagulation disorder c. Screening laboratory tests—bleeding time (prolonged), partial thromboplastin time (prolonged) 2. Most patients on above drugs without an additional platelet or coagulation problem will not bleed excessively following surgery

Treatment plan modifications	Oral complications	Emergency care
Depending on cause of DIC treatment plan should be altered: 1. Cases of acute DIC, no routine dental care until medical evaluation and correction of cause 2. Cases of chronic DIC, no routine dental care until medical evaluation and correction of cause when possible, if prognosis is poor based on underlying cause (advanced cancer), limited dental care would be indicated	1. Spontaneous gingival bleeding 2. Petechiae 3. Ecchymoses 4. Prolonged bleeding following invasive dental procedures	1. No invasive procedures unless direct medical support and preparation are available 2. Acetaminophen (Tylenol) with codeine can be used for pain relief 3. If invasive dental procedures must be done, prophylactic antibiotics can be considered to prevent postoperative infection
Usually no modifications indicated for patients who have no other platelet or coagulation disorder	1. Excessive bleeding may occur following surgery 2. Petechiae, ecchymoses, and hematomas may be found when other platelet or coagulation disorders are present	1. Avoid surgery in patients on these drugs and with history of another platelet or coagulation disorder unless screening tests are within normal limits 2. Treat pain in conservative manner—acetaminophen (Tylenol) with codeine 3. Treat infection by antibiotics; avoid incision and drainage (I&D) if possible

Dental Management: A Summary—cont'd

Medical problem	Potential problem related to dental care	Prevention of complications
Disorders of platelet release—cont'd		3. Patients with prolonged bleeding time and/or partial thromboplastin time should be referred for evaluation prior to any surgical procedures being performed 4. Elective surgery can be performed following withdrawal of drug and management of other platelet or coagulation disorder by appropriate means

Primary fibrinogenolysis *(p 427)*	Excessive bleeding following invasive dental procedures	1. Identification of patients
		  a. History—liver disease, cancer of lung, cancer of prostate, and heat stroke may develop this condition
		  b. Examination findings
		    (1) Jaundice
		    (2) Spider angiomas
		    (3) Ecchymoses
		    (4) Hematomas
		  c. Screening laboratory tests—platelet count (often normal), prothrombin time (prolonged), bleeding time (usually normal), partial thromboplastin time (prolonged), thrombin time (prolonged)
		2. Consultation and referral prior to any invasive dental procedure; epsilon-aminocaproic acid therapy will inhibit both plasmin and plasmin activators

Iron deficiency anemia *(pp 439-440)*	1. Usually none 2. In rare cases severe leukopenia and thrombocytopenia may result in problems with infection and excessive loss of blood	1. Detection and referral for diagnosis and treatment 2. In females most cases will be caused by physiologic process—menstruation or pregnancy 3. In males most cases will be secondary to underlying disease—peptic ulcer, carcinoma of colon, etc
G-6-PD deficiency *(pp 441, 453-454)*	Accelerated hemolysis of red blood cells	1. Control infection 2. Avoid drugs containing phenacetin 3. These patients often have increased sensitivity to sulfa drugs, aspirin, chloramphenicol
Pernicious anemia *(pp 440-441)*	1. Infection 2. Bleeding 3. Delayed healing	Detection and medical treatment (early detection and treatment can prevent permanent neurologic damage)

Treatment plan modifications	Oral complications	Emergency care
Patients with advanced cancer should have treatment limited to emergency dental procedures and preventive measures; complex dental restorations in general are not indicated; in other patients, once preparation to avoid excessive bleeding has occurred (epsilon-aminocaproic acid), most dental treatment can be rendered	1. Prolonged bleeding following invasive dental procedures 2. Jaundice of mucosa 3. Ecchymoses	1. Avoid surgical procedures 2. Conservative management of infection and pain, if possible; otherwise, patient must be prepared for surgery by consultation with hematologist
Usually none	1. Paresthesias 2. Loss of papillae from tongue 3. In rare cases infection and bleeding complications 4. Patients with dysphagia seem to have increased incidence of carcinoma of oral and pharyngeal area (Plummer-Vinson syndrome)	Usually as indicated (white blood cell count and platelet status should be checked)
Usually none unless anemia severe, then only urgent dental needs	Usually none	As indicated, unless patient is having hemolytic crisis; then conservative control of pain and infection
None once patient under medical care	1. Paresthesias of oral tissues (burning, tingling, numbness) 2. Delayed healing (severe cases), infection, red tongue, angular cheilosis 3. Petechial hemorrhages	Usually can be rendered without complications; in patient suspected of having pernicious anemia, suggest conservative treatment until medical diagnosis and therapy established

Dental Management: A Summary—cont'd

Medical problem	Potential problem related to dental care	Prevention of complications

Sickle cell anemia *(pp 441-442, 453-454)*	Sickle cell crisis	1. Avoidance of any procedure that would produce acidosis or hypoxia
		2. Drug considerations
		  a. Avoid excessive use of barbiturates and narcotics, as suppression of respiratory center can occur, leading to acidosis, which can precipitate acute crisis
		  b. Avoid excessive use of salicylates, as "acidosis" may result, again leading to possible acute crisis; codeine and acetaminophen in moderate dosage can be used for pain control
		  c. Avoid use of general anesthesia, as hypoxia can lead to precipitation of acute crisis
		  d. Nitrous oxide may be used, provided 50% oxygen is supplied at all times; critical to avoid diffusion hypoxia at termination of nitrous oxide administration
		  e. For nonsurgical procedures use local without vasoconstrictor; for surgical procedures use 1:100,000 epinephrine in anesthetic solution
		    (1) Aspirate before injecting
		    (2) Inject slowly
		    (3) Use no more than three cartridges
		3. Must avoid infection; if infection does occur, treat in aggressive manner:
		  a. Heat
		  b. I&D
		  c. Antibiotics
		  d. Corrective treatment—extraction, pulpectomy, etc
		4. Avoid dehydration in patients with infection or patients receiving surgical treatment

Agranulocytosis *(p 444)*	Infection	1. Referral for medical diagnosis and treatment 2. Drug considerations—avoidance of chloramphenicol for oral infection because of high incidence of agranulocytosis
Cyclic neutropenia *(p 444)*	Infection	1. Antibiotics to avoid infection 2. Serial white blood cell counts, to pick time in cycle when count is closest to normal level

Treatment plan modifications	Oral complications	Emergency care

Usually none unless symptoms of severe anemia present, and then only urgent dental needs should be met	1. Osteoporosis
	2. Loss of trabecular pattern
	3. Delayed eruption of teeth
	4. Hypoplasia of teeth
	5. Pallor of oral mucosa
	6. Jaundice of oral mucosa
		1. As indicated unless crisis present; then conservative control of pain (with drugs) and infection (with antibiotics)
		2. Treat infection in aggressive manner
		3. Avoid dehydration
		4. Avoid excessive use of barbiturates and narcotics
		5. Avoid excessive use of salicylates
		6. Avoid use of general anesthesia
		7. Moderate dose of codeine and acetaminophen can be used for pain control
		8. Use only small concentration of epinephrine (1:100,000) in local anesthetic
		  a. Aspirate before injecting
		  b. Inject slowly
		  c. No more than 3 cartridges

No dental treatment except emergency care and supportive therapy for oral lesions See Appendix B for specific treatment regimens	1. Oral ulcerations 2. Periodontitis 3. Necrotic tissue	Conservative pain control and control of infection
As indicated; if white cell count depressed severely, antibiotics to avoid postoperative infection	1. Periodontal disease 2. Oral infection 3. Oral ulceration similar to aphthous stomatitis	Depending on severity of disease, may limit to disease control and maintenance procedures

Dental Management: A Summary—cont'd

Medical problem	Potential problem related to dental care	Prevention of complications

Leukemia *(pp 445-450, 452-453, 455-456)*	1. Prolonged bleeding
	2. Infection
	3. Delayed healing
		1. Detection and referral for diagnosis and treatment
		2. Determination of platelet status on day of any surgical procedure, including scaling of teeth; bleeding time is within normal range, proceed; if not, postpone procedure (platelet count less than 80,000/mm^3)
		3. Avoidance of postoperative infection by prophylactic use of antibiotics can be considered; modification of AHA regimen for prevention of endocarditis can be used following medical consultation
		  a. Most situations
		    (1) Give 2 g penicillin V, orally, at least 30 minutes before procedure
		    (2) Give 500 mg penicillin V, orally, every 6 hours for remaining part of appointment day
		    (3) Give 500 mg of erythromycin, orally, every 6 hours for following 2 to 5 days
		  b. For patients allergic to penicillin
		    (1) Give 1 g of erythromycin, orally, 2 hours before procedure
		    (2) Give 500 mg of erythromycin, orally, every 6 hours for remaining part of appointment day
		    (3) Give 500 mg of erythromycin, orally, every 6 hours for following 2 to 5 days
		  c. Based on special conditions and medical consultation, other agents, dosage, and duration of treatment may be indicated

Multiple myeloma *(pp 451-452, 457)*	1. Excessive bleeding following invasive dental procedures 2. Risk of infection due to decrease in normal immunoglobulins 3. Risk of infection and bleeding in patients being treated by radiation or chemotherapy	1. See section on chemotherapy concerning prevention and management of medical complications 2. See section on radiation therapy concerning prevention and management of medical complications 3. Patients with oral soft tissue lesions and/or osseous lesions should be biopsied by dentist or referred for diagnosis and treatment as indicated 4. Medical history should identify patients with diagnosed disease; medical consultation is needed to establish current status

Treatment plan modifications	Oral complications	Emergency care
1. During acute stages of disease, avoidance of dental care of any kind if at all possible 2. When patient is in state of remission, all active dental disease should be treated and patient placed on good hygiene maintenance program 3. Avoidance of long, drawn-out dental procedures 4. Complex restorative procedures usually not indicated for patients with poor prognosis 5. See Appendix B for treatment regimens for oral complications of leukemia	1. Infection 2. Ulceration 3. Gingival bleeding 4. Ecchymoses 5. Petechiae 6. Gingival hyperplasia 7. Soft tissue and osseous lesions 8. Paresthesias—numbness, burning, tingling 9. Candidiasis 10. Lymphadenopathy	1. As indicated, during remission 2. Conservative otherwise (antibiotic sensitivity testing should be considered); antibiotics for infection; strong analgesics for pain 3. Drainage through pulp chamber rather than extraction
1. Supportive dental care only for patients in terminal stage 2. General prognosis is poor, so complex dental procedures are usually not indicated 3. If thrombocytopenia or leukopenia is present, special precautions needed to prevent bleeding and infection (platelet replacement, antibiotic therapy) when invasive dental procedures are performed 4. See sections on chemotherapy and radiation therapy for treatment plan modifications 5. Patients may be bleeders due to presence of abnormal immunoglobulin M macroglobulins, which form complexes with clotting factors, thus inactivating the clotting factors	1. Soft tissue tumors 2. Osseous lesions 3. Amyloid deposits in soft tissues 4. Unexplained mobility of teeth	1. Conservative for patients undergoing radiation or chemotherapy 2. Patients with "stable" disease can receive any indicated emergency treatment 3. Patients in terminal stage should receive only conservative treatment

Dental Management: A Summary—cont'd

Medical problem	Potential problem related to dental care	Prevention of complications
Lymphomas: Hodgkin's disease, non-Hodgkin's lymphoma, Burkitt's lymphoma *(pp 450-451, 456-457)*	1. Increased risk for infection 2. Risk of infection and excessive bleeding in patients receiving chemotherapy 3. Possible risk of osteonecrosis in patients treated by radiation to head and neck region (this usually does not occur because radiation dosage seldom exceeds 6000 rads) 4. Xerostomia may occur in patients treated by radiation to head and neck region 5. Non-Hodgkin's lymphoma can be found in patients with AIDS; hence transmission of infectious agents may be a potential problem	1. See section on chemotherapy concerning management and prevention of medical complications 2. See section on radiation for prevention and management of medical complications 3. Patients with generalized lymphadenopathy, extranodal tumors, and osseous lesions need to be identified and referred for medical evaluation and treatment 4. Dentist can biopsy extranodal or osseous lesions to establish a diagnosis; patients with lesions involving lymph nodes should be referred for needle biopsy 5. Medical history should identify patients with diagnosed disease; medical consultation will be needed to establish current status

Radiation-treated patients (radiation to head and neck) *(pp 471-472, 475, 476-479)*	1. Patients treated by radiation tend to develop the following problems during and just after completion of therapy
	  a. Mucositis
	  b. Xerostomia
	  c. Loss of taste
	  d. Constricture of muscles
	  e. Secondary infections—viral, bacterial, fungal (candidiasis)
	  f. Sensitivity of teeth
	2. Chronic problems caused by radiation therapy include
	  a. Xerostomia
	  b. Cervical caries
	  c. Osteonecrosis
	  d. Muscle trismus
	  e. Sensitivity of teeth
	  f. Loss of taste
		1. Before radiation therapy is started, dentist should be involved; and after a complete examination the following procedures should be done:
		  a. Extract all teeth that cannot be repaired
		  b. Extract all teeth with advanced periodontal disease
		  c. Perform all preprosthetic surgery
		  d. Restore all large carious lesions
		  e. Establish good oral hygiene
		  f. Start daily fluoride treatment using flexible tray and gel
		  g. All nonvital teeth should be endodontically treated or extracted
		  h. Chronic infection in jawbones should be treated
		2. During radiation treatment, dentist can be involved with
		  a. Symptomatic treatment of mucositis (Appendix B)
		  b. Management of xerostomia (Appendix B)
		  c. Prevention of trismus by having patient place tongue blades or bite block into mouth each day to maintain maximum opening.
		  d. Chlorhexidine rinses for plaque and candidiasis control (Appendix B)

Treatment plan modifications	Oral complications	Emergency care
1. Patients in terminal phase should receive only supportive dental treatment 2. Patient under "control" can receive any indicated treatment; however, complex restorative treatment may not be indicated in cases with poor prognosis 3. See sections on radiation and chemotherapy for treatment plan modifications 4. Platelet replacement may be needed for patients with thrombocytopenia	1. Extranodal oral tumors or osseous soft tissues 2. Xerostomia in patients treated by radiation; some of these patients may be prone to osteonecrosis 3. Burning mouth or tongue symptoms may occur 4. Petechiae or ecchymoses if thrombocytopenia present due to tumor invasion of bone marrow 5. Cervical lymphadenopathy 6. Mucositis in patients treated by radiation or chemotherapy	1. Conservative for patients undergoing radiation or chemotherapy 2. Patients with stable disease can receive any indicated emergency treatment 3. Patients in terminal stage should receive conservative treatment

1. Once radiation treatment has been completed and more than 6000 rads used, every effort must be made to avoid osteonecrosis
  a. Teeth should not be extracted
  b. Diseased teeth should be endodontically treated if indicated
2. Aggressive preventive measures are needed to prevent periodontal disease and cervical caries
3. Most dental procedures other than extractions and surgical procedures can be done
	1. Mucositis
	2. Candidiasis
	3. Xerostomia
	4. Loss of taste
	5. Trismus
	6. Sensitivity of teeth
	7. Cervical caries
	8. Osteonecrosis
		Must avoid extractions if at all possible in postradiation patients; other emergency care can be provided as needed

Dental Management: A Summary—cont'd

Medical problem	Potential problem related to dental care	Prevention of complications

Radiation-treated patients (radiation to head and neck)—cont'd		e. Diagnosis and treatment of secondary infection—candidiasis, etc (Appendix B)
		f. Continue daily fluoride treatment
		3. Following radiation treatment, dentist should
		  a. Have patient back for frequent recall appointments (every 3 to 6 months)
		  b. Continue emphasis on good oral hygiene
		  c. Treat carious lesions when first detected
		  d. Make every effort to avoid oral infection
		  e. Manage xerostomia (Appendix B)
		  f. Manage chronic loss of taste (Appendix B)

Patients receiving chemotherapy for cancer *(pp 472-473, 479-481)*	1. Excessive bleeding because of bone marrow suppression (thrombocytopenia)
	2. Prone to infection because of bone marrow suppression (leukopenia)
	3. Severe anemia from bone marrow suppression
	4. Thrombocytopenia, leukopenia, and anemia may also be complications of underlying cancer
		1. Prior to starting chemotherapy
		  a. Eliminate gross infection
		    (1) Periapical
		    (2) Periodontal
		    (3) Soft tissue
		  b. Treat advanced carious lesions
		  c. Provide oral hygiene instructions
		  d. In children and young adults
		    (1) Remove mobile primary teeth
		    (2) Remove gingival operculum
		2. During chemotherapy
		  a. Consult with oncologist prior to any invasive dental procedures
		  b. If invasive procedures must be performed
		    (1) Antibiotic prophylaxis if granulocyte count less than $2000/mm^3$
		    (2) Consider platelet replacement if platelet count less than $80,000/mm^3$
		  c. Culture and antibiotic sensitivity testing of exudate from areas of infection
		  d. Control spontaneous bleeding by gauze, periodontal packing, soft mouth guard
		  e. Topical fluoride for caries control
		  f. Chlorhexidine rinses for plaque and candidiasis control (Appendix B)
		  g. Symptomatic relief of mucositis and xerostomia (Appendix B)
		  h. If severe anemia is present, avoid general anesthesia
		  i. Home care instructions (may need to be modified based on oral status): reduce or stop flossing and brushing if excessive bleeding or tissue irritation result; can use damp gauze to wipe gingiva and teeth; use solution of water and baking soda to rinse mouth to clean ulcerated tissues

Treatment plan modifications	Oral complications	Emergency care

1. Perform only emergency dental treatment during chemotherapy
2. Based on prognosis of underlying disease, dental treatment may be limited to only immediate care needs for patients being treated in palliative sense; however, children and adults being treated for leukemia may have very good prognosis, and any indicated dental treatment can be performed; also many patients with lymphoma can have good prognosis
	1. Mucositis
	2. Excessive bleeding following minor trauma
	3. Spontaneous gingival bleeding
	4. Xerostomia
	5. Infection
	6. Poor healing
		1. Conservative emergency treatment during chemotherapy:
		  a. Pain medication
		  b. Antibiotics for infection
		  c. Avoid surgical procedures if possible
		2. When surgical procedure must be done
		  a. Consult with oncologist
		  b. Platelet replacement if indicated
		  c. Gelfoam and thrombin, microfibrillar collagen, and/or splints may be used
		  d. Prophylactic antibiotics may be indicated

Dental Management: A Summary—cont'd

Medical problem	Potential problem related to dental care	Prevention of complications

Patients receiving chemotherapy for cancer— cont'd		j. Avoid food aversion during chemotherapy— fast before treatment (4 hours), eat novel non-important food just before treatment, avoid nutritionally important foods during posttreatment nausea
		3. Following completion of chemotherapy
		  a. Monitor patient until all side effects of therapy have cleared
		  b. Place patient on dental recall program

Behavioral and psychiatric disorders: bipolar disorders, schizophrenia, major depression, Alzheimer's disease, posttraumatic stress disorder (PTSD), substance abuse *(pp 483-511)*	1. Patient may be difficult to communicate with
	2. Patient may be uncooperative or aggressive
	3. Significant drug side effects may occur in patients taking neuroleptic, antidepressant, or antianxiety medications
	4. Significant drug interactions may occur with agents used by dentist in treating patients taking neuroleptic, antidepressant, or antianxiety medications
	5. Patient may have little interest in maintaining good oral health
	6. Patient may not be able to maintain good hygiene due to inability to function
	7. Patients abusing cocaine may be at great risk if treated while "high"; danger is from myocardial ischemia and cardiac arrhythmias secondary to cocaine, which can be aggravated by medications used in dental care such as epinephrine
	8. Patient who is an IV substance abuser is at increased risk for hepatitis (HBV, HCV, HDV) and AIDS
		1. Identification of patients with behavioral or psychiatric disorders
		  a. History—illness that has been diagnosed by physician; taking medication used to manage behavioral or mental disorder
		  b. Examination findings
		    (1) Injuries that could be self-inflicted
		    (2) Observation of unusual behavior that could be associated with undetected mental disorders
		2. Referral for diagnosis and management—patient identified who may have a behavioral or mental disorder
		3. Consultation with patient's physician to confirm medications, determine current status, and review dental management plan
		4. No dental treatment should be provided to any patient who is "high" on cocaine; at least 6 hours should have elapsed since last administration of cocaine before dental treatment is considered
		5. Infection control procedures must be followed when treating any patient, but of particular concern are patients with history of IV substance abuse; dental personnel should be vaccinated for protection from hepatitis B

Treatment plan modifications	Oral complications	Emergency care

1. See section below for precautions regarding use of epinephrine, sedatives, hypnotics, narcotics, atropine, and phenylephrine
2. PTSD—extra important to attempt to develop trust and to establish communication with these patients
3. Dementia—establish good oral hygiene and dental repair early in course of disease
   a. Use empathetic approach
   b. Positive nonverbal communication
   c. Keep attention, short words and sentences
   d. Be repetitive
   e. Sedation may be needed, chloral hydrate or oxazepam
   f. Aggressive preventive program, 3-month recall
4. Manic disorder—often tendency to overbrush, may cause abrasion of teeth and injury to gingiva
5. Depression—little interest in dental health; often poor dental repair
6. Schizophrenia
   a. Have attendant or family member accompany patient
   b. Schedule morning appointments
   c. Avoid confrontational and authoritative attitude
   d. Elective care only if under good medical management

1. PTSD: poor hygiene increased incidence of caries and periodontal disease, glossodynia, bruxism
2. Dementia: oral injuries, poor hygiene, periodontal disease
3. Manic disorder: injury to soft tissue and abrasion of teeth from over-flossing or over-brushing
4. Depression: facial pain syndromes, glossodynia, poor hygiene, medications (see section below)
5. Oral lesions (may be self-inflicted in some cases)

Emergency dental care can be rendered as needed, provided
1. Phone consultation with physician if possible
2. Local anesthetic without vasconstrictor is used
3. Pain medication is selected with care
   a. Use nonnarcotic analgesics, or
   b. Use ¼ to ½ normal dose of narcotics
4. Patients who are uncooperative may have to be sedated
5. No dental treatment for patient who is high on cocaine (wait at least 6 hours)
6. Use infectious disease control procedures for *all* patients

Medical problem	Potential problem related to dental care	Prevention of complications
Behavioral and psychiatric disorders: bipolar disorders, schizophrenia, major depression, Alzheimer's disease, posttraumatic stress disorder (PTSD), substance abuse—cont'd		
Medications used for mental disorders 1. **Antipsychotic (neuroleptic) agents: chlorpromazine (Thorazine), fluphenazine (Permitil), trifluoperazine (Stelazine), mesoridazine (Serentil), haloperidol (Haldol), molindone (Moban)** 2. **Heterocyclics: amitriptyline (Elvavil), imipramine (Tofranil), amoxapine (Asendin), maprotiline (Ludiomil)** 3. **Monoamine oxidase inhibitors: phenelzine (Nardil), isocarboxazid (Marplan), tranylcypromine (Parnate)**	1. Drug side effects a. Xerostomia (MAO inhibitors, lithium, neuroleptics) b. Hypotension (MAO inhibitors, heterocyclics, neuroleptics) c. Tachycardia, arrhythmias (heterocyclics, neuroleptics) d. Bleeding, thrombocytopenia (neuroleptics) e. Infection, leukopenia (neuroleptics, lithium) f. Kidney failure (lithium) g. Stomatitis (lithium) h. Sedation, cognitive impairment, aggressive and impulsive behavior (benzodiazepines) 2. Drug interactions with agents used in dentistry a. Epinephrine—potential for hypertensive crisis, myocardial infarction, etc (neuroleptics, heterocyclics) b. Atropine—increased intraocular pressure (MAO inhibitors, heterocyclics) c. Sedatives, hypnotics, barbiturates, and narcotics—may cause respiratory depression (neuroleptics, MAO inhibitors, heterocyclics, benzodiazepines)	1. Identification of patients a. History—patients with bipolar disorder, schizophrenia, major depression, Alzheimer's disease, posttraumatic stress disorders, substance abuse disorders, and other behavioral or mental disorders may be taking neuroleptics, antidepressants, or anxiolytics b. History—ask patients to list or identify all medications they are taking c. Identification of patients with side effects of neuroleptics, MAO inhibitors, lithium, heterocyclic drugs, or benzodiazepines (1) Neuroleptics (a) Agranucytosis (b) Leukopenia (c) Thrombocytopenia (d) Dystonia (e) Akathisia (f) Tardive dyskinesa (2) MAO inhibitors and heterocyclics (a) Hypotension (b) Tachycardia (c) Arrhythmias (d) Orthostatic hypotension (3) Lithium (a) Renal failure (b) Stomatitis (c) Chorea (d) Seizures (4) Benzodiazepines (a) Sedation (a) Cognitive impairment (b) Impulsive and aggressive behavior 2. Referral of patients found to have significant side effects resulting from their medications 3. Consultation with physician to confirm medications, determine current status of patient, and review dental management plan

Treatment plan modifications	Oral complications	Emergency care

e. Consider sedation if patient difficult to manage
7. Treatment plan should attempt to
   a. Maintain oral health and comfort
   b. Prevent and control oral diseases
   c. Be realistic
   d. Be dynamic and flexible

Treatment plan modifications	Oral complications	Emergency care

1. See specific section above
2. Use local anesthetic without vasoconstrictor whenever possible; however, for surgical procedures or long complex restorative procedures an anesthetic with small amounts of epinephrine can be used
   a. 1:100,000 epinephrine
   b. Aspirate before injecting
   c. Use no more than three carpules
3. Do not use "topical" epinephrine to control bleeding or in retraction cord
4. Avoid use of atropine
5. Reduce dosage of sedatives, hypnotics, or narcotics

1. See above section for oral findings associated with certain mental conditions
2. No significant oral findings associated with medications unless drug side effects present
   a. Agranulocytosis—ulceration, infection
   b. Xerostomia
   c. Thrombocytopenia—bleeding
   d. Leukopenia—infection
   e. Stomatitis

Emergency dental care can be rendered as needed, provided
1. Phone consultation with physician if possible
2. Local anesthetic without a vasoconstrictor is used
3. Pain medication is selected with care and given in reduced doses
   a. Use nonnarcotic analgesics
   b. Use ¼ to ½ normal dose of narcotics

Dental Management: A Summary—cont'd

Medical problem	Potential problem related to dental care	Prevention of complications

Medications used for mental disorders—cont'd
4. Lithium
5. Benzodiazepines (antianxiety), chlordiazepoxide (Librium), diazepam (Valium), alprazolam (Xanax) *(pp 495-500, 508)*
	3. Difficult to manage during dental appointment
	4. Diffult for patient to follow preventive meaures—flossing, brushing, etc
		4. Reduce dosage or avoid agents used in dentistry that may cause drug interactions with medications patient is taking
		  a. Epinephrine (neuroleptics, heterocyclics)
		  b. Sedatives, hypnotics, narcotics, antihistamines (neuroleptics, MAO inhibitors, heterocyclics)
		  c. Atropine (MAO inhibitors, heterocyclics)
		  d. Antacids (neuroleptics)
		  e. Phenylephrine (MAO inhibitors)

Chronic obstructive pulmonary disease *(pp 235-238)*	Aggravation or worsening of compromised respiratory function	1. Use upright chair position 2. Avoid bilateral mandibular or palatal blocks 3. Avoid use of rubber dam in severe disease 4. Low-flow oxygen may be helpful 5. Nitrous oxide–oxygen sedation is best avoided 6. Low-dose oral diazepam is acceptable 7. Avoid barbiturates, narcotics, antihistamines, and anticholinergics 8. If taking steroids, may need supplementation 9. If patient taking theophylline, avoid erythromycin 10. Outpatient general anesthesia is contraindicated

Osteoarthritis *(pp 322-324)*	1. Joint pain, stiffness, and loss of mobility
	2. Bleeding tendency from aspirin or NSAIDs
		1. Short appointment
		2. Ensure physical comfort
		  a. Position changes
		  b. Comfortable chair position
		  c. Physical supports
		3. Pretreatment bleeding time if taking large dosage of aspirin or NSAIDs (less than 20 minutes)

Treatment plan modifications	Oral complications	Emergency care
None	None	Basic recommendations apply to emergency care
Dictated by severity of disability; if severe, extensive treatment not indicated; encourage and facilitate oral hygiene	Temporomandibular joint involvement	Follow normal recommendations

Dental Management: A Summary—cont'd

Medical problem	Potential problem related to dental care	Prevention of complications

Hypertension *(pp 161-173)*	1. Stress and anxiety related to dental visit may cause increase in blood pressure; angina, myocardial infarction, or cerebrovascular accident may precipitated
	2. Patients being treated with antihypertensive agents may become nauseated, may become hypotensive, or may develop postural hypotension
	3. Excessive use of vasopressors may cause significant elevation of blood pressure
	4. Many antihypertensive agents can potentiate sedative action of barbiturates
	5. Sedative medication used in patients taking certain antihypertensive agents may bring about hypotensive episode(s)
	6. If blood pressure is significantly elevated, excessive bleeding may occur following surgical or scaling procedure
		1. Detection and referral of patients with significant elevation of blood pressure for medical evaluation and treatment
		2. Patients being treated with antihypertensive agents
		  a. Reduce stress and anxiety of dental visit by premedication, short appointments, and open concerned atmosphere by dentist and staff; let patient talk about fears and concerns related to dental visit; nitrous oxide can be used, but hypoxia must be avoided
		  b. If patient becomes overly stressed, terminate appointment
		  c. Avoid orthostatic hypotension by changing chair position slowly and supporting patient when getting out of chair
		  d. Avoid stimulating gag reflex
		  e. Select sedative medication and dosage based on consultation with patient's physician
		3. Drug considerations
		  a. Use local anesthetics judiciously with minimal concentration of vasopressor (epinephrine 1:100,000 or 1:200,000) and no more than three cartridges; aspirate before injection and inject slowly
		  b. Do not use topical vasopressors to control local bleeding
		  c. Do not use gingival packing material that contains epinephrine
		  d. Reduce dosage of barbiturates and other sedatives whose actions are enhanced by many antihypertensive agents
		  e. Avoid use of general anesthesia
		  f. Epinephrine and levonordefrin may be used in patient being treated with MAO inhibitor

Asthma *(pp 238-241)*	Precipitation of acute asthma attack	1. Identification of asthmatic patient by history
		2. Determination of character of asthma
		  a. Type (allergic or nonallergic)
		  b. Precipitating factors
		  c. Age at onset
		  d. Frequency and severity of attacks
		  e. How usually managed
		  f. Medications being taken
		  g. Necessity for past emergency care
		3. Avoidance of known precipitating factors
		4. Consultation with physician for severe, active asthma

Treatment plan modifications	Oral complications	Emergency care
1. In severe, uncontrolled hypertensive patients (>200 systolic or >115 diastolic), emergency care only 2. In patients under good medical management with no complications, such as renal failure, any indicated treatment 3. In patients with complications, refer to appropriate section	1. Xerostomia secondary to diuretics and other antihypertensive 2. Mercurial diuretics may cause oral ulceration or stomatitis 3. Lichenoid reactions may be seen with thiazides, methyldopa, propranolol, and labetalol 4. Lupus-like reaction, rarely seen with hydralazine 5. Excessive bleeding could develop in uncontrolled hypertensive patient following surgical procedure	Basic management recommendations apply to necessary emergency care
None required	Oral candidiasis reported with use of inhaler without "spacer" but is rare	Basic recommendations also apply for emergency care

Dental Management: A Summary—cont'd

Medical problem	Potential problem related to dental care	Prevention of complications

Asthma—cont'd		5. Patient should bring medication inhaler to each appointment
		6. Drug considerations; avoid
		  a. Aspirin containing medications
		  b. NSAIDs
		  c. Narcotics and barbiturates
		  d. Erythromycin if patient taking theophylline
		7. May want to avoid sulfite-containing local anesthetic solution
		8. Chronic corticosteroid use may require supplementation
		9. Premedicate anxious patient (nitrous oxide or diazepam)
		10. Provision of stress-free environment

Tuberculosis
(pp 241-247)
	1. Tuberculosis may be contracted by dentist from actively infectious patient
	2. Patients and staff can be infected by dentist who is actively infectious
		Caveat: Many patients with infectious disease cannot be identified by history or examination; therefore all patients should be approached using universal precautions (Appendix A)
		1. Patient with active sputum-positive tuberculosis
		  a. Consultation with physician before treatment
		  b. Treatment limited to emergency care (over age 6 years)
		  c. Treatment in hospital setting with proper isolation, sterilization, mask, gloves, gown, ventilation
		  d. Patient under age 6 years—treatment as normal patient (noninfectious) after consultation with physician
		  e. Patient producing consistently negative sputum while undergoing chemotherapy—treat as normal patient
		2. Patient with past history of tuberculosis
		  a. Approach with caution; obtain good history of disease and its treatment; appropriate review of systems
		  b. Should give history of periodic chest x-rays and examination to rule out reactivation
		  c. Consult with physician and postpone treatment if
		    (1) Questionable history of adequate treatment
		    (2) Lack of appropriate medical supervision since recovery
		    (3) Signs or symptoms of relapse
		  d. If present status free of clinical disease, treat as normal patient

Treatment plan modifications	Oral complications	Emergency care

None required	1. Oral ulceration (rare), tongue most common
	2. Tuberculous involvement of cervical and submandibular lymph nodes (scrofula)
		1. If clinical disease present
		  a. Consultation with physician before treatment
		  b. Isolation of dental operatory (hospital)
		  c. Strict aseptic procedures
		  d. Gloves, gown, mask
		  e. Use of rubber dam when possible
		  f. Use of slow-speed handpiece when possible to minimize aerosol
		  g. Minimize use of air syringe
		  h. Only necessary work done
		  i. Scrubbing and sterilizing of all equipment after use
		2. If free of clinical disease, provide normal care as indicated

Dental Management: A Summary—cont'd

Medical problem	Potential problem related to dental care	Prevention of complications

Tuberculosis— cont'd		3. Patients with recent conversion to positive tuberculin skin test (purified protein derivative [PPD])
		   a. Should have been evaluated by physician to rule out clinical disease
		   b. May be receiving isoniazid (INH) for 6 months to 1 year prophylactically
		   c. Treatment as normal patient
		 4. Patients with signs or symptoms of tuberculosis
		   a. Refer to physician and postpone treatment
		   b. If treatment necessary, treat as in 1 above

Viral hepatitis, type B, delta, type C
 (pp 258-269)
	1. Hepatitis may be contracted by dentist from infectious patient
	 2. Patients or staff can be infected by dentist with active hepatitis or who is a carrier
	 3. With chronic active hepatitis may have bleeding tendency or altered drug metabolism
		Caveat: Because most carriers are undetectable by history, all patients should be treated using universal precautions (Appendix A); risk can be decreased by use of hepatitis B vaccine
		 1. Patient with active hepatitis
		   a. Consultation with physician
		   b. Treatment on emergency basis only
		 2. Patients with history of hepatitis
		   a. Consultation with physician
		   b. Probable type determination
		     (1) Age at time of infection (type B uncommon under age 15 years)
		     (2) Source of infection (if food or water, usually type A or E)
		     (3) If blood transfusion–related, probably type C
		     (4) If type indeterminate, radioimmunoassay (RIA) for hepatitis B surface antigen (HBsAg) may be considered
		 3. Patients in high-risk categories—consider RIA for HBsAg or anti-HCV
		 4. If HBsAg positive (carrier)
		   a. Consultation with physician
		   b. Minimize drugs metabolized by liver
		   c. Preoperative prothrombin time and bleeding time if chronic active hepatitis

Alcoholic liver disease (cirrhosis)
 (pp 269-275)
	1. Bleeding tendencies; unpredictable drug metabolism	1. Identification of alcoholic patients
		   a. History
		   b. Clinical examination
		   c. Detection of odor on breath
		   d. Information from friends or relatives
		 2. Consultation with physician to verify current status

Treatment plan modifications	Oral complications	Emergency care

None required	Bleeding	1. If active disease
		  a. Consult with physician
		  b. Minimize drugs detoxified by liver
		  c. If surgery necessary, obtain prothrombin time and bleeding time before surgery
		  d. Do only necessary work
		2. If no active disease, provide care as indicated

Since oral neglect is commonly seen in alcoholics, patients should be required to demonstrate interest in and ability to care for dentition before any significant treatment	1. Neglect 2. Bleeding 3. Ecchymoses 4. Petechiae 5. Glossitis 6. Angular cheilosis 7. Impaired healing	In addition to prior medical recommendations, abnormal laboratory values in surgical patients may suggest use of antifibrinolytic agents, platelets, fresh frozen plasma, and vitamin K

Medical problem	Potential problem related to dental care	Prevention of complications
Alcoholic liver disease (cirrhosis)— cont'd		3. Laboratory screening a. Complete blood count with differential b. AST, ALT c. Bleeding time d. Thrombin time e. Prothrombin time 4. Minimize drugs metabolized by liver 5. If screening tests abnormal for surgery, consider antifibrinolytic agents, fresh frozen plasma, vitamin K, platelets
End-stage renal disease *(pp 248-257)*	1. Bleeding tendency 2. Hypertension 3. Anemia 4. Intolerance to nephrotoxic drugs metabolized by kidney 5. Enhanced susceptibility to infection	1. Consultation with physician 2. Pretreatment screening for hematologic disorder (bleeding time, prothrombin time, partial thromboplastin time, hematocrit, hemoglobin) 3. Close monitoring of blood pressure before and during treatment 4. Avoidance of drugs excreted by kidney or nephrotoxic drugs 5. Meticulous attention to good surgical technique to minimize chances of abnormal bleeding or infection 6. Aggressive management of infection
Hemodialysis *(pp 252-257)*	1. Bleeding tendency 2. Hypertension 3. Anemia 4. Intolerance to nephrotoxic drugs metabolized by kidney 5. Bacterial endarteritis of arteriovenous fistula secondary to bacteremia 6. Hepatitis (active or carrier)	1. Consultation with physician 2. No dental treatment until off dialysis machine for at least 4 hours (because of heparin); best on day following 3. Pretreatment screening for bleeding disorder (bleeding time, prothrombin time, partial thromboplastin time) 4. Avoidance of drugs metabolized by kidney or nephrotoxic drugs 5. Consider antibiotic prophylaxis for dental work to minimize effects of bacteremia 6. Pretreatment screening for HBsAg
Gonorrhea *(pp 276-278, 285, 286)*	Remote possibility of transmission from oral or pharyngeal lesions of an infected patient	Caveat: Many patients with sexually transmitted disease cannot be identified by history or examination and therefore all patients must be approached using universal precautions (Appendix A) 1. Patients currently receiving treatment for gonorrhea—provide necessary care 2. Patients with past history of gonorrhea a. Obtain good history of disease and its treatment b. Provide necessary care 3. Patients with signs or symptoms suggestive of gonorrhea a. Refer to physician for evaluation b. Provide necessary care

Treatment plan modifications	Oral complications	Emergency care
	8. Parotid enlargement 9. Candidiasis 10. Oral cancer 11. Alcohol breath odor 12. Bruxism 13. Dental attrition 14. Xerostomia	
1. Major emphasis on oral hygiene and optimum maintenance care to eliminate possible sources of infection 2. No contraindications for routine dental care but would discourage extensive reconstructive crown and bridge procedures	Mucosal pallor Xerostomia Metallic taste Ammonia breath odor Stomatitis Loss of lamina dura Bone radiolucencies	Follow same management recommendations as for routine dental care but consider hospitalization for severe infection or major procedures
1. Major emphasis on oral hygiene and optimum maintenance care to eliminate possible sources of infection 2. No contraindications for routine dental care	Oral ulcerations and candidiasis	Follow same management recommendations as for routine dental care but consider hospitalization for severe infection or major procedures
None required	Rare but varied expression including generalized stomatitis, ulceration, and formation of pseudomembranous coating	1. If active oral disease present a. Provide necessary dental care b. Refer to physician 2. If free of disease, provide normal care as indicated

Dental Management: A Summary—cont'd

Medical problem	Potential problem related to dental care	Prevention of complications

Syphilis
(pp 279-282, 286-287)
	1. Syphilis may be contracted by dentist from actively infectious patient
	2. Patients or staff may be infected by dentist who has syphilis
		Caveat: Many patients with sexually transmitted disease cannot be identified by history or examination; therefore all patients must be approached using universal precautions (Appendix A)
		1. Patients currently receiving treatment for syphilis
		  a. Consultation with physician before treatment
		  b. Provide necessary care
		  c. Oral lesions of primary and secondary syphilis are infectious prior to initiation of antibiotic therapy
		2. Patients with past history of syphilis
		  a. Approach with caution; obtain good history of disease, its treatment, and negative serologic tests for syphilis (STS) test following therapy
		  b. If free of disease, treat as normal patient
		3. Patients with signs or symptoms suggestive of syphilis
		  a. Refer to physician and postpone treatment
		  b. May elect to order STS test before referral
		  c. If treatment necessary, treat as in category I

Genital herpes *(pp 282-285, 286, 287)*	Inoculation of oral cavity and potential transmission to dentist's fingers	Caveat: Many patients with sexually transmitted disease cannot be identified by history or examination; therefore all patients must be approached using universal precautions (Appendix A) 1. Localized genital infection poses no problem; however, be aware of possibility of autoinoculation to oral cavity by patient 2. Oral infection of type 1 or type 2—postpone elective dental care

Pregnancy and lactation
(pp 383-389)
	1. Dental procedures could harm developing fetus via
	  a. Radiation
	  b. Drugs
	2. Supine hypotension in late pregnancy
	3. Poor nutrition
	4. Transmission of drugs to infant via breast milk
		1. Women of childbearing age
		  a. Always use contemporary radiographic techniques including lead apron when performing radiographic examination
		  b. Avoid prescribing drugs that are known to be harmful to fetus or whose effects are as yet unknown (Table 20-3)
		  c. Encourage patients to maintain balanced, nutritious diet
		2. Pregnant women
		  a. Advisable to contact patient's physician to verify physical status, present management plan; ask for suggestions regarding patient's treatment especially relating to drug administration

Treatment plan modifications	Oral complications	Emergency care

None required	1. Chancre
	2. Mucous patch
	3. Gumma
	4. Interstitial glossitis
		1. If active disease present
		  a. Consult with physician before treatment
		  b. Provide necessary care
		2. If free of disease, provide normal care as indicated

None required	Autoinoculation of type 2 herpes to oral cavity	If oral herpetic lesions are present, avoid elective care; if care necessary, use gloves and wear protective eyeglasses; avoid contact with lesion
None, except that major reconstructive procedures, crown and bridge fabrication, or significant operations are best delayed until after delivery	1. Exaggeration of periodontal disease, "pregnancy gingivitis" 2. "Pregnancy tumor" 3. Tooth mobility	Essentially same as for routine care; advisable to consult physician before treatment

Medical problem	Potential problem related to dental care	Prevention of complications

Pregnancy and lactation— cont'd		b. Maintain optimum oral hygiene, including prophylaxis, throughout pregnancy
		c. Avoid elective dental care during first trimester; second trimester and most of third trimester are best times for elective treatment
		d. Avoid radiographs during first trimester; thereafter take only those necessary for treatment, always using lead apron
		e. Avoid administration of drugs known to be harmful to fetus or whose effects are unknown (Table 20-3)
		f. In advanced stages of pregnancy (late third trimester), avoid placing patient in supine position for prolonged periods; avoid aspirin
		5. Lactating mothers
		  a. Most drugs are of little pharmacologic significance to lactation
		  b. Avoid drugs known to be harmful (Table 20-3)
		  c. Administer drugs just after breast-feeding

Rheumatoid arthritis *(pp 316-322)*	1. Joint pain and immobility
	2. Bleeding tendencies secondary to aspirin and nonsteroidal anti-inflammatory drugs
	3. Bone marrow suppression from gold salts, penicillamine, sulfasalazine, or immunosuppressives—resulting in anemia, agranulocytosis, or thrombocytopenia
		1. Short appointments
		2. Physical comfort
		  a. Position changes
		  b. Comfortable chair position
		  c. Physical supports
		3. Management of drug complications
		  a. Aspirin or nonsteroidal antiinflammatory drugs (NSAIDs)—obtain pretreatment bleeding time (less than 20 minutes)
		  b. Gold salts, penicillamine, sulfasalazine, or immunosuppressives—obtain complete blood count with differential and bleeding time
		  c. Corticosteroids—possible need for supplements

Stroke *(pp 334-339)*	1. Dental treatment could precipitate stroke
	2. Bleeding secondary to drug therapy
		1. Identification of stroke-prone patient from history (hypertension, smoking, transient ischemic attacks [TIAs], etc)
		2. Reduce patient's risk factors for stroke
		3. For past history of stroke
		  a. For current TIAs—no elective care
		  b. Drug considerations
		    (1) Aspirin and dipyridamole—obtain pretreatment bleeding time (less than 20 minutes)
		    (2) Coumarin drugs—obtain prothrombin time under 35 seconds
		  c. Short, morning appointments
		  d. Monitor blood pressure
		  e. Use minimum amount of vasoconstrictor in local anesthetic
		  f. No epinephrine in retraction cord

Treatment plan modifications	Oral complications	Emergency care
Dictated by severity of disability and temporomandibular joint involvement; if severe, extensive treatment not needed; temporo-mandibular joint surgery may be indicated; encourage and facilitate oral hygiene	1. Temporomandibular joint involvement 2. Stomatitis secondary to gold salts, penicillamine and immunosuppressives	Follow normal recommendations
1. Dependent on physical impairment 2. All restorations should be easily cleansable 3. Modified oral hygiene aids may be needed	None	Follow normal recommendations

Dental Management: A Summary—cont'd

Medical problem	Potential problem related to dental care	Prevention of complications

Epilepsy
(pp 328-334)
	1. Occurrence of generalized tonic-clonic seizure in dental office
	2. Drug-induced leukopenia and thrombocytopenia (phenytoin, carbemazepine, valproic acid)
		1. Identification of epileptic patient by history
		   a. Type of seizure
		   b. Age at time of onset
		   c. Cause of seizures
		   d. Medications
		   e. Regularity of physician visits
		   f. Degree of control
		   g. Frequency of seizures
		   h. Last seizure
		   i. Precipitating factors
		   j. History of seizure-related injuries
		2. Well controlled—provide normal care
		3. Poorly controlled—consult with physician; may require medication change
		4. Be alert to adverse effects of anticonvulsants
		5. Patients taking valproic acid—obtain bleeding time; avoid aspirin and NSAIDs
		6. Avoid propoxyphene and erythromycin in patients taking carbemazepine
		7. Be prepared to manage seizure

Adrenal insufficiency
(pp 361-369)
	1. Inability to tolerate stress
	2. Delayed healing
	3. Susceptibility to infection
	4. Hypertension
		1. For routine dental procedures, including extractions, using local anesthetic
		   a. Patients currently taking corticosteroids—no additional supplementation generally required; be sure to obtain good local anesthesia and good postoperative pain control
		   b. Patients with past history of regular corticosteroid usage—if less than 2 weeks, give normal daily maintenance dose on day of procedure; if more than 2 weeks, none generally required
		   c. Patients using topical or inhalational steroids—generally no supplementation
		2. For extensive procedures or extreme patient anxiety, with local anesthetic
		   a. Patients currently taking corticosteroids—double normal daily dose on day of procedure; if postoperative pain is anticipated, double daily dose on first postoperative day
		   b. Patients with past history of regular corticosteroid usage—if less than 2 weeks, give double daily maintenance dose on day of procedure; if longer than 2 weeks, none generally required

Treatment plan modifications	Oral complications	Emergency care
1. Maintenance of optimum oral hygiene 2. Surgical reduction of gingival hyperplasia if indicated 3. Replace missing teeth with fixed prosthesis as opposed to removable 4. Choose metal over porcelain when possible	Gingival hyperplasia secondary to phenytoin (Dilantin)	Follow normal recommendations
None required	1. Primary—pigmentation of oral mucous membranes 2. Delayed healing 3. Susceptibility to infection	Basic recommendations apply to emergency care

Dental Management: A Summary—cont'd

Medical problem	Potential problem related to dental care	Prevention of complications

Solid organ transplantation *(pp 512-532, 517-520)* ▪ **Common problems found in all patients**	1. Infection from suppression of immune response by
	  a. Cyclosporine
	  b. Azathioprine
	  c. Prednisone
	  d. Antithymocyte globulin
	  e. Antilymphocyte globulin
	  f. Orthoclone (monoclonal antibody)
	2. Acute rejection, reversible
	3. Chronic rejection, nonreversible
	  a. Graft failure—end stage organ failure
	  b. Bleeding—liver, kidney
	  c. Drug overdosage—liver, kidney
	  d. Death or transplantation—heart, liver
	  e. Transplantation or hemodialysis—kidney
	  f. Transplantation or insulin—pancreas
	4. Cancer associated with use of immunosuppressants
	  a. Squamous cell carcinoma of skin
	  b. Squamous cell carcinoma of lip
	  c. Lymphoma
	  d. Kaposi's sarcoma
	5. Side effects of drugs used to suppress the immune response
	  a. Hypertension
	  b. Diabetes mellitus
	  c. Osteoporosis
	  d. Psychoses
	  e. Anemia
	  f. Leukopenia
	  g. Thrombocytopenia
	  h. Gingival hyperplasia
		1. Dental evaluation and treatment before transplantation
		  a. Establish stable oral and dental status free of active dental disease
		  b. Initiate aggressive oral hygiene program to maintain oral health
		  c. Medical consultation for patients with organ failure prior to performing needed dental treatment to establish
		    (1) Degree of failure
		    (2) Current status of patient
		    (3) Need for antibiotic prophylaxis
		    (4) Need to modify drug selection or dosage
		    (5) Need to take special precautions to avoid bleeding
		    (6) If surgery is indicated, access to recent prothrombin time, partial thromboplastin time, bleeding time, and white cell count or differential may be needed
		2. Dental treatment after transplantation
		  a. Immediate posttransplant period (6 months)
		    (1) Emergency dental care only
		    (2) Continue oral hygiene procedures
		  b. Stable graft period
		    (1) Maintain oral hygiene
		    (2) Recall every 3 months
		    (3) Use universal precautions
		    (4) Vaccination of dental staff against HBV infection
		    (5) Medical consultation
		      (a) Need for antibiotic prophylaxis
		      (b) Need for precautions to avoid excessive bleeding
		      (c) Need for supplemental steroids
		      (d) Selection of drugs and dosage
		    (6) Examine for clinical evidence of
		      (a) Organ failure or rejection
		      (b) Overimmunosuppression (tumors, infection, etc)
		    (7) Monitor blood pressure at every appointment

Treatment plan modifications	Oral complications	Emergency care

1. Prior to transplantation
  a. Patients with poor dental status, consider extractions and full dentures
  b. Patients with good dental status
    (1) Maintain dentition
    (2) Establish aggressive oral hygiene program
      (a) Toothbrushing, flossing
      (b) Diet modification if indicated
      (c) Topical fluorides
      (d) Plaque control, calculus removal
      (e) Chlorhexidine or Listerine mouth rinse
    (3) Treat all active dental disease
      (a) Extraction—nonrestorable teeth
      (b) Endodontics—nonvital teeth
      (c) Restore carious teeth
      (d) Defer complex dental prostheses, etc until after transplantation
  c. Patients with dental status in between above extremes
    (1) Decision to maintain natural dentition must be made on individual patient basis
    (2) Factors to be considered
      (a) Extent and severity of dental disease
      (b) Importance of teeth to patient
      (c) Cost of maintaining natural dentition
      (d) Systemic status of patient and prognosis
	1. Usually none
	2. Excessive immune suppression
	  a. Candidiasis
	  b. Herpes simplex
	  c. Herpes zoster
	  d. Hairy leukoplakia
	  e. Lymphoma
	  f. Kaposi's sarcoma
	  g. Aphthous stomatitis
	  h. Squamous cell carcinoma of lip
	3. Side effects of immunosuppressant drugs
	  a. Bleeding (spontaneous)
	  b. Infection
	  c. Ulceration
	  d. Petechiae
	  e. Ecchymoses
	  f. Gingival hyperplasia
	4. Graft failure
	  a. Uremic stomatitits (kidney)
	  b. Bleeding (liver)
	  c. Petechiae (liver, kidney)
	  d. Ecchymoses (liver)
		1. Medical consultation prior to performing invasive dental procedure
		2. Establish need for antibiotic prophylaxis
		3. Prior to surgical procedures patients with end-stage renal or liver disease will require special preparation (see Chapters 11 and 12)
		4. Conservative treatment as possible for patients with end-stage organ failure (prior to transplantation) or organ rejection
		5. Establish status regarding presence of side effects of immunosuppressant drugs and manage as indicated

Dental Management: A Summary—cont'd

Medical problem	Potential problem related to dental care	Prevention of complications

Solid organ transplantation—cont'd
■ **Common problems found in all patients—cont'd**
	i. Adrenocortical suppression
	j. Tumors (listed above)
	k. Poor healing
	l. Bleeding
	m. Infection
		(8) If evidence of drug side effects, graft rejection, or overimmunosuppression is found, refer patient to physician
		c. Chronic rejection period
		  (1) Immediate or emergency dental care only
		  (2) Follow guidelines for stable graft when treatment is performed

■ **Heart transplantation special considerations**	1. Patient may be on long-term anticoagulation therapy; excessive bleeding may occur with surgical procedures 2. Graft atherosclerosis may occur, increasing risk for myocardial infarction 3. There is no nerve supply to the transplanted heart; thus pain will not be symptom of an MI 4. Some patients require cardiac pacing; electrical equipment may interfere with pacemaker	1. Have physician modify degree of anticoagulation to 2½ normal prothrombin time or less if surgical procedures are planned 2. Consult with physician to establish status of coronary vessels of transplanted heart; if advanced graft atherosclerosis is present, manage as described under section on coronary atherosclerotic heart disease 3. Be aware of signs and symptoms of MI other than pain; if these occur, obtain immediate medical assistance for patient 4. Do not use Cavitron or electrosurgery in patients with pacemaker

Treatment plan modifications	Oral complications	Emergency care

(3) Physical ability to maintain good oral hygiene
2. Following transplantation
  a. Immediate posttransplantation period—limit dental care to emergency needs
  b. Stable graft period—treatment plan based on needs and desires of patient; recall every 3 to 6 months
  c. Chronic rejection period—limit dental care to immediate or emergency needs
  d. Maintain aggressive oral hygiene program throughout all periods
  e. Medical consultation to confirm patient's current status and need for special precautions		

1. AHA has stated that there is inconclusive evidence regarding need for antibiotic prophylaxis for prevention of endocarditis in patients with heart transplantation 2. AHA recommends that the need for prophylaxis be determined on an individual patient basis following consultation with physician 3. If prophylaxis is decided on, standard amoxicillin regimen of AHA would be appropriate	Usually none See above	See above

Dental Management: A Summary—cont'd

Medical problem	Potential problem related to dental care	Prevention of complications
Solid organ transplantation—cont'd		
▪ **Liver transplantation special considerations**	1. Drugs that may be toxic to liver must be avoided 2. Some patients may be on anticoagulation medication 3. Excessive bleeding could occur with surgical procedures	1. Avoid drugs that are toxic to liver 2. Have physician modify degree of anticoagulant to 2½ times normal prothrombin time or less
▪ **Kidney transplantation, special considerations**	Drugs that may be toxic to kidney must be avoided	Avoid drugs that are toxic to kidney
▪ **Pancreas transplantation—cont'd**	No special considerations	

Bone marrow transplantation *(pp 512-532, 520)*	1. Immune suppression and pancytopenia resulting from conditioning therapy
	  a. Total body irradiation
	  b. Cyclophosphamide
	  c. Busulfan
	2. Problems during conditioning phase and critical phase (until transplanted marrow become functional
	  a. Infection
	  b. Bleeding
	  c. Poor healing
		1. Avoid dental treatment during conditioning and critical phases of bone marrow transplantation
		2. If possible treat all active dental disease prior to bone marrow transplantation
		3. See solid organ transplantation (above) for details of hygiene program and dental management
		4. Antibiotic prophylaxis for invasive dental procedures
		  a. Indicated if procedures must be performed on emergency basis during conditioning or critical phases of bone marrow transplantation
		  b. Need should be determined by medical consultation

Treatment plan modifications	Oral complications	Emergency care
Need for prophylactic antibiotics for invasive dental procedures in patients with stable liver transplants should be determined on individual patient basis by medical consultation	See above	See above
Need for prophylactic antibiotics for invasive dental procedures in patients with stable kidney transplants should be determined on individual patient basis by medical consultation	See above	See above
Need for prophylactic antibiotics for invasive dental procedures in patients with stable pancreas transplants should be determined on individual patient basis by medical consultation	See above	See above
1. If possible, treat active dental disease prior to transplantation 2. Prognosis varies based on reason for transplantation, source of marrow to be transplanted, and techniques used to condition and maintain patient; other factors affecting prognosis include age and general health status; complex dental prostheses may not be indicated for many patients 3. See solid organ transplantation for other suggested treatment planning considerations 4. For management of soft tissue complications, see Appendix B	1. Mucositis 2. Gingivitis 3. Xerostomia 4. Candidiasis 5. Herpes simplex infections 6. Osteoradionecrosis 7. Gingival hyperplasia (with cyclosporine)	1. During conditioning, critical, and rejection phases — as conservative as possible treatment for dental emergency problems is indicated 2. During stable graft phase — emergency dental care as needed 3. Prior to dental emergency care — medical consultation should be obtained to establish patient's current status and need for antibiotic prophylaxis

Dental Management: A Summary—cont'd

Medical problem	Potential problem related to dental care	Prevention of complications

	3. Immune suppression resulting from maintenance medications used to prevent graft-versus-host disease and chronic rejection
	   a. Cyclosporine
	   b. Prednisone
	   c. Methotrexate
	4. Problems during maintenance phase
	   a. Infection
	   b. Others listed above under solid organ transplantation relating to medication(s) being used
	5. Graft-versus-host disease and chronic rejection
	   a. Infection
	   b. Bleeding	

Prosthetic devices (pp 533-541)
  ▪ **Artificial heart valves**
	1. Prosthetic valve endocarditis can occur following dental procedures that may cause transient bacteremias
	2. Prolonged bleeding may occur following scaling or surgical procedures in patients being treated with anticoagulants
		1. Medical consultation to determine patient's current status and presence of other medical problems and to confirm dental management plan
		2. Prophylactic antibiotic coverage to prevent prosthetic valve endocarditis for all dental procedures; use one of standard or special regimens recommended by the AHA
		   a. Patients not allergic to penicillin—3 g amoxicillin, orally, 1 hour before procedure, then 1.5 g amoxicillin 6 hours after initial dose; or, if practitioner desires, a parenteral regimen: 1 to 2 g ampicillin, IM or IV, followed by gentamicin 1.5 mg/kg, IM or IV, 30 minutes before procedure, followed by 1.5 g amoxicillin, orally, 6 hours after loading dose
		   b. Patients allergic to penicillin—clindamycin 300 mg, orally, 1 hour before procedure, then 150 mg 6 hours after initial dose; or, if practitioner desires, a parenteral regimen: 1 g vancomycin, IV infusion over 60-minute period just before dental procedure

Treatment plan modifications	Oral complications	Emergency care

1. Patients not allergic to penicillin
  a. No dental treatment is contraindicated, but patients with advanced periodontal disease should be encouraged to consider complete denture therapy rather than prolonged complicated periodontal-restorative treatment
  b. Oral hygiene should be improved before restorative dental procedures are performed
  c. As much dental treatment as possible should be done during each coverage period
  d. At least 1 week should elapse between coverage periods
  e. Use of chlorhexidine mouth rinse and sulcular irrigation before extractions and periodontal therapy can be considered
	Usually none unless patient is receiving anticoagulation therapy; these patients may have areas of ecchymosis or gingival bleeding	Antibiotic coverage to prevent prosthetic valve endocarditis needed for any dental treatment; conservative management of pain and infection if prothrombin time is greater than 2½ times normal

Medical problem	Potential problem related to dental care	Prevention of complications
Prosthetic devices—cont'd ■ **Artificial heart valve—cont'd**		3. In patients taking anticoagulant medication, if scaling or surgical procedures are planned, dosage of anticoagulant medication should be reduced by physician so that on day of procedure prothrombin time is 2½ times normal or less
■ **Synthetic vascular grafts**	Endothelial tissue may not completely line inside of graft material; potential for infection during transient bacteremia	Prophylactic antibiotics for invasive dental procedures?

Treatment plan modifications	Oral complications	Emergency care

f. Coverage period may have to be extended, using amoxicillin 500 mg, orally, qid, for 1 to 5 days, when healing is slow following surgical procedures
g. Patients needing pre-prosthetic surgery should receive appropriate prophylactic antibiotic regimen; otherwise, complete denture patients do not require antibiotic prophylaxis for denture construction; patients should be seen on day after insertion of new dentures to correct any over-extension and should be told to return anytime denture sores develop
2. Patients allergic to penicillin
  a. Poor dental status—should be counseled concerning problems and expense and directed toward complete dentures
  b. Option of using an oral regimen of clindamycin or an erythromycin avoids complications of parenteral vancomycin (cost, hospitalization); however, IV vancomycin may still be selected for certain patients based on medical consultation		

AHA has stated that there is inconclusive evidence regarding need for antibiotic prophylaxis for prevention of endarteritis in patients with synthetic arterial grafts; it recommends that the need for prophylaxis be determined on an individual patient basis following consultation with physician; if prophylaxis is decided on, standard amoxicillin regimen of the AHA would be appropriate	None	As needed; requirement for antibiotic prophylaxis must be determined by medical consultation

Dental Management: A Summary—cont'd

Medical problem	Potential problem related to dental care	Prevention of complications
Prosthetic devices—cont'd ■ **Synthetic patches for closing cardiac defects**	Again, endocardial tissue may not completely line graft material; potential for infection during transient bacteremia	Prophylactic antibiotics for invasive dental care?
■ **Cardiac pacemakers and defibrillators**	1. Infection of cardiac lead(s) 2. Electrical interface with cardiac defects	1. Prophylactic antibiotics for invasive dental procedures? 2. Avoid Cavitron or electrosurgery

■ **Joint prostheses**	Deep infection is possible secondary to bacteremia caused by acute infection elsewhere in body; there is no evidence that transient bacteremias caused by invasive dental procedures can infect these prostheses in patients free of complicating systemic factors; however, patients with active rheumatoid arthritis, severe type I diabetes mellitus, congenital or acquired immune deficiency, or hemophilia may be at increased risk for infection; patients with a loose prosthesis or history of infection of the prosthesis may also be at risk	1. Obtain good history
		2. Patients with stable joint prostheses and no history of infection who are in good systemic health do not need prophylaxis
		3. Prophylaxis should be considered for patients with
		  a. Unstable prosthesis
		  b. History of infection of prosthesis
		  c. Systemic conditions—rheumatoid arthritis, severe type I diabetes, congenital or acquired immune deficiency, hemophilia
		4. Use medical consultation to establish need for prophylaxis
		5. Current AHA regimens would be adequate or a cephalosporin; if a cephalosporin is selected, 1 g dose 1 hour before dental procedure, and 500 mg 6 hours later, is regimen most preferred by orthopedic surgeons

■ **Cerebrospinal fluid shunts**	Infection following transient dental bacteremias caused by invasive dental procedures	1. Antibiotic prophylaxis is indicated for ventriculoatrial shunts but not for ventriculoperitoneal shunts 2. Standard AHA regimens are recommended for patients with ventriculoatrial shunt when receiving invasive dental procedures

Treatment plan modifications	Oral complications	Emergency care
Again, AHA has stated that evidence is *inconclusive* regarding need for antibiotics to prevent endocarditis in patients with synthetic cardiac patches (Dacron patch to close ventricular septal defect); decide on individual patient basis following medical consultation; standard amoxicillin regimen of AHA would be appropriate if prophylaxis is selected	None	As needed; requirement for antibiotic prophylaxis must be determined by medical consultation
AHA *does not* recommend antibiotic prophylaxis for patients with cardiac pacemakers or defibrillators	None	As needed; avoid Cavitron and electrosurgery
None	None	1. Aggressive treatment of acute infection in these patients 2. Establish need for prophylactic antibiotics by medical consultation
Usually none	None	Antibiotic prophylaxis for patients with ventriculoatrial shunts

Dental Management: A Summary—cont'd

Medical problem	Potential problem related to dental care	Prevention of complications
■ Penile implants	There is *no* evidence suggesting that these implants are at risk for infection from transient dental bacteremias	Antibiotic prophylaxis is not indicated for these patients based on available evidence; however, need should be decided on individual patient basis following medical consultation
■ Intraocular lenses	No risks	No special precautions
■ Breast implants	No risks	No special precautions
■ Intravascular access devices (Uldall catheter, central IV line, Broviac-Hickman device)	High rate of infection but role of transient dental bacteremias causing these infections has not been established	Determine need for antibiotic prophylaxis on an individual patient basis following medical consultation

Treatment plan modifications	Oral complications	Emergency care
None	None	As needed, medical consultation to determine need for prophylaxis
None	None	As needed
None	None	As needed
Depends on reason for intravascular device	None	As needed, determine need for prophylaxis by medical consultation

1

Interrelationships of Medicine and Dentistry

Dentistry of today is far different from what was practiced only a decade or two ago, not only in techniques and procedures but also in the types of patients seen. As a result of advances in medical science, people are living longer and are receiving medical treatment for disorders that were considered to be fatal only a few years ago. For example, damaged heart valves are surgically replaced, occluded coronary arteries are surgically bypassed, organs are transplanted, severe hypertension is medically controlled, and many types of malignancies and immune deficiencies are being managed.

Because of the increasing numbers of dental patients with chronic medical problems, it is critical that the dentist remain knowledgeable about patients' medical conditions, for many disorders necessitate alterations in the provision of dental treatment. Failure to make appropriate treatment modifications can result in serious consequences.

The purpose of this chapter is to provide an overview of the interrelationships of medicine and dentistry and to provide insight and appreciation for the significance of various medical problems as they relate to the provision of dental care. The chapters that follow will provide details of specific disorders and make appropriate dental management recommendations.

PHYSICAL EVALUATION

The initial step in the dental management of medically compromised patients is an evaluation of their physical status. This evaluation includes a past medical history, limited physical examination, clinical laboratory testing, and medical consultation. The goals of the physical evaluation include the following:

1. Identification of a medical problem that could necessitate the modification of dental treatment
2. Identification of systemic disease that could pose a threat to dental personnel or other patients
3. Identification of drugs or medicine that could result in adverse interaction with drugs or treatment administered by the dentist
4. Establishment of good patient-dentist rapport by demonstrating concern about the patient's overall health problems and well-being
5. Facilitation of effective communication with the patient's physician
6. Provision of medicolegal protection for the dental staff

HEALTH HISTORY

It is mandatory that a medical history be taken on every patient who is to receive dental treatment. There are a number of techniques and instruments that may be used to obtain a medical history, ranging from an interview, in which the questioner records the patient's responses on a blank sheet, to a printed questionnaire that the patient fills out. The latter is most commonly used in dental practice. There are many types of questionnaires commercially available today, including one from the American Dental Association. It is also feasible to develop a questionnaire of your own to meet

MEDICAL HISTORY

PATIENT'S NAME _____ DATE_____

Please check the box for any condition that you have had in the past or have now. (PARENTS OR GUARDIAN: If you are completing this form for your child, please indicate your child's health status by checking the appropriate box.)

1 CARDIOVASCULAR

Heart failure ☐
Heart disease or attack ☐
Angina pectoris or chest pain ☐
High blood pressure ☐
Heart murmur ☐
Mitral valve prolapse ☐
Rheumatic fever ☐
Congenital heart defect or
  lesion ☐
Artificial heart valve ☐
Arrhythmias ☐
Heart pacemaker or defibrillator ☐
Heart surgery or transplant ☐
Other heart problems ☐
Stroke ☐
Aneurysm ☐

2 HEMATOLOGIC

Blood transfusion ☐
Anemia ☐
Hemophilia ☐
Leukemia ☐
Sickle cell (anemia) disease ☐
Tendency to bleed longer
  than normal ☐

3 NEURAL and SENSORY

Eye pain ☐
Visison problems ☐
Glaucoma or cataract ☐
Earaches, ringing in ears ☐
Hearing loss ☐
Severe headaches ☐
Fainting or dizzy spells ☐
Epilepsy, seizures, or convulsions ☐
Nervousness ☐
Psychiatric treatment ☐

4 GASTROINTESTINAL

Stomach or intestinal ulcers ☐
Gastritis ☐
Colitis ☐
Persistent diarrhea ☐
Hepatitis ☐
Liver disease ☐
Yellow jaundice ☐
Cirrhosis ☐

5 RESPIRATORY

Hay fever ☐
Sinus trouble ☐
Allergies or hives ☐
Asthma ☐
Chronic cough ☐
Emphysema ☐
Tuberculosis (TB) ☐
Breathing difficulties ☐

**6 DERMAL MUCOCUTANEOUS
MUSCULOSKELETAL**

Allergy to latex (rubber) ☐
Skin rash ☐
Dark mole(s) (recent changes
  in appearance) ☐
Night sweats ☐
Sore muscles ☐
Stiff joints ☐
Arthritis ☐
Artificial joint ☐
Fever blister ☐
Mouth ulcers or canker sores ☐
Colored or discolored areas
  in mouth ☐

7 ENDOCRINE

Diabetes ☐
Thyroid disease ☐

**8 URINARY—SEXUALLY
TRANSMITTED**

Urinate frequently ☐
Kidney, bladder problem ☐
Sexually transmitted disease
  (syphilis, gonorrhea, chlamydia,
  genital herpes) ☐
HIV-positive ☐

9 OTHER CONDITIONS

Frequent sore throats ☐
Enlarged lymph node or "gland" ☐
Use tobacco ☐
Use alcohol ☐
Drug addiction ☐
Tumor or cancer ☐
X-ray or cobalt treatment ☐
Chemotherapy ☐
Disease, problem or condition
  not listed ☐
If yes, list

_____

_____

_____

_____

FIG. 1-1 Health questionnaire.

MEDICAL HISTORY — cont'd

		YES	NO
10	Are you currently under the care of a physician?	☐	☐

Physician name _____ Address _____

Phone no. _____ Last appointment date _____

For what? _____

11	Are you taking (or supposed to be taking) any medicine, drugs, or pills of any kind?	☐	☐

If yes, what kind and dose?

_____

_____

_____

12	Have you taken cortisone or other steroids in the past 12 months?	☐	☐
13	Do you have reactions or allergies to drugs or medicines?	☐	☐
14	Have you had a reaction to dental or general anesthesia?	☐	☐
15	Have you ever had an operation or surgery? Describe the problem and any complications	☐	☐

_____

16	Have you ever been hospitalized?	☐	☐
17	When you walk up stairs or take a walk, do you ever have to stop because of pain in your chest, shortness of breath, or feeling tired?	☐	☐
18	Do your ankles swell during the day?	☐	☐
19	Do you sleep on two or more pillows?	☐	☐
20	Have you unintentionally lost or gained more than 10 pounds in the past year?	☐	☐
21	Are you on a special diet?	☐	☐
22	Does your occupation bring you into contact with blood, blood products, or needles?	☐	☐
23	WOMEN: Are you pregnant?	☐	☐

To the best of my knowledge, all of the preceding answers are true and correct. If I ever have any change in my health, abnormal laboratory test, or medicine change, I will inform the dentist at the next appointment without fail.

_____ _____
Date   Patient, parent, or
             guardian signature

_____
Student dentist signature

_____
Faculty member signature

∗∗∗

Height _____; Weight _____; BP _____; Pulse _____; Resp. _____; Temp. _____

HEALTH COMMENTS & SUMMARY: ASA I   II   III   IV

_____

_____

_____

_____

_____

_____

_____

_____

FIG. 1-1, cont'd   Health questionnaire.

the specific needs of your practice. Figure 1-1 is the health questionnaire that is currently being used at the University of Kentucky College of Dentistry. It provides a comprehensive review of a patient's medical history and a review of systems, and it also serves as a basis for teaching and discussion. One of the most effective methods is utilization of a questionnaire followed by a pertinent interview by the dentist to review selected questions or responses.

OVERVIEW OF THE MEDICAL HISTORY QUESTIONNAIRE

Although questionnaires will differ in organization and content detail, most will attempt to elicit information about the same problems. This particular form is organized into two sections—the first section composed of questions followed by the signatures of patient and dentist (or student and faculty member) and the second providing for the recording of vital signs, health comments and summary, and the American Society of Anesthesiologists (ASA) classification. The comments section is intended for an explanation of and treatment modifications for *significant* positive responses that the patient has made on the medical history form; it can then be referred to for a capsular summary of the patient's health status.

The following information is provided as a means of explaining (1) the rationale for asking certain questions and (2) the significance of positive responses to those questions. Detailed information concerning most of these medical problems will be found throughout the remainder of this book.

Cardiovascular diseases

This is a particularly important section, because patients with various forms of cardiovascular disease are potentially susceptible to physical or emotional challenges that may be encountered during dental treatment.

HEART FAILURE

This is not a disease but rather a symptom complex of an underlying cardiovascular problem—such as valvular deformity or an arrhythmia. As such the underlying problem should be identified and its potential significance assessed. Chair position is frequently a factor with these patients being unable to tolerate a supine or semisupine position. Vasoconstrictors should be used judiciously in patients taking digitalis glycosides since the combination may potentially precipitate arrhythmias.

MYOCARDIAL INFARCTION

A history of heart attack within the past 6 months usually precludes *elective* dental care, because during the immediate postinfarction period patients have an increased susceptibility to repeat infarctions, significant arrhythmias, ventricular aneurysms, or heart failure. Many patients may be taking various medications—such as antianginals, anticoagulants, adrenergic-blocking agents, antiarrhythmic agents, or digitalis. Several of these drugs may alter the dental management of these patients, due to potential interaction with vasoconstrictor in the local anesthetic, as well as drug side effects or other interactions.

ANGINA PECTORIS

Brief substernal pain due to myocardial ischemia commonly provoked by physical activity or emotional stress is a common and significant symptom of coronary heart disease. Patients with angina are candidates for arrhythmias, myocardial infarction, or unexpected sudden death. These patients may be taking a variety of vasoactive medications—such as nitroglycerin, beta-blocking agents, or calcium channel blockers—for the control of this problem. In patients with severe or progressive angina, local anesthetics containing vasoconstrictors should be used judiciously.

HIGH BLOOD PRESSURE

Patients with hypertension should be identified. It is important to find out if there has ever been a diagnosis of high blood pressure, because it is not uncommon for patients to stop taking their medications without the doctor's knowledge. Current blood pressure readings should be noted, as should any symptoms that may be associated with hypertension—such as dizziness or headaches. Some antihypertensive medications may require special consideration during dental treatment. Vasoconstrictors may potentially interact with some of these medications (e.g., the adrenergic inhibitors) and should be used judiciously.

HEART MURMUR

The presence of a heart murmur is of special significance in the dental patient. A heart murmur is caused by turbulence of blood flow producing vibratory sounds during the beating of the heart. This turbulence may be due to either physiologic or pathologic factors of the heart valves or vessels. The primary question that must be answered is what is the cause of the heart murmur. If a murmur is due to a pathologic condition, the patient may be susceptible to an infection inside the heart (on or near the heart valves) as a result of bacteria entering the bloodstream from dental treatment that caused bleeding. This infection is called infective or bacterial endocarditis and is a serious problem that can be fatal. If a patient is identified as having a heart murmur of pathologic origin, or of unknown origin, then he or she should be placed on prophylactic antibiotics in an attempt to prevent bacterial endocarditis. Currently amoxicillin is the drug of choice for this purpose and is administered orally 1 hour before an appointment and again 6 hours later.

MITRAL VALVE PROLAPSE (MVP)

This is a condition in which leaflets of the mitral valve are thickened (redundant). As a result, tight closure of the leaflets may not be possible, which can result in regurgitation of blood. Patients with MVP and regurgitation will require antibiotic prophylaxis for dental treatment likely to result in bleeding. Currently oral amoxicillin is the drug of choice for this purpose and is administered orally 1 hour immediately before an appointment and again 6 hours later.

RHEUMATIC FEVER

This is an autoimmune condition that can follow an upper respiratory tract, beta-hemolytic streptococcal infection and can lead to permanent damage of the heart valves. This condition is then called rheumatic heart disease. Patients with rheumatic heart disease are thought to be susceptible to bacterial endocarditis as a result of bacteria entering the bloodstream during the course of dental treatment that causes bleeding. Patients with rheumatic heart disease are provided with prophylactic antibiotics for all dental care likely to result in any bleeding, in an attempt to prevent bacterial endocarditis. Currently amoxicillin is the drug of choice for this purpose and is administered orally 1 hour before an appointment and again 6 hours later.

CONGENITAL HEART DEFECT OR LESION

Patients with most forms of persistent or unrepaired congenital heart defects are thought to be susceptible to bacterial endocarditis and are provided prophylactic antibiotics for dental care likely to result in bleeding. Currently amoxicillin is the drug of choice for this purpose and is administered orally 1 hour before an appointment and again 6 hours later.

ARTIFICIAL HEART VALVE

Patients with one or more artificial heart valves are considered to be highly susceptible to bacterial endocarditis from bacterial seeding resulting from bleeding during dental treatment. This is a significant problem in view of the fact that up to 50% of patients with artificial heart valves who get bacterial endocarditis may die. These patients are provided prophylactic antibiotics for dental care likely to result in any bleeding. Currently amoxicillin is the drug of choice for this purpose administered orally 1 hour before an appointment and again 6 hours later. However, there are also parenteral drugs, which some physicians may elect to administer in place of or in addition to the oral regimen.

ARRHYTHMIAS

These problems are frequently related to heart failure or coronary artery disease. Stress, anxiety, physical activity, and hypoxia can precipitate arrythmias. Vasoconstrictors in local anesthetics should be used judiciously, since arrhythmias can be precipitated by excessive or inappropriate use. Patients may be taking anti-arrhythmic drugs, some of which may have oral manifestations or other side effects. A patient with arrhythmias may require a pacemaker or defibrillator to artificially regulate heart rhythm. These patients generally do not require antibiotic prophylaxis, or any other significant management considerations.

HEART SURGERY OR TRANSPLANT

One of the most common forms of cardiac surgery performed today is the coronary artery bypass graft procedure. These patients do *not* require antibiotic prophylaxis following recovery, unless there are other accompanying conditions as have been previously described. Likewise, most patients with surgically repaired congenital defects do not require antibiotic prophylaxis. Heart transplant patients are not seen frequently; however, as with any organ transplant, the administration of powerful immunosuppressive drugs renders them susceptible to infection as well as causes other side effects. In addition, some physicians recommend antibiotic prophylaxis during dental treatment.

STROKE

Efforts should be made to minimize stress and hypoxia in patients with a history of stroke. It is important to identify those problems that may have predisposed to stroke, such as hypertension or diabetes, and to make appropriate management alterations. Vasoconstrictors should be used judiciously in many of these patients. Anticoagulant medications can result in prolonged hemostasis. Many stroke patients may have hemiplegia, speech difficulties, or other physically handicapping problems.

ANEURYSM

Patients with a known unrepaired aneurysm are not candidates for elective dental care. If care becomes necessary, stress, hypoxia, hypertension, and excessive physical exertion are to be avoided. Patients with a repaired aneurysm may require antibiotic prophylaxis for dental procedures likely to result in bleeding to prevent bacterial endarteritis.

Hematologic disorders
BLOOD TRANSFUSION

Patients with a history of blood transfusion are of concern from at least two aspects—first, to identify the underlying problem that necessitated the transfusion and, second, to recognize that patients who have had blood transfusions are at risk of having been unknowingly infected with hepatitis B or C or HIV. Laboratory screening or medical consultation may be appropriate.

ANEMIA

A significant reduction in red cell mass is the result of an underlying pathologic process such as blood loss, decreased production of RBCs, or hemolysis. Some anemias—such as G6PD (glucose-6-phosphate dehydrogenase) deficiency, aplastic anemia, and sickle cell disease—require dental management considerations. Oral lesions, infections, delayed wound healing, and adverse response to hypoxia are all potential concerns.

LEUKEMIA

Depending on the type of leukemia and its status of activity, some patients may have bleeding problems, delayed healing, or be prone to infection. Some effects can be due to powerful chemotherapeutic agents and require special management considerations.

TENDENCY TO BLEED LONGER THAN NORMAL

A potentially significant problem is patients who have a history of abnormal bleeding. This is of obvious concern if any surgical treatment is planned. Bleeding tendencies may be genetic or acquired. An example of a common genetic bleeding tendency is the patient with hemophilia (Factor VIII deficiency). Examples of acquired bleeding tendencies include some forms of leukemia or patients on various medications such as coumarin, some of the nonsteroidal antiinflammatory drugs, or aspirin. It should be recognized, however, that many complaints of abnormal bleeding are more apparent than real and that further historical information may serve to make this distinction.

Neural and sensory diseases

Responses in this section may signify that a patient has signs or symptoms related to a central nervous system disorder, perhaps contributing to other problems in the history. It is significant in that some of these problems may be unknown to the patient.

GLAUCOMA

Patients with closed-angle glaucoma can experience an acute increase in intraocular pressure if anticholinergic drugs are administered. Therefore, any dentally used or prescribed drug with anticholinergic effects should be avoided.

EPILEPSY, SEIZURES, OR CONVULSIONS

Epilepsy or grand mal seizures need to be identified and the degree of control determined. Etiologic factors of the seizures should be identified and avoided. Some medications used to control seizures may affect dental treatment due to actions or side effects. Gingival hyperplasia is a well-known side effect of phenytoin. Patients may discontinue the use of their antiseizure medication without the doctor's knowledge and therefore may be susceptible to seizures during dental treatment.

PSYCHIATRIC TREATMENT

Patients with a current or past history of psychiatric illness, and the nature of their problem, need to be identified. This may be important in explaining a patient's behavioral patterns or problems of which the patient may be complaining (i.e., unexplainable or bizarre pain). Additionally, some psychiatric drugs have the potential to interact adversely with vasoconstrictors in local anesthetic.

Gastrointestinal diseases

STOMACH OR INTESTINAL ULCERS, GASTRITIS, COLITIS

Patients with these problems should not be given drugs that are directly irritating to the GI tract—such as aspirin or nonsteroidal antiinflammatory drugs (NSAIDs) (Table 15-3). Patients with colitis or a history of colitis may not be able to take certain antibiotics. Drugs used to treat ulcers can cause dry mouth.

HEPATITIS, LIVER DISEASE, YELLOW JAUNDICE, CIRRHOSIS

Patients who have a history of viral hepatitis are of interest to dentistry since they may be carriers of the disease and as such could transmit the disease to dental personnel or to other patients. Of the three types of viral hepatitis, only B and C have carrier stages. Fortunately, laboratory tests are available to accurately identify these patients. Patients with chronic hepatitis or cirrhosis may have impaired liver-function, which could result in prolonged bleeding or the inability to efficiently metabolize certain drugs, including local anesthetic and analgesics.

Respiratory tract diseases

ALLERGIES OR HIVES

Patients with an allergic history may be allergic to some of the drugs or materials that are used in dentistry. Common drug allergens include antibiotics and analgesics. It is important to pursue an allergic history by specifically asking the patient how he or she reacts to the substance. This is necessary to establish a definite history of allergy rather than merely an intolerance or adverse side effect that has been incorrectly identified as an allergy. True allergic symptoms include itching, urticaria (hives), rash, swelling, wheezing, angioneurotic edema, rhinorrhea (runny nose), and tearing eyes. Isolated symptoms such as nausea, vomiting, palpitations, or fainting are generally not of an allergic basis but rather are psychogenic or examples of intolerance.

EMPHYSEMA

Patients with chronic pulmonary diseases—such as emphysema or chronic bronchitis—need to be identified to avoid medications or procedures that might further depress respiratory function. Chair position is frequently a factor, with patients being unable to tolerate a supine position. Use of a rubber dam may not be advisable.

TUBERCULOSIS

Patients with a past or current history of tuberculosis need to be identified for infection control purposes, and information concerning the diagnosis and treatment history of the disease needs to be defined. A history of follow-up care is also important. A positive skin test means that the person has been infected with TB, but it does not mean that the patient is actively infectious. Patients with AIDS have a high incidence of tuberculosis, and this relationship may need to be explored.

Dermal, mucocutaneous, and musculoskeletal diseases

ALLERGY TO LATEX (RUBBER)

Some patients may be allergic to latex or rubber gloves, rubber dam, or rubber-based impression material. If so, alternative materials should be used to avoid an adverse reaction.

SKIN RASH, DARK MOLES

Patients who have skin lesions need to be identified and the nature of these abnormalities defined. You may uncover allergic manifestations or you may identify autoimmune, malignant, or infectious problems. The history of occurrence and the behavior of the lesions are important. A mole that changes color, enlarges, or bleeds should be considered potentially malignant. The presence of oral lesions along with skin lesions may be significant.

NIGHT SWEATS

This is a symptom of one of several serious illnesses—such as AIDS, tuberculosis, bacterial endocarditis, or Hodgkin's disease.

SORE MUSCLES, STIFF JOINTS, ARTHRITIS

Patients with arthritis may be taking a variety of medications that may influence dental care. NSAIDs and steroids are two such examples. Chair position may become a factor in physical comfort. Patients may also have problems with manual dexterity. In addition, patients with arthritis of other joints in the body may have involvement of the temporomandibular joint.

ARTIFICIAL JOINT

Patients who have an artificial joint (or joints) are "potentially" at risk for infection of these prostheses and may need to be given prophylactic antibiotics for dental care likely to result in bleeding. It should be noted that the scientific evidence for this practice is lacking; however, it has become a standard recommendation of most orthopedic surgeons.

FEVER BLISTER, MOUTH ULCERS OR CANKER SORES, COLORED OR DISCOLORED AREAS IN THE MOUTH

These and similar intraoral lesions can be benign conditions of the oral soft tissues but may also be associated with systemic problems such as AIDS or malignancies.

Endocrine diseases

DIABETES

Patients with diabetes mellitus need to be identified in terms of the type of diabetes and how it is controlled. Some diabetics do not require insulin (non–insulin dependent diabetes mellitus, NIDDM) whereas others do require it (insulin-dependent diabetes mellitus, IDDM). Symptoms suggestive of diabetes are excessive thirst, hunger, and urination along with weight loss and frequent infections. Complications of diabetes include blindness, hypertension, and kidney failure. These need to be identified for management. Diabetics typically do not handle infections well. They may also have exaggerated periodontal disease. Patients taking insulin are prone to hypoglycemia in the dental office.

THYROID DISEASE

Patients with uncontrolled or unidentified hyperthyroidism are potentially sensitive to stress, and the use of vasoconstrictors is generally contraindicated. Patients with hyperthyroidism may be easily upset, intolerant of heat, and subject to tremors. Exophthalmos may be seen. Patients with hypothyroidism generally pose minimal management concerns.

Urinary tract and sexually transmitted diseases

URINARY FREQUENCY

This is a common sign of diabetes and should raise suspicion if present. Some drugs may also result in frequent urination.

KIDNEY AND BLADDER PROBLEMS

Patients with end-stage renal disease (ESRD) or a kidney transplant would be identified here. The potential for abnormal drug metabolism, immunosuppressive drug therapy, bleeding problems, hepatitis, infections, and blood pressure problems demands special management consideration.

SEXUALLY TRANSMITTED DISEASES

A variety of sexually transmitted diseases—such as syphilis and gonorrhea—can have manifestations in the oral cavity due to oral-genital contact or dissemination in the blood, and the dentist may be the first to identify their presence. In addition, many of these diseases (including AIDS and hepatitis B) can be transmitted to the dentist via direct contact with oral lesions or infectious blood.

HIV-POSITIVE STATE

AIDS and the various manifestations of AIDS may be identified through oral lesions or symptoms and may be the first indication of the presence of the disease. Candidiasis, hairy leukoplakia, Kaposi's sarcoma, and rapidly progressing periodontitis are some of the oral conditions commonly associated with AIDS.

Other conditions

This is a grab bag of symptoms not included under other sections.

FREQUENT SORE THROATS, ENLARGED LYMPH NODES OR "GLANDS"

Patients who complain of frequent sore throats, enlarged lymph nodes, persistent diarrhea, chronic cough, breathing difficulties, mouth ulcers, or discolored areas in the mouth may have AIDS. These symptoms may be the first indications that a patient has the disease.

TOBACCO, ALCOHOL

The use of tobacco products is a risk factor associated with malignancies, cardiovascular disease, and pulmonary disease. Excessive use of alcohol is a risk factor for malignancies and has the potential to cause liver disease and heart disease.

DRUG ADDICTION

Patients who have a history of IV drug abuse are at risk for infectious diseases such as hepatitis B or C and AIDS. Narcotic drugs should be prescribed cautiously in these patients.

TUMOR OR CANCER

Patients who have had cancer are at a proven high risk for the disease, and as such additional lesions or recurrences are always a possibility. Also, many chemotherapeutic agents necessitate significant management considerations.

X-RAY OR COBALT TREATMENT, CHEMOTHERAPY

Patients with previous x-ray treatment, especially around the head and neck area, need to be identified to avoid osteoradionecrosis. Radiation treatment in the head and neck can result in decreased saliva, mucosal irritation, and increased dental caries. Chemotherapy can produce many undesirable side effects.

Current physician

Information should be sought regarding why the patient requires medical care, the diagnoses made, and any treatment being received. If the reason for seeing a physician was for a physical examination only, the patient should be asked if any abnormalities were discovered and the date of the examination. The name, address, and phone number of the patient's physician should be recorded for future reference. The patient who answers no to this question may need a more cautious approach than the person who has had regular check-ups. This is especially true for the patient who has not seen a physician in several years. The patient may be perfectly healthy; however, he or she could also have an undetected problem. The response to this question also may provide insight into the priorities that the person assigns to health care.

Drugs, medicines, pills

Medications being taken for an illness may be the only clue to the patient's disorder. The patient may not have believed that it was important to mention a problem but may have included it in an answer to this question. An example might be the patient with long-standing stable angina pectoris who takes nitroglycerin but has not seen a physician recently. Drugs may also cause untoward reactions during dental treatment; thus the dentist should identify the various drugs that a patient may be taking and should become familiar with their actions and possible side effects and interactions. The dentist must be cautious not to administer any drug or medication that may interact adversely with the patient's medications. *Drug Information for the Health Care Professional, Accepted Dental Therapeutics,* and the *Physicians' Desk Reference (PDR)* are useful sources to aid in the identification of drugs and their actions and interactions. The *PDR* is helpful in the identification of unknown pills or capsules. The pill or capsule can be matched with pictures of various manufacturers' products. Once identified, the appropriate descriptive section can be consulted in the *PDR* or in one of the previously mentioned drug references. It is important to stress "drugs, medicine, or pills *of any kind,*" when questioning a patient because frequently people will not consider over-the-counter drugs as being legitimate medicine. For example, it is not unusual for a patient taking several aspirin tablets a day for arthritis to answer "none" to this question.

Steroids

Corticosteroid usage is of interest since chronic use of corticosteroid can render a patient unable to adequately respond to the stress of a dental procedure and could be a potentially life-threatening situation. Cortisone and prednisone are common examples of steroids used in the treatment of many diseases.

Allergies or reactions

This question should not be limited to allergies to medications because patients are exposed to other allergens in the dental office — such as cements, tape, stains, latex, or iodine. Also a person may be identified as "allergic" individual because of existing allergies to numerous substances and thus would be at risk to be or to become allergic to other medications or substances used in dentistry.

Operations or hospitalizations

A history of hospitalizations can give a good record of past serious illnesses that may have current significance. For example, a patient may have been hospitalized for cardiac catheterization, during which time a congenital septal defect was discovered. Another example would be a patient hospitalized for hepatitis. Neither patient might ever have received medical follow-up care for these problems, and the response to this question might be the only indication of the problems. It is important to learn as much as possible about hospitalizations — such as diagnosis, treatment, and complications. In addition to past hospitalizations, it is important to know what kind of operations the patient has had, the reason for the procedures, and any untoward events associated with them — such as anesthetic emergencies, unusual postoperative bleeding, or infections.

Cardiovascular or pulmonary signs and symptoms

These questions are designed to primarily discover a patient with signs or symptoms that could be associated with cardiovascular disease, pulmonary disease, or malignancy.

Diet

This may identify a patient who is on a diet due to an underlying systemic problem such as diabetes, hyperthyroidism, or cancer.

Blood contact

This question has significant implications since hepatitis, AIDS, syphilis, and other forms of communicable diseases can be transmitted via contact with infectious blood or blood products.

Pregnancy

This question identifies a woman's status in regard to pregnancy. It is important, in that women who are pregnant may need special consideration in the taking of radiographs, administration of drugs, or timing of dental treatment.

• • •

Signature

The patient is requested to date and sign the questionnaire, attesting to the accuracy of the information provided. The dentist should also sign, indicating that the form has been reviewed.

Vital signs

These are obtained by questioning (height, weight) and by direct measurement (blood pressure, pulse, respiratory rate). Temperature is usually recorded only when indicated. Abnormal readings may require further investigation or referral.

American Society of Anesthesiologists (ASA) classifications

ASA I: Normal healthy patient; no dental management alterations required

ASA II: Patient with mild systemic disease that does not interfere with day-to-day activity or that is a significant health risk factor (e.g., smoking, alcohol abuse, obesity); may or may not need dental management alterations
Examples: mild hypertension, NIDDM, heart murmur, asymptomatic rheumatic heart disease, allergy, well-controlled asthma, well-controlled epilepsy, hepatitis B surface antigen positive, HIV-positive, mild chronic obstructive pulmonary disease (COPD)

ASA III: Patient with moderate to severe systemic disease that is not incapacitating but that may alter day-to-day activity; may have significant drug concerns; may require special patient care; would generally require dental management alterations

Examples: IDDM, moderate to severe hypertension, angina pectoris, MI within past 6 months, congestive heart failure, ARC, AIDS, severe COPD, mild hemophilia

ASA IV: Patient with severe systemic disease that is a constant threat to life; definitely requires dental management alterations; best treated in special facility
Examples: severe cardiac disease, end-stage renal disease, liver failure, advanced AIDS, chemotherapy, severe hemophilia

Health comments and summary

This section is for comments on *only* those items to which the patient has positively responded *and* that have potential impact on the provision of dental care. It provides a quick reference and a capsular summary of the health status and treatment modifications required.

ASA I, II, III, IV

_____
_____
_____
_____
_____
_____
_____

DENTAL HISTORY

A thorough dental history is important for any patient who is to be treated from a comprehensive standpoint. It is important to know what has been done in the past, when it was done, and the outcome of the treatment. This would include restorative procedures, prosthetic devices, surgical procedures, orthodontic treatment, endodontic therapy, periodontal treatment, and radiographs. Any complications with the treatment, anesthetic, or medications prescribed should be noted. It is also helpful to learn how the patient feels about dentists and what the patient expects from the dentist. Also, dental problems will occasionally serve as a clue to an underlying systemic disease. For example, a patient with severe progressive periodontal disease may be found to have diabetes or leukemia.

PHYSICAL EXAMINATION

In addition to a comprehensive health history, the dental patient should be afforded the benefits of a simple abbreviated physical examination, which should include assessment of general appearance, pulse rate, blood pressure, respiratory rate, body temperature (if appropriate), and a head and neck examination.

GENERAL SURVEY

Much can be learned about a patient and his or her state of health from a purposeful but tactful visual inspection. Careful observation can lead to an awareness and recognition of abnormal or unusual features or conditions that may exist and could influence the provision of dental care. This survey consists of an assessment of the general appearance and inspection of specific exposed areas, including skin and nails, face, eyes and nose, ears, and neck. Each of these visually accessible areas may demonstrate peculiarities that could signal underlying systemic disease or abnormalities.

Overall appearance

The outward appearance of a patient can give an indication of the general state of health and well-being. Examples of possible trouble might include a wasted, cachectic appearance; lethargic demeanor; ill-kept, dirty clothing and hair; staggering or halting gait; extreme thinness or obesity; bent posture; and difficulty breathing. The dentist should also remain sensitive to breath and body odors such as acetone associated with diabetes, ammonia associated with renal failure, putrefaction of pulmonary infections, and alcohol possibly associated with liver disease.

Skin and nails

The skin is the largest organ of the body, and usually large areas are exposed and available for inspection. Changes in the skin and nails frequently are associated with systemic disease. For example, cyanosis can indicate cardiac or pulmonary insufficiency, jaundice may be caused by liver diseases, pigmentation may be associated with hormonal abnormalities, and petechiae or ecchymoses can be from a blood dyscrasia (Fig. 1-2). Alterations in the fingernails may be caused by infection (onychomycosis) or a chronic disorder—such as clubbing (seen in cardiopulmonary insufficiency, Fig. 1-3), whitening (seen in cirrhosis), yellowing

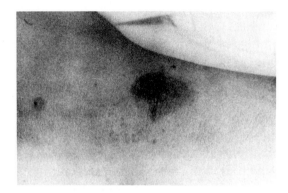

FIG. 1-2 Ecchymosis, which may be caused by a bleeding disorder.

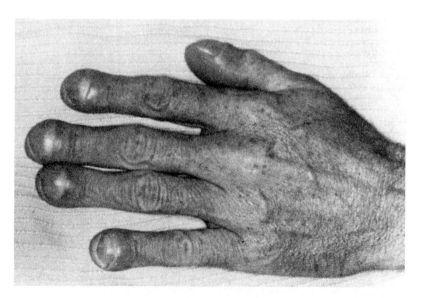

FIG. 1-3 Clubbing of digits and nails can be associated with cardiopulmonary insufficiency.

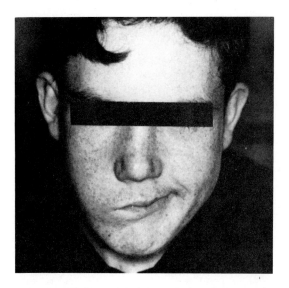

FIG. 1-4 Unilateral facial paralysis consistent with Bell's palsy.

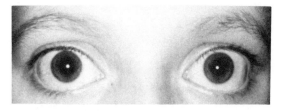

FIG. 1-5 Lid retraction caused by hyperthyroidism.

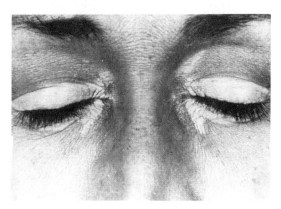

FIG. 1-6 Xanthomas of the periocular area can signal hypercholesterolemia.

(from malignancy), or linear (splinter) hemorrhages (from bacterial endocarditis).

Face

The shape and symmetry of the face are often abnormal in a variety of syndromes and conditions. Well-known examples include the coarse features of acromegaly, pale edematous features in the nephrotic syndrome, moon facies in Cushing's syndrome, dull puffy facies of myxedema, and unilateral paralysis of Bell's palsy (Fig. 1-4).

Eyes and nose

The eyes can be sensitive indicators of systemic disease and should be closely inspected. If a patient wears glasses, he or she should be requested to remove them during examination of the head and neck. Hyperthyroidism can produce a characteristic lid retraction, resulting in a wide-eyed stare (Fig. 1-5). Xanthomas of the lids are frequently associated with hypercholesterolemia (Fig. 1-6), as is arcus senilis in a young person. Scleral yellowing may be caused by hepatitis. Reddened conjunctivae may be from the sicca syndrome or allergy. The bridge of the nose and the eyelids are areas at risk for basal cell carcinoma.

Ears

The ears should be inspected for gouty tophi in the helix or anthelix. Also a lateral crease in the earlobe may be associated with an increased risk of coronary artery disease.

Neck

The neck should be inspected for enlargement and asymmetry. Depending on location and consistency, enlargement can be caused by goiter (Fig. 1-7), infection, cysts, swollen lymph nodes, or vascular deformities.

VITAL SIGNS

The benefits of measuring vital signs during an initial examination are twofold.

First, the establishment of baseline normal values ensures a standard for comparison in the event of an emergency during treatment. Were an emergency to occur, it would be necessary to know what was normal for that particular

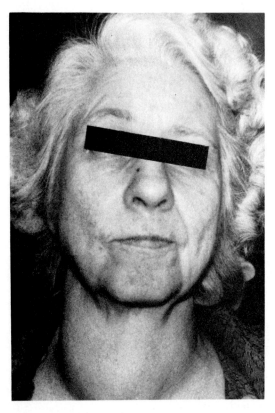

FIG. 1-7   Midline lower neck enlargement from goiter.

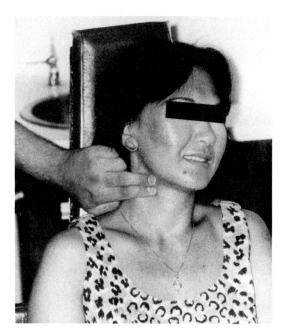

FIG. 1-8   Palpation of the carotid pulse.

patient to determine the severity of the problem. For example, if a patient lost consciousness unexpectedly and the blood pressure was 90/50, the concern would be entirely different for a patient whose blood pressure was normally 110/65 from what it would be for the hypertensive patient whose blood pressure was normally 180/100. The dentist would probably be dealing with simple syncope in the first patient, as opposed to a shock state in the second.

A **second** benefit of obtaining vital signs during an examination is screening to identify abnormalities, either diagnosed or undiagnosed. The adage "never treat a stranger" has good foundation. For example, if a person with severe, long-standing hypertension was not identified but was treated with no management alteration, the consequences could be serious. It should be kept in mind that the purpose of this examination is merely detection of an abnor-

mality, not diagnosis. This is the responsibility of the physician. If it is determined that the abnormal finding is significant, the patient should then be referred to a physician for further evaluation.

Pulse

In examining the pulse, it is standard procedure to palpate either the carotid artery (at the side of the trachea) or the radial artery (on the thumb side of the wrist) (Figs. 1-8 and 1-9). There are some advantages in using the carotid artery for pulse determination. First, the carotid pulse is accessible because the dentist is already working in the area. Second, it is reliable because the carotid is a central artery supplying the brain; therefore in emergency situations it may remain palpable when the peripheral arteries are not. Finally, it is easily palpated because it is large.

The carotid pulse can best be palpated along the anterior border of the sternocleidomastoid muscle at approximately the level of the thyroid cartilage. Displacing the sternocleidomastoid slightly posteriorly will allow palpation of the pulse with the first and middle finger. The pulse

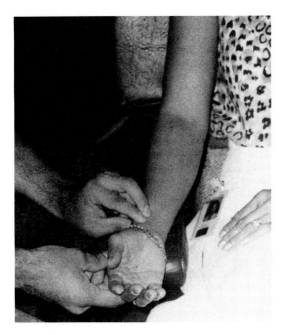

FIG. 1-9 Palpation of the radial pulse.

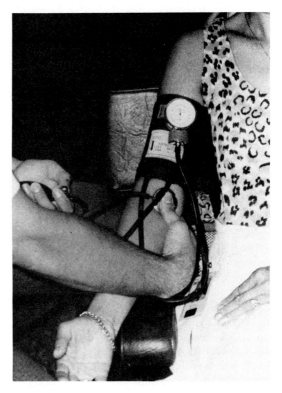

FIG. 1-10 Blood pressure cuff and stethoscope in place.

ideally should be monitored for a full minute to detect irregular patterns.

RATE

The average pulse rate in normal adults is 60 to 100 beats per minute. A pulse rate greater than 100 is termed *tachycardia* whereas an abnormally slow pulse of less than 60 is called *bradycardia*.

RHYTHM

The normal pulse is a series of rhythmic beats that follow each other at regular intervals. When they follow each other at irregular intervals, the pulse is termed irregular, dysrhythmic, or arrhythmic.

Blood pressure

Blood pressure is usually determined indirectly in the upper extremities by employing a blood pressure cuff and stethoscope (Fig. 1-10). The blood pressure cuff should be the correct width to give an accurate recording. The standard cuff width for an average adult arm is 12 to 14 cm. A cuff that is too narrow will yield falsely elevated values whereas one that is too wide will yield falsely low values. Narrower cuffs are available for use on children, and wider-than-average cuffs are available for obese or large patients. As an alternative in an obese patient, a standard-size cuff can be placed on the forearm below the antecubital fossa and the stethoscope placed over the radial artery for auscultation.

The stethoscope should be of good standard quality. It is recommended that the bell end (cup) be used to auscultate the brachial artery; however, use of the diaphragm (flat) is acceptable.

The auscultation method of obtaining blood pressure is widely used. The technique advocated by the American Heart Association[2] (AHA) will be described. The patient should be in a standard sitting position and the cuff placed on either the right or the left arm. Whenever it is necessary to repeat the procedure, the same position and arm should be used because blood pressure can vary between arms and positions. The cuff should be placed above the elbow in a snug fashion with the lower border about an inch above the antecubital fossa. The standard cuff has arrows designating the location of the brachial artery (at the medial aspect of the tendon of the biceps). Applying the cuff too loosely will give falsely elevated values.

It is possible to fail to recognize an "auscultatory gap." Sounds may disappear between the systolic and diastolic pressures and then reappear. If the cuff pressure is raised only to the range of the gap, the systolic reading will be falsely low. This error is eliminated by first determining the systolic level by the palpatory method.

The cuff is inflated until the radial pulse disappears, and it is then inflated about an additional 30 mm Hg. The stethoscope is placed over the previously palpated brachial artery at the bend of the elbow, in the antecubital fossa (not under the cuff). Nothing should be heard.

The pressure is then slowly released 2 to 3 mm Hg per second, and, as the needle falls, a point is reached at which beats become audible. This is recorded as the systolic pressure.

As the needle continues to fall, the sound of the beats becomes louder and then gradually diminishes until a point is reached at which there is a sudden marked diminution in intensity. The weakened beats are heard for a few moments more and then disappear altogether (Fig. 1-11). The most reliable index of diastolic pressure is the point where the sound completely disappears. Occasionally it will be pos-

sible to hear muffled sounds continuously far below the true diastolic pressure. When this occurs, the initial point of muffling should be used as the diastolic pressure.

In the average, healthy adult the normal systolic pressure varies from 90 to 140 mm Hg, generally increasing with age. The normal diastolic pressure is 60 to 90. Pulse pressure is defined as the difference between systolic and diastolic pressures. Hypertension in adults is generally equal to or greater than 140/90.[4] Table 1-1 shows the levels considered to be significant hypertension in children.

The anxious patient may have a falsely elevated blood pressure; therefore the dentist should not be satisfied with a single high reading. The cuff should be left in place and the pressure rechecked at periodic intervals, allowing at least 2 to 3 minutes between recordings.

Respiration

The rate and depth of respiration should be monitored by carefully observing the movement of the chest and abdomen in the quietly breathing patient. The respiratory rate in a normal resting adult is approximately 12 to 16 breaths per minute. The respiratory rate in infants may be double that of an adult.

Notice should be made of patients with labored breathing, rapid breathing, or irregular breathing patterns because all may be signs of systemic problems, especially cardiopulmonary disease.

A common finding in apprehensive patients is hyperventilation (rapid, prolonged, deep

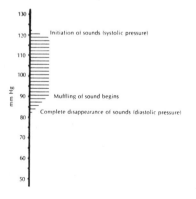

FIG. 1-11 Typical sound pattern obtained when recording blood pressure in a normotensive adult.

TABLE 1-1

Hypertension in Children (95th percentile for age)

	Systolic/diastolic blood pressure	
Age (years)	Pressure (mm Hg)
3 to 5	≥ 116/76
6 to 9	≥ 122/78
10 to 12	≥ 126/82
13 to 15	≥ 136/86
16 to 18	≥ 142/92

From Report of the Joint National Committee, *Arch Intern Med* 148:1023-1038, 1988.

breathing or sighing) that results in lowered carbon dioxide levels and may cause disturbing symptoms, including perioral numbness, tingling in the fingers and toes, nausea, and carpopedal spasms.

Temperature

Temperature is not usually recorded during a normal examination but rather when a patient has febrile signs or symptoms. Normal oral temperature is 98.6° F (37° C) although it may vary as much as ±1° F over the course of a day and is usually higher in the afternoon. Rectal temperature is about 1° F higher than oral, and axillary temperature 1° lower.

Weight

The patient should be questioned about any recent unintentional gain or loss of weight. A rapid weight loss may be a sign of malignancy, diabetes, tuberculosis, or other wasting diseases, whereas a rapid weight gain could be a sign of heart failure, edema, or neoplasm.

Head and neck examination

The examination of the head and neck region may vary in its comprehensiveness and may include inspection and palpation of the soft tissues of the oral cavity, maxillofacial region, and neck (Fig. 1-12) as well as an evaluation of

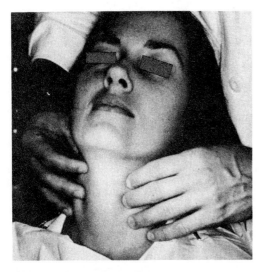

FIG. 1-12 Bimanual palpation of the anterior neck.

cranial nerve function. The reader is referred to standard texts on physical diagnosis or oral pathology for further descriptions.

LABORATORY EVALUATION

Laboratory evaluation for screening purposes is an important phase in the determination of a patient's health status. Fortunately, most patients do not require laboratory screening; however, it can be a useful tool for those patients who do require it. The dentist should know the indications for certain clinical laboratory procedures, how to order others from a laboratory, and how to interpret the results of the tests. It should be noted that tests such as biopsy, cytology, and culture and sensitivity are not included in this section but obviously are of great importance. The reader is referred to an oral pathology text for further information.

It is important that clinical laboratory tests be performed when indicated. Such indications for clinical laboratory testing in dentistry include the following:

1. Aiding in the diagnosis of suspected disease (e.g., diabetes, infection, bleeding disorders, leukemia, neutropenia)
2. Screening high-risk patients for undetected disease (e.g., hepatitis B, diabetes)
3. Establishing normal baseline values before treatment (e.g., anticoagulant status, chemotherapy, radiation therapy)
4. Medicolegal considerations (e.g., possible bleeding disorders, hepatitis B infection)

It is beyond the scope of this text to summarize all laboratory tests that a dentist might conceivably order; therefore, emphasis will be placed on only those that are more commonly used. Clinical laboratory tests ordered by dentists usually include a complete blood count (CBC) with differential, blood glucose, hemostasis, and hepatitis B or C. Each test or series of tests is discussed briefly in the following section.

Complete blood count with differential[1]

The CBC with differential series of tests examines the formed elements of the blood (red blood cells [RBCs], white blood cells [WBCs], platelets) and provides information about the number of each type of cell, the ratio of types of cells to others, and the morphology of cell types.

WBCs — total number of all types of white blood cells

per ml^3 of whole blood (normal range is 4500 to 11,000)

Differential WBC count — the number of each type of WBC expressed as a percentage of the total number of WBCs (normal mean percentages are 56% segmented neutrophils, 3% bands, 0.3% basophils, 2.7% eosinophils, 34% lymphocytes, 4% monocytes)

RBCs — total number of red blood cells per ml^3 of whole blood (normal for males is 4.6 to 6.2 × 10^6; for females 4.2 to 5.4 × 10^6)

Hemoglobin (Hgb) — the amount of hemoglobin (in grams) contained in 100 ml of whole blood (normal for males is 13.5 to 18.0; for females 12.0 to 16.0)

Hematocrit (Hct) — the volume percentage of packed red blood cells in 100 ml of whole blood (normal for males is 40% to 54%; for females 38% to 47%)

RBC indices — includes the mean corpuscular volume (MCV), the mean corpuscular hemoglobin (MCH), and the mean corpuscular hemoglobin concentration (MCHC) (normal MCV is 80 to 96 mm^3; normal MCH is 27 to 31 pg; normal MCHC is 32% to 36%)

Platelet count (PLT) — number of platelets per mm^3 (normal is 150,000 to 450,000)

Peripheral smear — size, shape, and morphology of the RBCs and WBCs

Blood glucose (blood sugar)[4]

The blood glucose measures the concentration of glucose in 100 ml of serum or plasma. For screening purposes, a fasting glucose (before breakfast) is generally the test of choice to minimize variables of diet (normal is 70 to 110 mg/100 ml).

Hemostasis[4]

Tests for hemostasis examine the ability to control bleeding by vasoconstriction, platelet aggregation and coagulation, and (indirectly) fibrinolysis.

Ivy bleeding time (BT[Ivy]) — the number of seconds required for a small stab wound to stop bleeding; platelet quantity and quality and vessel integrity are determinants (normal is 2 to 8 minutes depending on method)

Prothrombin time (PT) — the number of seconds required for coagulation via the extrinsic and common pathway (normal is 10 to 13 seconds depending on reagent)

Activated partial thromboplastin time (APTT) — the number of seconds required for coagulation via the intrinsic and common pathway (normal is 25 to 35 seconds depending on reagent)

Thrombin time (TT) — the number of seconds required to convert fibrinogen to fibrin; adversely influenced by the presence of fibrin split products (normal is 17 to 25 seconds depending on reagent)

Hepatitis B and C

These tests detect either past or current infection with the hepatitis B or C virus and are based on antigen-antibody reactions to the various viral segments.

Hepatitis B surface antigen (HBsAg) — detection of the surface coat antigen of a virus; implies either active disease or a chronic carrier state

Hepatitis B surface antibody (anti-HBs) — detection of antibodies to a surface antigen; implies past infection with immunity

Hepatitis C surface antibody (anti-HC) — detection of antibodies to the hepatitis C viral antigen; implies past or current infection.

Following are some examples of how clinical laboratory tests can be used in dental practice.

CASE 1 A 38-year-old man was going to be treated for a periodontal condition that would require surgery. During the history he mentioned that when he had had a tooth extracted about 3 years earlier he had bled for several days following the extraction. He had gone to a physician, who gave him an injection of vitamin K, after which the bleeding stopped. Before the periodontal surgery this patient was screened through a commercial laboratory for a possible bleeding condition. A BT, PT, APTT, and TT were ordered. These tests were necessary because there was no real insight into the possible cause of the bleeding problem, if indeed the patient had one. The possibilities to be ruled out included coagulation disorders, platelet deficiency, vascular wall defects, and defects of fibrinolysis. The screening tests for this patient were all normal, and he was treated with no complications.

CASE 2 A 40-year-old man with advanced periodontitis stated during the medical history that his mother had insulin-dependent diabetes mellitus. This placed the patient in a high-risk group for diabetes. A fasting glucose test was ordered for this patient, and the results were normal (100 mg/100 ml), but it was recommended to the patient that he be checked once a year in a similar manner.

CASE 3 A 30-year-old woman appeared for routine dental care. During the discussion of her past medical history, she revealed that she had had hepatitis a few years ago but did not know anything about the details of the disease and could not remember her physician's name. Therefore a screening test for HBsAg was ordered to rule out the possibility that she could be a carrier of hepatitis B. The test was positive for HBsAg, indicating that the patient was indeed a carrier of hepatitis B. She was referred to her physician for evaluation of her liver function before initiating any treatment, and plans were made to provide dental care with attention to asepsis, barrier techniques, and infection control.

When dealing with a commercial laboratory, the dentist should take the time to visit the laboratory facilities and meet the pathologist in charge. At this time the dentist should find out what tests of interest are performed by the laboratory, what the costs are for these tests, and what the normal ranges are for test results. Copies of the order sheets for these tests should also be obtained. If the patient is sent to the laboratory for collection of the sample to be tested (such as blood), the laboratory will send the results directly to the dentist for interpretation and will bill the patient. The dentist should inform the patient of the cost before referral to the laboratory.

If the dentist does not want to become involved with ordering laboratory tests, the patient should be referred to a physician for medical and laboratory screening.

REFERRAL TO A PHYSICIAN FOR CONSULTATION

Based on the medical history, physical examination, or results of laboratory screening, it may be necessary to contact the patient's physician for consultation or referral purposes. The usual methods are by phone, personal contact, or letter. Personal contact is common, particularly in a small community where physicians and dentists may socialize and may informally discuss a mutual patient. The main drawback to this type of "sidewalk consultation" is its lack of formality and of a legal record of the transaction. If this method is employed, a letter should be sent to confirm the conversation as soon as possible. A phone conversation also should have this type of formal follow-up documentation and confirmation. The principal advantage of the conversational approach is one of immediate information and the chance to gain additional information to questions that may not

have been included in the letter. If a patient needs work without delay, a phone call to find out the pertinent information from the physician will allow the dentist to proceed with the work; however, this should be followed with a chart entry and a letter to the physician stating the dentist's understanding of the conversation and requesting confirmation in writing. This should then be attached to the patient's chart, and it becomes a part of the legal document.

A letter to a physician should be kept concise and to the point; only pertinent information should be included, and questions or the reasons why the patient was referred should be specific. (See the examples of letters sent to physicians for various reasons.)

REFERRAL FOR EVALUATION OF SUSPECTED DIABETES

Re: Patient's name
Chart number

Dear Dr. _____:

Mr. A. Johnson, a 30-year-old white male, has presented to my office for comprehensive dental care. Examination revealed him to have generalized severe periodontal disease. Upon questioning, he reported weight loss, nocturia, and excessive thirst. A screening fasting blood sugar was 240 mg%. Based on these findings, I am referring Mr. Johnson to you for evaluation of possible diabetes. I would appreciate a summary of your findings at your convenience.

Sincerely,

_____, D.M.D.

An additional approach to the referral-consultation request is a printed form. Figure 1-13 is the request-for-medical-consultation form in use at the University of Kentucky College of Dentistry. The advantage of this approach is that it simplifies and standardizes the procedure for the dentist and physician.

Albert B. Chandler Medical Center College of Dentistry Lexington, Kentucky Department of Oral Diagnosis/Oral Medicine Phone (606) 233-5950 Medical consultation	Patient name: Number:	
Referred to	Patient's address	
Student		
Date	Age	Sex
Attending dentist	Family physician	

Patient history

Planned dental treatment

Reason for referral

Report of medical consultant

Date

Signature of consultant

FIG. 1-13 Request-for-medical-consultation form in use at the University of Kentucky College of Dentistry.

REFERRAL TO VERIFY THE PRESENCE OF RHEUMATIC HEART DISEASE

Re: Patient's name
    Chart number

Dear Dr. _____:

Mr. A. Smith, a 37-year-old white male, has reported to my office for comprehensive dental care. He reports a history of rheumatic fever at age 8 years but is unaware of any residual damage to his heart that would predispose to infective endocarditis. He denies any symptoms associated with heart disease and is a well-developed, well-nourished, athletic individual. We are planning to provide comprehensive dental care for Mr. Smith.

The purpose of this referral is to request an evaluation of his cardiac status to rule out the presence of rheumatic heart disease and the need for prophylactic antibiotics to prevent infective endocarditis or any additional medical problems of which I should be aware. If in your opinion antibiotics are required, I plan to follow the current recommendations of the American Heart Association.

I would appreciate receiving a summary of your findings at your earliest convenience. Thank you for seeing this patient.
    Sincerely,

_____D.M.D.

REFERRAL BECAUSE OF UNCONTROLLED HYPERTENSION

Re: Patient's name
    Chart number

Dear Dr. _____:

Mrs. A. Jones, a 50-year-old obese black female, has reported to my office for dental care. During the examination and history she reported frequent headaches and dizzy spells in addition to her "eyes bothering her." She has not seen a physician for several years but remembers taking a "water pill" for blood pressure at one time. In my office today her blood pressure was 215/125, right arm, sitting, at the beginning of the appointment and 210/125 at the termination of the appointment. At this point I have elected to discontinue any further dental work and have advised her to seek an immediate medical evaluation from you.

I would appreciate a summary of findings and treatment of this patient, if appropriate. I will plan to resume treatment when you believe that her condition has stabilized.

Thank you for seeing this patient.

    Sincerely,

_____D.M.D.

REFERENCES

1. Henry JB, editor: *Clinical diagnosis and management by laboratory methods,* ed 18, Philadelphia, 1991, WB Saunders.
2. *Recommendations for human blood pressure determination by sphygmomanometers*, Publ. no. 70-019-B, Dallas, 1980, American Heart Association.
3. Report of the Second Task Force on Blood Pressure Control in Children—1987, *Pediatrics* 79:1-25, 1987.
4. Report of the Joint National Committee on Detection, Evaluation, and Treatment of High Blood Pressure—1988, *Arch Intern Med* 148:1023-1037, 1988.

2

Infective Endocarditis

Infective endocarditis (IE) is a disease caused by microbial infection of the heart valves or endocardium, most often in proximity to congenital or acquired cardiac defects. A similar disease, infective endarteritis, may occur, involving a patent ductus arteriosus, coarctation of the aorta, surgical grafts of major vessels, and surgical arteriovenous shunts. This disease is most often caused by bacteria; however, in recent years fungi and other microorganisms have been identified as causative agents.

The dentist must make every attempt to identify patients with congenital or acquired cardiovascular defects before any dental manipulations are performed that could produce a transient bacteremia. In these patients the bacteremia could result in infective endocarditis or endarteritis. These infections were essentially 100% fatal before the antibiotic era. Even with the best of medical treatment, these diseases have about a 10% to 65% mortality rate.[25,30,48] It appears that infective endocarditis and endarteritis can be prevented in most cases by adequate prophylactic antibiotic therapy. This chapter will deal primarily with infective endocarditis and its prevention. The same principles of prevention apply to infective endarteritis. The terms shown in Table 2-1 should be reviewed, for they will be used in this chapter.

GENERAL DESCRIPTION
INCIDENCE AND PREVALENCE

The incidence of infective endocarditis is not positively known. A study by Porgrel and Welsby[62] in Scotland found 83 cases of bacterial endocarditis over a 15-year period from a population of about 500,000 people being served by the Aberdeen Royal Infirmary. This would suggest an incidence of much less than 1%. Mostaghim and Millard[48] reported 64 cases of bacterial endocarditis being treated at the University of Michigan Hospital over a 10-year period. Based on hospital admissions during that period, the incidence was, again, much less than 1%. Falace and Ferguson[30] reported 49 patients admitted to the University of Kentucky's University Hospital for bacterial endocarditis between 1963 and 1975. During this period there were 142,082 admissions to the hospital; again, the incidence was much less than 1% (0.034%). Thus the incidence of infective endocarditis appears to be between 0.3 and 3 cases per 1000 hospital admissions. From this standpoint it is clear that endocarditis is a rare or relatively rare disease in the population as a whole. It has been estimated[58] to occur in 11 to 50 persons per 1 million population.

However, when only the more susceptible portion of the population is considered, bacterial endocarditis becomes a much more common problem. The Bland and Jones study of rheumatic fever[10] in 1951 found that 10% of the deaths were caused by bacterial endocarditis. In that study 30 patients out of 1000 died of bacterial endocarditis. No mention was made of the number of patients who developed the disease and lived. Patients on hemodialysis have a 5% risk for endocarditis. Patients with a previous history of endocarditis have about a 3% to 10% risk of another endocarditis episode.[44,58] Thus the true incidence of bacterial endocarditis is still not known; however, it appears to be very low in the general population and to increase sharply in susceptible individuals.

Certain features of infective endocarditis (IE)

TABLE 2–1
Endocarditis Terminology

Term	Abbreviation	Definition
Infective endocarditis	IE	Microbial infection of heart valves or endocardium
Infective endarteritis		Microbial infection of endothelium of arteries
Bacterial endocarditis	BE	Bacterial infection of heart valve or endocardium
Alpha-hemolytic streptococcus endocarditis		Infecting organism identified
Nonbacterial thrombotic endocarditis	NBTE	Sterile vegetation formed by platelets and fibrin at sites of endocardial damage
Acute bacterial endocarditis	ABE	Sudden onset, fatal in less than 6 weeks if untreated, usually caused by *Staphylococcus aureus*; normal valves often involved
Subacute bacterial endocarditis	SBE	Slower onset, fatal in months, if not treated, most often caused by *Viridans* streptococci infecting damaged valves
Native valve endocarditis	NVE	Infection of native heart valves
Prosthetic valve endocarditis	PVE	Infection of prosthetic heart valves
Nosocomial infective endocarditis		Hospital-acquired endocarditis

have changed during the past 20 years. It is now more common in males (2 to 1 ratio), and the median age has increased from 30 to 50 years. There has been an increase in the number of acute cases and a slight decrease in the proportion of streptococcal cases. Also the number of cases caused by fungi and gram-negative bacteria has increased. The classic signs of IE are found less often. IE remains rare in children but has become more common in the elderly.[24,25,44,53] IE in patients over the age of 65 has increased from 30% (between 1944 to 1965) to 55% (between 1965 to 1983).[5]

The use of prophylactic antibiotics has not appeared to have reduced the number of cases of infective endocarditis being reported. This may be because fewer than 1 in 5 cases of subacute bacterial endocarditis (SBE) have been associated with medical or dental procedures, and very few of the acute cases are reported to be associated with medical or dental procedures.[24,25]

More than 200 cases of streptococcal endocarditis that followed dental and genitourinary tract procedures have been reported in the literature. In the vast majority of these cases, symptoms of the disease occurred within 2 weeks of the procedure.[24,25]

ETIOLOGY

Endocarditis occurs when bacteria enter the bloodstream and infect damaged endocardium or endothelial tissue located near high-flow shunts between arterial and venous channels. Other microorganisms—such as fungi—may rarely infect these sites. Other host factors must be important in the development of this disease, because a number of patients with congenital or acquired heart lesions have had dental extractions without antibiotic protection and have not developed bacterial endocarditis.

The report by Mostaghim and Millard[48] suggested that drug addicts, with or without cardiac lesions, may be more susceptible to the disease. Recent reports[22,24,43,61] have confirmed the increased risk of endocarditis in drug

TABLE 2–2

Conditions that May Lead to Infective Endocarditis in Patients with Normal Hearts or Those with Cardiac Defects

	Endocarditis	
Conditions	**Normal heart**	**Cardiac defect**
IV drug abuse	Usually	Uncommon
Hemodialysis	Usually	Uncommon
Genitourinary tract manip-ulation		
Cystoscopy	Uncommon	Usually
Urethral catheterization	Uncommon	Usually
Prostatectomy	Uncommon	Usually
Septic abortion	Uncommon	Usually
Pelvic infection		
Intrauterine contracep-tive device	Uncommon	Usually
Skin infections (staphylo-coccal	Sometimes	Usually
Cancer of colon	Rare	Usually
Dental treatment and den-tal infection	Rare	Usually
Nosocomial		
Surgery	Sometimes	Sometimes
Intracardiac pressure–monitoring devices	Usually	Uncommon
Ventriculoatrial shunts	Usually	Uncommon
Hyperalimentation lines into right ventricle	Usually	Uncommon
Severe burns	Usually	Uncommon

addicts. Intravenous drug abusers have a 30% risk for endocarditis within 2 years of drug use.[58] Bacteria are released directly into the bloodstream because of the use of nonsterile needles, or an infection develops at the injection site and bacteria gain access to the bloodstream. Over 50% of the cases of endocarditis in drug addicts are caused by *Staphylococcus aureus,* and about 50% involve the right side of the heart, usually the tricuspid valve.[24,25,27,44] Septic pulmonary infarcts are a common finding in these patients. Other conditions that may lead to IE in patients with or without cardiac defects are shown in Table 2-2.

Endocarditis may occur in patients who do not have cardiac defects. The disease has been reported[25,57] in young children, under the age of 2, who had no cardiac defects. Most studies reporting infective endocarditis will show that 60% to 80% of the patients have some type of predisposing heart or arterial disease[57] (Table 2-3). The remainder of the patients will have no known predisposing cardiovascular defects. About 30% of cases of infective endocarditis occur in patients with rheumatic heart disease, 10% to 20% occur in patients with congenital heart disease and 10 to 33% in patients with mitral valve prolapse.[44,57]

Streptococci and staphylococci are responsible for approximately 80% of the cases of endocarditis.* However, the percentage caused by streptococci is decreasing. During the 1960s gram-negative bacteria accounted for about 1.7% of cases of infective endocarditis. These organisms now cause about 7% of the cases.[4,16] They account for 13% to 20% of cases in drug

---

* References 24, 27, 43, 44, 61.

TABLE 2–3

Approximate Frequency in Percent of the Major Preexisting Cardiac Lesions
in Patients with Infective Endocarditis

Condition	Children under 2 (%)	Children 2 to 15 (%)	Adults 15 to 50 (%)	Adults over 50 (%)	IV drug abusers (%)
No known heart disease	50 to 70	10 to 15	10 to 20	10	50 to 60
Congenital heart disease*	30 to 50	70 to 80	25 to 35	15 to 25	10
Rheumatic heart disease	Rare	10	10 to 15	10 to 15	10
Degenerative heart disease	0	0	Rare	10 to 20	Rare
Previous cardiac surgery	5	10 to 15	10 to 20	10 to 20	10 to 20
Previous endocarditis	Rare	5	5 to 10	5 to 10	10 to 20

*Includes mitral valve prolapse.
From Durack DT: In Hurst JW, editor: *The heart, arteries, and veins,* ed 7, New York, 1990, McGraw-Hill,
p 1232.

addicts and for 10% to 20% in patients with
prosthetic heart valves.[25,27,44] Table 2-4 presents
a comparison of native valve and prosthetic
valve endocarditis with endocarditis in drug
addicts. Table 2-5 shows the frequency of the
various organisms causing IE.

The risk of endocarditis occurring in a patient
after he or she has received dental treatment is
not known. It has been estimated[57,62] to vary
from 0 to as high as 1 in 533. The number of
patients considered susceptible to endocarditis
has been estimated to be as high as 5% to 10%
of the general population.[62] This includes individuals with conditions such as rheumatic heart
disease or congenital heart disease and devices
such as prosthetic heart valves (Table 2-6).

TABLE 2–4

Comparisons Among Various Types of Endocarditis

	Native valve	Prosthetic valve	Drug abusers
Causative organism	Streptococci most common Streptococci and staphylococci, over 80% of cases When *Streptococcus bovis* found, look for carcinoma of colon	*Staphylococcus epidermidis* most common Gram-negative bacilli and fungi, up to 25%	*Staphylococcus aureus,* over 50% Gram-negative bacilli, about 15% of cases
Most common location	Mitral valve	Aortic valve	Tricuspid valve
Predeposing defect	Lesion, 60% to 68%	Prosthetic device at suture line	Most often on normal valves
Mortality rate	Streptococci, 10% Staphylococci, 40% Fungi, high	Early PVE, 40% to 80% Late PVE, 20% to 40%	Staphylococci, low (90% cure rate)

PVE, Prosthetic valve endocarditis.

TABLE 2–5

Frequency of Various Organisms Causing Infective Endocarditis

Organism	NVE (%)	IV drug abusers (%)	Early PVE (%)	Late PVE (%)
Streptococci	65	15	5	35
Alpha-hemolytic	35	5	Less than 5	25
S. bovis	15	Less than 5	Less than 5	Less than 5
S. faecalis	10	8	Less than 5	Less than 5
Staphylococci	25	50	50	30
Coagulase-positive	23	50	20	10
Coagulase-negative	Less than 5	Less than 5	30	30
Gram-negative bacilli	Less than 5	5	20	10
Fungi	Less than 5	5	10	5
Culture-negative endocarditis	5 to 10	5	Less than 5	Less than 5

NVE, Native valve endocarditis; *PVE,* prosthetic valve endocarditis.
From Durack DT: In Hurst JW, editor: *The heart, arteries, and veins,* ed 7, New York, 1990, McGraw-Hill, p 1233.

TABLE 2–6

Degree of Risk for Infective Endocarditis Posed by Various Cardiac or Vascular Lesions*

Relatively high

Prosthetic heart valve*
Aortic valve disease
Mitral insufficiency
Patent ductus arteriosus
Ventricular septal defect
Coarctation of aorta
Marfan's syndrome

Intermediate

Mitral valve prolapse with regurgitation
Pure mitral stenosis
Tricuspid valve disease
Pulmonary valve disease
Previous infective endocarditis*

Calcific aortic sclerosis
Hyperalimentation or pressure-monitoring line that reaches right atrium
Nonvalvular intracardiac prosthetic implant
Hypertrophic cardiomyopathy

Very low or negligible

Atrial septal defect
Arteriosclerotic plaques
Coronary artery disease
Syphilitic aortitis
Cardiac pacemaker
Surgically corrected cardiac lesion (without prosthetic implants, more than 6 months after surgery)

*Considered high-risk by the AHA.[12, 21]
From Durack DT: In Hurst JW, editor: *The heart, arteries, and veins,* ed 7, New York, 1990, McGraw-Hill, p 1232.

PATHOPHYSIOLOGY AND COMPLICATIONS

The lesions of bacterial endocarditis are divided into three groups—cardiac, embolic, and general.

Cardiac lesions are usually valvular, and the mitral valve is most often affected. Infection of the pulmonary valve is rare. Vegetative lesions occur on the line of contact of the damaged valve cusps and cover the valve. They generally consist of an amorphous mass of fused platelets, fibrin, and bacteria (Fig. 2-1).

Sterile vegetations may develop prior to

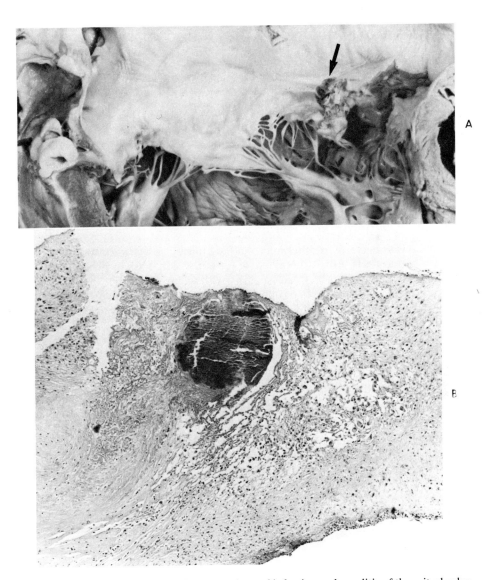

FIG. 2-1 **A,** Gross appearance of the vegetations of infective endocarditis of the mitral valve (*arrow*). **B,** Photomicrograph of the vegetations of bacterial endocarditis of the aortic valve (*arrow*). (**A** courtesy Jesse E. Edwards, M.D., St Paul Minn; **B** courtesy W. O'Connor, M.D., Lexington Ky.)

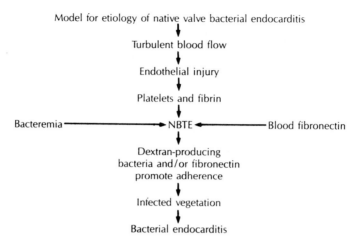

Model for etiology of native valve bacterial endocarditis

↓

Turbulent blood flow

↓

Endothelial injury

↓

Platelets and fibrin

↓

Bacteremia ——————————→ NBTE ←————— Blood fibronectin

↓

Dextran-producing
bacteria and/or fibronectin
promote adherence

↓

Infected vegetation

↓

Bacterial endocarditis

FIG. 2-2 Sequence of events in the formation of nonbacterial thrombotic endocarditis (NBTE).

becoming infected with bacteria or other micro-organisms. This condition is termed nonbacterial thrombotic endocarditis (NBTE). NBTE is now thought[27,44] to precede most cases of native valve bacterial endocarditis. The sequence of events involved with the formation of NBTE and bacterial endocarditis is shown in Figure 2-2. NBTE has been reported in about 50% of cases of systemic lupus erythematosus,[13] and it increases the risk for bacterial endocarditis in these patients.

Embolic lesions are common because the vegetations are friable and easily detached. Petechial hemorrhages on skin and mucous membranes may result from these emboli (Fig. 2-3). Osler nodes (small, raised, tender, vascular lesions) involving the skin may arise from emboli or may represent a reaction to bacterial endotoxins. Emboli may affect the kidneys, brain, eyes, and other tissues.

General lesions include an enlarged spleen, mycotic aneurysms, clubbing of the fingers, and arthritis. Other conditions that may be present in patients with bacterial endocarditis include cardiac failure, liver disease, and anemia. These effects may be a result of toxemia from the infection.[25]

As stated earlier, patients with bacterial endocarditis who do not receive antibiotic treatment will have a mortality rate of 100%.[25] The mortality rate for treated patients varies from 10% to 65%.[13,22] The morbidity rate is also significant, average hospital stays ranging from 4 to 6 weeks. Patients who recover are still faced with many potential complications—including reinfection, congestive heart failure, renal disease, and cerebrovascular accident. Early and effective treatment decreases both the death rate and the number of complications. Patients who have recovered from endocarditis often will have a scarred valve that may be perforated or ruptured. The valve may be functionally altered, and the patient is at increased risk for reinfection.[26]

CLINICAL PRESENTATION

SIGNS AND SYMPTOMS

Subacute bacterial endocarditis is caused most often by alpha-hemolytic streptococci. Its onset is often insidious. The patient may be unable to pinpoint when the disease first started. However, in retrospect, symptoms can usually be pinpointed to within 2 weeks of the precipitating event. Symptoms include weakness, weight loss, fatigue, fever, chills, night sweats, anorexia, and arthralgia. Emboli may produce paralysis, chest pain, abdominal pain, blindness, and hematuria. The fever may spike, with peaks often being noted in the afternoon or evening. Petechiae may be found on the skin or mucosal tissues. Linear hemorrhages may be found under the nails in about 20% of the patients, and Osler nodes (small, painful, tender, red or purplish nodules) may be found in

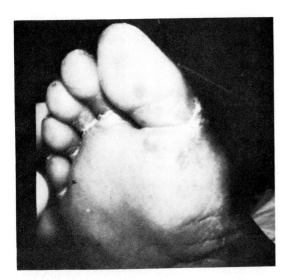

FIG. 2-3 Petechiae caused by septic emboli of bacterial endocarditis. (Courtesy H.D. Wilson, M.D., Lexington Ky.)

TABLE 2–7
Signs and Symptoms of Infective Endocarditis

Signs

  Petechiae
  Linear hemorrhage (nails)
  Osler nodes
  Janeway lesions
  Retinal hemorrhages
  Clubbing of fingers
  Murmurs

Symptoms (primary)

  Weakness
  Weight loss
  Fatigue
  Fever, chills, night sweats
  Arthralgia

Symptoms (secondary, caused by septic emboli)

  Paralysis
  Chest pain
  Abdominal pain
  Blindness
  Hematuria

various subcutaneous areas in 10% to 20% of the patients. Janeway lesions (flat, nontender, red spots) may be found on the palms and soles and will blanch on pressure. Retinal hemorrhages can be found in 10% to 25% of patients.[25,27,44]

Patients may appear pale because of the anemia that is often associated with endocarditis. In long-standing cases clubbing of the fingers may be found. Heart findings are related to the underlying cardiac disease, which is usually valvular. Thus almost all patients will have a murmur (Table 2-7). Heart failure is a most important finding and carries a poor prognosis. The spleen and liver may be enlarged.[24,25,27] Neurologic symptoms occur in about 40% to 50% of the cases of IE. Neurologic symptoms include confusional states, psychiatric manifestations, strokes, and cerebritis.[27]

Highly pathogenic microorganisms, such as *Staphylococcus aureus,* will cause a sudden appearance of symptoms, and a rapid course to death will result unless medical measures are taken. Acute bacterial endocarditis frequently involves normal hearts. Severe suppurative infections often precede the onset of this type of endocarditis. The study by Mostaghim and Millard[48] suggested that the number of cases of this type of endocarditis may be increasing.

More recent studies[27,44] have clearly shown that, although the total number of cases of endocarditis has not changed, there has been an increase in the proportion due to staphylococci, fungi, and gram-negative bacilli. There has also been a decrease in the proportion of cases caused by streptococci.

LABORATORY FINDINGS

Laboratory tests for the presence of active infection are usually positive in the patient with bacterial endocarditis (BE). Leukocytosis with neutrophilia is common. The erythrocyte sedimentation rate is increased, the C-reactive protein is positive, and serum immunoglobulins may be increased. A positive test for rheumatoid factor is found in about 50% of the cases of SBE and is rare in ABE.[27]

Blood for culture and antibiotic sensitivity testing is usually taken before specific therapy for the infection is begun. Blood culture is the most important step in the diagnosis of IE. Blood cultures should be obtained for all patients with fever and a heart murmur unless the cause is clear. Three samples of venous blood should be taken on the first day. If no growth occurs, then on the second day two more samples should be taken. If still no growth, then one venous and one arterial blood sample should be taken on the third day. Each sample is divided for aerobic and anaerobic culturing.[27,44] Patients who have been receiving penicillin to prevent recurrent attacks of rheumatic fever and who develop bacterial endocarditis may not show a positive blood culture for 7 or more days. The blood culture is positive in over 85% of the patients with bacterial endocarditis. Five to fifteen percent of the cases of IE may be culture-negative. Most cases of IE caused by *Aspergillus* are culture-negative. Thirty-three percent of the *Candida* cases are culture-negative. SBE of long duration may be culture-negative.[27]

Streptococcus viridans is the microorganism most commonly responsible for the form of endocarditis that has a slow onset (subacute). *Staphylococcus aureus* is the most common cause of a sudden onset of the disease. Recent studies[27,44] have shown an increase in the number of cases caused by *S. aureus* and a reduction in the number caused by *S. viridans*.

Echocardiography can be used to demonstrate valvular vegetations. However, PVE vegetations are difficult to show using this technique. Chest x-ray is useful to demonstrate increased heart size if heart failure is present. In general, cardiac catheterization with cineangiography is not needed for patients who respond to treatment and who do not develop heart failure. This technique may be used to determine the need for a prosthetic heart valve.[27] Gallium scintigraphy using single photon emission computed tomography (SPECT) has been shown[52] to be a noninvasive method to demonstrate PVE and associated valve ring abscess. Radionuclide imaging is used to confirm embolization to the liver or spleen.[52]

MEDICAL MANAGEMENT

The basic principles for the treatment of patients with bacterial endocarditis are as follows[25,27,45]: (1) treat as early as possible; (2) base therapy on culture and sensitivity findings whenever possible; (3) treat with bactericidal agents; (4) treat with adequate doses of antibiotics; (5) administer antibiotics IV; and

TABLE 2–8

Medical Management for Infective Endocarditis — Principles of Treatment

1. Treat early
2. Culture and sensitivity tests
3. Bactericidal agents
4. Adequate dosage
5. IV route
6. Treat long enough

(6) continue treatment long enough. (These are reiterated in Table 2-8.) The best prognosis for patients with endocarditis is if they are young, the diagnosis is made early, the causative agent is a penicillin-sensitive streptococcus, and treatment is started promptly.

Along with cultures and sensitivity testing, a serum bactericidal level is sometimes performed. This is an in vitro study in which the patient's serum containing the administered antibiotic is titered against the causative organism. If the serum is bactericidal for the causative organism at a 1 to 8 dilution or greater, the antibiotic dosage is thought to be adequate.

Penicillin G is the drug of choice for most cases of endocarditis caused by *Streptococcus viridans*. Four million units IV every 6 hours is usually an adequate starting dose for endocarditis caused by *S. viridans*. Gentamicin 1 mg/kg is given twice a day IV in addition to the penicillin [25,27,37,44,65] (Table 2-9).

For infections caused by *Staphylococcus aureus* nafcillin 2 g, IV, every 4 hours is used as the standard regimen. Gentamicin 1 mg/kg, IV, every 8 hours may be added for patients with severe disseminated staphylococcal disease. Patients allergic to penicillin can be treated with cefazolin 2 g, IV, every 8 hours or vancomycin 15 mg/kg, IV, every 12 hours. Treatment will last 4 weeks or longer (Table 2-9). Patients with signs and symptoms of endocarditis who are blood culture–negative are treated with ampicillin plus gentamicin or nafcillin, ampicillin, and gentamicin.[26,27,44]

Mycotic infections are usually treated with large doses of amphotericin B. The length of treatment is usually 4 to 6 weeks. Therapy for mycotic infections may be extended from 4 to 12 weeks. The prognosis is poor with mycotic

TABLE 2–9

Antibiotic Treatment for Infective Endocarditis*

Organism	Regimen	Duration (weeks)
S. viridans	Penicillin G, 4 million units, IV every 6 hours plus gentamicin 1 mg/kg, IV, every 12 hours	2
S. aureus	Nafcillin 2 g, IV, every 4 hours	4
Candida albicans	Amphotericin B, dose variable	4 to 12

*Includes only the standard regimen; special regimens are indicated for patients with complications, penicillin-resistant organisms, penicillin allergy, renal failure, eighth-nerve defects, or other causative organisms.

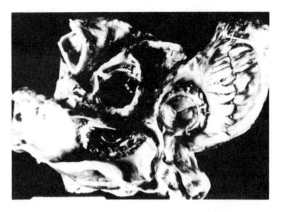

FIG. 2-4 Postmortem specimen from a patient with rheumatic heart disease who underwent surgical replacement of three valves. (Courtesy W. O'Connor, M.D., Lexington Ky.)

endocarditis, and patients who do not respond to amphotericin B may require surgery to remove the infected valve.

Patients with a history of mild allergic reactions to penicillin may still be given this drug following desensitization. Corticosteroids may be given before beginning the penicillin therapy. Start the penicillin by giving small (5-unit) subcutaneous injections and increasing the dose every 90 minutes (5, 10, 100, 1000, 10,000, 50,000 units). If no serious reaction occurs following these injections, then start the IV dosage. Another technique is to infuse 1 unit of aqueous penicillin in 250 ml of 5% glucose and water. If no immediate reaction occurs, increase the penicillin dosage sixfold to tenfold every 20 minutes until therapeutic levels are reached.[37,65] Anticoagulant therapy should be avoided in patients with IE if at all possible. If anticoagulants must be used, warfarin is recommended, but keep the prothrombin time at 1.5 times normal or less. Heparin is contraindicated for patients with IE. Antibiotic treatment should not include an IM regimen if the patient is on anticoagulant therapy.[27]

Surgical correction of infected valves is indicated when (1) severe, intractable heart failure is present; (2) systemic emboli recur; (3) the infecting organism is a fungus and the patient does not respond to medical therapy; or (4) endocarditis is superimposed on an artificial valve. Patients with congenital heart defects and endocarditis are best managed by corrective surgery following successful medical treatment of the endocarditis (Fig. 2-4). However, if the infection cannot be controlled, surgical repair

may be attempted.[25,27,44] Table 2-10 shows the estimated cure rates for endocarditis caused by different organisms and treated by antimicrobial agents and surgery.

Dacron and other prosthetic materials used in cardiovascular surgery to correct congenital or acquired lesions may become infected. Often under these circumstances a cure can be obtained only by removing the infected graft and replacing it. The surgical risk is high for the preceding procedures in patients with endocarditis, but the alternative is a very high mortality rate.

Patients with exteriorized transvenous cardiac pacemakers have on occasion developed an infection resembling endocarditis. For this condition the pacemaker and wire are replaced and moved to another location. The removed wire is cultured, and sensitivity tests are made from the cultured microorganisms. The patient is then treated as for endocarditis.

DENTAL MANAGEMENT

MEDICAL CONSIDERATIONS

The dentist's goal is to prevent endocarditis from occurring in susceptible dental patients. Any dental procedure that causes injury to the soft tissue or bone resulting in bleeding can produce a transient bacteremia that, in the susceptible patient, can result in endocarditis. Even minor dental manipulations such as the cleaning of teeth or the placement of a matrix band can result in a transient bacteremia (Table

TABLE 2–10

Estimated Microbiologic Cure Rate (in percent) for Various Forms of Endocarditis

	Antimicrobial therapy (%)		Antimicrobial therapy plus surgery (%)	
Native valve endocarditis (NVE)				
Alpha-hemolytic streptococci, group A streptocci *Streptococcus bovis,* pneumococci, gonococci	98		98	
S. faecalis	90		Greater than 90	
Staphylococcus aureus (young addicts)	90		Greater than 90	
S. aureus (elderly patients)	50		70	
Gram-negative aerobic bacilli	40		65	
Fungi	Less than 5		50	
	Early (%)	**Late (%)**	**Early (%)**	**Late (%)**
Prosthetic valve endocarditis (PVE)				
Alpha-hemolytic streptococci, group A streptococci, *S. bovis* pneumo-cocci, gonococci	Insufficient data	80	Insufficient data	90
S. faecalis	Insufficient data	60	Insufficient data	75
Staphylococcus aureus (young addicts)	25	40	50	60
S. aureus (elderly patients)	20	40	60	70
Gram-negative aerobic bacilli	Less than 10	20	40	50
Fungi	Less than 1	Less than 1	30	40

From Durack DT: In Hurst JW, editor: *The heart, arteries, and veins,* ed 7, New York, 1990, McGraw-Hill, p 1246.

2-11). In normal patients the body's defenses handle these bacteremias, and usually no serious problem develops. However, in the patient with a heart defect such as rheumatic heart disease, the anatomy and function of the affected valve are altered because of the scarring following the acute rheumatic fever attack.[70] When bacteremias occur the altered valvular tissue with NBTE provides an ideal location for attachment and growth of bacteria. Thus in patients with rheumatic heart disease or those with other types of cardiovascular defects (Table 2-6) there is a very real threat of endocarditis during every period of bacteremia.

Transient bacteremias have been reported to occur following normal physiologic activities involving the mouth. These bacteremias usually clear within 10 minutes. The chewing of paraffin was found to introduce bacteria into the blood-stream in about 50% of subjects investigated, toothbrushing resulted in transient bacteremias in 40%, oral irrigation produced bacteremias in up to 50%, and random testing of individuals with periodontal disease showed the presence of bacteria in the blood in 11% of the cases.[8,25,50,53,58] Guntheroth[35] estimated that with normal physiologic use of the mouth, there would be about 5376 minutes of transient bacteremia per month occurring in an individual (approximately 12% of the time).

Dental procedures resulting in injury to the oral tissues and bleeding can lead to transient bacteremias. The risk of transient bacteremia has been estimated[25,35,50] to be as high as 85% of the time when teeth are extracted, 88% with periodontal surgery, and less often for other procedures. Shafer et al.[68] reported, in a summary of 15 studies on the frequency of transient

TABLE 2–11

Frequency of Bacteremia Associated with Various Dental Procedures and Oral Manipulations

Extractions	51% to 85%
Periodontal surgery	88%
Periodontal scaling	8% to 80%
Dental prophylaxis	0% to 40%
Toothbrushing	0% to 40%
Chewing	17% to 51%
Random in patients with periodontal disease	11%
Random using anaerobic techniques	60% to 80%
Endodontic therapy (nonvital tooth)	0%
Wooden cleansing devices	20% to 40%
Irrigation devices	7% to 50%

Based on Bender IB, et al: *J Am Dent Assoc* 109:415–420, 1984; and Pallasch TJ: *J Calif Dent Assoc* 17(6):27–39, 1989.

TABLE 2–12

Nonstreptococcal and Nonstaphylococcal Bacterial Endocarditis: Relationship with Dental Treatment and Dental Disease

Organism	Reported cases	Cases reported to be related to dental treatment or disease
Haemophilus	81	28
Actinobacillus actinomycet-emcomitans	88	26
Cardiobacterium hominis	60	6
Eikenella corrodens	24	7
Capnocytophaga ochracea	5	4
Kingella denitrificans	6	2
Kingella kingae	22	7
Neisseria subflava	7	2
Neisseria mucosa	7	4
Lactobacillus	30	21
	330	107 (32.4%)

From Barco CT: *J Periodontol* 6:511, 1991 (with permission of The American Academy of Periodontology).

bacteremias following various dental procedures, that in 25% of the cases (302 of 1232) bacteria were released into the bloodstream.

Based on the high frequency of physiologic bacteremias and the low incidence of dental procedures preceding the onset of endocarditis, Guntheroth[35] suggested that the odds of any given case of endocarditis occurring from the physiologic "seeding" of oral bacteria was 1000 times greater than if it occurred following a given dental procedure. Most cases of IE are not related in time to medical or dental procedures. Only one out of five cases of SBE follows a medical or dental procedure that might cause transient bacteremias. Even fewer cases of ABE are associated with such procedures.[27]

Finch[32] estimated that less than 3% of 254 cases of SBE caused by oral bacteria could have been prevented by antibiotic prophylaxis. Other authors place this figure higher, but at best only at 15% to 20%. However, in a recent review of nonstreptococcal and nonstaphylococcal cases of BE[5] the authors found that 32.4% of 330 cases reviewed reported dental treatment or dental disease associated with the onset of BE (Table 2-12). By contrast, in a recent study involving eight patients with high-risk lesions who developed IE within 12 weeks of a dental procedure and 24 control subjects matched for lesion and age,[38] the authors estimated a 91% protective efficacy for antibiotic prophylaxis.

ANTIBIOTIC PROPHYLAXIS

Antibiotic prophylaxis should be considered for the following three clinical situations[59]: (1) when a complication is common but not fatal, (2) when it is rare but has a high mortality rate, and (3) when a single type of organism is usually involved. In practice, effective prophylaxis is complicated by several factors[59]: (1) often a number of different organisms may be involved; (2) these organisms have variable virulence; (3) organisms may originate from multiple sites; (4) they may have varying sensitivity to given antibiotics; (5) random physiologic bacteremias may occur; (6) there are no controlled studies showing the efficacy of antibiotic prophylaxis.

Several important general principles are involved in ideal antibiotic prophylaxis.[56,59] The specific organism involved should be known, and an antibiotic effective against that organism should be selected. The proper dosage of the antibiotic should be used, and the antibiotic should be given just before the procedure to provide maximum blood levels at the time of the injury. The antibiotic should be continued as long as bacteria can be released, which is usually for a short duration. The benefit/risk ratio must be considered for each procedure; in other words, does the risk of developing a problem outweigh the risks involved by the use of the antibiotic?

The American Heart Association guidelines for the prevention of BE meet most of the above principles for effective prophylaxis. IE, although a rare disease, has a significant mortality risk. Prophylaxis is designed against alpha-hemolytic streptococci. These organisms are by far the most common ones found in transient dental bacteremias. Amoxicillin is effective against these bacteria. High doses at the time of bacteremia are provided and continued for an adequate length of time. However, there are no clinical trials that show antibiotic prophylaxis in fact prevents IE in humans. The risk/benefit ratio is questioned for lesions that have moderate to low risk. In addition, using prophylaxis for patients with moderate- to low-risk lesions may not be cost-effective.

It becomes more difficult to support antibiotic prophylaxis for patients with organ transplants, blood dyscrasias, immune deficiencies, joint prostheses, or penile implants, and for patients undergoing chemotherapy or radiation therapy, when the above principles for effective antibiotic prophylaxis are applied. This is true despite the fact that antibiotic prophylaxis at the time of surgery has been shown[22,43,57,59] to reduce infectious complications of prosthetic heart valves, joint prostheses, penile implants, and organ transplants.

It has been estimated[63] that 25% to 50% of antibiotic use in hospitals is for prophylaxis (typically at the time of surgery). The complications associated with antibiotic use include toxicity, allergy, superinfections, resistant bacteria, high costs, and in some cases careless surgery. The problem with allergy alone is significant. About 5% to 10% of the patients who take penicillin will have an allergic reaction.[63] A small number of these patients (0.04% to 0.14%) will develop an anaphylactic reaction, and 10% of these individuals will die. Anaphylactic deaths caused by penicillin account for 400 to 800 deaths per year in the United States.[59,63]

There are still several problems with the current use of antibiotic prophylaxis against endocarditis. The risk of developing the disease in susceptible patients is not known. A number of different microorganisms are found to cause endocarditis; therefore no one antibiotic is effective in preventing the disease. The duration of coverage is not known for oral wounds healing by secondary intention. Bacterial resistance during a coverage period is becoming a problem, as is the presence of resistant strains in the oral flora before antibiotic prophylaxis is initiated. If the antibiotic regimen is too complicated and expensive, the patient may be discouraged from seeking needed dental treatment. The failure of prophylaxis to protect a patient (i.e., one who was given recommended antibiotic prophylaxis but still developed endocarditis) has also been reported. The benefit/risk ratio appears to differ depending on the nature of the underlying cardiac defect.[11,57,58,72]

Several studies[11,15,72] have been reported that question the benefit of antibiotic prophylaxis when considering the number of endocarditis deaths prevented by antibiotic prophylaxis and the number of deaths caused by severe allergic reactions.

In one study[11] it was estimated that 47 cases of endocarditis would occur in 10 million dental visits by patients with mitral valve prolapse if no antibiotic prophylaxis were given. Two deaths could be predicted in the 47 cases of endocarditis. If penicillin prophylaxis were given for each visit, the number of cases of endocarditis would be reduced to 5, with no deaths occurring. However, it was estimated that 175 penicillin-allergy–related deaths would occur (Table 2-13).

In another study,[72] using rheumatic fever as the model, it was estimated that for a population of 100 million there would be about 26 deaths per year caused by endocarditis associated with dental treatment. If the estimated 3.4 million individuals with rheumatic heart disease in this population each received one dental visit per year and were covered by penicillin prophylaxis, there would be about 136 deaths from anaphylactic shock (Table 2-14).

Based on the above studies the use of antibiotic prophylaxis for noncomplicated mitral valve prolapse and other low-risk conditions does not appear to be supported. It also can be

TABLE 2–13

Estimated Death Rates Associated with Mitral Valve Prolapse With and Without Penicillin Prophylaxis (10 Million Dental Patient Visits)

Status	Prophylaxis	No prophylaxis
Number of infective endocarditis cases	5	47
Number of deaths caused by infective endocarditis	0	2
Number of allergy-related deaths	175	0
Total number of deaths	175	2

From Bor DH, Himmelstein DF: *Am J Med* 76:711-717, 1984.

TABLE 2–14

Estimated Yearly Death Rate in a Population of 100 Million Caused by Infective Endocarditis of Dental Origin Versus Yearly Death Rate Attributable to Prophylactic Antibiotics in Patients with Rheumatic Heart Disease Receiving Dental Treatment

Status	Infective endocarditis	Rheumatic heart disease
Prevalence or incidence	1900 (0.0019%)	3,400,000 (3.4%)
Known susceptible patients	1092 (57.5%)	3,400,000
Probability of infective endocarditis caused by dental care	39 (3.6%)	?
Patients with anaphylactic reaction	–	1360 (0.04%)
Deaths from anaphylactic shock	–	136 (10%)
Deaths from infective endocarditis of dental origin	26 (67%)	–

From Tzukert AA, et al: *Oral Surg* 62:276-280, 1986.

questioned whether their use for moderate-risk conditions such as rheumatic heart disease is indicated. The models used in the above studies—decision-tree analytic analysis—do show a benefit for high-risk groups such as patients with prosthetic heart valves or a previous history of endocarditis. Although these studies question the value in terms of risk/benefit for antibiotic prophylaxis in low to moderate at-risk patients, we are not prepared at this time to recommend the discontinuance of prophylaxis for these patients when receiving dental treatment. If after a thorough discussion among the physician, dentist, and patient it is decided that antibiotic prophylaxis is not indicated or desired, we see no problem in proceeding thus with low-risk patients and some moderate-risk patients. There is no question that all high-risk patients receiving dental treatment should be given prophylactic antibiotic coverage as recommended by the American Heart Association.

Even when antibiotic prophylaxis is used, however, it is not 100% effective in preventing endocarditis.[41] In 1981 the American Heart Association formed a national registry to record prophylaxis failures for endocarditis.[9,24,25,41] As of 1983, there had been 52 cases reported involving the development of endocarditis in patients given antibiotic prophylaxis. Most of these patients had cardiac lesions, and ten had prosthetic heart valves. The vast majority had received dental treatment. They had been given either penicillin or erythromycin prophylaxis.

However, only 6 of the 52 cases reported had received one of the standard regimens recommended by the American Heart Association.[24] These data are interesting from two aspects. First, the majority of failures received improper coverage. Second, six cases involved patients who were covered as recommended and still developed the disease. A number of questions remain unanswered concerning this topic. To find the answers and determine the real need for antibiotic prophylaxis, it has been estimated[57] that a double-blind placebo study involving 6000 at-risk patients would be needed. This of course will not be done because of the serious nature of the disease and the moral and ethical problems involved in conducting an investigation on human subjects.

Thus, current practice involves the identification of at-risk patients and the use of antibiotic prophylaxis before dental procedures are performed on any individual in whom a transient bacteremia could induce infective endocarditis.

TABLE 2–15
Summary of American Heart Association Guidelines: 1955–1984

Year	Oral	Parenteral-oral	Parenteral	Penicillin allergy protection	Special
1955	Low loading dose Low dosage Day before, day of, 4 days following	None	Single IM injection	None	None
1960	None	Oral, 2 days before, day of, 2 days following IM loading dose*	IM injections (procaine) one on each of 2 days before and 2 days following IM loading dose (aqueous and procaine) on day of procedure	Erythromycin for penicillin allergy	None
1965	Start 1 hour before Low dosage 3 days	None	Single IM injection	Erythromycin for penicillin allergy	None
1972	Start 1 hour before Extra loading dose* Low dose 3 days following	None	Three IM injections, reduced aqueous dosage, 1 hour before and 2 days following	Erythromycin for penicillin allergy or patients on penicillin for rheumatic fever protection	None
1977	High loading dose* Moderate dosage About 2 days	High IM loading dose* Moderate oral dose About 2 days	None	Erythromycin High loading dose Moderate following dose	IM penicillin and streptomycin plus oral penicillin IV or vancomycin plus oral erythromycin*
1984	High loading dose Single following dose* Less than 1 day	None	High IM loading dose followed by IM dose 6 hours later Only aqueous*	Erythromycin High loading dose Single following dose Less than 1 day	IM or IV ampicillin, Gentamicin plus single-dose oral penicillin IV Vancomycin only

*Significant change or new recommendation.
From Barco CT: *J Periodontol* 6:511, 1991 (with permission of The American Academy of Periodontology).

The problem of bacterial endocarditis has been the subject of six sets of recommendations by the American Heart Association.[22,24,61] As can be seen from Table 2-15, the changes tended to be empirical.

1955

In 1955 the American Heart Association[1] made the first of what proved to be a series of recommendations. Its Committee on Prevention of Rheumatic Fever and Bacterial Endocarditis consisted of seven members, all of whom were physicians. The original recommendations were for either an oral or a parenteral route using penicillin G. The oral regimen consisted of 250,000 units of penicillin G given 4 times on the day before the procedure, 250,000 units of penicillin G given 4 times on the day of the procedure, and an additional 250,000 units of penicillin G given just before the procedure, followed by administration of the same dosage 4 times a day on each of the 4 days following the procedure. The parenteral regimen (which was preferred) consisted of a single IM injection of 600,000 units of aqueous penicillin G plus 600,000 units of procaine penicillin G 30 minutes before the procedure.

1960

The American Heart Association[2] made its next recommendations in 1960. The members of the committee were not identified; however, dentistry did not appear to be represented. The recommendations were modified by (1) eliminating the oral regimen; (2) extending the parenteral regimen to include injections 2 days before, on the day of, and 2 days following the dental procedure; and (3) introducing a combined oral and parenteral regimen (500,000 units of penicillin V, four times a day, 2 days before, on the day of, and 2 days following the procedure, with an IM injection of 600,000 units of aqueous penicillin G 1 hour before the procedure). In addition, the committee recommended for the first time that erythromycin should be used if a history of penicillin allergy was found.

1965

In 1965 the American Heart Association[3] changed its recommendations to again include an oral regimen and reduced the parenteral regimen to a single IM injection of 600,000 units of aqueous penicillin G and 600,000 units of procaine penicillin G given 1 to 2 hours before the dental procedure. The oral regimen consisted of 250 mg of penicillin V starting 1 hour before the dental procedure and continuing on a 4-times-a-day basis for the rest of that day and the next 2 days. The erythromycin regimen for patients allergic to penicillin was modified by starting with 250 mg given 1 hour before the dental procedure and continuing on a 4-times-a-day basis for the rest of that day and the next 2 days. The committee membership had been expanded to 12, with dentistry still not being represented.

1972

In 1972 the American Heart Association[4] made its next recommendations. The committee for the first time had a dentist, Dr. Dean Millard, as a member, and as of this writing he continues to be the sole dental representative. The oral regimen was modified by increasing the initial dose of penicillin to 500 mg given 1 hour before the dental procedure. The parenteral regimen was once again extended to include injections on each of the 2 days following the dental procedure. The dose for each of the 3 injections was reduced by decreasing the aqueous component from 600,000 to 200,000 units of penicillin G. The erythromycin regimen for patients allergic to penicillin was modified by increasing the initial dose to 500 mg. However, the committee for the first time recommended that this regimen be used for patients on continual oral penicillin prophylaxis for prevention of rheumatic fever (the low dose is ineffective in endocarditis prevention). Past committees had suggested increasing the penicillin dosage or using other antibiotics for patients on penicillin prophylaxis for rheumatic fever prevention.

1977

In 1977 the American Heart Association[17] made major changes in the recommendations for endocarditis prevention. These changes were based on the results of studies in animals.[25,34,65] The animal studies had shown that endocarditis could be prevented by very high blood levels of antibiotics if present before the release of bacteria into the bloodstream and if maintained for at least 9 hours. Therefore the initial dose of all regimens was greatly increased. In addition, a regimen was recommended for patients considered to be at greatest risk — recent open heart surgery, history of endocarditis, prosthetic heart valves.

The oral penicillin regimen recommended consisted of 2 g of penicillin V given 30 to 60 minutes before the procedure followed by 500 mg of penicillin V every 6 hours for 8 doses. A combined parenteral-oral regimen was also suggested using 1 million units of aqueous penicillin G and 600,000 units of procaine penicillin G, IM, 30 to 60 minutes before the dental procedure followed by 500 mg penicillin V every 6 hours for 8 doses. This regimen was preferred by the committee. However, we recommend selection of the oral route whenever possible — the reason being that when penicillin is given by injection about 1% to 2% of the patients will develop an allergy to the drug, but when given by the oral route, this is reduced to about 0.1% to 0.2%. Hence, with reliable patients, the oral regimen is preferable. (See Chapter 19.)

Patients at high risk (i.e., prosthetic heart valves) were recommended to be given a special regimen for prophylaxis. Those not allergic to penicillin were to be given a parenteral-oral regimen consisting of 1 million units of aqueous penicillin G and 600,000 units of procaine penicillin G, IM, 30 to 60 minutes before the dental procedure along with 1 g of streptomycin, IM, followed by 500 mg penicillin V, orally, every 6 hours for 8 doses. High-risk patients allergic to penicillin were to be given 1 g of vancomycin by IV infusion over a 30-minute period just before the dental procedure followed by 500 mg of erythromycin, orally, every 6 hours for 8 doses.

1984

The American Heart Association's next recommendations were made in December 1984.[18] Several important changes were made in the recommendations. A clear preference was suggested for the use of an oral regimen for low to moderate at-risk patients. The other major change was to reduce the duration of coverage following the dental procedure. The standard regimen recommended for most patients consisted of 2 g of penicillin V, orally, 1 hour before the dental procedure followed 6 hours later by

1 g penicillin V (i.e., 6 hours following the loading dose). Patients allergic to penicillin or on a low dose of oral penicillin for prevention of rheumatic fever or who were taking penicillin for other reasons were given 1 g of erythromycin, orally, 1 hour before the procedure followed by 500 mg erythromycin 6 hours later. (It may be best to allow 1½ to 2 hours to elapse following the loading dose to ensure maximum blood levels of erythromycin.) For the few patients at low to moderate risk for endocarditis who could not take oral penicillin, the committee recommended 2 million units of aqueous penicillin G, IM, 30 to 60 minutes before the dental procedure followed by 1 million units of aqueous penicillin G, IM, 6 hours later.

For patients at high risk of developing endocarditis (i.e., prosthetic heart valves), the committee recommended a special regimen. Those patients not allergic to penicillin were given 1 to 2 g of ampicillin, IM or IV, and, in a separate dose, gentamicin 1.5 mg/kg, IM or IV, ½ hour before the dental procedure followed by 1 g penicillin V, orally, 6 hours later. Patients allergic to penicillin were given, as recommended in 1977, 1 g of vancomycin given by IV infusion over the 60 minutes before the dental procedure. However, the erythromycin following this dose was eliminated. The committee made no mention of the high-risk patient taking anticoagulation medication. Parenteral injection may be contraindicated in these patients.

CURRENT AHA RECOMMENDATIONS (1990)

The current recommendations of the AHA[19] were made in December of 1990. These recommendations demonstrated the concern of the AHA regarding the low compliance rate reported for the 1984 special regimens among high-risk patients.[44,49,51,64] The current recommendations suggest the use of amoxicillin as the standard regimen for all at-risk patients (Table 2-16). The British Society for Antimicrobial Chemotherapy (BSAC), the European Society of Cardiology (ESC), and the Scandinavian Society for Antimicrobial Chemotherapy (SSAC) also recommend amoxicillin as the standard regimen for IE prophylaxis.[32] However, these organizations recommend a single dose of amoxicillin. By contrast, the AHA recommends two doses. The other organizations also recommend a single 600 mg dose of

TABLE 2–16
American Heart Association Recommended Standard Prophylactic Regimen for Dental Procedures*

Adults	Amoxicillin 3 g orally 1 hour before procedure, then 1.5 g 6 hours after initial dose
Children	Amoxicillin 50 mg/kg orally 1 hour before procedure, then half initial dose 6 hours later
	or
	Children less than 15 kg (33 lb): initial dose, 750 mg amoxicillin
	Children 15 to 30 kg (33 to 66 lb): initial dose, 1500 mg amoxicillin
	Children over 30 kg (66 lb): initial dose, 3000 mg amoxicillin
	Given 1 hour before procedure followed 6 hours later with half initial dose

*Used in all at-risk patients, including those with prosthetic heart valves. Children's doses should not exceed adult dose. From *JAMA* 264:22, 1990 (with permission of the AHA and the AMA). Copyright 1990, American Medical Association.

TABLE 2–17
Recommended Standard Prophylactic Regimen for Dental Procedures in Patients Allergic to Amoxicillin/Penicillin or Who are on Long-Term Penicillin Therapy for Rheumatic Fever Prevention

Adults	Erythromycin ethylsuccinate 800 mg
	or
	Erythromycin stearate 1 g orally 2 hours before procedure, then half dose 6 hours after initial dose
Children*	Erythromycin ethylsuccinate or stearate 20 mg/kg 1 hour before procedure, then half dose 6 hours after initial dose

*Children's doses should not exceed adult doses. From *JAMA* 264:22, 1990 (with permission of the AHA and the AMA). Copyright 1990, American Medical Association.

TABLE 2–18
Recommended Standard Prophylactic Regimen for Dental Procedures in Patients Allergic to Penicillin and Intolerant of Erythromycin

Adults	Clindamycin 300 mg 1 hour before procedure, then 150 mg 6 hours after initial dose
Children*	Clindamycin 30 mg/kg 1 hour before procedure, then half dose 6 hours after initial dose

*Children's doses should not exceed adult doses. From *JAMA* 264:22, 1990 (with permission of the AHA and the AMA). Copyright 1990, American Medical Association.

clindamycin for patients who are allergic to amoxicillin.

The AHA prefers using erythromycin or clindamycin in patients who are allergic to penicillins (Tables 2-17 and 2-18). Two forms of erythromycin are suggested. The time of the loading dose has been extended to 2 hours to allow for proper blood levels to be reached before the dental procedure is performed. In 1984 the AHA had recommended a 1-hour loading time. Other preparations of erythromycin can be selected, but the dentist should be aware of what dosage and loading time are needed for effective blood levels. Patients who are allergic to penicillin and unable to tolerate erythromycin can be given clindamycin according to the current AHA guidelines (Table 2-18). Patients who are taking penicillin for prevention of rheumatic fever or who are being treated with penicillin for other reasons can be protected with erythromycin. If these patients are intolerant of erythromycin, then clindamycin can be used.[21] High-risk patients who are allergic to

amoxicillin should be given clindamycin if an oral regimen is selected.

Dental patients undergoing general anesthesia for surgical treatment should be given IM ampicillin according to the current AHA guidelines.[21] The following dosage is given with IM ampicillin if the patient is not yet awake. Oral amoxicillin is suggested if the patient is awake. Clindamycin is recommended for patients undergoing general anesthesia if they are allergic to penicillin (Table 2-19).

Parenteral-oral regimens are still available

TABLE 2–19

Alternate Prophylactic Regimen for Patients Given General Anesthesia for Oral Surgical or Dental Procedures or Who Are Unable to Use Oral Medications*

Ampicillin 2 g, IV or IM, 30 min before procedure, then 1.5 g amoxicillin 6 hours after initial dose if patient is awake and stable; if patient unable to take oral medication, then 1 g ampicillin IV or IM 6 hours after initial dose

Allergic to Penicillin

Clindamycin 300 mg, IV, 30 min before procedure and 150 mg orally 6 hours after initial dose; if patient still unable to take oral medication, then 150 mg clindamycin IV 6 hours after initial dose

Pediatric dosages. Follow-up oral doses should be half initial dose. Total pediatric dose should not exceed total adult dose:
　　Ampicillin, 50 mg/kg
　　Clindamycin, 10 mg/kg
From *JAMA* 264:22, 1990 (with permission of the AHA and the AMA). Copyright 1990, American Medical Association.

TABLE 2–20

Alternate Prophylactic Regimens for High-Risk Patients for Whom the Practitioner Desires to Use a Parenteral Regimen*

Ampicillin 2 g IV or IM plus gentamicin 1.5 mg/kg IV or IM (not to exceed 80 mg), ½ hour before procedure followed by 1.5 g oral amoxicillin 6 hours after initial dose; alternatively, parenteral regimen may be repeated 8 hours after initial dose.

Allergic to Penicillin

Vancomycin 1 g, IV, administered over 1 hour, starting 1 hour before procedure; no repeat dose is necessary

Initial pediatric dosages. Follow-up oral doses should be half initial dose. Total pediatric dose should not exceed total adult dose:
　　Ampicillin, 50 mg/kg
　　Gentamicin, 2 mg/kg
　　Vancomycin, 20 mg/kg
　　Follow-up dose for amoxicillin, 25 mg/kg
From *JAMA* 264:22, 1990 (with permission of the AHA and the AMA). Copyright 1990, American Medical Association.

for use in selected patients (Table 2-20). Also penicillin-V is still available for use as an alternate oral regimen. The AHA did not speak directly to the issue of changing the regimen for patients taking oral penicillin-V to amoxicillin. The following statement was made:

The choice of the 1984 penicillin V oral regimen for standard risk patients against alpha-hemolytic streptococcal bacteremia following dental and oral procedures is still rational and acceptable.

However, high-risk patients and patients allergic to penicillin should receive one of the 1990 AHA regimens.[19] From a practical standpoint it would seem appropriate to leave patients on the penicillin-V regimen who have been on it for some time. New patients should be placed on the amoxicillin regimen. For patients with high-risk lesions who have been on parenteral-oral regimens a medical consultation is suggested before switching to the amoxicillin regimen. If the patient's physician feels strongly that the patient should remain on a parenteral-oral regimen and the patient agrees, then the dentist would be best advised to do so. However, the advantages of the new amoxicillin regimen

and its recommendation by the AHA should be discussed with the physician and patient.

PREVENTION OF MEDICAL COMPLICATIONS

Current dental management for the prevention of endocarditis involves the identification of at-risk patients and the use of antibiotic prophylaxis before dental procedures according to the 1990 American Heart Association recommendations. Excellent oral hygiene, the prevention of dental disease, and the treatment of existing disease in susceptible patients are the first line of defense in prevention of endocarditis.

PATIENT IDENTIFICATION

The first step in management is the identification of susceptible patients. A list of susceptible patients based on the degree of risk is presented in Table 2-6. Tables 2-21 to 2-23 show the conditions that the AHA recommends for antibiotic coverage, those that it does not, and those for which there is insufficient information to make specific recommendations. A careful health history will identify most of these pa-

TABLE 2-21

Conditions for Which the American Heart Association Recommends Antibiotic Prophylaxis for Endocarditis Prevention

---

Prosthetic cardiac valves
  Bioprosthetic
  Homograft
Previous bacterial endocarditis
Sugically constructed systemic-pulmonary shunts
Most congenital cardiac malformations
Rheumatic and other acquired valvular dysfunction, even after surgery
Hypertrophic cardiomyopathy
Mitral valve prolapse with regurgitation

From Dajani AS, et al: *JAMA* 264:2919–2922, 1990.

TABLE 2-22

Conditions for Which the American Heart Association Does Not Recommend Antibiotic Prophylaxis for Endocarditis Prevention

---

Isolated secundum atrial septal defect
Surgical repair without prosthetic materials 6 months or more after surgery
Previous coronary bypass graft surgery
Mitral valve prolapse without valvular regurgitation
Physiologic, functional (or innocent) heart murmurs
Previous Kawaskaki disease without valvular dysfunction
Previous rheumatic fever without valvular dysfunction (RHD)
Cardiac pacemakers and implanted defibrillators

From Dajani AS, et al: *JAMA* 264:2919–2922, 1990.

TABLE 2-23

Conditions for Which the American Heart Association Believes There Are Insufficient Data to Support Specific Recommendations for Endocarditis Prevention*

Cardiac transplantation
Synthetic arterial grafts
Cardiac lesions corrected with synthetic materials (does not include valves) 6 months or more after surgery

---

*The dentist is advised to consult with the patient's surgeon and cardiologist concerning the need for antibiotic prophylaxis in patients with these conditions.
From Dajani AS, et al: *JAMA* 264:2919–2922, 1990.

tients. Medical consultation should be used to clarify or confirm a patient's current status and the need for antibiotic prophylaxis. Two groups of patients present the greatest problem to the dentist in trying to determine whether the patient may be susceptible to endocarditis: (1) those with a history of rheumatic fever and (2) those who state that they have a heart murmur. (See Chapter 3.)

A single attack of rheumatic fever results in residual heart damage (rheumatic heart disease) in about 66% of the cases. If the patient has had more than one attack of rheumatic fever, there is a nearly 100% chance that rheumatic heart disease is present (Chapter 3).

A patient with a history of a single episode of rheumatic fever who needs emergency dental care must be assumed to have rheumatic heart disease unless it is very clear that the heart was not damaged or the patient's current status can be confirmed by a telephone consultation with the physician. If the patient is not sure of his or her current status and/or medical consultation does not substantiate the absence of rheumatic heart disease, prophylactic antibiotics should be given for the procedure.

A patient needing routine dental care who has a history of a single attack of rheumatic fever should have a medical consultation to establish the presence or absence of rheumatic heart disease. If the patient is not aware of his or her current status and does not have a physician, referral to an internist or cardiologist for evaluation is indicated. This would include auscultation, an echocardiogram, an ECG, and an AP chest radiograph. If the patient is found to be free of rheumatic heart disease, no antibiotic coverage is recommended for future dental treatment.

A patient needing routine dental care who has a history of more than one attack of rheumatic fever can be assumed to have rheumatic heart disease. However, as a matter of professional courtesy, consultation with his or her physician to confirm the current status and need for prophylaxis is recommended. Such patients nearly always require antibiotic prophylaxis for dental treatment.

A patient may report having a heart murmur but not know if it is functional or pathologic. The murmur must be considered pathologic until proven otherwise. Thus the patient needing emergency dental care who has a history of murmur may be given prophylactic antibiotics unless the functional nature of the murmur is confirmed or a telephone consultation establishes that it is functional.

Medical consultation should be initiated for the patient needing routine dental care who gives a history of having a murmur. If the murmur is found to be functional in nature, no antibiotic prophylaxis will be needed. A patient with a pathologic or organic murmur should be covered by antibiotics for dental treatment.

PREVENTIVE DENTISTRY, DENTAL REPAIR, AND ANTIBIOTIC PROPHYLAXIS

The major means by which endocarditis can be minimized in the susceptible dental patient is to reduce the probability of bacteremia, reduce its magnitude when it does occur, and use the most effective antibiotic in proper dosage for prophylaxis.[25,35,58,72,73]

Patients with no active dental disease experience fewer physiologic bacteremias from brushing, flossing, chewing, and other oral functions. When bacteremias occur in patients with healthy clean mouths, the magnitude of any bacteremia will be minimal. Therefore the primary goal of the physician and dentist dealing with patients susceptible to endocarditis is to encourage excellent dental repair and effective preventive dental procedures[35,58,73] — including regular dental check-ups, fluoridation, diet modification to reduce the risk of caries and periodontal disease, and daily oral hygiene (with effective brushing and flossing of the teeth).[35,58,73]

Patients with active dental and/or periodontal disease who are susceptible to endocarditis should be encouraged to upgrade the general health of their gingival tissues by improved oral hygiene procedures before having elective dental procedures performed.[73] By helping a patient reduce the amount of gingival inflammation, the dentist can lower the risk for bacteremias associated with dental treatment procedures. In addition, when bacteremias occur, their magnitude should also be reduced.[8,72,73]

Most authors would agree with the above approach for preventing endocarditis in susceptible dental patients. However, general agreement has not existed for some of the other suggested methods used to reduce the risk of endocarditis in susceptible dental patients. These methods include (1) using an antibacterial mouth rinse,[65] (2) using sulcular irrigation with antibacterial solutions,[8] (3) using an antibiogram[73] of the individual's oral flora for the selection of antibiotics to be used in prophylaxis, and (4) performing a minimum amount of dental treatment during each coverage period.[8,73]

Antibacterial mouth rinses have been shown to reduce the frequency and possibly the magnitude of dental bacteremias, but their use in the past has not generally been accepted. In addition, some authors[8,66,67] have recommended both antibacterial mouth rinses and sulcular irrigation before extracting teeth or performing periodontal therapy. A 1% povidone-iodine solution has been suggested[8] for rinsing and sulcular irrigation. A 0.2% or 1% solution of chlorhexidine also has been recommended.[73] However, there is no direct evidence showing that these procedures reduce the risk of endocarditis in susceptible patients. Nevertheless, the logic of their use is understandable. The 1990 AHA guidelines for the first time suggest the use of antibacterial mouth rinses prior to performing invasive dental procedures.

Tzukert et al.[73] recommend the use of an *antibiogram* (antibiotic sensitivity testing) of the individual patient's oral flora to base the selection of antibiotics to be used for prophylaxis. The antibiogram is an in vitro method for the determination of susceptibility of bacterial samples to specific antibiotics. It indicates the presence of significant numbers of resistant bacterial strains and the antibiotics that may be most effective against them. In addition, a series of antibiograms from a patient undergoing multiple coverage periods may indicate a change in the composition of the oral flora and the need to select a different antibiotic for prophylaxis. The use of this technique, again, makes sense and is understandable, although in the paper of Tzukert et al. they state that "in our experience penicillin is the drug of choice in most instances. . . ."[73]

For most patients requiring antibiotic prophylaxis, the use of an antibiogram does not seem cost-effective nor does it alter the decision that the most appropriate antibiotic is a penicillin in most cases. In the management of high-risk patients in hospital settings, the antibiogram can be useful for identifying patients with resistant bacteria and thus altering the selection of antibiotics to be used for prophylaxis. However, current practice in the United States does not include the use of an antibiogram when managing patients susceptible to endocarditis in the dental office.

We do not recommend the routine use of antibiograms in the management of patients susceptible to endocarditis. In certain high-risk patients this procedure can be considered on an individual basis. The patient, physician, and dentist should discuss the advantages and disadvantages involved with the incorporation of this procedure into the management plan. If it is considered advisable to include it in the plan, then this should be done.

Several authors[8,73] have recommended that a limited amount of dental treatment be planned for each prophylactic coverage period. The basis for this is the assumption that the larger the magnitude of the bacteremia the greater will be the risk for endocarditis. This point, however, has not been proven by any clinical investigations involving humans. The more coverage periods needed, the greater is the risk for allergic reactions and the development of resistant bacterial strains. In addition, it makes it more costly and difficult for the patient to obtain needed dental treatment. The 1990 AHA guidelines[19] speak to this issue and suggest that the maximum amount of dental treatment be performed during each coverage period.

Recent animal studies[22,24-26,34] have demonstrated that a high loading dose is necessary to prevent endocarditis. The dental procedures planned during a given coverage period should be performed after the loading dose has been given. It would appear that procedures performed during an extended coverage period (e.g., 5 to 7 days) would carry increased risk to the patient, because the longer the patient is receiving antibiotic prophylaxis the greater will be the risk of releasing resistant strains of bacteria.[12,23,28,54,60,69]

Based on these considerations we recommend that all routine dental procedures be performed once the loading dose has been given and the appropriate waiting time has elapsed. The next 1 to 2 hours of the coverage period should be used to do as much dental treatment as possible. It is during this period that the patient is best protected. If additional coverage periods are needed, at least 1 week should elapse before another coverage period is initiated. This will allow the oral flora to return to normal. There is some confusion on this point. Several studies[28,69] have suggested that resistant bacteria may remain as long as 6 months after the use of penicillin. By contrast, other studies[36,40] have shown that penicillin V and ampicillin had no effect on the oral, throat, and fecal flora. In one study[36] the agents were given for 10 days and the various flora examined each day and for 19 days following termination of the antibiotics. No resistant strains were found; both aerobic and anaerobic testing was done.

A recent study[33] demonstrated that individuals given penicillin-V prophylaxis on three consecutive Mondays developed resistant oral streptococci, but these represented only 0.0003% to 0.41% of the total cultivable streptococcal population. The authors concluded that the use of penicillin-V prophylaxis on three consecutive occasions 1 week apart should not result in the development of clinically significant levels of resistance among oral streptococci.[33] If the dentist is concerned about the presence of resistant bacteria, the next coverage period may use erythromycin rather than penicillin. In our opinion this is not necessary if at least 1 week has elapsed before the next coverage period is started.

Patients needing complete dentures should receive antibiotic coverage when preprosthetic surgery is performed. The current AHA guidelines[19] do not recommend antibiotic coverage during the construction of dentures or to cover the susceptible patient during denture insertion. The patient should be seen on the next day, and any irritations or ulcerations caused by overextended areas of the denture should be corrected. All denture patients who are at risk for IE should be rescheduled if any sore spots develop any time following the insertion period.

Another problem that often comes up is how to deal with the surgery patient in whom the tissues are healing by secondary intention. The standard duration of coverage may not be adequate, particularly if secondary infection develops in the wound area. The only option in this situation is to extend the coverage period using 500 mg of amoxicillin 4 times a day during the extended period. If the coverage must be extended further, erythromycin can be used.

Patients who are having orthodontic bands adjusted do not require prophylactic coverage, and patients undergoing exfoliation of their deciduous teeth do not appear to need coverage.

Children requiring endocarditis prophylaxis because of conditions such as congenital heart defects should not routinely be given antibiotics for initial or periodic dental examinations. The examination, radiographs, and fluoride treatment can be done without antibiotic coverage. When dental prophylaxis and/or other treatment procedures are indicated, then antibiotic prophylaxis should be used[20] (Tables 2-16 to 2-19).

Based on the above considerations our recommendations for the dental management of the patient susceptible to endocarditis include encouraging effective preventive dental procedures; providing emergency dental care as needed; providing routine dental procedures only after the patient has reduced gingival inflammation as much as possible by conscientious oral hygiene; encouraging needed complex restorative therapy; performing as much dentistry as possible during each antibiotic coverage period; using antibacterial mouth rinses prior to invasive dental procedures and to irrigate the gingival sulcus prior to extracting teeth; performing all dental treatment procedures under antibiotic prophylaxis as recommended by the American Heart Association (Tables 2-16 to 2-18); and allowing at least 1 or 2 weeks to elapse before starting a new coverage period.

TREATMENT PLANNING CONSIDERATIONS

The treatment-planning considerations for patients susceptible to endocarditis are covered in Chapters 3 and 6.

ORAL COMPLICATIONS

There are no specific oral complications associated with infective endocarditis.

REFERENCES

1. American Heart Association Committee on Prevention of Rheumatic Fever and Bacterial Endocarditis: Prevention of rheumatic fever and bacterial endocarditis through control of streptococcal infections, *Circulation* 11:317-320, 1955.
2. American Heart Association Committee on Prevention of Rheumatic Fever and Bacterial Endocarditis: Prevention of rheumatic fever and bacterial endocarditis through control of streptococcal infection, *Circulation* 21:151-155, 1960.
3. American Heart Association Committee on Prevention of Rheumatic Fever and Bacterial Endocarditis: Prevention of rheumatic fever and bacterial endocarditis through control of streptococcal infection, *Circulation* 31:953-955, 1965.
4. American Heart Association Committee on Rheumatic Fever and the Committee on Congenital Cardiac Defects: Prevention of bacterial endocarditis, *Circulation* 46(suppl): 3-5, 1972.
5. Barco CT: Prevention of infective endocarditis: a review of the medical and dental literature, *J Periodontol* 6:510-523, 1991.
6. Barnett ML, Friedman D, Kastner T: The prevalence of mitral valve prolapse in patients with Down's syndrome: implications for dental management, *Oral Surg* 66:445-447, 1988.
7. Bayliss R, Clarke C, Oakley CM, et al: The teeth and infective endocarditis, *Br Heart J* 50:506-512, 1983.
8. Bender IB, Naidorf IJ, Garvey GJ: Bacterial endocarditis: a consideration for physician and dentist, *J Am Dent Assoc* 109:415-420, 1984.
9. Bisno AL, Durack DT, Fraser DW, et al: Failure of prophylaxis for bacterial endocarditis: American Heart Association Registry, *J Fam Pract* 19:16-20, 1980.
10. Bland EF, Jones TD: Rheumatic fever and rheumatic heart disease, *Circulation* 4:836-843, 1951.
11. Bor DH, Himmelstein DV: Endocarditis prophylaxis for patients with mitral valve prolapse: a quantitive analysis, *Am J Med* 76:711-717, 1984.
12. Bornfield M: Bacterial endocarditis, *J Am Dent Assoc* 96:27, 1978.
13. Bulkley BH, Humphries JO: The heart and collagen vascular disease. In Hurst JW, editor: *The heart, arteries, and veins,* ed 6, New York, 1986, McGraw-Hill.
14. Ciancio SG: The impact of chemotherapeutic agents on treatment planning, *J Can Dent Assoc* 56(7, suppl): 37-39, 1990.
15. Clemens JD, Ransohoff J: A quantitive assessment of pre-dental antibiotic prophylaxis for patients with mitral valve prolapse, *J Chronic Dis* 37:531-544, 1984.
16. Cohen PS, Maguire JH, and Weinstein L: Infective endocarditis caused by gram-negative bacteria: a review of the literature, 1945-1977, *Prog Cardiovasc Dis* 22(4):205-242, 1979.
17. Committee on Rheumatic Fever and Bacterial Endocarditis of the Council on Cardiovascular Disease in the Young of the American Heart Association: Prevention of bacterial endocarditis, *Circulation* 56: 139A-143A, 1977.
18. Committee on Rheumatic Fever and Bacterial Endocarditis of the Council on Cardiovascular Disease in the Young of the American Heart Association: Prevention of bacterial endocarditis, *Circulation* 70: 1123A-1127A, 1984.

19. Council on Dental Therapeutics and American Heart Association: Preventing bacterial endocarditis: a statement for the dental professional, *J Am Dent Assoc* 122:87-92, 1991.

20. Crespi PV, Friedman RB: Dental examination guidelines for children requiring infective endocarditis prophylaxis, *J Am Dent Assoc* 7:931-933, 1985.

21. Dajani AS, Bisno AL, Chung KJ, et al: Prevention of bacterial endocarditis: recommendations by the American Heart Association, *JAMA* 264:2919-2922, 1990.

22. Dascomb HE: The current status of prophylaxis against infective endocarditis, *J La State Med Soc* 132:91-99, 1980.

23. Drucker DB, Jolly M: Sensitivity of oral microorganisms to antibiotics, *Br Dent J* 131:442-444, 1971.

24. Durack DT: Infective and non-infective endocarditis. In Hurst JW, editor: *The heart, arteries, and veins,* ed 5, New York, 1983, McGraw-Hill.

25. Durack DT: Infective and non-infective endocarditis. In Hurst JW, editor: *The heart, arteries, and veins,* ed 6, New York, 1986, McGraw-Hill.

26. Durack DT, Petersdorf RG: Changes in the epidemiology of endocarditis. In Kaplan EL, Taranta AV, editors: *Infective endocarditis,* American Heart Association Monograph no. 52, pp 45-54, 1977.

27. Durack DT: Infective and noninfective endocarditis. In Hurst JW, editor: *The heart, arteries, and veins,* ed 7, New York, 1990, McGraw-Hill, pp 1230-1254.

28. Elliot RH, Dunbar JM: Antibiotic sensitivity of oral alpha-hemolytic streptococcus from children with congenital and acquired cardiac disease, *Br Dent J* 142:283-285, 1977.

29. Enffmeyer JE: Penicilin allergy, *Clin Rev Allergy* 4: 171-186, 1986.

30. Falace D, Ferguson T: Bacterial endocarditis, *Oral Surg* 40:189-195, 1976.

31. Felder RS, Nardone D, Phlac R: Prevalence of predisposing factors for endocarditis among an elderly institutionized population, *Oral Surg* 73:30-34, 1992.

32. Finch R: Chemoprophylaxis of infective endocarditis, *Scand J Infect Dis* (suppl) 70:102-110, 1990.

33. Fleming P, Feigal RJ, Kaplan EL, et al: The development of penicillin-resistant oral streptococci after repeated penicillin prophylaxis, *Oral Surg* 70:440-444, 1990.

34. Garrison PK, Freedman LR: Experimental endocarditis. I. Staphylococcal endocarditis in rabbits resulting from placement of a polyethylene catheter in the right side of the heart, *Yale J Biol Med* 42:394-410, 1970.

35. Guntheroth WG: How important are dental procedures as a cause of infective endocarditis, *Am J Cardiol* 54:797-801, 1984.

36. Hermdahl A, Nord CE, Weilander K: Effect of phenoxymethylpenicillin bacampicillin and clindamycin on the oral, throat, and colon microflora of man, *Swed Dent J* 4:39-52, 1980.

37. Hurst JW, editor: *The heart, arteries, and veins,* ed 4, New York, 1978, McGraw-Hill.

38. Imperiale TF, Horwitz RI: Does prophylaxis prevent post dental infective endocarditis? A controlled evaluation of protective efficacy, *Am J Med* 88(2):131-136, 1990.

39. International Rheumatic Fever Study Group: Allergic reactions to long-term benzathine penicillin prophylaxis for rheumatic fever, *Lancet* 337:1308-1310, 1991.

40. Istre GR, et al: Susceptibility of group A beta-hemolytic streptococcus isolates to penicillin and erythromycin, *Antimicrob Agents Chemother* 20:244-246, 1981.

41. Kaplan EL: Personal communications, 1986.

42. Kaplowitz GJ, Reifler JR: Compliance with AHA guidelines for preventing bacterial endocarditis: report of a study, *J Acad Gen Dent* 31:56-59, 1983.

43. Kaye D: Infective endocarditis. In Rose LF, Kaye D, editors: *Internal medicine for dentistry,* St Louis, 1983, CV Mosby.

44. Kaye D: Infective endocarditis. In Wilson JD, et al, editors: *Harrison's Principles of internal medicine,* ed 12, New York, 1991, McGraw-Hill pp 508-513.

45. Little JW: Prosthetic implants: risk of infection from transient dental bacteremias, *Compendium* 12(3): 160-164, 1991.

46. Longman LP, Martin MV: The use of antibiotics in the prevention of postoperative infection: a reappraisal, *Br Dent J* 170:257-262, 1991.

47. MacGregor AJ: Letter to the editor: The use of antibiotics in the prevention of post-operative infection: a reappraisal, *Br Dent J* 170:290, 1991.

48. Mostaghim D, Millard HO: Bacterial endocarditis: a retrospective study, *Oral Surg* 40:219-234, 1975.

49. Murrah VA, Merry JW, Little JW, Jaspers MT: Compliance with guidelines for management of dental school patients susceptible to infective endocarditis, *J Dent Educ* 51(5):229-232, 1987.

50. Murray M, Moosnick F: Incidence of bacteremia in patients with dental disease, *J Lab Clin Med* 26:801, 1941.

51. Nelson CL, Van Blaricum CS: Physician and dentist compliance with American Heart Association guidelines for prevention of bacterial endocarditis, *J Am Dent Assoc* 118(2):169-173, 1989.

52. O'Brien K, Barnes D, Martin RH, Rae JR: Gallium-spect in the detection of prosthetic valve endocarditis and aortic ring abscess, *J Nucl Med* 32(9) 1791-1793, 1991.

53. Okell CC, Elliott SD: Bacteraemia and oral sepsis, with special reference to the aetiology of subacute endocarditis, *Lancet* 2:869-872, 1935.

54. Oill PA, Kalmanson GM, Freedman LR, Guze LB: Choice of antibiotics for prophylaxis for treatment of group D streptococcal endocarditis. (Abstract.) *N Engl J Med* 305:101, 1981.

55. Overholser CD, Moreillon P, Glauser MP: Experimental endocarditis following dental extractions in rats with periodontitis, *J Oral Maxillofac Surg* 46:857-861, 1988.

56. Pallasch TJ: Principles of antibiotic therapy: principles

of antimicrobial chemoprophylaxis, *Dent Drug Serv Newsletter* 3:12, December 1982.

57. Pallasch TJ: Principles of antibiotic therapy: prevention of infective endocarditis, *Dent Drug Serv Newsletter* 4:1, January 1983.

58. Pallasch TJ: A critique of antibiotic prophylaxis, *Can Dent Assoc J* 52:28-36, 1986.

59. Pallasch TJ: Antibiotic prophylaxis: theory and reality, *J Calif Dent Assoc* 17(6):27-39, 1989.

60. Parrillo JE, Borst GC, Mazur MH, et al: Endocarditis due to resistant viridans streptococci during oral penicillin chemoprophylaxis, *N Engl J Med* 300:296-300, 1979.

61. Pelletier LL Jr, Petersdorf RG: Infective endocarditis. In Petersdorf RG, et al, editors: *Harrison's Principles of internal medicine,* ed 10, New York, McGraw-Hill, pp 1418-1423, 1983.

62. Porgrel MA, Welsby PD: The dentist and prevention of infective endocarditis, *Br Dent J* 139:12-16, 1975.

63. Requa-Clark B, Holroyd SV: Antimicrobial agents. In Holroyd SV, Wynn RL, editors: *Clinical pharmacology in dental practice,* ed 3, St Louis, 1983, CV Mosby, pp 245-278.

64. Sadowsky D, Kunzel C: "Usual and customary" practice versus the recommendations of experts: Clinical noncompliance in the prevention of bacterial endocarditis, *J Am Dent Assoc* 118:175-180, 1989.

65. Scheld WM, Sande MA: Endocarditis and intravascular infections. In Mandell GL, et al, editors: *Principles and practice of infectious disease,* New York, 1979, John Wiley & Sons.

66. Scopp IW: Gingival degerming: bacteremia reduction in dental procedures. In Kaplan EL, Taranta AV, editors: *Infective endocarditis,* American Heart Association Monograph no. 52, pp 55-60, 1977.

67. Scopp IW, Orvietto LD: Gingival degerming by povidone-iodine irrigation: bacteremia reduction in extraction procedures, *J Am Dent Assoc* 83:1294-1296, 1971.

68. Shafer WG, Hine MK, Levy BM: *Textbook of oral pathology,* ed 4, Philadelphia, 1983, WB Saunders.

69. Sprunt K: Role of antibiotic resistance in bacterial endocarditis. In Kaplan EL, Taranta AV, editors: *Infective endocarditis,* American Heart Association Monograph no. 52, pp 17-19, 1977.

70. Stollerman GH: Rheumatic fever. In Thorm GW, et al, editors: *Harrison's Principles of internal medicine,* ed 8, New York, 1977, McGraw-Hill.

71. Thyme GM, Ferguson JW: Antibiotic prophylaxis during dental treatment in patients with prosthetic joints, *J Bone Joint Surg* 73B(2):191-194, 1991.

72. Tzukert AA, Leviner E, Benoliel R, Katz J: Analysis of the American Heart Association's recommendations for the prevention of infective endocarditis, *Oral Surg* 62:276-280, 1986.

73. Tzukert AA, Leviner E, Sela M: Prevention of infective endocarditis: not by antibiotics alone, *Oral Surg* 62:385-389, 1986.

3

Rheumatic Fever, Rheumatic Heart Disease, and Murmurs

Patients who have a history of rheumatic fever may have residual cardiac damage and rheumatic heart disease. These patients need to be given prophylactic antibiotic therapy during dental treatment to prevent infective endocarditis. For patients who have a history of rheumatic fever but no evidence of rheumatic heart disease there is no need for prophylactic antibiotics because these patients are not susceptible to infective endocarditis.

To be able to detect and manage the patient who has rheumatic heart disease, the dentist must be aware of the basic pathogenesis and clinical manifestations of rheumatic fever and heart disease. Because of the close relationship between these two entities in the clinical situation that usually confronts the dentist, they are covered in sequence in this chapter. Other conditions that render the patient susceptible to infective endocarditis or endarteritis are discussed in Chapters 2, 4, and 5.

Rheumatic fever

Rheumatic fever is an acute inflammatory condition that develops in some individuals as a complication following group A streptococcal infections. Just how these streptococci initiate rheumatic fever is not known. A popular but unestablished concept[9,13,15] is that rheumatic fever results from an autoimmune reaction between normal tissues that have been altered by products of the bacteria and antibodies that have been produced by the host in response to these altered tissues.

GENERAL DESCRIPTION
INCIDENCE AND PREVALENCE

Acute rheumatic fever is a sequela of group A streptococcal infection. The rheumatic fever attack rate in patients with proven streptococcal infection varies from 0.3% to 3.0% and is related to the virulence of the strain causing the infection.[9,14,15]

Rheumatic fever is principally a childhood disease, with about 75% of the cases occurring before the age of 20 years. It is rare in children under 3 years of age. Most cases occur in children 5 to 15 years of age.[8,15] Rheumatic fever and its sequelae account for about 95% of all cases of heart disease in children.[14,15]

In developing countries of South America, Africa, the Middle East, and Asia, rheumatic fever is the leading cause of death in the first five decades of life. It accounts for 25% to 40% of all cardiovascular diseases in all age groups.[9] Rheumatic fever is found in these countries with the frequency that it was seen in the United States about 100 years ago.[8]

The incidence and severity of rheumatic fever attacks have been decreasing in developed countries. Between 1950 and 1986 there has been an 87% decline in the age-adjusted death rate from rheumatic fever.[8] About 100,000 cases are still being reported per year in the United States. The current annual mortality rate from rheumatic fever is about 6500 per year. In addition, the incidence of carditis associated with recent attacks of rheumatic fever has been decreasing and is now less than 20% of acute cases.[8]

Rheumatic fever and rheumatic heart disease are found at the rate of 7 cases per 1000 in persons of all ages. They are found at the rate of 12 per 1000 in persons over 45 years.[8] Rheumatic fever alone is found at the rate of 0.7 case per 1000 schoolchildren and 6 to 9 cases per 1000 college freshmen.[8,9,11,14]

Although rheumatic fever is now uncommon in the United States, it still occurs with a much higher frequency in economically disadvantaged Americans including blacks, Puerto Ricans, Mexican-Americans and American Indians.[8] During the 1980s a number of local outbreaks of rheumatic fever occurred in military personnel, school children, and middle-class communities in the United States.[9,15]

It is estimated[14] that 1% to 6% of the population of the United States exhibits specific valvular defects of the heart. This may give some clue as to the real incidence of rheumatic fever in this country. Many cases of rheumatic fever are probably unrecognized but leave behind a damaged heart valve. To support this concept, various studies have shown that only about 60% of the patients with mitral valve disease give a history of having had acute rheumatic fever.

Age does not alter susceptibility to rheumatic fever. However, streptococcal infections are much less likely to be acquired in adult life, thus explaining the lower incidence of rheumatic fever in adults.

ETIOLOGY

Group A streptococcal infection of the pharynx precedes the onset of rheumatic fever. Infection at other sites, such as skin, by these organisms does not result in rheumatic fever.[15] Strains of group A streptotocci that have high virulence properties, type-specific M protein and large hyaluronate capsules, are most often involved. M-serotypes 3, 5, 18, 19, and 24 have all been reported in patients who develop rheumatic fever. Just how these group A streptococci initiate the disease process is not known.[9,15] *Streptococcus*-induced autoimmunity remains popular but is an unestablished concept for the etiology of rheumatic fever.[15] Group A streptococci, M-types 3 and 18, were responsible for the outbreaks of rheumatic fever that occurred during the 1980s in the United States.[15]

The clinical sequence of events usually starts with a sore throat that, if cultured, often will reveal group A streptococci (Fig. 3-1). The presence of a streptococcal infection, however, must be established by detecting an increase in antibody titer to one of the various antigens found on the bacteria, because group A *Streptococcus* can be cultured from throats of individuals who do not have streptococcal infection.

The most important clinical finding that supports the diagnosis of rheumatic fever is an elevated titer of antibodies, which confirms a recent streptococcal infection. Bacterial cultures of the throat may even be negative in some of these patients.[9,14,15]

Not all patients who develop rheumatic fever will have complained of a sore throat. Also, all patients with sore throats do not have streptococcal infection. Any number of other bacteria or viruses can cause this symptom.

About 3% of individuals who have a symptomatic exudative streptococcal pharyngitis will develop rheumatic fever. This incidence falls to about 0.3% in persons who have a less severe streptococcal pharyngitis.[9,13,15] The incidence of rheumatic fever following streptococcal pharyngitis increases to 5% to 50% in patients with a history of rheumatic fever.[9,14,15]

In individuals who develop rheumatic fever following a streptococcal infection, a latent period of 2 weeks to as long as 6 months occurs. Once an attack of rheumatic fever has developed, the patient is much more susceptible to recurrent attacks than is the rest of the population to a first attack.

Because the streptococcal organisms do not

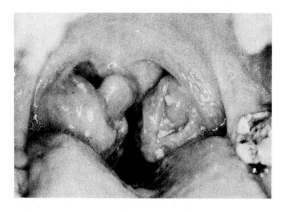

FIG. 3-1 Hypertrophied tonsils with areas of purulent exudate.

directly invade the heart or joints, rheumatic fever is not an infectious disease from that standpoint. According to the autoimmune concept, group A streptococcal throat infection is believed to sensitize the tissues of areas such as the heart and joints by prosthetic groups from the organism that unite with connective tissue protein to form an antigen. The prosthetic groups may be endotoxins or exotoxins. The antigen complex then stimulates the production of specific antibodies. Once these antibodies are in circulation, they combine with the antigens at the various tissue locations and cause an allergic necrosis that is accompanied by a characteristic cellular response to the allergic reaction.

Factors affecting the incidence and severity of pharyngeal streptococcal infection are important in the development of rheumatic fever. Overcrowded, poor, undernourished populations who live in damp climates appear to be much more susceptible to rheumatic fever. Crowding that occurs in military barracks, closed institutions, and large families living in small quarters has been reportedly associated with recent outbreaks of rheumatic fever in the United States.[15] Individuals with a history of rheumatic fever have about a 5% to 50% risk of developing rheumatic fever following a streptococcal infection. This risk is greatest in individuals who have had carditis with the initial rheumatic fever attack.[15] The reduced frequency of severe streptococcal throat infections in developed countries explains their reduced incidence of rheumatic fever.[8,9,14,15]

PATHOPHYSIOLOGY AND COMPLICATIONS

Based on the most popular hypothesis for the cause of rheumatic fever, as mentioned previously, it is considered an immune-related disease associated with group A streptococcal throat infections. Products from the bacteria are thought to sensitize connective tissue, forming antigens that stimulate antibody production. Antigen-antibody complexes then occur and produce local tissue necrosis and an inflammatory reaction. The connective tissue of the heart, including the valves, is very susceptible to the disease. In addition, the connective tissue of the larger joints and the lungs and the subcutaneous tissues are susceptible.

The major manifestations of the disease, from a clinical standpoint, are signs and symptoms relating to the inflammatory reactions that take place in the heart, larger joints, and skin. Pulmonary involvement may be an important part of the clinical picture in some patients.[9,15] The acute attack of rheumatic fever leaves no permanent skin or joint damage or functional impairment. The primary complication of the disease relates to its cardiac and pulmonary effects. The patient may develop congestive heart failure and die during an acute attack, or the heart may be so damaged that complications occur following recovery. These complications include constrictive pericarditis, valve damage resulting from scarring, and congestive heart failure. In addition, the patient with damaged valves is susceptible to endocarditis. In a few cases lung involvement during the acute attack may be so severe that the patient dies.[9,15]

CLINICAL PRESENTATION
SIGNS AND SYMPTOMS

The major manifestations of rheumatic fever are arthritis, carditis, chorea, erythema marginatum, and subcutaneous nodules. Minor manifestations include fever, arthralgia, abnormal erythrocyte sedimentation rate, presence of C-reactive protein, and possibly ECG changes (Table 3-1).

The diagnosis of rheumatic fever is based on the presence of at least two major manifestations and one minor manifestation or one major and two minor manifestations and a history of preceding throat infections with elevation of the anti–streptolysin O (ASO) titer.[9,14,15]

The acute attack of rheumatic fever will abate within 6 weeks in about 75% of the cases, within 12 weeks in about 90%, and longer than 6 months in about 5%.[15]

The arthritis associated with rheumatic fever develops rapidly and lasts for about 2 or 3 weeks. The large joints of the knees and ankles are commonly affected. The small joints of the hands and feet are uncommonly involved. The spine and TMJ are rarely affected. Pain is the first symptom, followed by redness, heat, and then swelling of the joint. Joint involvement is transient and migratory, and usually no permanent deformities result. Severe joint involvement is much more common in adults than in children.[9,15]

Chorea is a spasmodic, nonrepetitive motion

TABLE 3–1
Revised Jones Criteria for the Diagnosis of
Rheumatic Fever

Major manifestations

Carditis
Polyarthritis
Chorea
Erythema marginatum
Subcutaneous nodules

Minor manifestations

Fever
Arthralgia
Elevated erythrocyte sedimentation rate,
  C-reactive protein
Prolonged PR (time from beginning of atrial
  contraction to beginning of ventricular contrac-
  tion) interval on ECG

From Stollerman GH: In Hurst JW, editor: *The heart,
arteries, and veins,* ed 6, New York, 1986, McGraw-Hill, p
1311. By permission of the American Heart Association.

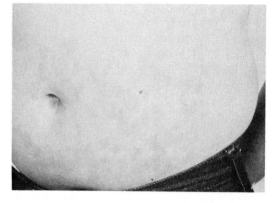

FIG. 3-2   Erythema marginatum as a manifestation
of rheumatic fever. (Courtesy C. Cottrill, M.D.,
Lexington Ky.)

involving voluntary muscles that does not occur
when the patient is asleep. The onset of chorea
is variable and may be several months after the
streptococcal infection. The patient may first
develop problems with being able to write or
draw. Things may be dropped. In small children
the movements may become so violent that the
crib must be padded.[15]

Erythema marginatum is a nonpruritic, flat
skin rash that occurs in about 5% of patients
who have rheumatic fever (Fig. 3-2). It usually
coexists with arthritis, chorea, or carditis. When
it occurs, it lasts for about 2 or 3 days.[9,15]

Subcutaneous nodules are firm, painless,
colorless subcutaneous swellings that occur in
about 5% of patients with rheumatic fever (Fig.
3-3). They usually coexist with carditis. They
occur most commonly on the skin over the
elbows and persist for 1 to 2 weeks.[9,15]

The carditis associated with rheumatic fever
reveals itself clinically as an abnormal murmur,
a pericardial rub, cardiac enlargement, congestive heart failure, or a combination of these. The
murmur results from dilation of the valvular
ring, destruction of the valvular substance, or
contraction of the chordae tendineae. The
mitral valve is affected most often, followed by
the aortic valve. The pericardial rub is caused by

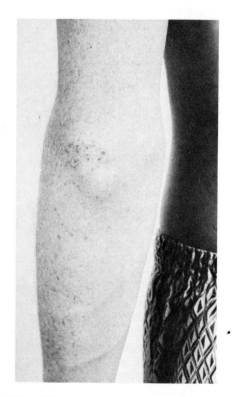

FIG. 3-3   Subcutaneous nodules as a manifestation
of rheumatic fever.

an acute inflammatory pericarditis. Congestive heart failure, when present, develops rapidly. The patient will have dyspnea with rales. An ache in the upper right quadrant of the abdomen may develop as a result of liver congestion and distention of the hepatic capsule. Pulmonary congestion may cause a nonproductive cough. Swelling of the ankles and distention of neck veins can occur. About 5% to 10% of patients will have epistaxis secondary to cardiac involvement.[9,14,15]

In the past, definite evidence of carditis occurred in about 40% to 50% of patients having their first attack of rheumatic fever. Carditis now occurs in only about 20% of the patients who develop rheumatic fever. Patients who have carditis during the first attack are much more prone to develop recurrent attacks of rheumatic fever than are those with no carditis. Patients who did not develop carditis during the first attack usually remain free of rheumatic heart disease thereafter unless they suffered additional attacks of rheumatic fever. Patients with no carditis during the acute rheumatic fever attack when examined 10 years later are 95% free of evidence of rheumatic heart disease. Only 30% of those with mild carditis are found 10 years later to have rheumatic heart disease. Totally 40% of those with a basal diastolic murmur are found 10 years later to have rheumatic heart disease, and 70% of those with heart failure or pericarditis are found 10 years later to have rheumatic heart disease.[9,15]

The incidence of significant cardiac damage (rheumatic heart disease) following the initial attack of rheumatic fever varies from 30% to 80%. In recent years there has been a decline in the severity of rheumatic fever attacks, the incidence of associated carditis, and the frequency of residual cardiac disease.[2,9,14,15]

Patients who develop an abnormal heart murmur during the initial attack of rheumatic fever must be considered to have rheumatic heart disease until proven otherwise. Patients who have both a murmur and congestive heart failure during the initial attack will have significant rheumatic heart disease. About 20% of them will die within 10 years after the initial rheumatic fever attack.[2] In general, the susceptibility to recurrent attacks of rheumatic fever is in direct relation to the severity of heart damage, and it decreases as the patient becomes older. During the first attack of rheumatic fever, carditis is often not detected because of its own clinical manifestations but is found by the physician because the patient seeks medical attention for arthritis, chorea, or fever.

LABORATORY FINDINGS

The urine is usually normal in rheumatic fever, although trace amounts of albumin may be found during the febrile period. If the acute attack of rheumatic fever is prolonged, anemia as well as leukocytosis may be present. The sedimentation rate of the blood usually increases during the acute phase of the disease. As clinical improvement is made, the sedimentation rate decreases and usually returns to normal. The C-reactive protein content of the blood is measured. Its appearance and increase in amount correlate with the presence of a bacterial infection and are not specific for rheumatic fever. The C-reactive protein level is very useful for judging the degree of rheumatic activity.

Streptococcal antibody titers are used to confirm the occurrence of a preceding streptococcal infection. A high ASO titer that falls during the convalescent period is an important finding that confirms the presence of a previous group A streptococcal infection. Anti–DNase B (anti–deoxyribonuclease B) streptococcal titers can also be used to confirm a previous streptococcal infection when the ASO titer is borderline. The antistreptozyme test can be used in patients with isolated polyarthritis to rule out rheumatic fever as the cause.[15] Throat culture for group A streptococcal organisms is also helpful. However, as mentioned previously, a negative culture does not rule out the presence of rheumatic fever. Throat cultures are less satisfactory than antibody tests as supporting evidence for recent streptococcal infection.[15]

No single laboratory test establishes the diagnosis of rheumatic fever. The most important factors are the presence of various combinations of the following clinical manifestations: polyarthritis, carditis, chorea, erythema marginatum, subcutaneous nodules, and recurrent attacks supported by positive laboratory tests (increased sedimentation rate, presence of C-reactive protein, ASO titer above 250 Todd units).[15]

MEDICAL MANAGEMENT

Medical treatment of rheumatic fever usually starts with a single large dose of benzathine penicillin given by injection to eradicate group A streptococcal bacteria from the throat, even if these have not been cultured. Bed rest has no proven value and in many cases may be psychologically deleterious. Patients will, in general, limit their own activity. Those with severe congestive heart failure may be placed on bed rest.[9,14,15]

Patients without carditis are treated by codeine or salicylates if they have symptoms of arthritis. The symptoms of arthritis respond quickly to salicylate therapy. In patients with arthritis who do not respond to salicylates another diagnosis should be considered.[9] Salicylates are given until they produce clinical effects or until toxic symptoms (tinnitus, headache) occur. Aspirin is recommended because it is cheap and effective.[9] Diazepam or chlorpromazine is used to treat chorea.[9,15] Patients with evidence of carditis are treated with large doses of either salicylates or corticosteroids. Some physicians will start with salicylates and, if symptoms do not improve, change to corticosteroids. Other physicians begin directly with the steroids. Most physicians will use steroids if congestive heart failure is present.

Following recovery from the acute phase of rheumatic fever patients are placed on prophylactic antibiotics to prevent recurrent streptococcal infection, which could trigger another attack of rheumatic fever. For patients with no evidence of rheumatic heart disease the secondary prophylaxis is continued for at least 5 years and until the 18th birthday. Patients with RHD will have a more prolonged period of prophylaxis, in some cases for the rest of their life.[5,9,15] Consistent secondary prophylaxis to prevent recurrent attacks of rheumatic fever is probably the single most effective measure the physician has to offer patients with a history of rheumatic fever.[9]

The prophylactic regimen used to prevent recurrent streptococcal infection in patients who have had a recent attack of rheumatic fever consists of one of the following[9]:

1. Benzathine penicillin, 1.2 million units, IM, once a month
2. Oral penicillin V, 250 mg bid

3. Patients allergic to penicillin: oral sulfadiazine, 1 g qd
4. Patients allergic to both penicillin and sulfadiazine: oral erythromycin, 250 mg bid

These dose levels, however, are not sufficient to prevent endocarditis in patients who have cardiac damage resulting from a rheumatic fever attack. These patients will require additional antibiotics during dental manipulations to protect them from infective endocarditis.

An important issue for patients on long-term penicillin prophylaxis is the possibility of increased risk for allergic reactions to penicillin. A prospective study involving 1790 patients from 11 countries[7] was conducted to answer this important question. After 32,430 injections, 57 of the 1790 patients (3.2%) had an allergic reaction. Four patients had anaphylactic reactions (0.2%), and one died (0.05%). These rates were similar to those for patients without rheumatic fever who received short-term treatment with parenteral penicillin. The study concluded that there was no increased risk of allergy for rheumatic fever patients on long-term penicillin prophylaxis. Another important finding was the demonstration of the effectiveness of this treatment. Rheumatic fever recurred in only 8 of the patients (0.45%) who received prophylaxis. In 96 patients who did not comply with the prophylaxis, 11.5% (11 of 96) developed recurrence of rheumatic fever.[7]

Rheumatic heart disease

The cardiac damage that results from an acute attack of rheumatic fever is called rheumatic heart disease. It usually involves damage of the mitral or aortic valve. The scarring and calcification that occur in the affected valve may result in stenosis or regurgitation.

GENERAL DESCRIPTION
INCIDENCE AND PREVALENCE

Bland and Jones[2] give one of the best insights into the incidence of rheumatic heart disease following acute rheumatic fever attacks. In this study 1000 patients were followed for at least 20 years or until they died. These patients were admitted to the Good Samaritan Hospital in Boston with acute rheumatic fever. The study was started in 1921, and the last new patient was added in 1931. The study was concluded in 1951.

The most common symptom of rheumatic fever found in these patients was carditis — followed by chorea, arthritis, arthralgia, subcutaneous nodules, and erythema marginatum. By the end of the study 301 patients were dead. The most common causes of death were congestive heart failure (231) and infective endocarditis (30).

Patients who had symptoms of either an enlarged heart or congestive heart failure during the acute attack of rheumatic fever had the poorest prognosis. Of the 70 patients who had heart enlargement, 56 were dead within 10 years and 57 within 20 years. Of the 207 patients who had initial congestive heart failure, 148 were dead within 10 years and 152 within 20 years.

However, patients who developed chorea during the acute attack had a much better prognosis. Only 63 of the 518 patients who had this symptom were dead by the end of 20 years.

Following the initial acute rheumatic fever attack, 653 patients showed clinical evidence of rheumatic heart disease. By contrast, 347 patients showed no early evidence of rheumatic heart disease, although at the end of the study 154 of these showed clinical evidence of the disease. An interesting observation was that chorea was a prominent feature in most of these 154 patients.

Thus by the end of the study 301 patients were free of any clinical evidence of rheumatic heart disease; 193 of these patients never developed any clinical evidence of the disease, and 108 had clinical evidence at one time but by the end of the study showed no evidence of the disease. Depending on how one looks at these data, the incidence of rheumatic heart disease could be said to be as low as 69% (based on patient status at the end of the study) or as high as 81% (based on presence of rheumatic heart disease at any time during the study). More recent studies already cited would suggest a much lower incidence of rheumatic heart disease following acute attacks of rheumatic fever. However, from the dentist's viewpoint, it is impossible to know for a given patient with a history of rheumatic fever whether rheumatic heart disease is present without medical evaluation.

Another interesting question that these data raise is whether there is significant scarring in the heart valves of those patients who have lost any clinical evidence of rheumatic heart disease. In other words, would these individuals be susceptible later to infective endocarditis even though they showed no clinical evidence of rheumatic heart disease?

ETIOLOGY

Rheumatic heart disease develops as a sequela of acute rheumatic fever. The primary lesion in rheumatic heart disease is valvular deformity with associated compensatory changes in the size of the cardiac chambers and the thickness of their walls. Primary myocardial lesions occur but usually are of no clinical significance. A history of an acute attack of rheumatic fever is not obtained from all patients who have rheumatic heart disease. This may be explained by the subclinical attacks that some patients experience or by a missed diagnosis of the rheumatic fever episode.

PATHOPHYSIOLOGY AND COMPLICATIONS

The basic lesions in rheumatic heart disease consist of valvular changes, myocardial changes, and pericardial changes. Rheumatic nodules may involve just the endocardium of the valve or its entire thickness. The eventual outcome of the valve disease is accumulation of scar tissue and deformity of the valve. This interferes with function and, if the interference is significant, can lead to congestive heart failure. The edges of valve cusps may be fused together, with resulting stenosis of the valve opening (Figs. 3-4 and 3-5). All four heart valves may show microscopic evidence of rheumatic activity; however, functional impairment is most common in the mitral valve, followed by the aortic valve, and (much less often) the tricuspid valve. Calcification of the injured cusps is common.[1,3,12]

The most common valvular defect resulting from rheumatic fever is mitral stenosis. Incompetence of the aortic valve is the next most common. Aortic stenosis is less common. Lesions of the valves are more severe on the left side of the heart because of the greater strain placed on these valves. Mitral valve lesions are seen more often in women, and aortic valve

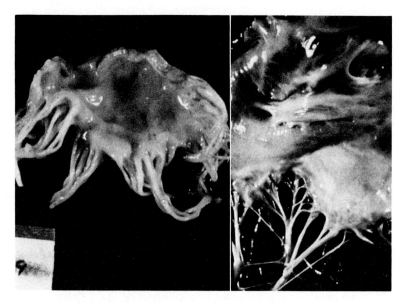

FIG. 3-4   Normal mitral valve. Compare this with the diseased valve in Fig. 3-5.

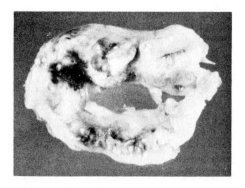

FIG. 3-5   Stenosis of the mitral valve as a result of rheumatic fever.   (Courtesy W. O'Conner, M.D., Lexington Ky.)

lesions in men. The damaged valves are susceptible to infective endocarditis.

The typical myocardial lesion is the Aschoff nodule (a focus of fibrinoid degeneration surrounded by a granulomatous inflammatory response) (Fig. 3-6). Depending on the amount of inflammation during the attack of rheumatic fever, there will be varying degrees of myocardial destruction. If inflammation is great, the myocardial destruction will be great and congestive heart failure may develop. If destruction is less, the damage will be repaired by fibrous connective tissue.

Rheumatic fever is the most common cause of acute pericarditis, which is serofibrinous inflammation of the pericardium. If the reaction is severe, a chronic adherent pericarditis may develop.

CLINICAL PRESENTATION
SIGNS AND SYMPTOMS

The clinical signs and symptoms found in patients who have rheumatic heart disease are usually associated with the valve disease and its effect on the heart. A murmur may be heard if the valve disease is sufficient to alter function of the valve. This may be the only sign of rheumatic heart disease for a number of years. As the compensatory ability of the heart is exceeded, chamber dilation and hypertrophy may occur. Exertional dyspnea, angina pectoris, epistaxis, blood in the sputum, and congestive heart failure may then occur[1,3,12] (Table 3-2).

LABORATORY FINDINGS

The diagnosis of rheumatic heart disease is made at two levels. At the first is the patient who is asymptomatic but has a murmur indicative of valvular damage. This type of patient also may

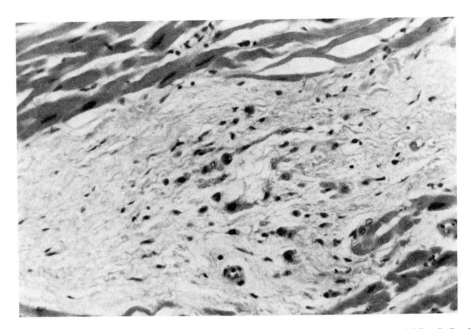

FIG. 3-6   Photomicrograph of an Aschoff nodule. (Courtesy Jesse E. Edwards, M.D., St Paul Minn.)

show cardiac enlargement on chest radiographs, abnormal valve by echocardiography, and ECG changes that suggest hypertrophy of the left ventricular wall. The patient may or may not give a history of rheumatic fever. The second type of patient has clinical symptoms of rheumatic heart disease and is usually much easier to identify.

Any patient with a history of rheumatic fever needs to be evaluated for the presence of rheumatic heart disease before dental treatment is begun. This evaluation may consist of communication with the physician who has followed up on the patient since the rheumatic fever attack or evaluation by a physician to whom the patient is now going or would like to be referred. The presence or absence of rheumatic heart disease in the patient who has a history of rheumatic fever is best established by (1) history of symptoms, (2) AP chest radiographs, (3) ECG, (4) echocardiography, and (5) good physical evaluation, including auscultation of the heart.

MEDICAL MANAGEMENT

The patient who has asymptomatic rheumatic heart disease requires no medical treatment other than prevention of recurrent attacks of rheumatic fever and prevention of infective endocarditis. The patient who has congestive heart failure is managed as described in the section on congestive heart failure (Chapter 9). This patient may be treated by surgical removal of the damaged valve and the placement of an artificial valve.

DENTAL MANAGEMENT
MEDICAL CONSIDERATIONS

The basic problem that confronts the dentist in dealing with patients who have a history of rheumatic fever is whether or not rheumatic heart disease is present. If the patient has

TABLE 3–2
Signs and Symptoms of Rheumatic
Heart Disease

Exertional dyspnea
Angina pectoris
Congestive heart failure
Epistaxis
Blood in sputum
Murmur
ECG changes (T wave flattening) (Fig. 8-2)
Enlarged heart

rheumatic heart disease, antibiotic prophylaxis is indicated to prevent infective endocarditis. If rheumatic heart disease is not present, the patient is not considered susceptible to endocarditis and does not require antibiotic prophylaxis.

DETECTION OF PATIENTS WITH RHEUMATIC HEART DISEASE

A medical history should be obtained from each patient before any dental manipulations are performed. Patients are asked if they are under the care of a physician. If they are, the nature of the problem and the way it is being treated are established. Patients are asked if they have ever had rheumatic fever, rheumatic heart disease, or a heart murmur. The medical history is reviewed to see, among other things, if the patient has ever had a condition suggestive of rheumatic fever for which medical attention was not sought. An inquiry is made concerning the presence of signs or symptoms suggestive of rheumatic fever, rheumatic heart disease, and congestive heart failure.

The name, address, and phone number of the patient's physician are recorded in the dental record. Any medications the patient is taking or has taken during the past year also are recorded. Of particular interest is the patient who may be taking prophylactic antibiotics to prevent recurrent upper respiratory streptococcal infections and thereby reduce the risk of recurrent rheumatic fever attacks.

The dentist usually is not qualified by training to examine a patient for many of the signs of rheumatic heart disease other than the gross ones associated with congestive heart failure — distention of neck veins and swelling of the ankles. These signs, however, seldom develop until later in the course of the disease. Therefore, in general, the physical examination will be of little aid to the dentist in identifying the patient with rheumatic heart disease.

GROUPING OF PATIENTS ACCORDING TO RISK OF RHEUMATIC HEART DISEASE

Based on the findings of the medical history interview and, to a limited extent, the physical examination, three separate groups of patients can be identified who have or may have had rheumatic heart disease. These patients will require additional attention before examination or treatment procedures are begun. The three groups are described here and summarized in Table 3-3.

GROUP 1

Patients have a history of an illness that could have been rheumatic fever but a physician was not sought at the time. The patient is asymptomatic but should be referred for medical evaluation concerning the presence of rheu-

TABLE 3–3
Management of the Dental Patient with a History of Rheumatic Fever

Group 1	History of illness that could have been rheumatic fever but physician was not sought at time of illness
	a. Refer for medical evaluation
	b. If rheumatic heart disease is present, use standard regimen for antibiotic prophylaxis
Group 2	History of illness diagnosed by physician as rheumatic fever
	a. If no medical follow-up is available, refer for evaluation for presence of rheumatic heart disease
	b. If medical follow-up is available, consult with patient's physician to confirm current status
	c. If rheumatic heart disease is present, use standard regimen for prophylaxis
Group 3	Treated for symptoms of rheumatic heart disease by physician
	a. Consult with physician to determine patient's current status and need for prophylaxis
	b. Use standard regimen for history of congestive failure
	c. Use special regimen for prosthetic heart valve or history of infective endocarditis
	d. Manage congestive heart failure as described in Chapter 9
	e. Manage prosthetic heart valve as described in Chapter 5

matic heart disease. If this is found, then prophylactic antibiotics should be given before any invasive dental procedure. The standard regimen of the American Heart Association is used. (See Chapter 2.)

GROUP 2

Patients have a history of illness that was diagnosed by the physician as rheumatic fever. When no medical follow-up care has occurred since the attack, the patient should be referred for medical evaluation concerning the presence of rheumatic heart disease. When the patient is under active medical follow-up care, the physician should be contacted to confirm the presence or absence of rheumatic heart disease. All patients established to have rheumatic heart disease should be given prophylactic antibiotics before any invasive dental procedure, again using the American Heart Association standard regimen (Chapter 2).

GROUP 3

Patients have been treated for symptoms of rheumatic heart disease by a physician. The patient's current status and need for antibiotic prophylaxis should be established by medical consultation. Patients who have rheumatic heart disease with a history of congestive heart failure should be given the standard amoxicillin regimen for prophylaxis before invasive dental procedures; management should follow the principles described in Chapter 9. Patients with prosthetic heart valves should be given the standard amoxicillin regimen or a special parenteral regimen (Chapter 2) for prophylaxis before invasive dental procedures; management should follow the principles described in Chapter 5. The patient with a history of infective endocarditis should be given the standard amoxicillin regimen or a special parenteral regimen for prophylaxis as described in Chapter 2.

SPECIFIC DENTAL MANAGEMENT

No dental examination or treatment procedures should be performed on patients suspected of having rheumatic heart disease without antibiotic coverage or until they have been determined free of the disease by medical consultation or referral. Dental procedures should not be performed on patients with rheumatic heart disease who show signs and

symptoms of congestive heart failure until consultation with a physician.

Once the need for prophylactic antibiotics has been determined and the patient is free of significant evidence of congestive heart failure, the standard regimen is recommended for patients receiving either routine or emergency dental care. Patients with prosthetic heart valves or a history of infective endocarditis can be given the standard amoxicillin regimen or a special parenteral regimen. (See Chapter 2.)

In general, we suggest that the oral route of administration for antibiotics be selected whenever possible because of the lower incidence of allergic sensitivity.[16] (See Chapter 21.)

TREATMENT PLANNING MODIFICATIONS

Patients with rheumatic heart disease who show no evidence of congestive heart failure can receive any indicated dental care as long as they are protected by antibiotics against infective endocarditis. The most important aspects of dental care are dental education, preventive dentistry procedures, and the maintenance of good dental repair. Active gingival disease should be treated and good periodontal health obtained before performing extensive restorative procedures are undertaken. The dentist should plan to do as much treatment as possible during each coverage period so the patient's dental treatment will not be spread over too long a time and thus the number of necessary coverage periods can be kept to a minimum. One to two weeks or more should elapse between coverage periods (Chapter 2).

The patient should receive prophylactic antibiotic coverage for all dental procedures, including certain examination procedures—such as periodontal probing. With proper planning, crowns and bridges can be constructed for patients with rheumatic heart disease. During one coverage period the preparations can be made, impressions taken, and temporaries placed. Then a new coverage period can be used for the insertion of the crowns or bridges.

Orthodontic patients who have rheumatic heart disease should be given antibiotic coverage during the placement and removal of bands, but they do not need coverage for adjustment when already wearing the bands. If tissue injury may occur during the adjustment of orthodontic appliances prophylaxis should be considered. However, in most cases this should not be necessary.[5]

Children with rheumatic heart disease who are in the process of naturally losing deciduous teeth are not given antibiotic coverage. They need coverage only if the teeth are being extracted.

Edentulous patients who have rheumatic heart disease should be given antibiotic coverage during surgical procedures needed to prepare the mouth for dentures. Overextended areas should be corrected immediately and sore spots allowed to heal. Antibiotic prophylaxis at the time of initial denture insertion is not indicated.[5]

Heart murmurs

One of the more confusing problems that can face a dentist is evaluating a patient who has a history of a heart murmur and deciding when antibiotic prophylaxis is necessary. Dentists, for the most part, are not trained to detect or evaluate heart murmurs; therefore it is necessary to rely on a physician colleague to perform these tasks. The ensuing information is presented to enhance understanding of what murmurs are and to facilitate communication with physicians on the subject.

Murmurs are nothing more than the sound caused by turbulence in the circulation through the valves and chambers of the heart. The turbulence is usually due to an increased flow rate, a change in viscosity, stenotic or narrowed valves or vessels, dilated valves or vessels, or a vibration of membranous structures such as the valve leaflets.[4] Innocent, or functional, murmurs are sounds caused by turbulence in the absence of any cardiac abnormality; they do not require antibiotic prophylaxis. Organic murmurs are sounds caused by a pathologic abnormality in the heart; they do require antibiotic prophylaxis.

Murmurs are described on the basis of their occurrence during the cardiac cycle (systolic, diastolic, or continuous), their loudness or intensity (on a scale of I to VI), the location on the chest wall in which they are best heard, and whether they radiate or are localized. Therefore a common description of a functional murmur would be a grade II/VI ("two over six") systolic ejection murmur best heard at the pulmonic area that does not radiate.

Interpretation of murmurs is not always easy. A combination of history, physical examination, AP chest radiograph, ECG, echocardiogram, and laboratory tests may be needed. Diastolic murmurs are almost always organic in nature and therefore pathologic. Systolic murmurs may be organic or functional.[4] The physician must make that judgment. Two examples of common innocent (or functional) murmurs that require no antibiotic prophylaxis are murmurs that occur only during childhood development and murmurs that occur only during pregnancy.

Murmurs discovered during **childhood** are extremely common, and in fact almost every child will have one at some time. They are usually detected between the ages of 3 and 7 years and subsequently disappear (by adolescence).[6,10] It is thought that they probably result from an increase in flow rate combined with a thin chest wall that enhances normal flow sounds.

Murmurs occurring during **pregnancy** are usually caused by a significant increase in blood volume and resulting cardiac output. They disappear shortly after delivery as the cardiovascular system returns to its normal status.

In both cases an innocent murmur is classically reported only during that period, with disappearance on subsequent examinations. Preexisting murmurs or murmurs that have persisted (into adulthood or beyond pregnancy) may be organic and require prophylactic antibiotics.

Whenever a patient reports a history of heart murmur, it is recommended that the physician (preferably a cardiologist) be consulted for a definitive judgment, even in cases of murmurs that are probably innocent.

If the murmur is considered innocent, or nonpathologic, no antibiotic prophylaxis is indicated. If it is considered organic, or pathologic, the standard regimen of the American Heart Association should be used for antibiotic prophylaxis. In patients needing emergency dental care and for whom the dentist is unable to establish the nature of a reported heart murmur, antibiotic prophylaxis is recommended. (See Chapter 2 for management.)

REFERENCES

1. Barrett MJ: Valvular heart disease. In Rose LF, Kaye D, editors: *Internal medicine for dentistry,* St Louis, 1983, CV Mosby.
2. Bland EF, Jones TD: Rheumatic fever and rheumatic heart disease, *Circulation* 4:836-843, 1951.
3. Braunwald E: Valvular heart disease. In Petersdorf RG, et al, editors: *Harrison's Principles of internal medicine,* ed 10, New York, 1983, McGraw-Hill.
4. *Cardiovascular disease in dental practice,* Publ. no. 71-0009, Dallas, 1991, American Heart Association, pp 2-5.
5. Dajani AS, Bisno AL, Chung KJ, et al: Prevention of bacterial endocarditis: recommendations of the American Heart Association, *JAMA* 264:2919-2992, 1990.
6. Delp MH, Manning RT: *Major's Physical diagnosis: an introduction to the clinical process,* ed 9, Philadelphia, 1981, WB Saunders.
7. International Rheumatic Fever Study Group: Allergic reactions to long-term benzathine penicillin prophylaxis for rheumatic fever, *Lancet* 337:1308-1310, 1991.
8. Kannel WB, Thom JJ: Incidence, prevalence, and mortality of cardiovascular diseases. In Hurst JW, editor: *The heart, arteries, and veins,* ed 7, New York, 1990, McGraw-Hill, pp 627-639.
9. Kaplan EL: Acute rheumatic fever. In Hurst JW, editor: *The heart, arteries, and veins,* ed 7, New York, 1990, McGraw-Hill, pp 1523-1529.
10. Kulangara RJ, Strong WB, Miller MD: Differential diagnosis of heart murmurs in children, *Postgrad Med* 72:219-228, 1982.
11. Levy RI: Prevalence and epidemiology of cardiovascular disease. In Wyngaarden JB, Smith LH, editors: *Cecil textbook of medicine,* ed 17, Philadelphia, 1985, WB Saunders.
12. Rackley CE: Valvular disease. In Hurst JW, editor: *The heart, arteries, and veins,* ed 7, New York, 1990, McGraw-Hill, pp 795-871.
13. Rose LF, Godfrey P, Steinberg BJ: Dental correlations. In Rose LF, Kaye D, editors: *Internal medicine for dentistry,* St Louis, 1983, CV Mosby.
14. Santoro J, Ingerman MJ: Streptococcal infections and rheumatic fever. In Rose LF, Kaye D, editors: *Internal medicine for dentistry,* ed 2, St Louis, 1990, Mosby–Year Book, pp 194-200.
15. Stollerman GH: Rheumatic fever. In Wilson JD, et al, editors: *Harrison's Principles of internal medicine,* ed 12, New York, 1991, McGraw-Hill, pp 933-938.
16. Weinstein L: Chemotherapy of microbial diseases. In Goodman LS, Gilman A, editors: *The pharmacological basis of therapeutics,* ed 5, New York, 1975, Macmillan Publishing.

4

Congenital Heart Disease

There are three major types of congenital heart malformation.[3-5,9,10] One type includes malformations with initial left-to-right shunting of blood — atrial septal defect, ventricular septal defect, patent ductus arteriosus. The second consists of malformations with initial right-to-left shunting — transposition of the great vessels, persistent truncus arteriosus, tetralogy of Fallot. The third includes malformations that obstruct blood flow — pulmonary stenosis, coarctation of the aorta.

In general, lesions that shunt blood from left to right do not produce clinical evidence of cyanosis unless myocardial failure or pulmonary hypertension develops.[3,4] Conditions that shunt blood from right to left will cause significant cyanosis. Thus it is important to differentiate between cyanosis that has been present since birth and cyanosis that developed following cardiac failure or pulmonary hypertension. Patients with either type will develop polycythemia to compensate for the recirculation of desaturated hemoglobin.[1]

The prime concern of the dentist in dealing with a patient who has congenital heart disease is the prevention of infective endocarditis and endarteritis, because many of the defects are susceptible to these complications. Patients with polycythemia may be thrombocytopenic and have depleted plasma coagulation factors as a result of thrombosis in small vessels. They may have significant bleeding problems following scaling or surgical procedures and must be identified and given special attention before any dental treatment. In addition, the patient with congenital heart disease should be evaluated for the presence of pulmonary edema and cardiac failure and, if these are present, should be referred to a physician.

GENERAL DESCRIPTION
INCIDENCE AND PREVALENCE

The incidence of congenital heart disease has remained stable, with the exception of an unexplained increase in the number of cases of ventricular septal defect (twofold increase) and patent ductus arteriosus (threefold increase).[8] Congenital heart disease occurs in about 8 to 10 per 1600 live births annually. The incidence increases to over 1% in newborns, if stillborn infants and those with multiple defects who do not survive the first month are included.[3,4,6,8] Most infants born alive with cardiac defects will have anomalies that do not represent a threat to life, at least during infancy. However, a third of the infants born alive with congenital heart disease will have critical disease that leads to cardiac catheterization, cardiac surgery, or death in the first year.[9] About 60% of the infants with critical disease can be expected to survive the first year.[9] Congenital heart disease constitutes 1% to 3% of all cases of heart disease after infancy.[4] When the complexity of the development of the heart and great vessels is considered, it is a wonder that the incidence of abnormal development is so low.

There are approximately 4 to 5 million live births per year in the United States, and about 25,000 new cases of congenital heart disease occur.[3,8,10] There does not appear to be much difference in its incidence between blacks and whites.

The defect that most commonly causes cyanosis at birth and in infancy is tetralogy of

Fallot—which consists of a high ventricular septal defect, pulmonary stenosis, dextrapositioned aorta, and right ventricular hypertrophy. About 70% of blue babies have tetralogy of Fallot.[4,9,10]

Patency of the foramen ovale is clinically the least important of all congenital cardiac anomalies. The foramen ovale, an embryonic opening in the atrial septum, remains patent in about 25% of people, although in most cases it is very small and oblique; thus little blood flows through it.[4,9,10] Large defects are much more rare, and are found in females some four times as often as in males.

The most common congenital defect of the heart is bicuspid aortic valve. Excluding this lesion, the incidence of specific congenital heart defects is as shown in Table 4-1.[9] Note that ventricular septal defect is nearly 3 times as common as pulmonary stenosis and patent ductus arteriosus.

ETIOLOGY

The etiology of congenital heart disease involves complex multifactorial genetic and environmental causes.[5] However, the etiology in a number of cases remains unknown. Single mutant genes account for about 3% of the cardiac malformations found in humans.[8] Cardiac defects are associated with Down's, Turn-er's, and trisomy syndromes and may also be found in patients with enzyme disorders such as Hurler's syndrome and type II glycogen storage disease.[5] The incidence among siblings of patients with congenital heart disease is 17 per 1000 live births, compared to 7.6 per 1000 for the general population.[8]

Drugs, certain infections, and excessive radiation have been reported to cause cardiac defects. Alcohol, phenytoin, thalidomide, and lithium ingested during the early phase of pregnancy can result in cardiac malformations. Teratogens account for about 5% of the cardiac malformations. Rubella during pregnancy also can result in cardiac defects in the fetus.[5,8,9]

The number of cases of cardiac defects caused by rubella and Down's syndrome has decreased.[8] More women are now protected with vaccine against rubella. Older women are having fewer babies, thus reducing the risk for Down's syndrome.[8]

Fetal hypoxia, fetal endocarditis, immunologic abnormalities, and vitamin deficiencies have all been suggested[3,4,6] as causes of congenital heart defects. With few exceptions, patients who have congenital heart disease also have a negative familial history for congenital cardiac malformations. However, patent ductus arteriosus has been reported[4] to occur in successive generations.

Defects of the atrial septum and patency of the ductus arteriosus are more common in females. Pulmonary stenosis and ventricular septal defects show little sex predilection. Coarctation of the aorta and congenital aortic stenosis are much more common in males.

Pathophysiology and complications

The fetal circulation bypasses the uninflated lungs by flowing through the foramen ovale and ductus arteriosus. Oxygen is supplied by the placental circulation. The fetal circulation also bypasses the liver through the ductus venosus. At birth the lungs become inflated and blood flow is changed by increased left atrial pressure, which results in functional closure of the foramen ovale. Permanent closure occurs in most cases in 1 to 3 months. Prostaglandins maintain the patency of the ductus arteriosus prior to birth. The ductus functionally closes about 10 to 15 hours after birth, with complete closure usually in 10 to 21 days. Prior to birth the right

TABLE 4–1
Incidence of Specific Congenital Heart Defects

	Percent of cases (averaged)*
Ventricular septal defect	28.3
Pulmonary stenosis	9.5
Patent ductus arteriosus	8.7
Ventricular septal defect with pulmonary stenosis†	6.8
Atrial septal defect, secundum type	6.7
Aortic stenosis	4.4
Coarctation of aorta	4.2
Others (each less than 3.5%)	14.3

*Total number of cases, 103,590
†Includes tetralogy of Fallot.
Based on Nugent EW, et al. In Hurst JW, editor: *The heart, arteries, and veins*, ed 7, New York, 1990, McGraw-Hill, p 657.

and left ventricular pressures are about equal, and the ventricular walls are about the same thickness. At birth the left ventricular pressure increases and the wall of the left ventricle begins to thicken.[9] Many cardiac defects result in the maintenance of a pattern of circulation similar to that found in the fetus.

The physiologic effects of most congenital cardiac defects are a result of the shunting of blood. Left-to-right shunts cause a recirculation of blood that has flowed through the lungs. The blood that reaches the systemic capillaries is saturated with oxygen; thus cyanosis is not present. Under these conditions the pulmonary blood flow is about 12 to 15 liters per minute, and the systemic flow 4 to 5 liters per minute. The ratio of pulmonary to systemic flow can reach as high as 20:1 with a large left-to-right shunt (Figs. 4-1 and 4-2).

When the shunt is at the atrial or ventricular level, the right ventricle must work much harder, and this may lead to ventricular dilation and hypertrophy. If the shunt is at the pulmonary artery level, as with patent ductus arteriosus (without pulmonary hypertension), the left ventricle must work harder and will eventually undergo dilation and hypertrophy. If pulmonary hypertension develops, right ventricular dilation and hypertrophy may also occur.

When venous blood from the systemic circulation enters the left heart chambers before passing through the lung, as in the right-to-left shunt, the functional effect is to reduce the partial pressure of oxygen in the arterial systemic blood. This leads to a need for greater blood flow and increases the work of both ventricles. The clinical results of right-to-left shunting of blood are primarily caused by oxygen undersaturation of the arterial blood.

If the arterial blood contains 5 g/100 ml or more of unsaturated hemoglobin, cyanosis will be present. In congenital heart disease early cyanosis indicates right-to-left shunting of blood.

The body attempts to compensate for low oxygen content in the arterial system by polycythemia (increased numers of red blood cells) and increased blood flow. Polycythemia may result in a hematocrit of 50% to 80% and increases the total blood volume and viscosity. This leads to increased work for the heart. Patients with severe polycythemia are most prone to thromboses and must avoid dehydration. Thromboses can cause infarctions in vital

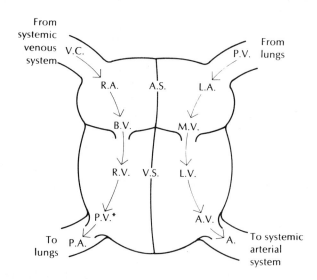

FIG. 4-1 Normal blood flow through the chambers of the heart, valves, and great vessels. *VC,* Vena cava; *RA,* right atrium; *BV,* bicuspid valve; *RV,* right ventricle; *PV*,* pulmonary valve; *PA,* pulmonary artery; *PV,* pulmonary vein; *LA,* left atrium; *MV,* mitral valve; *LV,* left ventricle; *AV,* aortic valve; *A,* aorta; *AS,* atrial septum; *VS,* ventricular septum.

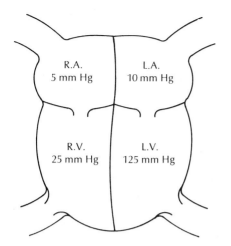

FIG. 4-2 Normal atrial and ventricular pressures.

TABLE 4–2
Complications of Congenital Heart Disease

Infective endocarditis (or endarteritis)
Pulmonary edema
Cardiac failure
Decreased oxygen content of arterial blood
Thromboses
Bleeding, fibrinogen depletion, thrombocytopenia
Brain abscess
Cyanosis
Pulmonary arterial hypertension
Retardation of growth
Exertional intolerance

organs. Red blood cell precursors may replace platelet precursors in the bone marrow, thus leading to thrombocytopenia. Thromboses also can lead to depletion of the fibrinogen level; therefore the patient may have bleeding tendencies as a result of either or both thrombocytopenia and hypofibrinogenemia.

Many patients with long-standing right-to-left shunts develop clubbing of the fingers and, in some cases, the toes. The origin of clubbing is unknown, but it may be caused by the increased blood flow in patients with cyanotic congenital heart disease. The terminal phalanges and nail beds are affected.

Pulmonary hypertension can develop in patients with congenital heart disease because of the increased pulmonary blood flow or increased puulmonary arteriolar resistance. In left-ro-right shunts pulmonary flow may increase more than five times the normal amount. The significance of pulmonary hypertension depends on the duration, site, and size of the cardiovascular defect and the amount of vasoconstriction present in the lung fields.

Pulmonary hypertension can lead to right ventricular hypertrophy, enlargement of the pulmonary artery, and development of cyanosis in patients with shunts that were initially left to right but changed to right to left because of the increased pulmonary resistance, myocardial failure, or both.

The complications of congenital heart disease are many and significant[3,4,5,9] (Table 4-2). Pa-

tients tend to have a lowered resistance to infection. Of all cases of infective endocarditis, 10% are found in patients with congenital heart disease. Patients with ventricular septal defects and deformities of the aortic valve are most prone to endocarditis. Patients with patent ductus arteriosus and coarctation of the aorta are prone to endarteritis, which carries the same grave prognosis as endocarditis. Patients with small atrial septal defects do not appear to be prone to endocarditis.

Patients with right-to-left shunting of blood are likely to develop thromboses and may have bleeding tendencies, as indicated previously. They also are susceptible to increased frequency of brain abscesses because infectious materials are not filtered by the lungs. Any patient with congenital heart disease who develops unexplained fever and headaches should be evaluated for a possible brain abscess.

Congestive heart failure is one of the major complications of congenital heart disease. It occurs in 20% of children with congenital heart disease, generally appearing at about 6 months of age. It involves critical lesions in approximately 80% of the children. When it occurs during the first 12 to 18 hours of life, it is due to volume overload or valvular regurgitation. When it occurs later (in the first week of life), it is due to a critical obstruction of flow such as coarctation of the aorta. When it occurs after the first week, it is usually due to ventricular septal defect.[9] If associated with congenital heart disease, the onset of congestive heart failure in an adult is usually due to atrial septal defect.[1]

Another major complication of congenital heart disease can be retardation of growth and development. Patients with mild congenital heart disease usually have near normal growth. Growth retardation becomes more severe in patients with overt cyanosis or with large left-to-right shunts.[9]

SPECIFIC CONGENITAL HEART DEFECTS
Bicuspid aortic valve

Bicuspid aortic valve is the most common form of congenital heart disease. It usually does not manifest signs or symptoms, however, until adulthood. Its incidence is about 2% in the general population. A bicuspid aortic valve may be found associated with other lesions such as coarctation of the aorta or interruption of the aortic arch. It is more common in males (2.5:1).[9]

The main complication of bicuspid aortic valve is fibrosis and calcification of the valve. This can occur in children, but it is usually found in individuals 15 to 65 years of age. Studies have shown that 85% of the cases of calcific aortic stenosis occur in bicuspid aortic valves. These valves result in aortic regurgitation and are susceptible to infective endocarditis. Some individuals with a bicuspid aortic valve do not develop calcification. The reasons for this are not clear.[9]

Because it is usually not found until adulthood, bicuspid aortic valve is seldom included in the frequency rates for congenital heart defects. Therefore understanding the frequency of the following lesions is based on excluding bicuspid aortic valve.

Atrial septal defects

Atrial septal defects, which include patent foramen ovale, are the most common congenital lesions of the heart (Figs. 4-3 and 4-4). The clinical effects depend on the size of the defect and the volume of blood shunted. Growth and development of the affected person usually are normal. Cyanosis and pulmonary hypertension develop only late in the course of the disease, if at all. Early symptoms are dyspnea, fatigue, and paroxysmal atrial tachycardia. Blood is usually shunted from left to right. The right atrium and ventricle may become enlarged, and right ventricular hypertrophy may develop. The pulmonary artery usually becomes dilated.

Ventricular septal defect

Ventricular septal defect is the second most common congenital heart lesion, after patency of the foramen ovale (Fig. 4-5). Nine out of every ten patients with a ventricular septal defect will have some other cardiac anomaly, usually pulmonary stenosis. Blood is shunted from left to right unless pulmonary hypertension, pulmonary stenosis, or myocardial failure is present.

About 75% of ventricular septal defects close

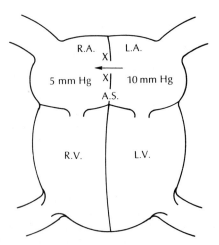

FIG. 4-3 Atrial septal defect resulting in a left-to-right shunt; *x* indicates the area most prone to infective endocarditis.

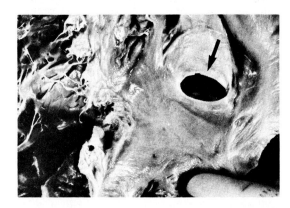

FIG. 4-4 Postmortem specimen of a heart with a large atrial septal defect. (Courtesy W. O'Conner, M.D., Lexington, Ky.)

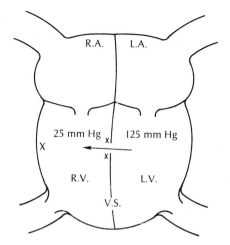

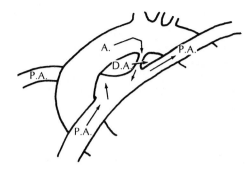

FIG. 4-6 Patent ductus arteriosus. *DA,* The ductus — connecting the aorta, *A,* and the pulmonary artery, *PA* — allows blood to flow from the aorta into the pulmonary artery.

FIG. 4-5 Ventricular septal defect resulting in a left-to-right shunt; *x* indicates the area most prone to infective endocarditis.

spontaneously by 10 years of age. Thus patients with this lesion are usually not operated on early unless the lesion is large and there are symptoms.[9]

Patent ductus arteriosus

The fetal connection between the pulmonary artery and aorta that allows fetal blood to bypass the lungs usually closes by the age of 2 years. This connection arises at the bifurcation of the pulmonary artery and ends in the aorta, usually just beyond the opening of the left subclavian artery.

If the ductus remains patent, left-to-right shunting occurs (Fig. 4-6). A temporary reversal of blood flow may occur with crying or violent physical activity. If pulmonary hypertension or heart failure develops, right-to-left shunting occurs, with the development of cyanosis.

Transposition of the great vessels

In transposition of the great vessels the aortic root opens into the right ventricle and the pulmonary artery into the left ventricle. If no other anomaly is present to allow for blood flow from one circulation to the other, this condition is not compatible with life.

Persistent truncus arteriosus

In persistent truncus arteriosus a high ventricular septal defect is present, with blood flowing from both ventricles into a common trunk. The pulmonary artery branches from the common trunk. Patients with this defect will be cyanotic from birth.

Tetralogy of Fallot

Tetralogy of Fallot is one of the most common cardiac defects causing cyanosis. About 75% of patients over the age of 2 years with cyanosis and not yet requiring surgery have tetralogy of Fallot.[9] Without surgery 75% of them die before the age of 10. Less than 5% survive past 30.[9]

Tetralogy of Fallot consists of pulmonary stenosis, ventricular septal defect, dextroposition of the aorta, and right ventricular hypertrophy (Fig. 4-7). With extreme pulmonary stenosis the ductus arteriosus must remain patent for life. If it does not, the Blalock-Taussig operation can be performed to bypass the obstructive lesion by making an artificial ductus. The preferred treatment, when possible, is to correct the ventricular septal defect and pulmonary stenosis.

Pulmonary stenosis

Pure pulmonary stenosis reduces the pulmonary blood flow and leads to right ventricular dilation and hypertrophy with eventual myocardial failure. Exertional dyspnea usually precedes the appearance of cyanosis. Once cyanosis has appeared, the entire symptom complex becomes much more severe.

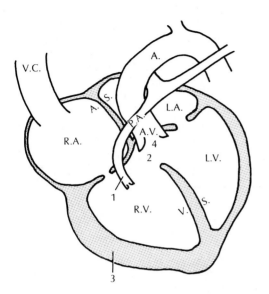

FIG. 4-7 Anatomic relationships in tetralogy of Fallot. *1*, Pulmonary stenosis; *2*, high ventricular septal defect; *3*, hypertrophied right ventricle; *4*, dextropositioned aorta (over the septum).

Coarctation of the aorta

Coarctation of the aorta consists of a narrowing of the aorta in the region where it is joined by the ductus arteriosus. Two types of coarctation are found. In the infantile type, which usually is not compatible with life, the aortic constriction is proximal to the ductus arteriosus (between the ductus and the left subclavian artery). In the adult type the constriction is at or distal to the ductus, which is usually obliterated. The adult type of coarctation causes severe hypertension in the upper body and may lead to cardiac failure or cerebral hemorrhage. Endarteritis may develop at the site of coarctation. Aneurysms may form near the coarctation, and the aorta may rupture. The lower body obtains its blood flow by way of a greatly dilated collateral system. Half the patients with the adult form of coarctation will die by the age of 40 years unless they have surgery.

CLINICAL PRESENTATION

Dyspnea is the most common symptom in patients with congenital heart disease. It may be caused by overloading of the pulmonary circu-

TABLE 4–3
Signs and Symptoms of Congenital Heart Disease

Dyspnea
Cyanosis
Ruddy color, polycythemia
Clubbing of fingers and toes
Murmurs
Congestive heart failure
Distention of neck veins
Enlarged liver
Ascites
Weakness
Dizziness, syncope, coma

lation, as occurs in large atrial septal defects, or by the large amount of unoxygenated blood shunted into the systemic circulation in anomalies with right-to-left shunts.

Cyanosis occurs late in lesions that produce initial left-to-right shunting of blood. When it occurs, it results either from pulmonary hypertension or from myocardial failure. Lesions that initially produce right-to-left shunting of blood will be accompanied by cyanosis as an early sign.

Polycythemia is a condition that develops as a result of the decreased oxygen-carrying capacity of blood that has been shunted from right to left and thus has not passed through the lungs. This causes a need for increased red blood cells to compensate for the decreased oxygen content.

Cerebral symptoms are common and consist of faintness, dizziness, syncope, and coma. In most cases they are caused by anoxia or thrombosis (complication of polycythemia). Weakness is a symptom that may be secondary to the other causes of dyspnea or myocardial failure (Table 4-3).

Patients with congenital heart disease may appear ruddy if significant polycythemia is present. Those with long-standing right-to-left shunting of blood may have clubbing of the fingers or toes (Fig. 4-8). Patients with high-velocity shunts will demonstrate murmurs and often associated thrills. Those who have developed myocardial failure may show distention of the neck veins, cyanosis, enlarged and tender liver, ascites, or other signs.

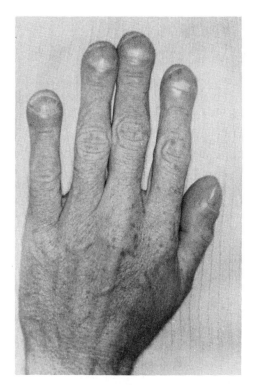

FIG. 4-8 Clubbing of the fingers secondary to congenital heart disease.

LABORATORY FINDINGS

Patients with polycythemia will have decreased hemoglobin and hematocrit values. Platelet counts may be normal or decreased. Fibrinogen levels may also be decreased, as reflected in longer prothrombin times. The bleeding time will be prolonged with significant thrombocytopenia. In severe cases the white blood cell count may be decreased.[9]

Chest radiographs can be used to demonstrate the increased heart size and dilation of pulmonary vessels in cases of congestive heart failure and pulmonary hypertension. An echocardiogram is used to demonstrate anatomic changes such as ventricular septal defects and valvular lesions. Angiocardiography is used to visualize the chambers of the heart, aorta, and pulmonary artery so abnormal flow patterns can be identified. Cardiac catheterization is performed to study the pressure and oxygen content of the various heart chambers and great vessels. Electrocardiography is used to evaluate the degree of dominance of right versus left ventricle. Under normal conditions the QRS axis switches to left dominance by 1 year of age. With certain congenital heart defects this does not occur.[1,9]

Controlled exercise tests are used to establish values for work heart rate, blood pressure, and ECG changes. Patients with significant cardiac defects often will have changes in these values.[1]

MEDICAL MANAGEMENT

Successful treatment by surgical means is now available for patent ductus arteriosus, pulmonary valvular stenosis, coarctation of the aorta, atrial septal defect, ventricular septal defect, transposition of the great vessels, and valvular anomalies involving the tricuspid, mitral, and aortic valves. [1,7,9] The frequency of these complications increases with the order in which they are listed. The surgical mortality rate for elective closure of uncomplicated patent ductus arteriosus is now virtually zero.[9]

Generally patients with physical signs of congenital heart disease who do not have symptoms should not undergo corrective surgery. Exceptions are patent ductus arteriosus, ventricular septal defect, and coarctation of the aorta because of the high risk of infective endocarditis or endarteritis if the deformation is not corrected. All infants with symptoms associated with coarctation of the aorta should be treated surgically. All others should be operated on between the ages of 4 and 6 years.[9]

Digitalis is the keystone to therapy for patients with right or left ventricular failure. Patients with polycythemia are protected against thrombosis by anticoagulation therapy or venisection and by prevention of dehydration. (For more details concerning the management of congestive heart failure and endocarditis and endarteritis, see Chapters 2 and 9.)

The surgical correction of adult-type coarctation of the aorta occasionally can be complicated by gangrene of the small intestine as a result of the pressure caused by rapid filling and distention of the branches of the abdominal aorta, with resulting necrosis of the tissues supplied by these vessels.[7]

Patients with tetralogy of Fallot may be

helped by the Blalock-Taussig operation, which makes an artificial ductus arteriosus that bypasses the pulmonary stenosis. However, the preferred treatment is to correct the ventricular septal defect and pulmonary stenosis surgically if the clinical situation allows. Surgical treatment of some of the major lesions may not solve all the problems. Residual effects such as pulmonary valve insufficiency are common after surgical correction of the right ventricular outflow tract of tetralogy of Fallot.[1] An important surgical advance for the treatment of absent or hypoplastic valves is the establishment of an extracardiac conduit. These conduits contain a valve.[1]

Medical management includes dealing with the complications of congenital heart disease—brain abscesses, infective endocarditis or endarteritis, cerebrovascular problems, congestive heart failure, acute pulmonary edema, bleeding problems, and associated emotional problems.

Women with congenital heart disease and resulting pulmonary vascular obstructive disease who become pregnant have a high risk of dying during delivery. Early abortion should be considered in these cases. The barrier method of birth control is the only option available to these women since intrauterine devices and oral contraceptives are contraindicated due to the risk of bleeding, infection, or thrombosis.[5]

DENTAL MANAGEMENT

The prime concern with the asymptomatic patient who has congenital heart disease is the prevention of infective endocarditis (IE) or endarteritis following dental procedures that produce transient bacteremias. Patients with patent ductus arteriosus, ventricular septal defect, coarctation of the aorta, or valvular anomalies are most prone to these infections, and patients who have undergone surgery to correct congenital lesions also are susceptible during the healing phase. It would appear that most patients who have had surgery to correct a congenital heart lesion would not be susceptible to IE if no synthetic materials were used and at least 6 months had elapsed since the surgery. (See Chapters 5 and 27.) However, before any dental treatment is performed on these patients, their physician or surgeon should be consulted regarding their status and the need for pro-phylactic antibiotic coverage to prevent endocarditis.

MEDICAL CONSIDERATIONS

Most patients with congenital heart disease are susceptible to IE. Prophylactic antibiotics are required when invasive dental treatment is to be performed. Patients with a small atrial septal defect do not require prophylaxis.[2] For those patients needing prophylaxis, the AHA standard regimen of amoxicillin is recommended. Erythromycin or clindamycin can be used for those allergic to penicillin. (See Chapter 2.) The management of patients with surgically corrected lesions is covered in Chapters 5 and 27.

No routine dental procedures should be done on a patient who has symptomatic congenital heart disease without complete consultation with the patient's physician. Patients with polycythemia may have clinical bleeding tendencies, and this should be evaluated before any surgery is attempted. A patient who has bleeding

TABLE 4–4
Dental Management of the Patient with Congenital Heart Disease

---

Medical consultation
Drugs—confirmation
Current status
Presence of congestive failure
Prevention of infective endocarditis (or endarteritis)
1. Standard regimen for most patients
2. Standard or special regimen for patients just following corrective surgery
3. After healing (6 months) patients whose defect was corrected using synthetic materials should receive American Heart Association standard regimen (oral amoxicillin) if indicated by consultation
4. After healing (6 months) patients whose defect was corrected without using synthetic materials will not require prophylaxis
Prevention of excessive blood loss if surgery performed
1. Anticoagulation medication
2. Depletion of fibrinogen
3. Thrombocytopenia

---

problems should not be operated on until the proper steps have been taken to avoid this complication. This will involve working with the patient's physician or a hematologist. Patients receiving anticoagulants should be managed as described in Chapter 22.

The patient with congestive heart failure secondary to congenital heart disease should not receive any routine dental care until the heart failure has been dealt with (Chapter 9), and then only after consultation with the patient's physician (Table 4-4).

Treatment planning considerations

The patient with congenital heart disease who is asymptomatic can receive any indicated dental treatment as long as antibiotics are used to prevent infective endocarditis. The patient with symptoms secondary to the congenital heart disease may have to have an altered plan of treatment, depending on the complication and its severity. Some patients may be able to receive only urgent dental care, and even then with some risk.

Oral complications

There are usually no oral complications directly related to congenital heart disease. The facial skin and oral mucosa may appear bluish in patients with the central type of cyanosis. Patients with significant polycythemia may have a ruddy color to the face and oral mucosa. If thrombocytopenia is present, patients may show evidence of small hemorrhages secondary to minor trauma in the oral mucosa. If significant leukopenia is present, patients may develop oral infection out of proportion to the etiologic factor(s) involved.

REFERENCES

1. Black IFS: Congenital heart disease. In Rose LF, Kaye D, editors: *Internal medicine for dentistry,* ed 2, St Louis, 1990, Mosby–Year Book, pp 442-452.
2. *Cardiovascular disease in dental practice,* Publ. no. 771-0009, Dallas, 1991, American Heart Association, pp 6-7.
3. Fortuin NJ, Kelly DT, Ross RS: Cardiac murmurs and other manifestations of valvular and acyanotic congenital heart disease. In Harvey A, et al, editors: *The principles and practice of medicine,* ed 19, New York, 1976, Appleton-Century-Crofts.
4. Friedman WF, Braunwald E: Congenital heart disease. In Thorn GW, et al, editors: *Harrison's Principles of internal medicine,* ed 8, New York, 1977, McGraw-Hill.
5. Friedman WF, Child JS: Congenital heart disease in the adult. In Wilson JD, et al, editors: *Harrison's Principles of internal medicine,* ed 12, New York, 1991, McGraw-Hill, pp 923-933.
6. Hurst JW, editor: *The heart, arteries, and veins,* ed 4, New York, 1978, McGraw-Hill.
7. Julian OC: *Cardiovascular surgery,* ed 2, Chicago, 1970, Year Book Medical.
8. Kannel WB, Thom TJ: Incidence, prevalence, and mortality of cardiovascular diseases. In Hurst JW, editor: *The heart, arteries, and veins,* ed 7, New York, 1990, McGraw-Hill, pp 627-638.
9. Nugent EW, Plauth WH, Edwards JE, Williams WH: The pathology, abnormal physiology, clinical recognition, and medical and surgical treatment of congenital heart disease. In Hurst JW, editor: *The heart, arteries, and veins,* ed 7, New York, 1990, McGraw-Hill, pp 655-794.
10. Silber EN, Katz LN: *Heart disease,* New York, 1975, Macmillan Publishing.

5

Surgically Corrected Cardiac and Vascular Disease

There is general agreement among physicians and dentists that patients who have congenital heart disease and rheumatic heart disease are more susceptible than the general population to infective endocarditis or infective endarteritis. These infections can develop following dental procedures that cause transient bacteremias. It is current practice to protect a susceptible patient with prophylactic antibiotics just before and after all dental procedures to minimize the chance of endocarditis or endarteritis.

The risk of these diseases occurring after dental treatment in a patient who has a surgically corrected cardiovascular lesion is less clearly defined, and the guidelines for prevention are more vague.

This chapter considers the risk of endocarditis or endarteritis in a patient who has undergone corrective surgery for various cardiac or vascular disorders and suggests guidelines for the dental management of such patients with respect to the need for protection against endocarditis or endarteritis. The following surgical procedures will be considered: (1) closure of an atrial or ventricular septal defect, (2) ligation or resection of a ductus arteriosus, (3) commissurotomy for diseased cardiac valve(s), (4) prosthetic replacement of diseased cardiac valve(s), (5) coronary artery bypass graft, (6) arterial graft, (7) implantation of a transvenous pacemaker, (8) implantation of a cardioverter-defibrillator, and (9) heart transplantation (Chapter 26).

GENERAL DESCRIPTION, CLINICAL PRESENTATION, AND SURGICAL MANAGEMENT
SURGICALLY CLOSED SEPTAL DEFECT

Three anatomic defects are found that involve the atrial septum. They are, in order of frequency, ostium secundum, sinus venosus, and ostium primum.

For an ostium secundum defect (atrial septal defect at the fossa ovalis) in an asymptomatic infant with left-to-right shunting greater than 2:1,* surgical closure usually is postponed until the child is about 6 years old. The operation is recommended even in older individuals who have pulmonary hypertension, as long as the left-to-right shunting of blood exists. Systemic pulmonary hypertension with a balanced shunt or right-to-left shunting is a contraindication for surgery. Usually a patient with an ostium secundum defect is treated if the heart is enlarged, heart failure is imminent, an arrhythmia is present, or the shunt is large. The patient is not treated if the shunt is small or if the patient is asymptomatic, has a normal heart size, or has developed pulmonary hypertension with reversal of the shunt. The defect is closed with sutures.[9,21,22,26]

A sinus venosus defect is located high in the

---

*Pulmonary-to-systemic flow ratio. Measured by a catheter inserted into the femoral vein (inside of the thigh) and run up to the heart through the inferior vena cava.

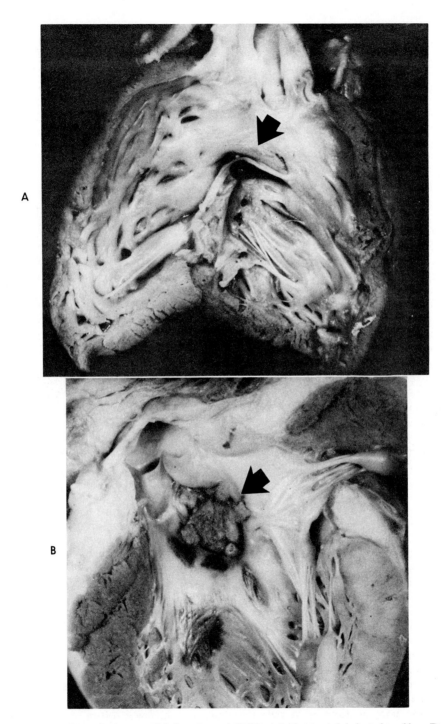

FIG. 5-1 **A,** Ventricular septal defect *(arrow)*. **B,** Ventricular septal defect closed by a Dacron patch *(arrow)*. (Courtesy Jesse E. Edwards, M.D., St Paul Minn.)

septum near the opening of the superior vena cava. The indications for surgical repair are the same as for ostium secundum defect. The defect is often larger than the ostium secundum type and requires a patch graft of pericardium or Dacron.[9,21,22]

The ostium primum defect is a more serious lesion than an ostium secundum or sinus venosus defect. Most patients who have ostium primum defect will not survive into adulthood without surgical repair of the defect. Ostium primum is a round defect located low in the septum and often is associated with malformations of the atrioventricular valves. One complication of surgery is injury to the conduction system, which can result in a heart block and necessitate a permanent pacemaker. The defect is closed with a patch graft of pericardium or Dacron.[9,24,26]

A small ventricular septal defect is compatible with a relatively normal life expectancy and may close spontaneously, particularly during infancy and childhood. Large defects eventually lead to increased pulmonary vascular resistance and right-to-left shunting. Once a left-to-right shunt has changed to right-to-left, it may be inoperable.[21,22,26] A child who has a small defect and normal pulmonary artery pressure does not require an operation unless there is a history of endocarditis.[9,21,22] Most patients who have large septal defects are operated on before they reach adulthood. Small lesions are treated by primary closure, larger lesions by a Dacron or pericardial patch[9,21,22,26] (Fig. 5-1).

LIGATED OR RESECTED DUCTUS ARTERIOSUS

Endarteritis and pulmonary hypertension are two complications found in untreated patients who have patent ductus arteriosus (Fig. 5-2). A 17-year-old patient with a patent ductus now has about half the life expectancy of an unaffected individual. The operative risks are small for patients who have a patent ductus without cardiac failure, and the mortality rate under these circumstances is less than 0.5%. If patients with cardiac failure are included, however, the operative mortality rate increases to about 2% or 3%. When the complications of a patent ductus arteriosus and the shortened life expectancy and low operative risk of patients with the condition are considered, corrective surgery is indicated in asymptomatic children or young adults. A patient over the age of 30 years with a patent ductus who is asymptomatic and has a normal-sized heart is commonly not treated. Repair is complicated in adults because of the enlargement of adjacent vessels and the presence of atherosclerotic lesions. The operative risk rises greatly in a patient with right-to-left shunting and/or pulmonary hypertension, to the point where surgery is contraindicated. Repair is performed by cutting the ductus and suturing the cut ends closed or by suturing the ductus closed without resection.[9,21,22,28]

COMMISSUROTOMY FOR DISEASED CARDIAC VALVE(S)

Mitral valve disease has a poor prognosis without surgical treatment. Twenty percent of patients with mitral stenosis die within a year, and 60% die within 10 years following the diagnosis. In pure mitral stenosis, commissurotomy is the procedure of choice. Operation is indicated if symptoms interfere with productivity or the quality of life, if atrial fibrillation is present, or if the patient has a history of thromboembolism. A pliable valve is required. Patients with nonpliable valves or previous valve surgery are best treated by prosthetic valve replacement.[23]

Closed mitral commissurotomy may be selected for a patient who has isolated noncalcific mitral stenosis without regurgitation. However, it is now an unusual operation in the United States,[23] although it may be done for pregnant patients with pliable mitral valves who are developing cardiac disability.[23] When performed, the appendage of the left atrium is opened, a finger is inserted into the atrium, and an attempt is made to separate the valve leaflets. If this fails, a small hole is made in the left ventricle and a transventricular dilator is inserted and guided to the mitral valve, separating the leaflets.[1]

Open commissurotomy involves open heart surgery using a bypass pump. The left atrium is opened, the mitral valve is examined, and a final decision is made for commissurotomy or valve replacement. Patients who have had open commissurotomy will often require reoperation within 5 to 20 years. The reoperation rate is about 5% per year.[23]

Patients with mitral regurgitation are not

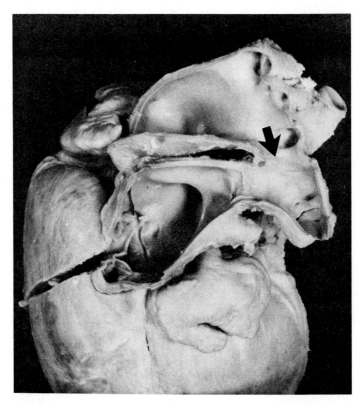

FIG. 5-2 Patent ductus arteriosus *(arrow)*. (Courtesy Jesse E. Edwards, M.D., St Paul Minn.)

treated by commissurotomy. Treatment of this condition involves either valve reconstruction or prosthetic replacement. Mitral valve prolapse is now the most common cause of mitral regurgitation.[23] Patients with aortic valve disease are not treated by commissurotomy. Surgical management for these cases requires prosthetic valve replacement.[24]

PROSTHETIC REPLACEMENT OF DISEASED CARDIAC VALVE(S)

A patient who has significant functional alteration of one or more cardiac valves is a candidate for the surgical placement of a prosthetic valve(s). Prosthetic valve replacement is indicated in a patient with a defective valve or valves who has developed (1) progressive congestive heart failure, (2) systemic emboli from the left atrium, and/or (3) endocarditis.[1,8]

The first aortic prosthetic valve was inserted in 1960. The first mitral prosthetic valve was placed in 1961, and the first tricuspid valve prosthesis in 1963.[10] The prognosis for patients receiving prosthetic heart valves has improved because of improved surgical techniques and valve design. The surgical mortality rate is now 2% to 5% for aortic valves, 3% to 8% for mitral valves, and 5% to 15% for multiple valves.[10] The 5-year survival rate is 80% to 85% for aortic valves, 70% to 85% for mitral valves, and 50% to 60% for multiple valves.[10]

Porcine or pericardial bioprostheses have a low thromboembolism rate, and long-term durability remains a question. In young adults (less than 35 years of age) these valves last for about 7 years. In older adults the valves can last for 10 years. A faster deterioration occurs in children. Anticoagulation is not needed for these valves if the patient has a normal sinus rhythm.

Two types of mechanical valves are in general use now. The *Bjork-Shiley* tilting disk valve has excellent long-term durability but a higher rate of thromboembolism (1 per 100 patient years). The rate of thromboembolism is higher for mitral valve replacement than for aortic. The other mechanical valve in general use is the *Starr-Edwards* ball valve. This valve also has excellent long-term durability and a moderate rate of thromboembolism (4 to 9 per 100 patient years). One limitation of the Starr-Edwards valve in the mitral position is that a large ventricle is required. The risk of hemorrhage in patients receiving anticoagulation medication is 2 per 100 patient years. This risk must be added to the risk for thromboembolism when selecting tissue versus mechanical valve.[10]

The use of cryopreserved human homografts in the aortic position is now strongly advocated.[10] They have a low incidence of reoperation, are free of thromboembolism, and do not need anticoagulation. Difficulty with anticoagulation is a strong argument against mechanical prostheses. Patients under 35 years should have a mechanical prosthesis because of the rapid deterioration of bioprostheses.[10] Occasionally a young woman who wants children is given a bioprosthesis to avoid the complication of anticoagulation therapy, but she must be aware that the valve will have to be replaced in about 10 years.[10]

Replacement of bioprostheses on an elective basis carries a low risk. However, when done on an emergency basis, the surgical mortality rate can be up to 50%. Mechanical valve dysfunction,

when it occurs, is usually catastrophic, requiring emergency replacement (with a high mortality rate).[10]

Several prosthetic valves have been designed and tested in laboratory animals and humans.[8,14] Two general types are now being used: mechanical valves and tissue valves (Table 5-1). Both types have a number of variations in design and materials used in their construction (Figs. 5-3 and 5-4). During open heart surgery the diseased valve is removed and the prosthetic valve attached to the surrounding tissues, using nonabsorbable sutures. Prosthetic valve failure involves (1) excessive thrombosis on and around the valve, leading to systemic emboli, (2) infection at the site of attachment to cardiac tissues, and (3) mechanical failure of the valve components (Table 5-2).

CORONARY ARTERY BYPASS GRAFT

Over 200,000 coronary bypass operations are performed annually in the United States. Coronary bypass surgery has been extremely successful. The procedure, coupled with medical therapy, has enormously improved the treatment of patients with coronary atherosclerotic heart disease.[25] Before a coronary artery bypass graft (CABG) procedure is selected for a patient who has significant coronary artery disease, the natural history of the disease must be considered (Fig. 5-5). The available reports[6,25] have shown that symptoms do not always correlate with risk of death or myocardial infarction. A person may have a myocardial infarction or die suddenly without a history of pain. Thus angiography may be indicated by reasonable suspicion for the presence of coronary disease in the absence of clinical symptoms.

TABLE 5–1

Types of Prosthetic Valves Now in Use

Mechanical valves

Caged ball
  Cloth-covered
  Non–cloth-covered
Central disk and conical occluder
Tilting disk

Tissue valves

Aortic valve homograft
Porcine aortic valve xenograft
Bovine pericardial xenograft
Dura mater homograft

From Lefrak EA, Starr A: *Cardiac valve prostheses,* New York, 1979, Appleton-Century-Crofts.

TABLE 5–2

Operative Mortality and 5-Year Survival Rates for Patients with Prosthetic Heart Valves

Valve	Operative mortality rate (%)	5-Year survival rate (%)
Aortic	2 to 5	80 to 85
Mitral	3 to 8	70 to 85
Multiple	5 to 15	50 to 60

Based on Guyton RA, Hatcher CR: In Hurst, JW, editor: *The heart, arteries, and veins,* ed 7, New York, 1990, McGraw-Hill, p 2205.

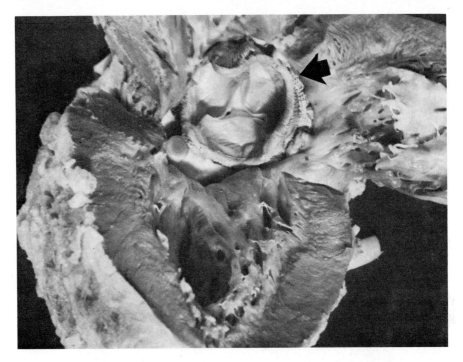

FIG. 5-3 Tissue prosthetic heart valve *(arrow)*. (Courtesy Jesse E. Edwards, M.D., St Paul Minn.)

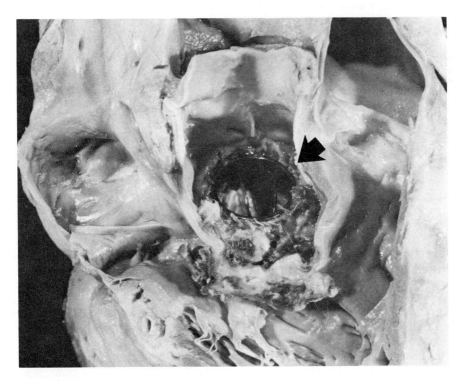

FIG. 5-4 Mechanical prosthetic heart valve with prosthetic valve endocarditis *(arrow)*. (Courtesy Jesse E. Edwards, M.D., St Paul Minn.)

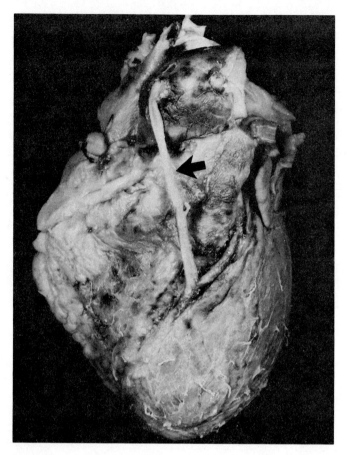

FIG. 5-5 Coronary artery bypass graft *(arrow).* (Courtesy Jesse E. Edwards, M.D., St Paul Minn.)

In a study of 112 patients who were advised to undergo a CABG procedure and refused,[6] the following observations were reported: (1) data available at the time of catheterization correlated poorly with subsequent death or survival; (2) 55% of the patients were dead within 2 years; (3) a symptom complex or crescendo of pain was associated with an increased mortality rate; (4) major stenosis of the proximal left coronary artery was the most significant predictor of early death; and (5) the absence of symptoms or the number of infarcts did not correlate with either survival or death.

Indications for CABG surgery are (1) tight stenosis of the proximal left coronary system, (2) severe vessel disease, and (3) crescendo-type anginal pain. As the number of coronary vessels involved by atherosclerotic narrowing increases, the death rate increases and surgery becomes more advisable.[6]

Single, nondominant coronary disease is not associated with early death and often is successfully treated by medical means.[6] A patient with poor ventricular function is a candidate for coronary artery surgery only when severe, life-threatening coronary atherosclerosis is present. Smoking is an important factor in the patient who develops pulmonary complications during the postoperative period. Some physicians will not perform elective surgery for the patient who continues to smoke.

CABG is a surgical procedure that requires a quiet heart. It is an open heart procedure using the heart bypass pump. Hypothermia is used to arrest the heart in diastole and to lessen the myocardial oxygen need. The choice of graft material is usually the saphenous vein. In some cases the lesser saphenous vein, cephalic vein, or internal mammary (thoracic) artery is used. The graft needs at least a 2 mm diameter to be effective. The choice for the coronary anastomotic site has been moved to a more distal location to avoid obstruction, which occurs usually more proximally in the coronary arteries. Once the coronary anastomoses have been completed, rewarming is started. The heart is electrically defibrillated if spontaneous conversion has not occurred. Then the proximal ends of the grafts are sutured to the aorta. As many as six separate grafts may be attached to the side of the aorta.[11]

Closure of the graft after surgery is one of the major concerns with coronary artery bypass surgery. The skill of the surgical team and the graft flow rate at the time of surgery are two other important factors in determining the long-term patency of the graft.

ARTERIAL GRAFT

Arterial grafts are used to replace segments of large arteries, such as the aorta, that have developed an aneurysm secondary to severe atherosclerotic disease. The material most commonly used for the graft is Dacron. Autogenous tissues also may be used for replacement of segments of large or small arteries.

Infections of arterial grafts are not common; nevertheless, one major cause of infection appears to be wound contamination from the skin or infected lymph nodes. Hematogenous bacteria also may appear on the uncovered surface of a graft following transient bacteremias after surgical manipulation of the genitourinary tract or oral cavity.[15,20,29]

IMPLANTATION OF A TRANSVENOUS PACEMAKER

When significant blockage has occurred in the conduction system of the heart, a pacemaker may have to be inserted to maintain a relatively normal cardiac rhythm. Temporary and permanent pacemakers are used (Chapter 8).

There are three types of temporary pacemakers: *External pacemakers* are the simplest and are used in emergency situations. Electrodes are placed at the scapula and right sternal border on the skin. Care must be taken to avoid pain, severe muscle spasms, and burns. *Percutaneous pacemakers* consist of a wire passed through the skin into the left ventricle and then attached to the skin by a suture. *Transvenous pacemakers* consist of a bipolar catheter inserted, under fluoroscopic control, through the external jugular vein into the right ventricle with a battery-operated pacemaker attached to the catheter. If a "soft" catheter is used, the fluoroscope is not needed for insertion.[2,4] A patient with a fixed complete heart block usually has a transvenous pacemaker inserted. This is then replaced by a permanent pacemaker implant.[7]

The most common permanent pacemaker is the transvenous type. At the time of implantation prophylactic antibiotics are often given to reduce the risk of postoperative infection from wound contamination. Fluoroscopy is needed for placement of the lead. A pacing system analyzer and ECG are also needed. Resuscitative equipment including a defibrillator must be available.[18] Under local anesthesia, a 4 to 5 cm incision is made in the chest wall just below the clavicle. The cephalic vein is isolated and a small incision is made in it. A catheter introducer is used to insert the pacing lead with stylet into the vein. The pacing lead is then passed into the subclavian vein and on to the right atrium. The tip of the lead is passed across the tricuspid valve and positioned at the apex of the right ventricle. The stylet is retracted 2 to 3 cm, and the electrode remains at the apex. Lead fixation devices are then activated.

Lead testing is performed to determine the optimal electrode stimulation and sensing site. The R wave size, slow rate (maximum rate of voltage change), stimulation threshold, pacing threshold, and impedance are measured. A small lithium pulse generator is then implanted in the subclavicular area. In this site it is accessible for magnet testing and reprogramming. The indifferent plate of a unipolar system is placed against the subcutaneous tissues to avoid muscle stimulation. Immediate postoperative care includes ECG monitoring for 24 hours, a 12-lead ECG recording, and discharge of the patient (usually on the next day). The patient needs regular checkups in a pacemaker clinic if possible. Routine ECGs are obtained to document function. Electric testing is done to determine repetition rate and pulse duration. Changes in the repetition rate and pulse duration are indicators of impending power source depletion. Telemetry is often used with dual chamber pacemakers. Patients with syncope, dizziness, or palpitations may be monitored with a Holter ambulatory system.[18]

Chung[4] reports that only 5% to 6% of patients who have transvenous pacemakers implanted develop a problem with infection. The mortality rate is low, about 2%. Endocarditis is uncommon but can occur. Most of the infections with pacemakers, however, involve the local area around the generator, which is remote from the heart. Infections involving the electrode catheter can lead to endocarditis.

IMPLANTATION OF A CARDIOVERTER-DEFIBRILLATOR

Patients with ventricular fibrillation or unstable ventricular tachycardias require a strong electric countershock to the heart to prevent death. An automatic implantable cardioverter-defibrillator (AICD) is available for use in patients with ventricular arrhythmias. This is a self-contained diagnostic-therapeutic system that monitors the heart and delivers the correct electric shock to restore normal rhythm when fibrillation or tachycardia of the ventricle is detected.[16]

The AICD Ventak weighs 250 g and is 148 cm^3 in size, with a 5-year monitoring life or 100 discharges. It has two pairs of electrodes. One serves as an epicardial patch electrode. The other is an epicardial screw-in electrode for rate determination and to synchronize R-wave signals. By 1987 over 2500 AICD units had been placed in patients who had survived arrhythmic arrest or had a history of ventricular fibrillation or ventricular tachycardia not controlled by antiarrhythmic therapy.[16]

The AICD unit is placed through a subxiphoidal approach or thoracotomy and implanted subcutaneously in the left paraumbilical pocket. It is 99% reliable in detecting ventricular tachycardias. The conversion effectiveness is excellent, and one 25-joule discharge usually works.[16]

Surgical complications and other risks with the AICD include infection, thromboembolism, lead dislodgement or fracture, battery depletion, and component failure. Patients selected

for implantation would have a 27% to 66% chance of death in 1 year without it. The death rate for those with it is less than 2%.[16]

HEART TRANSPLANTATION

Transplantation of organs presents a number of problems related to graft rejection and immunosuppressive therapy that are independent of the organ being transplanted. Because of these common problems, heart transplantation is discussed in Chapter 26.

DENTAL MANAGEMENT
MEDICAL CONSIDERATIONS

Patients who have had surgical procedures to correct cardiac or vascular defects are left with varying degrees of susceptibility to endocarditis and endarteritis—depending on the location of the surgery, the material used for the correction or replacement, and in some cases the length of time since surgery.

Experimental work with dogs has shown that cardiac and arterial grafts made of Dacron that become completely covered by repair tissue (endocardium or endothelium) are not susceptible to endocarditis or endarteritis once this has occurred. However, a significant number of Dacron grafts never become completely covered, and small defects remain that are susceptible to endocarditis or endarteritis.[19] By contrast, procedures that use autogenous tissues to close or replace the defect remain susceptible to endocarditis only until healing has occurred at the surgical site.

Prosthetic valve replacements are susceptible to infective endocarditis (IE) or prosthetic valve endocarditis (PVE), because they are attached to surrounding cardiac tissues by numerous nonabsorbable sutures. Thus the site of attachment remains susceptible to infection from transient bacteremias. The incidence of PVE is about the same for mechanical valves and tissue valves.

In general, tissue valves have a low thromboembolism rate and only moderate durability. They last about 7 years in young adults and 10 years in older patients.[8,10,23,24] Anticoagulants usually are not needed in patients with tissue valves and normal sinus rhythm. By contrast, mechanical valves have a higher thromboembolism rate and much longer durability.[8,10,23-25] Patients with mechanical valves usually require long-term anticoagulation therapy. Mechanical valves are usually selected for young individuals because of their excellent long-term durability.

The 5-year survival rate for patients with mechanical heart valves (Starr-Edwards) is now about 85%. The 5-year embolus-free rate for mechanical valves is 96% for mitral valve replacements and 85% for aortic valve replacements.[8,10,29] (See Table 5-2.)

When mechanical valves fail, the results are usually sudden and catastrophic. Failure of tissue valves, on the other hand, is a much slower process, with clinical deterioration occurring over an extended period. This reduces the risk for reoperation to replace a failing tissue valve.[8,23,24,25]

Each of the surgical procedures discussed in this chapter will be reviewed concerning its degree of susceptibility to infection from transient dental bacteremias and the type of antibiotic coverage that would best protect the patient from developing endocarditis or endarteritis.

Surgically closed septal defect

The type of septal defect and the material used to close it must be determined by medical consultation. Small septal defects closed by absorbable sutures are susceptible to endocarditis only during the immediate postoperative period. Once healing has occurred, the patient who had a septal defect closed by absorbable sutures is no longer susceptible to endocarditis and does not require antibiotic coverage for dental treatment. The patient with a septal defect that has been repaired by a patch of autogenous pericardial tissue also is susceptible to endocarditis only during the immediate postoperative period. Once healing has occurred, this individual is no longer considered susceptible to the disease.

Although healing usually is complete in 1 to 3 weeks, the patient is given antibiotic prophylaxis for any dental treatment received during the first 6 months after surgery. This practice is recommended by the American Heart Association.[3] The AHA also recommends the standard oral amoxicillin regimen for these patients.[3] Patients who are allergic to amoxicillin can be given either erythromycin or clinamycin (Tables 5-3 to 5-5). We prefer clindamycin because it comes in only one form and is better tolerated by most patients.

TABLE 5–3
American Heart Association Recommended Standard Prophylactic Regimen for Dental Procedures*

Adults	Amoxicillin 3 g orally 1 hour before procedure, then 1.5 g 6 hours after initial dose
Children*	Amoxicillin 50 mg/kg orally 1 hour before procedure, then half initial dose 6 hours later

or

Children less than 15 kg (33 lb): initial dose, 750 mg amoxicillin
Children 15 to 30 kg (33 to 66 lb): initial dose, 1500 mg amoxicillin
Children over 30 kg (66 lb): initial dose, 3000 mg amoxicillin
Given 1 hour before procedure followed 6 hours later with half initial dose

*Used in all at-risk patients, including those with prosthetic heart valves. Children's doses should not exceed adult doses. From *JAMA* 264:22, 1990 (with permission of the AHA and the AMA). Copyright 1990, American Medical Association.

TABLE 5–4
American Heart Association Recommended Standard Prophylactic Regimen for Dental Procedures in Patients Allergic to Amoxicillin and Penicillin or Who Are on Long-Term Penicillin Therapy for Rheumatic Fever Prevention

Adults	Erythromycin ethylsuccinate 800 mg

or

Erythromycin stearate 1 g orally 2 hours before procedure, then half dose 6 hours after initial dose

Children*	Erythromycin ethylsuccinate or stearate 20 mg/kg 1 hour before procedure, then half dose 6 hours after initial dose

*Children's doses should not exceed adult doses. From *JAMA* 264:22, 1990 (with permission of the AHA and the AMA). Copyright 1990, American Medical Association.

TABLE 5–5
American Heart Association Recommended Standard Prophylactic Regimen for Dental Procedures in Patients Allergic to Penicillin and Intolerant of Erythromycin (Can Also Be Used in Patients Allergic Only to Penicillin)

Adults	Clindamycin 300 mg 1 hour before procedure, then 150 mg 6 hours after initial dose
Children*	Clindamycin 30 mg/kg 1 hour before procedure, then half dose 6 hours after initial dose

*Children's doses should not exceed adult doses.
From *JAMA* 264:22, 1990 (with permission of the AHA and the AMA). Copyright 1990, American Medical Association.

The patient who has had a septal defect closed with a Dacron patch is considered susceptible to endocarditis during the immediate postoperative period and remains potentially susceptible thereafter because of incomplete coverage of the Dacron patch by endocardial tissues. The AHA advises prophylaxis during the 6-month postoperative period for invasive dental procedures. The regimens shown in Tables 5-3 to 5-5 are recommended.[3] The AHA[3] has also stated that the evidence for prophylaxis after the 6-month healing period is inconclusive, and hence the need for continued prophylaxis should be determined by medical consultation.

Ligated or resected ductus arteriosus

The patient with a surgically corrected ductus arteriosus remains susceptible to endarteritis during the immediate postoperative period (i.e., for the first 6 months after surgery) and should receive antibiotic coverage by the standard AHA regimen (Tables 5-3 to 5-5) during any dental treatment. After the 6-month postoperative period this individual is no longer considered susceptible to endarteritis and is not given antibiotic prophylaxis when receiving dental treatment.

The patient whose patent ductus arteriosus was closed by sutures will be given a standard regimen (Tables 5-3 to 5-5) for the 6 months after surgery when receiving any dental treat-

ment. After that time, no coverage is indicated. In rare cases the ductus may become patent again because of defective sutures, etc. If this occurs, the patient becomes susceptible to endarteritis again. Thus it is important to determine by medical consultation the method used to correct the ductus arteriosus, the patient's current status, and the need for antibiotic prophylaxis.

Commissurotomy for diseased cardiac valve(s)

The patient who has had either an open or a closed commissurotomy to improve cardiac valvular function remains susceptible to endocarditis and should be given the standard regimen (Tables 5-3 to 5-5) before and after all dental procedures. The dentist is advised to consult with the patient's physician whenever possible before rendering dental care.

Prosthetic replacement of diseased cardiac valve(s)

Table 5-2 shows the operative mortality and 5-year survival rates for patients with prosthetic heart valves.[10] The incidence of PVE is 0.5% to 1.3%, with an average among the various reports of about 1% (expressed as percent per patient year).[8,27] There is no relationship of PVE to valve type or design. The mortality rate for PVE ranges from 38% to 88%.[8,27]

A number of articles have demonstrated the problems with PVE in patients with prosthetic heart valves.

Wilson[30] reported on 4586 patients in whom 4706 prosthetic valves had been placed. In this series 45 cases of PVE occurred, representing an incidence of 0.98%. PVE was described as either early or late. The early cases occurred within 2 months of surgical implantation of the prosthetic valve and had an 88% mortality rate (14 of 16 patients). Early PVE is thought to be caused by contamination at the time of surgery. Late PVE occurred 2 months or longer after surgery and had a mortality rate of 38% (11 of 29 patients). Late cases of PVE are thought to be caused by transient bacteremias. One late case of PVE followed dental manipulation; others followed urinary tract infections, wound infections, surgical procedures, and trauma. In 22 cases no apparent portal of entry for the infecting agent was identified. The overall mortality rate of this group (early and late PVE) was 56% (25 of 45 patients).

Karchmer et al.[13] reported on 43 cases of late PVE in which the mortality rate was 53% (23 of 43 patients). Nine patients had had dental procedures performed before the onset of PVE symptoms. In addition, two patients had had severe periodontal disease. Thus a total of 11 patients may have had a dental cause for their PVE. The authors reported that three of the nine patients who received dental treatment before the onset of PVE had been given prophylactic antibiotics, but the drug or dosage was not described.

Dismukes[5] reported on 38 cases of PVE, 19 early and 19 late, with an overall mortality rate of 50%. Four patients with late PVE appeared to have an associated dental cause, and one of these patients had received prophylactic antibiotics.

These reports show that (1) PVE is associated with a significant mortality and (2) dental procedures may serve as a source of infection. A patient with a prosthetic heart valve(s) must be given antibiotic coverage before and after all dental procedures. The coverage recommended by the American Heart Association[3] now is the standard oral amoxicillin regimen (Table 5-3) or, in cases of allergy to amoxicillin, the oral clindamycin regimen shown in Table 5-5. Patients with significant periodontal disease may still be best protected by using the special oral-parenteral regimen shown in Table 5-6. The AHA[3] leaves the special oral-parenteral regimen as an option available to dentists. It should be noted that any patient unable to take oral medication, such as a patient being prepared for general anesthesia, should be given the special AHA regimen shown in Table 5-7.

Ideally, a patient who is going to receive a prosthetic heart valve should have all indicated dental treatment performed before the valve is placed. Whenever possible, the patient's physician should be consulted prior to any dental treatment.

Coronary artery bypass graft

Except for the immediate postoperative period, CABG patients do not appear to be susceptible to endarteritis[19] and therefore require no prophylactic antibiotic coverage for dental procedures. One of the standard regi-

TABLE 5–6

Alternate Prophylactic Regimens for High-Risk Patients for Whom the Practitioner Desires to Use a Parenteral Regimen*

Ampicillin 2 g, IV or IM, plus gentamicin 1.5 mg/kg, IV or IM (not to exceed 80 mg), ½ hour before procedure, followed by 1.5 g oral amoxicillin 6 hours after initial dose; alternatively, parenteral regimen may be repeated 8 hours after initial dose

Allergic to Penicillin

Vancomycin 1 g, IV administered over 1 hour, starting 1 hour before procedure; no repeat dose is necessary

*Initial pediatric dosages. Follow-up oral doses should be half initial dose. Total pediatric dose should not exceed total adult dose.
  Ampicillin, 50 mg/kg
  Gentamicin, 2 mg/kg
  Vancomycin, 20 mg/kg
  Follow-up dose for amoxicillin, 25 mg/kg
From *JAMA* 264:22, 1990 (with permission of the AHA and the AMA). Copyright 1990, American Medical Association.

TABLE 5–7

Alternate Prophylactic Regimen for Patients Given General Anesthesia for Oral Surgical or Dental Procedures or Who Are Unable to Take Oral Medications*

Ampicillin 2 g, IV or IM, 30 minutes before procedure, then 1.5 g amoxicillin 6 hours after initial dose if the patient is awake and stable; if patient is unable to take oral medication, then 1 g ampicillin IV or IM 6 hours after initial dose

Allergic to penicillin

Clindamycin 300 mg, IV, 30 minutes before the procedure and 150 mg orally 6 hours after initial dose; if patient still is unable to take oral medication, then 150 mg clindamycin IV 6 hours after initial dose

*Pediatric dosages. Follow-up oral doses should be half initial dose. Total pediatric dose should not exceed total adult dose:
  Ampicillin, 50 mg/kg
  Clindamycin, 10 mg/kg
From *JAMA* 264:22, 1990 (with permission of the AHA and the AMA). Copyright 1990, American Medical Association.

mens (Tables 5-3 to 5-5) is recommended when dental treatment must be done during the immediate postoperative period. The patient's current cardiac status and the need for prophylactic antibiotics should be established through consultation with the patient's physician before any dental treatment is performed.

Arterial graft

From 1963 to 1974, 859 vascular grafts were placed in patients at the Virginia Medical Center.[14] There were 22 cases of graft infection (2.5%). A review of the literature by Liekweg et al.[15] showed 153 cases of graft infection, which represented an incidence of infection ranging from 0.25% to 6%. There were 52 deaths (a 34% mortality rate). The longest interval from implantation to symptoms of infection was 87 months, with a mean of 27 weeks. Synthetic grafts appeared to be much more susceptible to infection than autogenous grafts.

The AHA[3] has stated that the evidence regarding the need for prophylaxis in this group of patients is inconclusive. It therefore suggests that the decision to use prophylaxis be made on an individual patient basis, in consultation with the patient's physician. We suggest prophylaxis for invasive dental procedures in patients less than 6 months postoperative. The standard regimen shown in Tables 5-3 to 5-5 should be used. We also suggest that after 6 months patients with autogenous grafts not be covered.

Implantation of a transvenous pacemaker and cardioverter-defibrillator

Bryan et al.,[2] in a report on endocarditis related to transvenous pacemakers, concluded that the problem is rare and does not support the use of prophylactic antibiotic therapy during procedures that are likely to cause transient bacteremias. The 1990 AHA guidelines for endocarditis prevention[3] stated that prophylaxis is not recommended for patients with pacemakers or implanted defibrillators. If prophylaxis is recommended by the patient's physician, the new guidelines should be discussed with the physician. If the physician still wants prophylaxis to be used, one of the standard regimens in Tables 5-3 to 5-5 is recommended. (See Chapters 2 and 27.) Electrical equipment (e.g., a Cavitron, an electric vitalometer, or electric cautery) equipment should not be used on a

patient who has a cardiac pacemaker because of possible interference with the function of the pacemaker. (See Chapter 8.)

TREATMENT PLANNING MODIFICATIONS

A patient being prepared for surgery to correct a cardiac or vascular defect should be referred for an evaluation of dental status. A patient found to have active dental disease should receive dental care before surgery to correct the cardiovascular defect. This is most important for a patient who is going to receive a prosthetic heart valve. The 1990 AHA guidelines allow for the use of oral regimens in patients with prosthetic heart valves (Chapter 2). This represents a major change from the 1984 guidelines, which recommended oral-parenteral or parenteral regimens. The parenteral regimens had led to very poor dentist compliance and served as a major roadblock to patients obtaining needed dental treatment. The 1990 guidelines should lead to better dental care for patients with high-risk lesions such as prosthetic heart valves.

The basic problem faced when dental treatment is planned for a patient who is about to have or has already undergone cardiovascular surgery (especially placement of a prosthetic heart valve or heart transplant) relates to the retention of teeth when the level of dental repair is moderate to poor. A patient with advanced periodontal disease may be best advised to have his or her teeth extracted and dentures constructed. This would be most advisable for the patient with a prosthetic heart valve or transplanted heart who is allergic to penicillin. The same consideration would be involved for patients who have extensive caries and have shown little interest in improving their level of oral hygiene or diet.

Patients with good dental health should be encouraged to keep their teeth, but they must be advised of the problems involved when dental care is provided after cardiovascular surgery.

Recommendations concerning the retention of teeth for patients with a dental status that falls between the extremes of poor and good are more difficult to make. The risks involved regarding endocarditis or endarteritis, the steps needed to prevent these complications, and the costs involved must be discussed with the patient and his or her cardiovascular surgeon. Then the patient can make an informed decision based on the value he or she places on the retention of natural teeth. A patient with poor oral hygiene who has failed to become motivated to improve the level of home care should be more strongly encouraged to become edentulous and have dentures constructed.

Once an antibiotic coverage period is started, as much dental treatment as possible should be performed during this period. Under very special circumstances, such as extensive surgical procedures, the coverage may be extended to 5 to 7 days. At least 1 week should elapse after completion of a coverage period before another is started (Chapter 2).

REFERENCES

1. Boake WC, Kroncke GM: Pacemaker complications. In Varriale P, Naclerio EA, editors: *Cardiac pacing: a concise guide to clinical practice,* Philadelphia, 1979, WB Saunders, pp 229-238.
2. Bryan CS, Sutton JP, Saunders DE Jr, et al: Endocarditis related to transvenous pacemakers: syndromes and surgical implications, *J Thorac Cardiovasc Surg* 75:758-762, 1978.
3. Council of Dental Therapeutics and American Heart Association: Prevention of endocarditis: a statement for the dental professional, *J Am Dent Assoc* 122:87-92, 1991.
4. Chung EK: Complications and malfunctions of artificial cardiac pacing. In Chung EK, editor: *Artificial cardiac pacing: a practical approach,* Baltimore, 1978, Williams & Wilkins, pp 327-346.
5. Dismukes WE: Prosthetic valve endocarditis, *Circulation* 48:365-377, 1973.
6. Eleland WP: Closed mitral valvotomy. In Longmore DB, editor: *Modern cardiac surgery,* Baltimore, 1978, University Park Press, pp 45-47.
7. Feola M: Techniques of permanent pacing. In Chung EK, editor: *Artificial cardiac pacing: a practical approach,* Baltimore, 1978, Williams & Wilkins, pp 223-239.
8. Fernandez J: Surgical aspects of valve implantation. In Morse D, Steiner RM, Fernandez J, editors: *Guide to prosthetic cardiac valves,* New York, 1985, Springer-Verlag, pp 101-171.
9. Friedberg CK: *Diseases of the heart,* ed 3, vol. II, Philadelphia, 1976, WB Saunders, pp 1187-1299.
10. Guyton RA, Hatcher CR: Techniques of valvular surgery. In Hurst JW, editor: *The heart, arteries, and veins,* ed 7, New York, 1990, McGraw-Hill, pp 2200-2207.
11. Jones EL, Hatcher CR: Techniques for the surgical treatment of atherosclerotic coronary artery disease and its complications. In Hurst JW, editor, *The heart, arteries,*
and veins, ed 7, New York, 1990, McGraw-Hill, pp 2217-2223.
12. Kaplan EL: Prevention of bacterial endocarditis, *Circulation* 70:1123A-1127A, 1984.
13. Karchmer AW, Dismukes WE, Buckley MJ, Austen WG: Late prosthetic valve endocarditis, clinical features influencing therapy, *Am J Med* 64:199-206, 1977.
14. Lefrak EA, Starr A: *Cardiac valve prostheses,* New York, 1979, Appleton-Century-Crofts, pp 41-67.
15. Liekweg WG, Levinson SA, Greenfield LJ: Infections of vascular grafts: incidence, anatomic location, etiologic agents, morbidity, and mortality. In Duma RJ, editor: *Infections of prosthetic heart valves and vascular grafts: prevention, diagnosis, and treatment,* Baltimore, 1977, University Park Press, pp 239-252.
16. Mirowski M: The implantable cardioverter-defibrillator. In Hurst JW, editor: *The heart, arteries, and veins,* ed 7, New York, 1990, McGraw-Hill, pp 2110-2111.
17. Mond HG, Sloman JG: The indications for and types of artificial cardiac pacemakers. In Hurst JW, editor: *The heart, arteries, and veins,* ed 7, New York, 1990, McGraw-Hill, pp 561-580.
18. Mond HG, Strathmore NF: The technique of using cardiac pacemakers: implantation, testing, and surveillance. In Hurst JW, editor: *The heart, arteries, veins,* ed 7, New York, 1990, McGraw-Hill, pp 2100-2110.
19. Moore WS: Experimental studies relating to sepsis in prosthetic vascular grafting. In Duma RJ, editor: *Infections of prosthetic heart valves and vascular grafts: prevention, diagnosis, and treatment,* Baltimore, 1977, University Park Press, pp 267-287.
20. Moore WS: Infection in prosthetic vascular grafts. In Rutherford RB, et al, editors: *Vascular surgery,* Philadelphia, 1977, WB Saunders, pp 385-397.
21. Nugent EW, Plauth WH, Edwards JE, Williams WH: The pathology, abnormal physiology, clinical recognition, and medical and surgical treatment of congenital heart disease. In Hurst JW, editor: *The heart, arteries, and veins,* ed 7, New York, 1990, McGraw-Hill, pp 655-794.
22. Perloff JK: Congenital heart disease. In Beeson PB, et al, editors: *Cecil textbook of medicine,* ed 15, Philadelphia, 1979, WB Saunders, pp 1149-1172.
23. Rackley CE, Edwards JE, Karp RB: Mitral valve disease. In Hurst JW, editor: *The heart, arteries, and veins,* ed 7, New York, 1990, McGraw-Hill, pp 820-851.
24. Rackley CF, Edwards JE, Wallace RB, Katz NM: Aortic valve disease. In Hurst JW, editor: *The heart, arteries, and veins,* ed 7, New York, 1990, McGraw-Hill, pp 795-819.
25. Rackley CE, Katz NM, Wallace RB: Artificial valve disease. In Hurst JW, editor: *The heart, arteries, and veins,* ed 7, New York, 1990, McGraw-Hill, pp 871-876.
26. Rosenthal A: When to operate on congenital heart disease. In Chung EK, editor: *Controversy in cardiology: the practical clinical approach,* New York, 1976, Springer-Verlag, pp 136-152.

27. Schoen FJ: Pathology of cardiac valve replacement. In Morse D, Steiner RM, Fernandez J, editors: *Guide to prosthetic cardiac valves,* New York, 1985, Springer-Verlag, pp 209-232.

28. Szarnicki RJ: Results of patent ductus arteriosus ligation in infants and children. In Longmore DB, editor: *Modern cardiac surgery,* Baltimore, 1978, University Park Press, pp 163-167.

29. Szilagyi DE: Antibiotic prophylaxis in vascular grafting. In Duma RJ, editor: *Infections of prosthetic heart valves and vascular grafts: prevention, diagnosis, and treatment,* Baltimore, 1977, University Park Press, pp 323-342.

30. Wilson WR: Prosthetic valve endocarditis: incidence, anatomic location, cause, morbidity, and mortality. In Duma RJ, editor: *Infections of prosthetic heart valves and vascular grafts: prevention, diagnosis, and treatment,* Baltimore, 1977, University Park Press, pp 3-17.

6

Hypertension

Hypertension is an abnormal elevation of arterial pressure that, if sustained and untreated, is associated with a significant increase in morbidity and mortality. Hypertension may remain an asymptomatic disease for long periods but ultimately leads to damage, with resultant symptoms, in several organs—including kidneys, heart, brain, and eyes. It is generally accepted that a sustained diastolic blood pressure of 90 mm Hg or greater is abnormal, as is a sustained systolic blood pressure of 160 or greater. Table 6-1 is a classification of hypertension in adults, and Table 6-2 is a classification of hypertension in children.

Most diagnostic and treatment decisions are based on diastolic pressures for two reasons[3,17]: (1) diastolic hypertension is fundamentally related to enhanced peripheral vascular resistance whereas systolic hypertension reflects increased cardiac output and/or large vessel stiffness and (2) the treatment of systolic hypertension is not clearly associated with a reduction of cardiovascular complications whereas the control of diastolic hypertension in older as well as younger patients results in clinical benefit.

Although the diagnosis of hypertension is rather straightforward, the decision of when to initiate treatment, especially in mild hypertension, is frequently unclear. Treatment decisions are made on an individual basis and take into consideration such factors as the absolute value of the blood pressure, physical and laboratory findings, family history, race, diet, life-style, age, and patient reliability. Generally speaking, the closer to normal the blood pressure is maintained the lower will be the morbidity and mortality.

The dentist can play a significant role in the detection of hypertension and in monitoring effective control. If a patient is unaware of his or her condition, the dentist may be the first to detect an elevation of blood pressure or symptoms of hypertensive disease or both. In addition, a patient who is aware of his or her condition and may be receiving treatment often may not be adequately controlled, because of poor compliance or inappropriate selection of drug therapy, in which case the dentist can provide a valuable monitoring service. It should be noted that the Joint National Committee on Detection, Evaluation, and Treatment of High Blood Pressure[15] specifically encourages the active participation of health care professionals in the detection of hypertension and the surveillance of treatment compliance. The diagnosis of hypertension and treatment decisions are made only by the physician; however, the dentist should and must make determinations of abnormal readings, which then become the basis for referral.

The dental patient with hypertension poses some significant management considerations. These considerations include identification, monitoring, stress and anxiety reduction, avoidance of drug interactions, and management of drug effects on the oral tissues. The remainder of this chapter addresses these concerns.

GENERAL DESCRIPTION
INCIDENCE AND PREVALENCE

It is currently estimated that as many as 58 million people in the United States have hypertension. Most adults now are aware of their blood pressure or have had it measured, thanks to the success of nationwide education and screening programs.[15] In one white, suburban

TABLE 6–1
Classification of Hypertension in Adults

Range (mm Hg)	Category
Diastolic	
<85	Normal blood pressure
85 to 89	High normal blood pressure
90 to 104	Mild hypertension
105 to 114	Moderate hypertension
≥115	Severe hypertension
Systolic (when diastolic is <90)	
<140	Normal blood pressure
140 to 159	Borderline isolated systolic hypertension
≥160	Isolated systolic hypertension

From Joint National Committee on Detection, Evaluation, and Treatment of High Blood Pressure. *NIH Publication* 84-1088, June 1984.

TABLE 6–2
Classification of Significant Hypertension in Children (95th percentile for age)

Systolic and diastolic blood pressures	
Age (yr)	Pressure (mm Hg)
3 to 5	≥116/76
6 to 9	≥122/78
10 to 12	≥126/82
13 to 15	≥136/86
16 to 18	≥142/92

From Second Task Force on Blood Pressure Control in Children. *Pediatrics* 79:1–25, 1987.

population (Framingham, Massachusetts)[19] a fifth of the adults were found to have blood pressure above 160/95 and almost half to have a blood pressure above 140/90. In a random nationwide screening of approximately 160,000 people in 14 different communities as part of the Hypertension Detection and Follow-up Program,[7,8] 10,940 individuals were found to be hypertensive (7%). Mild hypertension (diastolic pressure less than 105) was found in 71% of these persons and moderate to severe hypertension in 28.5%.[7,8]

A similar hypertension detection project was undertaken by dentists in Bergen County, New Jersey.[1] During the project, 1071 adult dental patients were screened for hypertension. Of these, 126 (12%) were found to have sustained hypertension; 68 of these patients knew of their condition, and 58 were unaware of the problem. Of the 58 patients who had possible hypertensive disease, 7 were lost to follow-up. Of the remaining 51 patients, 44 had hypertensive disease and were placed under medical treatment.[1]

About 5% of individuals with hypertension have an associated underlying condition that explains the presence of the hypertension. This form of hypertension is called *secondary hypertension.* The other 95% of the people with hypertension have what is termed *essential hypertension,* the exact cause of which is undetermined.[15,19]

The prevalence rate for hypertension increases with age; however, it occurs earlier in a higher percentage of blacks than whites. The incidence of hypertension in American blacks is significantly higher than in whites. Women develop hypertension slightly more commonly than men but appear to tolerate it better.[3a,8,19]

ETIOLOGY

As stated earlier, the vast majority of patients with hypertension have no cause established for their disease (essential hypertension). The small remainder of patients have an underlying systemic disease that produces hypertension as a secondary complication (secondary hypertension). The majority of conditions that cause secondary hypertension lead to an elevation of both diastolic and systolic blood pressure. These conditions include renal disease, endocrine disorders, and neurogenic problems. A few systemic conditions result only in an increase of the systolic blood pressure, including aortic regurgitation, thyrotoxicosis, arteriovenous fistula, and patent ductus arteriosus.[15,19]

Patients who have secondary hypertension resulting from unilateral renal disease such as renal artery obstruction or pyelonephritis can, once detected, be cured of the hypertension by surgical correction of the defect or removal of the diseased kidney. In a few patients with secondary hypertension, a tumor of the adrenal medulla (pheochromocytoma) has been found to be responsible. This lesion is surgically treatable. Hyperfunction of the adrenal gland caused by a tumor of the adrenal cortex or by cortical hyperplasia may cause secondary hypertension in a few cases. These conditions also are surgically treatable. Weight gain has been demonstrated[3a] to cause an increase in blood pressure. The most common cause of secondary hypertension is oral contraceptives.[19]

PATHOPHYSIOLOGY AND COMPLICATIONS

Blood pressure is measured by the use of a sphygmomanometer, an instrument that indirectly records the diastolic and systolic pressures (Fig. 6-1). The diastolic pressure represents the total resting resistance in the arterial system following passage of the pulsating force produced by contraction of the left ventricle. The pulsating force is modified by the degree of elasticity of the walls of larger arteries and the resistance of the arteriolar bed. The pressure at the peak of ventricular contraction is the systolic blood pressure. The difference between the diastolic and systolic pressures is termed *pulse pressure.*

Many factors may transiently alter the blood pressure. Increased viscosity of the blood can cause an elevation of blood pressure as a result of an increase in the resistance to flow. A decrease in blood volume or tissue fluid volume will reduce blood pressure, and an increase in blood volume or tissue fluid volume will increase blood pressure. Increased cardiac output associated with exercise, fever, and thyrotoxicosis will increase the blood pressure.

In sustained hypertension, however, the basic underlying defect is a failure in the regulation of vascular resistance. Control of vascular resistance is multifactorial, and abnormalities may exist in one or more areas. Mechanisms of control include neural reflexes and ongoing maintenance of sympathetic vasomotor tone, neurotransmitters (e.g., norepinephrine), extracellular fluid and sodium stores, the renin-angiotensin-aldosterone pressor system, and locally active hormones and substances such as prostaglandins, kinins, adenosine, and hydrogen ions. In isolated systolic hypertension, commonly seen in the elderly, the underlying defect is loss of elasticity of the aorta.[15,17]

Blood pressure increases normally with age, from under 110/75 in children less than 6 years of age to 140/90 in adults (Tables 6-1 and 6-2). A sustained blood pressure in excess of 140/90 in adults is considered abnormal. In about one third of the population a transient period of increased blood pressure may occur in early adulthood. On an individual basis such increases may be of little significance, but data based on large numbers of people indicate that occasional rises in the resting blood pressure are associated with shortening of the life span. Untreated sustained elevations in blood pressure carry an even greater risk in terms of shortening the life span. This is true for systolic as well as diastolic pressures.[18,19]

It has been estimated[15,17,19] that untreated hypertension reduces the life span by 10 to 20 years. Even mild hypertension that has not been treated for 7 to 10 years increases the risk of complications such as stroke and heart attack.

Sustained hypertension eventually results in arterial damage and in multiple complications—including renal failure, cerebrovascular accident, coronary insufficiency, myocardial infarction, congestive heart failure, and blindness. Hypertension precedes the onset of vascular changes in the kidney, heart, brain, and retina that then lead to these clinical complications.

About 1% of hypertensives develop malignant hypertension, which is a medical emergency and is characterized by severe blood

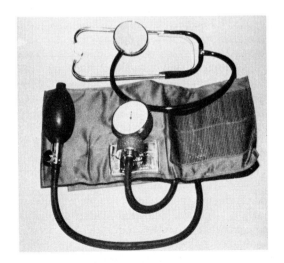

FIG. 6-1 Standard sphygmomanometer and stethoscope.

pressure elevation, papilledema, retinal hemorrhages, exudates, and frequently encephalopathy. This condition requires immediate medical treatment.[19]

CLINICAL PRESENTATION
SIGNS AND SYMPTOMS

Most cases of essential hypertension follow a chronic course. Elevated blood pressure measurements may be the only sign present for a number of years. Patients with intermittently elevated blood pressure are said to have labile hypertension. Isolated diastolic hypertension is very rare, and when it occurs it is found in children or young adults. Isolated systolic hypertension is generally found in older patients.[3,15] The patient with hypertension is usually asymptomatic at first and is unaware of any problem. The "early" symptoms of hypertension are occipital headache, vision changes, ringing ears, dizziness, and weakness and tingling of the hands and feet.[19] If there is significant kidney, brain, heart, or eye involvement, there will be other signs and symptoms related to these organ systems (Table 6-3).

Funduscopic examination of the eyes may show early changes of hypertension consisting of hemorrhages, narrowed arterioles, exudate, and in more advanced cases papilledema. Also in more advanced cases, the left ventricle may be enlarged and a tapping left ventricular apical beat can often be observed in thin individuals.

TABLE 6–3
Signs and Symptoms of Hypertensive Disease

Signs	Symptoms
Early	Occipital headache
Increased blood pressure	Failing vision
Narrowing of retinal	Ringing ears
arterioles	(tinnitus)
Retinal hemorrhages	Dizziness
Advanced	Weakness
Papilledema	Tingling of hands and
Cardiac enlargement—	feet
left ventricle	(paresthesias)
Hematuria	Congestive heart
Proteinuria	failure
	Angina pectoris
	Renal failure

Renal involvement can result in hematuria, proteinuria, and renal failure. Hypertensive persons may complain of fatigue and coldness of the legs as a result of peripheral artery changes that occur in advanced hypertension.[19]

These findings may be seen in patients who have essential hypertension as well as in patients who have secondary hypertension. However, additional signs or symptoms may be present in secondary hypertension that are associated with the underlying disease.

LABORATORY FINDINGS

The 1988 report of the Joint National Committee on Detection, Evaluation, and Treatment of High Blood Pressure[15] recommended that patients who have sustained hypertension be screened with hemoglobin, hematocrit, urinalysis, serum potassium, calcium, creatinine, plasma cholesterol, plasma glucose, and serum uric acid. An electrocardiogram also was suggested. These tests serve as the baseline laboratory values that should be obtained before initiating therapy. If clinical and laboratory findings suggest the presence of an underlying cause for the hypertension, then additional tests should be ordered.

MEDICAL MANAGEMENT

The management of a patient with hypertension necessarily begins with detection. Since hypertension is generally asymptomatic for many years, the only sign of trouble may be an elevated blood pressure. Since most adults with hypertension are already aware of it, the Joint National Committee on Detection, Evaluation, and Treatment of High Blood Pressure[15] recommends that efforts be directed toward maintenance and surveillance in known hypertensives and in high-risk groups (blacks, obese individuals, blood relatives of hypertensives).

Measurement of blood pressure should be accomplished in a standard manner with a relaxed patient. (See Chapter 1.) If the blood pressure is elevated, the dentist should tell the patient the numeric value of the blood pressure, that it is abnormal, and that further evaluation by a physician may be required. The dentist should not make a diagnosis of hypertension.

When referral to a physician occurs, a medical history is obtained including family history, identification of risk factors, associated disorders, and history of known hypertension and its treatment.

A thorough physical examination is performed, with particular emphasis on identification of causes of secondary hypertension and for evidence of target organ changes from hypertension (eyes, kidneys, brain, heart). Included in this evaluation are a few simple laboratory tests previously mentioned. Additional tests may be warranted based on clinical judgment. For example, many physicians now advocate the use of continuous 24-hour monitoring of blood pressure for definitive diagnosis.

There is not agreement among physicians on when to treat varying degrees of hypertension.

Factors *favoring* early medical treatment of patients with essential hypertension include the following[15,17,19]: a minimal elevation of either systolic or diastolic blood pressure increases morbidity and mortality; labile hypertension is associated with an increase in morbidity and mortality; and effective drugs with minimal side effects are now available to treat hypertension. Also, some data suggest that early treatment decreases the incidence of vascular complications and increases longevity. Adequate therapy also may reverse cardiac and retinal changes. The incidence of death from heart failure secondary to hypertension has been reported to be greatly decreased since the advent of drug therapy for hypertension.[15,17,19]

Factors *contraindicating* early treatment of patients with essential hypertension include the following[15,17,19]: drugs are expensive and produce a financial burden on patients; some of the drugs have significant side effects; when severe renal damage is present, therapy is difficult and less effective and may be dangerous; and if significant cerebral or coronary artery disease is present, therapy may be dangerous because of a decrease in perfusion pressure and a reduction in arterial flow.[15,17,19]

The ultimate decision to begin treatment is made on an individual basis between the physician and patient and is based upon the absolute blood pressure value and the presence of risk factors and physical complications. If the decision to begin treatment is made, nonpharmacologic measures are generally begun first

that may be definitive in and of themselves or may be used in addition to drug therapy. The goal of antihypertensive therapy is to achieve and maintain the diastolic blood pressure at or lower than 90 mm Hg if feasible.

Nonpharmacologic measures include weight loss for obese patients, restriction of dietary sodium, moderation of alcohol intake, reduction of dietary saturated fats and cholesterol, avoidance of smoking, encouragement of regular aerobic exercise, and initiation of relaxation therapy and stress reduction.[15] These measures alone may prove to be effective in the control of high normal and mild hypertension for long periods. However, moderate and severe hypertension almost always will require additional drug therapy to effectively decrease the blood pressure.

Isolated systolic hypertension in middle-aged and older patients is usually due to atherosclerosis of the aorta and its major branches; however, due to a paucity of definitive data, categorical recommendations for drug therapy cannot be made at this time.[3] Although controversy exists regarding initiation of the pharmacologic treatment for diastolic blood pressure between 90 and 94 mm Hg, for diastolic blood pressure of 95 mm Hg and above the benefits of drug therapy far outweigh the risks. When drug therapy does become necessary to control hypertension, drugs are usually chosen and administered according to a stepped-care approach as suggested by the Joint National Committee on Detection, Evaluation, and Treatment of High Blood Pressure.[15] The stepped-care approach begins by initiating therapy with a small dosage of an antihypertensive drug, increasing the dosage of that drug, and then adding or substituting one drug after another in gradually increasing doses as needed until the goal blood pressure is reached, side effects become intolerable, or the maximum dose of each drug is reached.[15] Once drug therapy becomes necessary, it usually must continue for the rest of the patient's life. Table 6-4 is a list of commonly used antihypertensive agents with their usual dosage ranges.

The Joint National Committee[15] has made the following recommendations concerning the choice and sequencing of stepped-care pharmacologic management of hypertension:

Step 1. Initial therapy is begun with a di-

TABLE 6–4
Antihypertensive Agents—Usual Dosage Ranges

Type of drug	Dosage range, mg per day	
	Minimum	Maximum
Diuretics		
Thiazides and related sulfonamide diuretics		
Bendroflumethiazide	2.5	5
Benzthiazide	12.5 to 25.0	50
Chlorothiazide	125.0 to 250.0	500
Chlorthalidone	12.5 to 25.0	50
Cyclothiazide	1.0	2
Hydrochlorothiazide	12.5 to 25.0	50
Hydroflumethiazide	12.5 to 25.0	50
Indapamide	2.5	5
Methyclothiazide	2.5	5
Metolazone	1.25	10
Polythiazide	2.0	4
Quinethazone	25.0	100
Trichlormethiazide	1.0 to 2.0	4
Loop diuretics		
Bumetanide	0.5	5
Ethacrynic acid	25.0	100
Furosemide	20.0 to 40.0	320
Potassium-sparing agents		
Amiloride	5.0	10
Spironolactone	25.0	100
Triamterene	50.0	150
Adrenergic inhibitors		
Beta-adrenergic blockers		
Acebutolol	200.0	1200
Atenolol	25.0	150
Metoprolol	50.0	200
Nadolol	40.0	320
Penbutolol sulfate	20.0	80
Pindolol	10.0	60
Propranolol hydrochloride	40.0	320
Propranolol, long acting (LA)	60.0	320
Timolol maleate	20.0	80
Central adrenergic inhibitors		
Clonidine	0.1	1.2
Clonidine transdermal therapeutic system (TTS)	0.1	0.3
Guanabenz	4.0	64
Methyldopa	250.0	2000
Peripheral adrenergic antagolists		
Guanadrel sulfate	10.0	100
Guanethidine monosulfate	10.0	150
Rauwolfia alkaloids		
Rauwolfia (whole root)	50.0	100
Reserpine	0.1	0.25

TABLE 6–4

Antihypertensive Agents — Usual Dosage Ranges — cont'd

Type of drug	Dosage range, mg per day	
	Minimum	Maximum
Alpha₁–adrenergic blockers		
Prazosin hydrochloride	1.0 to 2.0	20
Combined alpha– and beta–adrenergic blockers		
Labetalol hydrochloride	200.0	1800
Vasodilators		
Hydralazine hydrochloride	50.0	300
Minoxidil	2.5	80
Angiotensin-converting enzyme inhibitors		
Captopril	25.0 to 50.0	300
Enalapril maleate	2.5 to 5.0	40
Calcium Antagonists		
Diltiazem hydrochloride	60.0	360
Nifedipine	30.0	180
Nitrendipine	5.0	40
Verapamil	120.0	480
Verapamil SR	120.0	480

From Joint National Committee. *Arch Intern Med* 148:1023–1037, 1988.

uretic, beta–adrenergic blocking agent, angiotensin-converting enzyme (ACE) inhibitor, or calcium antagonist.

Step 2. After 1 to 3 months, if control has not been achieved, one of three options is recommended: increase the dose of the first drug; add an agent from a different class; or discontinue the first drug and substitute a drug from another class.

Step 3. If control has not been achieved, either add a third drug from a different class or discontinue the second drug and substitute another drug from a different class.

Step 4. If control has not been achieved, add a third or fourth drug from a different class or refer the patient for further evaluation.

Since lack of compliance is the single greatest problem in treating patients with hypertension, it is extremely important that patients be monitored periodically. Health care professionals are strongly encouraged to measure the blood pressure at each patient visit.

DENTAL MANAGEMENT
MEDICAL CONSIDERATIONS

It is important to identify the patient with severe undiagnosed or uncontrolled hypertension before starting dental treatment. The stress and anxiety associated with dental procedures potentially may raise a patient's already elevated blood pressure to dangerous levels and result in a cerebrovascular accident or myocardial infarction. In addition, the dentist may use an excessive amount of local anesthetic containing a vasoconstrictor, which can result in a significant rise in blood pressure. The dentist also may use a vasoconstrictor to control gingival bleeding or to retract gingival tissues in preparation for taking impressions. These procedures can result in a significant elevation of the blood pressure, which in an undetected or uncontrolled hypertensive patient could be life threatening.

The first task of the dentist is to identify, through history and measurement of blood pressure, those patients who may qualify as

History
    Past diagnosis of hypertension
    Signs and symptoms (Table 6–3)
    Medications
        Physicians' Desk Reference
        Drug Information for the Health Care
           Professional
        Physician, pharmacist
Blood pressure measurement
    Baseline for emergency management
    Screen for hypertensive disease
    Medicolegal necessity

hypertensive (Table 6-5). A complete medical history should be obtained from each patient. (See Chapter 1.) Included in the history are questions concerning the presence of signs or symptoms associated with hypertension or its sequelae. Many known hypertensive patients may be receiving medical treatment for complications of hypertensive disease — such as cardiac failure or myocardial infarction. These problems must be identified since they may necessitate modification of the dental management plan.

The patient should be asked if he or she is taking (or should be taking) any medications. If the patient does not know the name of the drug, the pictoral section of the *Physicians' Desk Reference (PDR)* can be used to identify it or the pharmacist may be consulted. It is important for the dentist to identify patients who are being treated with antihypertensive medications. Many of these drugs have significant side effects and may interact with vasoconstrictors or have oral manifestations or other side effects (Table 6-6).

Two blood pressure recordings separated by several minutes should be taken on all hypertensive patients during the first dental appointment, and the results averaged. To avoid erroneous results, the measurement should be taken not immediately upon entering the office but after the patient has relaxed. This average figure represents the blood pressure for that day. The blood pressure is recorded for three reasons.

First, it serves as a baseline from which to make decisions for the emergency management of the patient should an untoward reaction occur during dental treatment. Second, it is used to screen patients (along with a medical history) to identify those who have or may have hypertension. Finally, it is a medicolegal necessity.

Based on information obtained from a patient during the first dental examination appointment, the Joint National Committee on Detection, Evaluation, and Treatment of High Blood Pressure[15] makes recommendations for follow-up action in adults (recommendations for dental care are also made) (Table 6-7). Once the patient has been referred to a physician for evaluation, diagnosis, and treatment, the dentist should contact the physician to discuss the following:

1. Patient's current medical status and medications
2. Planned dental treatment in general terms (cleaning, filling, extractions, root canal, "gum" surgery)
3. Suggestions for modifications of management approach

MANAGEMENT CONSIDERATIONS (TABLE 6-8)

An attempt should be made by the dentist to develop an approach to the management of all patients that will reduce the stress and anxiety associated with dental treatment as much as possible. This is of particular importance in dealing with the hypertensive patient. A critical factor in providing an "anxiety-free" situation is the relationship established among the dentist, office staff, and patient. An attempt should be made to establish an atmosphere in which patients are encouraged to express and discuss their fears, concerns, and questions about dental treatment.

Anxiety can be reduced for many patients by premedication with a benzodiazepine such as diazepam (Valium). An effective approach is to prescribe 5 mg at bedtime the night before and 5 mg 1 hour before the dental appointment. Nitrous oxide–oxygen inhalation sedation is an excellent intraoperative anxiolytic for use in hypertensive patients. Care should be used to ensure adequate oxygenation at all times and especially at the termination of nitrous oxide administration. Hypoxia is to be avoided be-

TABLE 6–6
Dental Management of the Hypertensive Patient: Drug Considerations

Drug	Vasoconstrictor interactions	Oral manifestations	Other considerations
Diuretics			
Thiazides (Esedrix, Diuril)	None	Dry mouth, lichenoid reaction	Orthostatic hypotension; precipitate gout (TMJ); NSAIDs may reduce effects
Loop (Lasix, Edecrin, Bumex)			
Potassium sparing (Aldactone, Triamterene)			
Combination (Dyazide, Aldactazide)			
Adrenergic inhibitors			
Beta blockers Nadolol (Corgard) Propanolol (Inderal) Metoprolol (Lopressor) Atenolol (Tenormin)	Potential hypertension and bradycardia; use judiciously	Dry mouth, change in taste, lichenoid reaction (propranolol)	Orthostatic hypotension; NSAIDs may reduce effects
Central adrenergic inhibitors Clonidine (Catapres) Guanabenz (Wytensin) Guanfacine (Tenex) Methyldopa (Aldomet)	None (except potential with methyldopa; use judiciously)	Parotid swelling/pain, dry mouth (clonidine), lichenoid reaction (methyldopa)	Orthostatic hypotension; enhance CNS depressants; NSAIDs may reduce effects
Peripheral adrenergic antagonists Guandrel (Hylorel) Guanethidine (Ismelin) Rauwolfia (Reserpine)	Potential hypertension and arrhythmia; use judiciously	Dry mouth	Orthostatic hypotension; enhance CNS depressants; NSAIDs may reduce effects
Alpha₁ blockers Prazosin (Minipress) Terazosin (Hytrin)	Potential hypotension and tachycardia; use judiciously	None	Orthostatic hypotension; NSAIDs may reduce effects

Continued.

TABLE 6–6
Dental Management of the Hypertensive Patient: Drug Considerations — cont'd

Drug	Vasoconstrictor interactions	Oral manifestations	Other considerations
Combination alpha and beta blockers Labetalol (Trandate, Normodyne)	Potential hypertension and bradycardia; use judiciously	Dry mouth, change in taste, lichenoid reaction	Orthostatic hypotension; NSAIDs may reduce effect
Vasodilators Hydralazine (Apresoline) Minoxidil (Loniten)	None	Systemic lupus-like lesions (hydralazine), Stevens-Johnson syndrome (minoxidil)	NSAIDs may reduce effects
Angiotensin-converting enzyme (ACE) inhibitors Captopril (Capoten) Enalapril (Vasotec) Lisinopril (Zestril) Remipril (Altace) Fosinopril (Monopril) Benazepril (Lotensin)	None	Microbial infection, delayed healing or gingival bleeding secondary to neutropenia, angioedema, loss of taste	NSAIDs may reduce effects
Calcium antagonists Nifedipine (Procardia) Diltiazem (Cardizem) Nicardipine (Cardene) Verapamil (Calan, Isoptin) Isradipine (Dynacirc) Nimodipine (Nimotop) Felodipine (Plendil)	None	Gingival hyperplasia	NSAIDs may reduce effects

cause of the resultant elevation of blood pressure that can occur.

Hypertensive patients ideally should be scheduled for treatment in the morning rather than in the afternoon, when they may be stressed from the day's activities. Long appointments are best avoided. If the patient becomes anxious or apprehensive during the appointment, it should be terminated and the patient scheduled for another day.

Since many antihypertensive agents have the tendency to produce orthostatic hypotension, sudden changes in chair position during dental treatment routinely should be avoided. In ad-

TABLE 6–7

Dental Management of the Hypertensive Patient: Follow-up and Treatment Recommendations

Blood pressure	Follow-up	Dental treatment
Diastolic		
<85	Recheck at recall (within 2 years)	No restrictions
85 to 89	Recheck at recall (within 1 year)	No restrictions
90 to 104	Recheck within 2 months; if still elevated, refer to physician promptly	No restrictions
105 to 114	Refer promptly to physician (within 2 weeks)	Limited elective care or emergency care
≥115	Immediate referral to physician	Emergency care only
Systolic		
<140	Recheck at recall (within 2 years)	No restrictions
140 to 199	Recheck within 2 months; if still elevated refer to physician promptly (within 2 months)	No restrictions
≥200	Refer promptly to physician (within 2 weeks)	Limited elective care or emergency care

Adapted from Joint National Committee. *Arch Intern Med* 148:1023–1037, 1988.

TABLE 6–8

Dental Management of the Hypertensive Patient: Reduction of Stress and Anxiety

Establish honest, supportive relationship with patient

Discuss patient's questions, concerns, fears

Schedule morning appointments

Avoid long appointments

Use premedication as needed — diazepam

Use nitrous oxide as needed (avoid hypoxia)

Provide gradual changes of position to avoid postural hypotension

Avoid stimulating gag reflex

Dismiss patient if he or she appears to be overstressed

dition, when the patient is dismissed the dental chair should be returned to an upright position slowly and the patient physically supported as he or she gets out of the chair until it is clear that the patient has obtained good balance.

Ambulatory (outpatient) general anesthesia administered in the dental office is generally recommended only for patients who fit into the American Society of Anesthesiologists classifications ASA-I (healthy, normal patient) or ASA-II (mild systemic disease). This would tend to exclude many patients whose blood pressure is being controlled by drugs or is greater than 104 (diastolic) or 200 (systolic).

Vasoconstrictors and local anesthetic (Table 6-6)

One of the most common concerns encountered when planning dental treatment for patients with hypertension or other cardiovascular disorders concerns the use of epinephrine or other vasoconstrictors in the local anesthetic solution. It is well to recall the purposes for including a vasoconstrictor in the local anesthetic. These are (1) to delay systemic absorption of the solution, which increases the duration and profoundness of anesthesia as well as decreases the chances of toxicity, and (2) to provide local hemostasis, which improves working conditions in the operative field. These properties allow for enhanced quality and duration of pain control and markedly facilitate the technical procedures to be performed. Without these advantages the local anesthetic is of much shorter duration, of possibly less profoundness, and is absorbed more quickly, thus enhancing the possibilities of toxicity and increased bleeding into the operative field. Therefore the advantages of including a vasoconstrictor in the local anesthetic are obvious.

The potential danger in administering epinephrine or other vasoconstrictors to a patient with hypertension is an untoward increase in the blood pressure from a large quantity of vasoconstrictor injected over a short period and/or the inadvertent intravascular administration of a bolus of vasoconstrictor. In both cases the dentist is concerned with the amount of *exogenous* epinephrine, typically in amounts ranging from 0.018 to 0.054 mg (one to three cartridges respectively containing 1:100,000 epinephrine).

It is important to remember that the adrenal medulla of a 70 kg adult at rest (nonstressed) produces epinephrine at the rate of 0.007 to 0.014 mg per minute.[4,13] This is approximately equal to the amount of epinephrine contained in a half to one cartridge of local anesthetic containing 1:100,000 epinephrine. If an individual is stressed, however, the endogenous production of epinephrine can approach 0.280 mg per minute, an amount far in excess of the typical small amounts of exogenously administered epinephrine during dental treatment.[12] Therefore it becomes clear that the safety and advantages of administering typically minute physiologic amounts of epinephrine during dental treatment far outweigh any perceived or potential dangers or disadvantages. This conclusion is supported by several professional organizations[10,17,20] — including the American Heart Association, the American Dental Association, and the New York Heart Association.

An additional concern when treating patients with hypertension is the potential for adverse drug interactions between vasoconstrictors and antihypertensive drugs, especially the adrenergic blockers. The basis for concern with the beta–adrenergic blocking agents like propranolol is that the normal compensatory vasodilation of skeletal muscle vasculature is inhibited by these drugs, and an injection of epinephrine or other pressor agent could lead to uncompensated peripheral vasoconstriction, resulting in a significant elevation of blood pressure. An unusual case report involving this reaction has been published[5]; however, it involved the use of epinephrine in quantities several times those utilized in normal dental practice.

The peripheral adrenergic antagonists — such as reserpine and guanethidine — also present the potential for adverse interaction with vasoconstrictors because of the enhanced receptor sensitivity to direct-acting sympathomimetics, resulting in reports of enhanced systemic response to vasoconstrictors.[6]

Although the *potential* exists for adverse interaction between vasoconstrictors and adrenergic blocking agents, clinical experience suggests that the judicious use of epinephrine or other vasoconstrictor agent in the local anesthetic can safely be recommended for most patients.[9,13]

Although not considered antihypertensive drugs, monoamine oxidase (MAO) inhibitors are used occasionally to treat hypertension and there has been great concern about the interaction between MAO inhibitors and vasoconstrictors, especially epinephrine. This concern, however, for the most part has been unfounded. Epinephrine and levonordefrin are not greatly potentiated by MAO inhibitors, because these exogenous agents are primarily metabolized by catechol-O-methyltransferase (COMT) and not by MAO; therefore the inhibition of MAO has minimal effect on epinephrine and levonordefrin. Phenylephrine, however, is metabolized by MAO, and its use with an MAO inhibitor could lead to significant potentiation of the pressor effects. Therefore phenylephrine is the only vasoconstrictor used in dentistry that should be avoided in patients taking MAO inhibitors.[9]

Topical vasopressors, likewise, should generally not be used to control local bleeding in the hypertensive patient. When doing crown and bridge procedures for hypertensive patients, the dentist should avoid using gingival retraction cord that contains a vasoconstrictor; alternatively, a recent study[2] has reported, tetrahydrozoline (Visine), oxymetazoline (Afrin), and phenylephrine (Neosynephrine) can be used, with minimal systemic effects.

Many antihypertensive agents also can potentiate the actions of barbiturates or other sedatives. These drugs can still be used in patients who are taking antihypertensive medications, but the usual dosage should be reduced. In addition, sedative medications may cause hypotensive episodes in patients who are taking antihypertensive agents and must be used with care. Once again, the specific antihypertensive drug(s) that a patient is taking should be looked up, any significant side effects and drug interactions noted, and the appropriate action taken.

Many antihypertensive agents can produce a tendency for nausea and vomiting. Excessive stimulation of the gag reflex during dental treatment in patients taking these drugs may bring on nausea and vomiting and should be avoided.

TREATMENT PLANNING MODIFICATIONS

No elective dental procedures should be performed on the patient with severe uncontrolled hypertension. Patients who are receiving good medical management and have no systemic complications can receive any indicated dental treatment. If complications are present, the treatment plan may have to be modified.

Oral manifestations (Table 6-6)

There are very few oral complications associated with hypertension itself. Patients who have malignant hypertension have been reported to develop facial palsy on occasion.[3a] Patients with severe hypertension have been reported to bleed excessively following surgical procedures or trauma; however, excessive bleeding in hypertensive patients is not common and its significance is controversial.[11] Patients who are taking antihypertensive drugs, especially diuretics, may complain of a dry mouth.

The mercurial diuretics may cause oral lesions on an allergic or toxic basis. Lichenoid reactions have been reported with thiazides, methyldopa, propranolol, and labetalol. ACE inhibitors can cause neutropenia, resulting in delayed healing or gingival bleeding. Calcium antagonists (especially nifedipine) can cause gingival hyperplasia.

REFERENCES

1. Berman CL, Guarino MA, Giovannoli SM: High blood pressure detection by dentists, *J Am Dent Assoc* 87:359-363, 1973.
2. Bowles WH, Tardy SJ, Vakedi A: Evaluation of new gingival retraction agents, *J Dent Res* 70(11):1447-1449, 1991.
3. Brest AN: Antihypertensive therapy in perspective. I, *Mod Conc Cardiovasc Dis* 57(12):65-69, 1988.
3a. Drizd T, Dannenberg AL, Engel A: Blood pressure levels in persons 18-74 years of age in 1976-80, and trends in blood pressure from 1960 to 1980, *Vital Health Stat [11]*, no. 234, July 1986.
4. Guyton AC: *Textbook of medical physiology,* ed 4, Philadelphia, 1971, WB Saunders.
5. Hansbrough JF, Near A: Propranolol-epinephrine antagonism with hypertension and stroke, *Ann Intern Med* 92:717, 1980.
6. Hansten PD: Drug interactions affecting the cardiovascular response to sympathomimetics, *Drug Interact Newslett* 1:21-26, 1981.
7. Hypertension Detection and Follow-up Program Cooperative Group: Five-year findings. I. Reduction in mortality of persons with high blood pressure, including mild hypertension, *JAMA* 242:2562-2571, 1979.
8. Hypertension Detection and Follow-up Program Cooperative Group: Five-year findings. II. Mortality by race, sex, and age, *JAMA* 242:2572-2577, 1979.
9. Jastak JT, Yagiela JA: Vasoconstrictors and local anesthesia: a review and rationale for use, *J Am Dent Assoc* 107:623-630, 1983.
10. Kannel WB: Some lessons in cardiovascular epidemiology from Framingham, *Am J Cardiol* 37:269-282, 1976.
11. Knapp, JF, Fiori, T: Oral hemorrhage associated with periodontal surgery and hypertensive crisis. *J Am Dent Assoc* 108:49-51, 1984.
12. Malamed SF: *Handbook of medical emergencies in the dental office,* ed 3, St. Louis, 1987, CV Mosby.
13. Malamed SF: *Handbook of local anesthesia,* ed 3, St Louis, 1990, CV Mosby.
14. Reference deleted in proofs.
15. Report of the Joint National Committee on Detection, Evaluation, and Treatment of High Blood Pressure—1988, *Arch Intern Med* 148:1023-1037, 1988.
16. Scully C, Clawson RA: Cardiovascular disease. In Scully C, Clawson RA, editors: *Medical problems in dentistry,* London, 1982, Wright.

17. Smith WM: The case for treating hypertension in the elderly, *Am J Hypertens* 1:1735-1785, 1988.

18. Special Committee of the New York Heart Association: Use of epinephrine in connection with procaine in dental procedures, *J Am Dent Assoc* 50:108, 1955.

19. Williams GH: Hypertensive vascular disease. In Wilson JD, et al, editors: *Harrison's Principles of internal medicine,* ed 12, New York, 1991, McGraw-Hill.

20. Working Conference of the American Dental Association and American Heart Association: Management of dental problems in patients with cardiovascular disease, *J Am Dent Assoc* 68:333, 1964.

7

Ischemic Heart Disease

Coronary atherosclerotic heart disease may be asymptomatic or symptomatic. When it is symptomatic, it is referred to as ischemic heart disease. The symptoms result because of oxygen deprivation consequent to reduced perfusion of a portion of the myocardium. Other conditions—such as embolism, coronary ostial stenosis, coronary artery spasm, and congenital abnormalities—may cause ischemic heart disease. In this chapter coronary atherosclerosis and its myocardial complications are considered. The clinical spectrum of atherosclerotic coronary heart disease is shown in Table 7-1.

GENERAL DESCRIPTION
INCIDENCE AND PREVALENCE

It is estimated[15,16] that over 50 million Americans (25% of the population) have one or more of the cardiovascular diseases: 57 million have hypertension, 6.9 million have coronary heart disease, 1.7 million have rheumatic heart disease, and 2.8 million have stroke. The mortality rate per year from cardiovascular disease has been declining since 1950. A 42% decline in deaths caused by cardiovascular disease has occurred during the last 20 years.[15,16] In 1979 cardiovascular disease accounted for more than 50% of deaths in the United States. Even now, 1 out of every 3 men and 1 out of every 10 women will develop significant cardiovascular disease before the age of 60. Coronary heart disease is still the leading cause of death after the age of 40 years in men and 50 years in women. Over 524,000 Americans die of heart attacks each year.[16] Myocardial infarction and cardiac-related sudden death account for about 20% of the deaths due to coronary heart disease.[16] Since 1950, there has been a universal decline of cardiovascular disease in the United States. Fifty-eight percent of this decline has occurred in the years 1972 to 1986. This has included all races, both sexes, all age groups, and all geographic areas of the country. In recent years the largest absolute decline has been in coronary heart disease.[16] The incidence and severity of coronary heart disease increase with age. The process starts as coronary atherosclerosis, with the appearance of fatty streaks in the walls of the coronary vessels.[10,11] Essentially any American may have fatty streaks in the coronary vessels.[28] A raised fibrous plaque may be found in as many as 80% of American men and 65% of American women over the age of 40.[12,25,32]

Autopsies of American military personnel killed during the Korean War showed that 15% had significant coronary artery disease. The mean age for this study was 22.1 years. During the Vietnam War, autopsies of military personnel killed during battle showed 45% to have significant coronary artery disease. Again, the mean age was 22.1 years. It is clear from these two studies that a significant increase in the incidence of asymptomatic coronary artery disease occurred in young American adults during approximately a 20-year period.[32]

Studies on autopsied patients in the United States[7,10,25,32] have shown that by the age of 30 to 39 years just less than 20% of the patients have had more than 50% occlusion of one or more coronary arteries. By age 40 to 49 years this increases to over 40% of the patients. The Framingham study[7] revealed that 8% of the men between ages 30 and 44 years and 18% between 55 and 62 years had coronary atherosclerotic heart disease. These data also show the inci-

TABLE 7–1

Clinical Spectrum of Atherosclerotic Coronary Heart Disease

Coronary atherosclerosis without angina
Coronary atherosclerosis with reversible myocardial ischemia
Stable subsets
Stable angina pectoris
Positive exercise test
Silent myocardial ischemia
Unstable subsets
Unstable angina pectoris
Post–myocardial infarction angina
Prinzmetal's angina pectoris
Silent myocardial ischemia
Coronary atherosclerosis with irreversible myocardial ischemia and necrosis
Evolving infarction
Uncomplicated completed infarction
Complicated infarction
Silent myocardial ischemia
Cardiac arrhythmias
Sudden death
Syncope
Ischemic cardiomyopathy
Coronary atherosclerotic heart disease in combination with other conditions

From Hurst JW, editor: *The heart, arteries, and veins,* ed 7, New York, 1990, McGraw-Hill, p 994.

dence of coronary artery disease and the prevalence of coronary atherosclerotic heart disease to have increased with age in American men and, to some extent, in American women.

ETIOLOGY

The cause of coronary atherosclerosis is not known at present. It appears to be related to a variety of risk factors.[10,12,28]

The major risk factors most often mentioned are age, sex, familial history, serum lipid levels, diet, hypertension, cigarette smoking, and abnormal glucose tolerance.

The incidence of coronary atherosclerosis increases with age. However, this may reflect the effects of other risk factors acting for a longer time rather than the direct effects of aging.

Men are much more prone to clinical manifestations of coronary atherosclerosis than are women of childbearing age. Between the ages of

35 and 44 years the risk is 5.2 times higher for men.[36] Infarction and sudden death are rare in premenopausal women.[12,28] After menopause there is rapid reduction in this sex difference; between the ages of 65 and 74 the risk falls to only 2.3 times higher for men.[36] The sex difference in incidence of coronary atherosclerotic heart disease is more marked in whites than in blacks.

Recent studies[11] have confirmed that individuals with either parents or siblings affected by coronary atherosclerotic heart disease before the age of 50 have a greater risk of developing the disease at a younger age than do those without such a history. This risk factor may be as high as 5:1.

Elevation of serum lipid levels has been demonstrated to be a risk factor. Individuals with total cholesterol levels greater than 300 mg/dl have a 4 times greater risk of developing coronary atherosclerotic heart disease than do those with a cholesterol level below 200. Increased levels of low-density lipoprotein (LDL) cholesterol carry the greatest risk for atherosclerosis. Increased levels of high-density lipoprotein (HDL) cholesterol have been shown to reduce the risk for coronary atherosclerosis. Individuals with elevated triglyceride or beta-lipoprotein levels also have shown an increased risk for the disease. A diet rich in one or more of the following increases the risk: total calories, saturated fats, cholesterol, sugars, and salts.*

Thus, for a total cholesterol reading of less than 200 mg/dl the HDL fraction should normally be between 35 and 70 and the LDL fraction below 130 mg/dl. A ratio of HDL to total cholesterol approaching 70/200 (0.35 or higher) can be considered desirable from the standpoint of minimizing the risk of atherosclerotic heart disease.

Some patients have familial hypercholesterolemia, which greatly increases their risk for coronary heart disease. Heterozygotes are found in those who have high cholesterol levels at birth and as children. There is a dominant transmission pattern through families. These individuals have a twofold to threefold increase in LDL cholesterol levels. Their total blood cholesterol level as adults is in the 350 to 400

---

*References 3, 8, 10, 12, 14, 28.

mg/dl range. They usually have clinical evidence of atherosclerotic heart disease before the age of 40.[12]

Individuals who are homozygous for familial hypercholesterolemia have total cholesterol levels above 600 mg/dl at birth. These persons have severe coronary atherosclerosis in childhood and often have had a myocardial infarction by the age of 10. The marriage of two people having LDL receptor genes and hypercholesterolemia will result in one fourth of their offspring being homozygotes.[12]

A condition known as dysbetalipoproteinemia (type III familial hyperlipoproteinemia) is passed on as a recessive trait. It is more rare than familial hypercholesterolemia. The blood triglyceride levels are greater than 350 mg/dl. The LDL cholesterol is not elevated, and children are not affected.[12]

The most common form of hypercholesterolemia is termed *multifactorial* or *primary polygenic hypercholesterolemia*. This condition is due to unknown genetic abnormalities and environmental factors. There is no definite autosomal dominant pattern, although relatives of affected individuals may have slightly elevated blood cholesterol levels. Children show no increase in blood cholesterol. Adults often will have total blood cholesterol levels between 250 and 350 mg/dl. Other causes of hypercholesterolemia—such as hypothyroidism, diabetes mellitus, nephrotic syndrome, obstructive liver disease, Cushing's disease, and multiple myeloma—must be excluded before this condition can be established.[12]

Increased blood pressure appears to be one of the most influential risk factors in coronary atherosclerotic heart disease. The Framingham study[7] showed that angina, myocardial infarction, and nonsudden death were all significantly correlated with elevated blood pressure (greater than 140/90 mm Hg). Sudden death in men was related only to elevation in systolic blood pressure, and no correlation of sudden death in women was found with increased blood pressure. The evidence suggests that hypertension has its impact primarily on the rate of development of coronary atherosclerosis rather than acting as a primary cause in its development.

The risk of developing coronary atherosclerotic heart disease or the risk of death from the disease is from 2 to 6 times higher in cigarette smokers than in nonsmokers. The increased risk appears to be proportional to the number of cigarettes smoked per day. In a 5-year study of 4165 smokers with coronary atherosclerotic heart disease,[35] the death rate was reduced if the individual stopped smoking. The death rate was 22% for the 2675 individuals who continued smoking and was reduced to 15% for the 1490 who stopped smoking. Pipe smoking and cigar smoking carry little risk for developing the disease.[3,5,11]

Patients with diabetes mellitus have been found to have a greater incidence of coronary atherosclerotic heart disease, to have more extensive lesions, and to develop the condition at an earlier age than persons who do not have diabetes. Patients who receive radiation to the mediastinum have been reported[12] to develop coronary atherosclerosis at an accelerated rate. Accelerated coronary atherosclerosis has also been reported in patients with transplanted hearts, in patients receiving renal dialysis, and in patients with coronary artery bypass grafts.[12] Minor risk factors are obesity, sedentary living pattern, personality type, and psychosocial tensions.

It would appear that no single risk factor is responsible for the development of coronary atherosclerosis but that many factors contribute to its development. The evidence suggests that modification of those risk factors that can be controlled—such as smoking, hypertension, blood cholesterol level, and diabetes—will reduce or modify the clinical effects of the disease. For example, the Oslo Heart Study, the Lipid Research Clinic's Coronary Primary Prevention Trial, and three smaller studies involved with the role of lipoproteins in the progression of coronary atherosclerosis demonstrated that for every 1% reduction in serum cholesterol there was a 2% reduction in clinical events.[18,21]

PATHOPHYSIOLOGY AND COMPLICATIONS

Coronary atherosclerosis appears to begin with the accumulation of lipid-laden cells in the intima of a blood vessel. A "fibrous" reaction to the presence of fatty material or to growth factors then occurs, causing the intima to increase in thickness. The lipid-laden cells then rupture, releasing additional lipid material into the extracellular areas of the intima. This

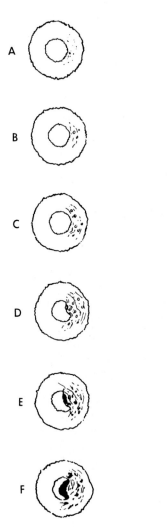

FIG. 7-1 Pathologic sequence in coronary atherosclerotic heart disease. **A,** Lipid-laden macrophages in the intima. **B,** Fibrous tissue reaction in the intima. **C,** Macrophages rupture, releasing additional lipids into the vessel wall. **D,** Increased fibrous connective tissue response to the lipid material decreases luminal size. **E,** Calcification of plaque in the vessel wall. **F,** Endothelial cells become damaged, and thrombosis occurs that may obstruct coronary blood flow.

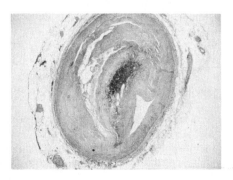

FIG. 7-2 Photomicrograph of a cross section of a coronary artery partially occluded as a result of coronary atherosclerotic disease. (Courtesy W. O'Connor, M.D., Lexington, Ky.)

reduced and atrophy of the medial portion of the vessel may occur (Figs. 7-1 and 7-2). There is a tendency for the greatest changes to occur at areas of arterial bifurcation, which suggests that mechanical factors may stimulate the atherosclerotic process.

Recent research findings have resulted in further insights into the cellular and tissue interactions involved following direct or indirect injury to the endothelial cells of affected arteries. Figure 7-1 demonstrates a modified response-to-injury hypothesis for atherogenesis. It suggests that at least two pathways may lead to the formation of intimal smooth muscle proliferative lesions. One pathway, demonstrated in hypercholesterolemia, involves monocyte, endothelial, and platelet interactions, with resulting smooth muscle proliferation and fibrous plaque formation. The second pathway involves direct stimulation of the endothelium, which may release growth factors that induce smooth muscle migration and proliferation and the release of a platelet-like growth factor leading to fibrous plaque formation. The second pathway may be important in diabetes, hypertension, cigarette smoking, or other circumstances associated with an increased incidence of atherosclerosis[27] (Fig. 7-3).

Three types of plaque can be found associated with atherosclerosis of coronary arteries. *Fatty streaks* consisting of lipid-laden myointimal cells are benign but serve as precursors of the two more advanced lesions. Fatty streaks are found in individuals of any age or sex, at

material then undergoes crystallization and calcification, and an additional fibrous tissue response follows in an attempt to encapsulate the lipid mass. As the thickness of the intima increases, the size of the vessel lumen may be

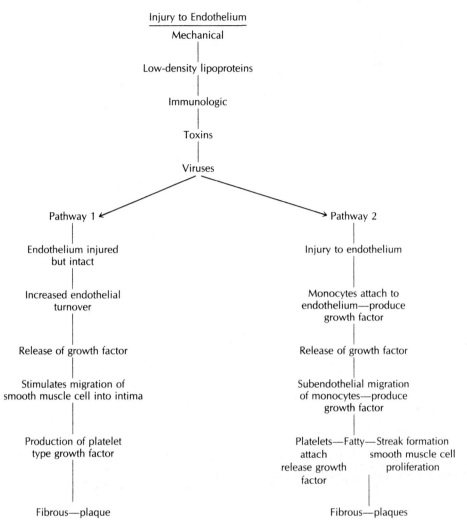

Injury to Endothelium

Mechanical

Low-density lipoproteins

Immunologic

Toxins

Viruses

Pathway 1

Endothelium injured
but intact

Increased endothelial
turnover

Release of growth factor

Stimulates migration of
smooth muscle cell into intima

Production of platelet
type growth factor

Fibrous—plaque

Pathway 2

Injury to endothelium

Monocytes attach to
endothelium—produce
growth factor

Release of growth factor

Subendothelial migration
of monocytes—produce
growth factor

Platelets—Fatty—Streak formation
attach   smooth muscle cell
release growth   proliferation
factor

Fibrous—plaques

FIG. 7-3 Pathogenesis of atherosclerosis, the revised response-to-injury hypothesis. (From Ross R. *N Engl J Med* 314:488-497, 1986.)

branching points of the coronary arteries. The second type of lesion is the *fibrous plaque.* This consists of lipid-laden myointimal cells plus fibrous connective tissue. Smooth muscle cells migrate into the lesion and secrete a protein, which becomes the collagen matrix. The third type of lesion is the *complicated plaque.* This is a degenerative lesion consisting of fibrin, fibrous tissue, calcium, lipid, blood, and necrotic debris.

The complicated plaque may enlarge acutely by hemorrhage or degeneration in its core or by a thrombus on its surface.[9]

Three theories have been presented for the origin of the lesions of atherosclerosis in coronary arteries[9]:

1. The *lipogenic* or insudation theory states that lipids initiate and cause the progression of an atheroma.

2. The *thrombogenic* or encrustation theory states that recurrent mural thrombosis over existing plaque accounts for the atheroma. Any intimal injury can trigger formation of the thrombus and its progression. Platelets, by releasing a growth factor, can stimulate smooth muscle cell proliferation in addition to releasing thromboxane and serotonin, which cause local vasoconstriction.

3. The *monoclonal* theory suggests that a single precursor cell proliferates, as in tumor growth, to cause the lesion.

All three theories most likely play a role in coronary atherosclerosis. It is clear that lipids play a central role. Lipid accumulation leads to internal injury, which leads to thrombosis and proliferation. Some proliferating thrombi may have been shown[9] to possess monoclonal properties. One suggested sequence[28] is plaque formation, fissuring, hemorrhage, and thrombosis.

Coronary atherosclerosis is usually a focal disease affecting the proximal portions of the coronary vessels. This fact allows for the success of bypass grafts and balloon angioplasty. However, in about 10% of the patients with severe coronary atherosclerosis the disease is diffuse.[9] Most cases of acute myocardial infarction are due to the abrupt interruption, by a thrombus, of the blood flow in an area of a coronary artery containing a complicated plaque. Plaque rupture, hemorrhage, or erosion can lead to thrombosis; and spasm of the coronary artery may trigger these events.[9]

The lumen of the artery with atherosclerosis may be circumferentially narrowed evenly or eccentrically depending on the location and extent of the lesion. Microthrombi may develop on the endothelial surface overlying the developing lesion, which can lead to thrombosis and total occlusion of the vessel or to embolism.

The intraarterial complications of coronary atherosclerosis are luminal narrowing, intramural hemorrhage, thrombosis, embolism, and aneurysm (Fig. 7-4). Intramural hemorrhage occurs because of a weakening of the intimal tissues and may lead to thrombosis. It also may serve as an irritant and cause a reflex reaction that results in spasm of the collateral vessels.

Coronary thrombosis is usually found in the segment of the artery that contains an advanced

FIG. 7-4 Postmortem specimen demonstrating atherosclerotic changes in the wall of the aorta on the left side. On the right is a normal aorta. (Courtesy W. O'Connor, M.D., Lexington Ky.)

atherosclerotic lesion. Once a thrombus has formed, it may become encapsulated and undergo fibrous organization and reconciliation.

Narrowing of the lumen of a coronary artery may lead to decreased blood flow to a portion of the heart muscle, resulting in myocardial ischemia. Myocardial ischemia may be manifested clinically as brief pain (angina pectoris), prolonged pain (myocardial infarction), or sudden death.

Patients with brief pain (angina pectoris) usually have coronary atherosclerotic disease. However, angina may occur in patients with hypertension, valvular heart disease, and anemia. Patients who have coronary atherosclerosis will demonstrate brief episodes of pain more often if hypertension also is present. In one study of 177 patients with a history of brief chest pain,[12] only 16% had coronary atherosclerosis alone; most had a combination of coronary atherosclerosis and hypertension and/or valvular heart disease.

Sudden death in the absence of demonstrable acute myocardial infarction is the largest single cause of death from coronary atherosclerosis. Some type of underlying heart disease is found in about 90% of the cases of sudden death. This approaches 100% if death occurs within 1 hour after the onset of symptoms. The predominant symptoms that most often precede sudden death include chest pain, cough, shortness of breath, fainting, dizziness, and palpitations and/or fatigue. Sudden death accounts for about

15% to 30% of all natural deaths. The incidence of sudden death is highest in the early morning hours.[12,18] Pathologic examinations of sudden death patients who died outside of a hospital have shown that acute coronary occlusion and demonstrable acute myocardial infarction are uncommon, and that signs of old subendocardial infarctions (infarction of the myocardium under the endocardium of the left ventricle) are common. The cause of sudden death appears to be ventricular fibrillation resulting from interruption of the electrical conduction system.

If the degree of ischemia resulting from coronary atherosclerosis is significant, the myocardium supplied by that vessel may undergo necrosis. The reduced blood flow may result from thrombosis in the affected artery, the effects of a hypotensive episode, an increased demand for blood, or emotional stress. The infarction, or area of necrosis, may be subendocardial or transmural (Fig. 7-5)—the latter involving the entire thickness of the myocardium. The cellular sequence that takes place is shown in Figures 7-6 to 7-8. This type of infarction is termed *coagulation necrosis*. With the increased use of thrombolytic agents in the

treatment of acute myocardial infarction, another type of necrosis has been found. This is described as contraction band necrosis and is the type of cell death that occurs when lethal myocardial ischemia is followed by reperfusion. A third type of infarction occurs that is called myocytolysis. In this type ("mini-infarction") focal nests of cells in the subendocardial region undergo balloonlike degeneration and death. These small infarcts heal leaving small scars.[9]

The causes of death in patients who have had an acute myocardial infarction include ventricular fibrillation, cardiac standstill, congestive heart failure, and rupture of the heart wall (Fig. 7-9). Rupture of the heart secondary to infarction most often takes place during the third or fourth day postinfarction. The rupture usually occurs at the periphery of the infarction, at the junction of necrotic and healthy muscle. Rupture of the heart wall occurs only in transmural infarctions. Depending on the location of the infarction, the ventricular septum may rupture or papillary muscles may tear.

Death also may be caused by thromboembolic complications. The embolism may originate from the left ventricle or from systemic veins. In the case of embolism from a mural thrombus in the left ventricle, the site of damage may be the brain, coronary arteries, or mesenteric arteries.

Transmural infarctions may cause a pericarditis, which usually is of only passing interest. However, if a hemorrhagic effusion occurs during an episode of fibrinous pericarditis secondary to a transmural infarction, cardiac tamponade and death may result.

The prognosis in patients who have a healed myocardial infarction varies. In one study of 329 patients with healed infarction at autopsy,[10] about a third were found to have died of noncardiac causes; the other patients died of cardiovascular causes. Among the patients who died of cardiovascular causes, 38% had sudden death without recurrent acute myocardial infarction, 27% had congestive heart failure, and 34% died as a result of complications of an acute myocardial infarction.

CLINICAL PRESENTATION
SYMPTOMS

A most important symptom of coronary atherosclerotic heart disease is pain. The pain may be brief, as in angina pectoris resulting from

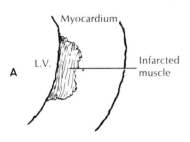

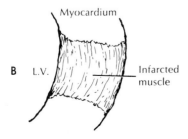

FIG. 7-5 Myocardial infarction. **A**, Subendocardial; **B**, transmural.

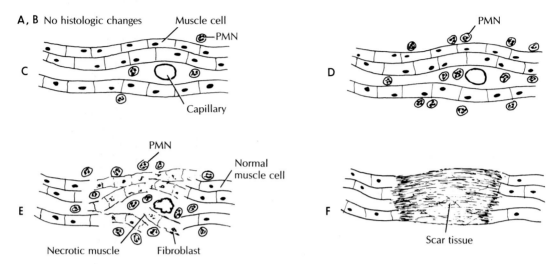

FIG. 7-6 Cellular sequence in myocardial infarction (times approximate): **A**, 1 to 11 hours, no histologic changes; **B**, 12 hours, eosinophilic appearance of muscle fibers; **C**, 18 hours, clumping of cytoplasm, dilation of capillaries, and infiltration of polymorphonuclear leukocytes (PMNs); **D**, 24 hours, a marked infiltration of PMNs; **E**, 72 hours, removal of necrotic tissue and formation of scar; **F**, 3 weeks, scar formed.

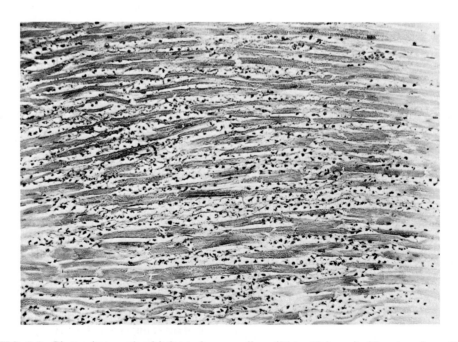

FIG. 7-7 Photomicrograph of infarcted myocardium (24 to 48 hours). (Courtesy Jesse E. Edwards, M.D., St. Paul, Minn.)

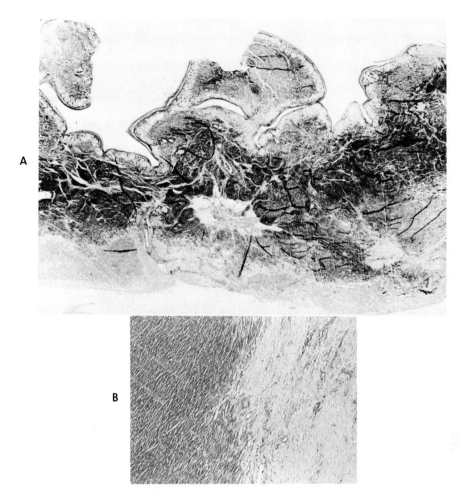

FIG. 7-8 **A,** Gross appearance of healed infarcted myocardium. **B,** Photomicrograph of healed myocardium. (**A** courtesy Jesse E. Edwards, M.D., St Paul Minn; **B** courtesy W. O'Connor, M.D., Lexington Ky.)

temporary ischemia of the myocardium, or it may be prolonged, as in myocardial infarction. Ischemic myocardial pain results when there is an imbalance between the oxygen supply to the muscle and the oxygen demand of the muscle. Atherosclerotic narrowing of the coronary arteries is an important cause of this imbalance. If the imbalance is severe enough, necrosis of the involved portion of the heart muscle may result. The exact mechanism or agents involved in producing the cardiac pain are not known.

Ischemic myocardial pain of a brief nature is usually described as an aching, heavy, squeezing pressure or tightness in the midchest region. The area of discomfort is about the size of the fist. The pain may radiate down the left or right arm, to the neck, to the lower jaw, to the palate, or to the tongue. In rare cases it may be present in only one of these distant sites, and the patient will be free of central chest pain. The pain is usually brief in duration, lasting only 1 to 3 minutes if the provoking stimulus is reduced or stopped (Table 7-2).

Patients with initial pain, progressive pain, or pain at rest are described as having an unstable form of angina. Patients with pain that has not

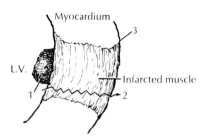

FIG. 7-9 Complications of a transmural infarction; *1*, a mural thrombus may give rise to an embolism to the brain, coronary arteries, or mesenteric arteries; *2*, the myocardial wall may rupture; *3*, a pericarditis may lead to tamponade.

TABLE 7–2

Predictive Value of Chest Discomfort Thought to be Caused by Myocardial Ischemia Secondary to Coronary Heart Disease

	Percent
Overall predictive value	70 to 75
Middle-aged men, effort-produced discomfort	90
Middle-aged men, relation to effort not clear	80
Women over 50, effort-produced discomfort	70
Women 50 years or younger, chest discomfort	50

From Hurst JW, editor: *The heart, arteries, and veins,* ed 7, New York, 1990, McGraw-Hill, p 965.

changed in frequency or severity over a period have stable angina.

Patients with a brief pain caused by myocardial ischemia who have a stable pattern for the pain attacks have a relatively good prognosis. Patients with unstable angina have a poor prognosis and often develop myocardial infarction within a short period.

A form of angina, Prinzmetal's variant angina, occurs at rest and is related to spasm of a coronary artery, usually with varying amounts of atherosclerosis. The prognosis depends on the degree of arterial disease.[36] It has been demonstrated[30] that patients with spasm of a coronary artery have morphologic changes in the endothelium at the site of the spasm. Angina has also been reported in individuals with normal coronary vessels.[36]

Patients with coronary atherosclerosis who develop prolonged pain resulting from myocardial ischemia usually are having an infarction of the myocardium. There may or may not be objective clinical evidence of infarction. The pain resulting from infarction is usually more severe and lasts longer — ½ to 1 hour or more — but has the same character as that described previously for angina. Its location is the same, and it may radiate in the same pattern as the brief pain resulting from temporary myocardial ischemia. With infarction there is no relief of pain by the administration of vasodilators or the cessation of activity. Neither brief nor prolonged pain resulting from myocardial ischemia is aggravated by deep breathing.

The differential diagnosis of chest pain should include acute dissection of the aorta, acute pericarditis, pulmonary embolism, and anxiety.

1. Acute dissection of the aorta produces severe pain in the anterior chest that lasts for hours and often has its maximum intensity at the onset. It may radiate to the back and is not aggravated by deep breathing.
2. Acute pericarditis produces a sharp pain usually located in the pericardial region that is aggravated by deep breathing. Its onset and severity are not related to effort.
3. Small pulmonary emboli usually do not cause pain. The pain produced by larger emboli may be similar to that resulting from myocardial infarction. The presence of acute, distressing dyspnea may be the only clue to pulmonary embolism as the cause of the pain.
4. Anxiety is the most common cause of chest pain. The pain may consist of a short series of "sticks" or "stabs" or be a prolonged and dull ache. The pain rarely radiates, is not initiated by effort, is not aggravated by breathing, and is usually associated with other signs of anxiety such as deep sighing, fatigue, or hyperventilation.

Palpitations of the heart may be present in patients with coronary atherosclerotic heart disease. The rhythm may be normal or abnormal. The complaint (disagreeable awareness of the heartbeat) is not directly related to the seriousness of the underlying cardiac problem. Syncope, a transient loss of consciousness resulting from inadequate cerebral blood flow, may occur in patients with coronary atherosclerotic heart disease.

If congestive heart failure develops as a complication of coronary atherosclerotic heart disease, then dyspnea, orthopnea, paroxysmal nocturnal dyspnea, edema, hemoptysis, fatigue, weakness, and cyanosis may be present. Fatigue and weakness may be present early in the course of the disease, before the onset of congestive failure. (See Chapter 8.)

SIGNS

The clinical signs of early coronary atherosclerotic heart disease are few and may reflect the anxiety felt by the patient concerning the episodes of brief cardiac pain rather than be directly related to the underlying disease process. The skin may be moist and ashen. The patient may be losing weight, and some irregularity in the rhythm of the pulse may be detected.

Signs associated with advanced coronary atherosclerotic heart disease usually reflect the presence of congestive heart failure. Distention of neck veins, peripheral edema, cyanosis, ascites, and enlarged liver may be present.

LABORATORY FINDINGS

Three tests are used most often for patients presenting with symptoms of angina pectoris. The selection of the tests depends on the clinical picture. These tests are a stress electrocardiogram, a stress thallium-201 test, and a coronary arteriogram.[12]

Coronary atherosclerosis may be detected by coronary arteriograms before the development of coronary atherosclerotic heart disease. Also, an abnormal electrocardiogram may be detected before the development of symptomatic coronary atherosclerotic heart disease. An exercise electrocardiogram is being used with increased frequency to detect patients with coronary atherosclerotic heart disease.[24]

Other tests used to diagnose coronary atherosclerotic heart disease include a chest radiograph, fluoroscopy, cinefluoroscopy, resting ECG, cardiac enzymes, radionuclide angiography (technetium 99m), and echocardiography.[12,28] Several new techniques are being tested for effectiveness in detecting coronary heart disease. These include magnetic resonance imaging, positron emission tomography, and single photon emission computed tomography[33] (Table 7-2).

The exercise stress test is performed using a treadmill or bicycle ergometer. The subject has a 12-lead ECG taken before, during, and after the exercise. A target heart rate of 85% of maximum for individuals of similar age and size is set before the test is started. The test is stopped at the onset of chest discomfort, shortness of breath, dizziness, fatigue, or ST-segment depression greater than 2 mm, a fall in systolic blood pressure of 15 or more mm Hg, or the development of ventricular tachycardia.

When compared to the gold standard coronary arteriogram, the exercise stress test has about a 15% rate of false-negative and 15% rate of false-positive results. The risk for death during the test is very small (1 per 10,000), and the risk for nonfatal complications is also very small (2 per 10,000). Ninety-eight percent of the patients with typical angina symptoms due to coronary disease will have a positive stress test. Eighty-eight percent of the patients with atypical chest pain, 44% of the patients with nonanginal chest pain, and 33% of asymptomatic individuals will have a positive test.[28] IV thallium-201 can be given right after exercise and again 2 to 4 hours later. By using a gamma camera the physician can assess myocardial perfusion. Areas with no initial uptake would indicate myocardial ischemia, infarction, or scarring. Later images showing areas perfused that were not seen in the initial images would support the interpretation of reversible ischemia. Areas that were nonperfused in both initial and later images would support the interpretation of infarction or a healed infarction (scar).[28]

Coronary arteriography is an invasive procedure that carries some risk. A catheter is placed into the coronary vessels and can cause thrombosis, embolism, and lethal arrhythmias. These complications can cause acute myocardial infarction, stroke, or death. The complications reported in 200,000 patients in whom the procedure was performed[12] were a 0.15% death rate, a 0.09% infarction rate, and a 0.5% vascular malformation rate. Coronary arteriography is not recommended in the absence of clinical problems. It is not recommended for patients with severe left ventricular dysfunction since they are not candidates for coronary artery bypass graft surgery. The procedure is usually performed in patients who have just completed thrombolytic therapy to determine the degree of stenosis of the affected coronary artery. Coronary arteriography and the related procedure left ventriculography allow the physician to map the coronary circulation, determine the location and degree of stenosis, estimate the size and quality of coronary vessels, and determine the status of the left ventricle.[12]

The electrocardiogram is used to aid in the diagnosis of acute myocardial infarction. It is of most diagnostic value when the infarction is large, transmural, and located in the anteroseptal position and when intraventricular conduction is normal. The electrocardiographic diagnosis of acute myocardial infarction is most difficult when the infarction is small, subendocardial, or located on the lateral wall of the left ventricle and when the left bundle branch conduction system is blocked. The electrocardiogram may also be used to determine the presence of old infarctions[6,11,23,36] (Table 7-3).

Serum enzyme determinations are often very helpful in establishing the presence of an acute myocardial infarction and the extent of infarction. This method is not specific for myocardial infarction, however, because any injured or necrotic tissue will release many of the enzymes that are released following infarction of heart muscle. Thus serum enzyme results must be evaluated in light of the patient's clinical picture to be meaningful from a diagnostic standpoint.

TABLE 7–3
Laboratory Tests for Coronary Heart Disease

Angina

Electrocardiography
Exercise electrocardiography
Thallium-201 imaging
Echocardiography
Arteriography

Myocardial Infarction

Electrocardiography
Increased serum enzymes
Technetium-99m stannous pyrophosphate
  and thallium-201 imaging
Echocardiography

Experimental Procedures

Indium-111 labeled platelet imaging
Measurement of prostaglandins
Radiolabeled myosin-specific antibody
Positron imaging
Photon emission imaging

The principal enzymes that are measured are creatine phosphokinase (CPK) and lactic dehydrogenase (LDH).[10,11,25] The CPK level increases above normal at about 6 to 8 hours following infarction. It reaches a peak value in approximately 24 hours and returns to normal in 3 to 4 days. The LDH level increases above normal approximately 24 to 48 hours after the infarction, peaks at 3 to 6 days, and returns to normal by 8 to 14 days (Table 7-4).

CPK and LDH are not specific for heart

TABLE 7–4
Laboratory Tests to Measure Serum Enzyme Levels for Evaluation of Myocardial Tissue Injury or Death*

Enzyme	Level increases above normal (hr)	Peak value (hr)	Level returns to normal (days)
Creatine phosphokinase (CPK)	6 to 8	24	3 to 4
Lactic dehydrogenase (LDH)	24 to 48	72 to 144 (3 to 6 days)	8 to 14

*Enzyme results must be looked at in light of the total clinical picture. Results are not specific for myocardial infarction.

tissue. These enzymes can also be released when necrosis of other tissues occurs. Peak enzyme levels do not correlate closely with infarct size. The enzyme levels have weak specificity but strong sensitivity. In other words, an increase in CPK and LDH indicates that necrosis is occurring but does not identify which organ or tissue is involved. An isoenzyme of CK, CK-MB, is much more specific for heart tissue. Radioimmunoassay and gel electrophoresis are used to measure the CK-MB level in blood. Increased levels of CK-MB usually indicate necrosis of the myocardium. Serial samples of CK-MB can reduce the errors of interpretation and allow for a CK-MB time curve to be calculated. The area under the CK-MB time curve correlates with the size of the infarct.[12,23] Massive injury to skeletal muscle can also increase CK-MB levels. Ninety-five percent of the patients with a myocardial infarction will show an increase in CK, CK-MB, or LDH.[23]

Thallium-201 and technetium-99m stannous pyrophosphate scintigraphy can be used to evaluate patients for acute myocardial infarction. "Hot-spot" imaging with technetium-99m stannous pyrophosphate can be positive for 2 to 5 days following an infarction. The area of infarction takes up the labeled material, but the normal myocardium does not. "Cold-spot" imaging with thallium-201 can also be done to evaluate the patient thought to have an acute MI. The thallium-201 is taken up by viable myocardium, but areas of new infarction have no uptake. However, old healed infarctions cannot be differentiated from the new infarcts since neither takes up the thallium-201 label.

MEDICAL MANAGEMENT

The patient with coronary atherosclerotic heart disease who has a history of brief pain (angina pectoris) is medically managed by a combination of approaches (Table 7-5). The patient may need to be aided in adjusting to the emotional impact of the presence of the disease. The disease should be explained, with reassurances given that a productive life can still be led. Management also may include general measures — an exercise program, weight control, diet alteration (with restriction of sodium chloride, cholesterol, and saturated fatty acids), cessation of smoking, and control of exacerbating conditions (anemia, hypertension, and hy-

TABLE 7–5
Medial Management of the Patient with Angina Pectoris

Explanation and reassurance
Reduction of risk factors
Elimination or control of coexisting illness
  (e.g., hypertension or hyperthyroidism)
Adaptation activities
Drug therapy
  Nitrates
  Beta-blockers
  Calcium-channel antagonists (blockers)
  Aspirin
Mechanical revascularization
  Percutaneous transluminal coronary angioplasty
    (PTCA)
  Coronary artery bypass grafting

perthyroidism). Drug therapy includes nitrates (nitroglycerin or long-acting nitrates), beta–adrenergic blockers, and calcium-channel blockers (Table 7-6). Cardiac glycosides and diuretics also may be prescribed.

The nitrates are vascular dilators, predominantly venodilators. In addition, nitrates may alleviate coronary artery spasm.[31] Nitroglycerin is placed under the patient's tongue; the long-acting nitrates usually are taken orally, but some can be placed sublingually. A nitroglycerin ointment may be applied to the skin or long-acting transdermal nitrate patches can be used. Beta-blockers are effective in the treatment of about 75% of patients with angina. The selection of a particular beta-blocker is dependent on a number of clinical factors[31] (Tables 7-6 and 7-7). Beta-blockers can increase the tone of vascular smooth muscle, causing vasoconstriction of peripheral vessels. Beta-blockers may also cause contraction of bronchial smooth muscle and are contraindicated in patients with a history of asthma, etc.

Calcium-channel blockers (e.g., diltiazem, nifedipine, and verapamil) are preferable to beta-blockers in patients with coronary atherosclerosis and coronary vasospasm or patients with coronary vasospasm alone. The pain of unstable angina has been found to be equally controlled by propranolol and nitrates as by nifedipine alone. Because of its marked effect on vessels (causing vasodilation), nifedipine

TABLE 7–6
Drugs Used in the Treatment of Angina Pectoris

Class	Drug	Route of administration	Daily dose (mg)	Doses per day
Nitrates	Nitroglycerin	Sublingual	0.15 to 0.6	As needed
	Long-acting nitrates	Oral	80	Four
	Nitroglycerin ointment	Topical	One to four applications of 2% ointment	
	Long-acting transdermal nitrate patches	Topical	5 to 30	One to six patches
Blocking agents	Propranolol	Oral	160 to 480	Two to four
	Metoprolol	Oral	100 to 200	Two to three
	Atenolol	Oral	50 to 200	One
	Nadolol	Oral	40 to 320	One
Calcium-channel blockers	Nifedipine	Oral	30 to 120	One
	Verapamil	Oral	240 to 360	Three
	Diltiazem	Oral	120 to 360	Three to four
Combination therapy	Nitrates and blockers Verapamil or diltiazem and nitrates Nifedipine and blockers			

TABLE 7–7
Physiologic Effects of Agents Used to Treat Angina

	Vasodilation	Decrease cardiac oxygen demand	Decrease cardiac contractility	Decrease atrioventricular conduction
Nitrates	Yes	Yes	No	No
Beta-blockers	No (vasoconstriction)	Yes	Yes	No
Calcium-channel blockers	Yes (most marked with nifedipine)	No	Yes (verapamil but little effect with others)	Yes (avoid verapamil and diltiazem)

TABLE 7–8
Physiologic Effects of Calcium-Channel Blockers

	Verapamil	Nifedipine	Diltiazem
Vasodilation	Moderate	Marked	Moderate
Decreased contractility	None or mild	None	None or mild
Decreased atrioventricular (A-V) conduction	Mild	None	Mild

may produce skin flushing, headache, and dizziness. Nifedipine and nitrates are seldom used in combination, because both agents cause vasodilation and the above side effects are common. Verapamil or diltiazem is usually avoided in patients with atrioventricular conduction abnormalities, because they tend to decrease atrioventricular conduction. In some patients verapamil may cause constipation as a side effect[31] (Tables 7-6 to 7-8).

If calcium-channel blockers or lipophilic beta-blockers are used to manage angina in patients with liver disease, the usual daily dose may have to be reduced since these agents are metabolized by the liver. Calcium-channel blockers are preferred to beta blockers in the management of angina in insulin-dependent diabetics. The beta-blockers are not used because they tend to mask symptoms associated with hypoglycemia, and they also inhibit glycogenolysis and thus may prolong periods of hyperglycemia. Beta-blockers are generally not used in treating angina in patients with severe depression or patients with sexual dysfunction.[31]

Percutaneous transluminal coronary angioplasty (PTCA) or coronary dilation employing a small balloon is being used for the nonoperative dilation of stenotic coronary arteries.[1,36] A 2-to-3-day hospital stay is required for PTCA. Patients with proximal stenosis of the epicardial vessels are candidates for PTCA. This procedure can also be done for patients who have had bypass grafts that have developed stenosis. The major risks are dissection and thrombosis. The mortality rate associated with PTCA is less than 1%. Myocardial infarction occurs in about 3% of the cases, and minor complications occur in 5% to 10% of the cases. PTCA results in 85% to 90% adequate dilation and relief of angina. However, stenosis recurs within 6 months in 20% to 40% of the patients and angina recurs in 6 to 12 months in 25% of the patients. If restenosis or angina has not occurred within 1 year, the prognosis for the next 4 years is excellent.[28] Laser devices are now being used to destroy the atheroma.[17]

A patient with significant obstruction of the proximal portions of two or more of the major coronary arteries or obstruction of the left proximal anterior descending coronary artery is a candidate for a coronary bypass operation. The surgical mortality rate for the procedure is less than 1%. About 60% of the patients who undergo this procedure will obtain complete relief of symptoms, and 20% to 30% will have major or partial relief. Bypass of the left main coronary artery in patients with atherosclerotic disease has been shown[1,36] to prolong life. It is not clear if the other bypass procedures prolong survival. Patients with unstable angina treated by medical or surgical means show no difference in mortality or myocardial infarction rates at the end of 3 years. However, pain relief is more complete in those treated by surgery.[36]

Occlusion of the graft occurs in 10% to 20% of cases during the first year. It occurs at a rate of 2% per year for the next 5 to 7 years and at 5% thereafter. Each patient has a limited supply of autogenous graft material; synthetic material does not work. Thus, reoperation is possible only two or three times. In addition, scarring makes any reoperation more difficult. Internal mammary (thoracic) artery grafts appear to be sturdier and less susceptible to graft atherosclerosis than vein grafts. They are preferred for the first bypass procedure when possible.[9]

Rest is an important part of the therapeutic approach. If activity brings on chest pain, the patient is instructed to stop and rest for several minutes or longer until the pain goes away. Nitroglycerin tablets also may be taken. Bed rest (10 to 14 days) usually is recommended only when the angina syndrome first appears. A period of bed rest also is suggested for patients with the stable type of angina that for no reason begins to occur more frequently and severely.

Patients who have significant angina are encouraged to avoid long hours of work, to take rest periods during the working day, to obtain adequate rest at night, to use mild sedatives, to take frequent vacations, and in some cases to change their occupation or retire.

Patients who have coronary atherosclerotic heart disease should avoid any of the precipitating factors that may bring on cardiac pain—such as cold weather, hot humid weather, big meals, emotional upsets, cigarette smoking, and drugs (e.g., amphetamines, caffeine, ephedrine, cyclamates, and alcohol).

The treatment of patients with an acute myocardial infarction is far from ideal at present. Since about two thirds of the deaths from acute myocardial infarction occur outside of a hospital (50% of these are sudden deaths),[10,11] it is clear that there is now no effective system or therapy to deal with this problem. Several strategies have been proposed by which a potential victim might be identified and a fatal myocardial infarction possibly prevented. These include the following:

1. Identification and control of risk factors
2. Periodic ECG monitoring of high-risk patients using an isometric stress test; monitoring and control of patients with cardiac arrhythmias
3. Long-term use of antiarrhythmic drugs for individuals with frequent ventricular premature beats, etc.; however, at present, available drugs have side-effects that discourage this approach
4. Mass educational programs to reduce the time between recognizing early symptoms and seeking medical care
5. Establishment of fixed and mobile life-support stations

Patients with an acute myocardial infarction are hospitalized as soon as possible. The basic management goal is to minimize the size of the infarction and to prevent death from lethal arrhythmias. As a general rule, the patient with an uncomplicated myocardial infarction is kept in the coronary intensive care unit for 4 to 5 days. If the infarction is complicated by a serious dysrhythmia, heart failure, or shock, the stay in the coronary unit is extended.

As stated above, one of the major goals in managing acute myocardial infarction is to limit the size of the infarct. If more than 40% of the left myocardium is lost, heart failure and cardiogenic shock will result. Recent findings[2,23,28] using thrombolytic therapy have shown that the hospital mortality rate can be reduced by 50% if thrombolytic therapy is given during the first hour of infarction. Good benefits can still be gained if it is started 1 to 3 hours after infarction, but early thrombolytic therapy reduces infarct size and limits left ventricular dysfunction. The best results occur in patients with large thrombi and good collateral circulation. Streptokinase or tissue plasminogen activator (a thrombus-specific lytic agent) are injected IV over a 1-hour period. Additional doses of tissue plasminogen activator are given at hours 2 and 3. Heparin is usually given at the start of the therapy and continued for 2 to 5 days. Aspirin also is given, 325 mg per day.[2,23,28]

Thrombolytic therapy is contraindicated in patients with a recent history (2 weeks) of stroke or surgery, the presence of marked hypertension (greater than 180/100), or an active peptic ulcer and in pregnant women. If significant coronary stenosis is found, then coronary angioplasty or coronary artery bypass grafting must be considered.[22,23]

The other major goal in the management of a patient with acute myocardial infarction is to prevent lethal arrhythmias. Beta-blocking agents, lidocaine, and amiodarone are used for this purpose. Beta-blocking agents have been shown[2] to reduce post-MI deaths by 24% 9 to 36 months after the infarction; and amiodarone reduced mortality by 60% and arrhythmic events by 74% in the first year following infarction.

In the past about 30% of hospital "coronary" deaths occurred in patients just after they were transferred from the coronary unit to standard care facilities in the hospital. This has led some hospitals to develop halfway or intermediate coronary care units. Current studies[36] show a significant reduction in hospital "coronary" deaths after transfer from the coronary intensive care unit. The length of stay in the intermediate coronary unit is 7 to 12 days.

The present trend is for early ambulation of the patient who has had a myocardial infarction in the hospital. In some uncomplicated cases this occurs at about the eighth day of hospitalization. For most patients ambulation is started around the twelfth to fifteenth day.

Pain relief is an important part of the early medical management of patients with an acute myocardial infarction. Morphine sulfate is the drug of choice for acute pain relief. Sedatives and hypnotic medications also are used to calm the patient and ensure adequate periods of rest.

Oxygen is used during the acute period to increase the degree of oxygen saturation of the blood and keep the work load for the heart at a minimum. However, 100% oxygen should be avoided since it may cause hypoxia, which can reduce coronary blood flow. Oxygen usually is best administered by nasal cannula.

Most studies of patients with myocardial infarction have shown a significant reduction in mortality rate and thromboembolic complications by the use of anticoagulants. Patients may be given anticoagulants during the acute phase of infarction and for as long as 2 years thereafter.

The development of dysrhythmias in patients who have had an acute myocardial infarction constitutes an emergency problem that must be treated aggressively. During the first 6 months after an infarction, the conduction system of the heart may be unstable. Patients are very prone to serious arrhythmias during this period. Therefore elective dental procedures should be avoided. (See Chapter 8.)

The primary purpose of the rehabilitation program for a patient who has had a myocardial infarction is to return him or her to as normal a life as possible. If this cannot be done because of medical restrictions, an attempt is made to alter the patient's life-style in a way that is consistent with his or her cardiac reserve but still allows full use of the person's physical and emotional capacities.

The primary concerns of many patients that must be dealt with effectively during rehabilitation are the possibilities of returning to their occupation and resuming an active sex life. The physical status of the individual patient and his or her emotional reaction to the events must be considered in developing the rehabilitation program. Patients with an uncomplicated first myocardial infarction usually can return to an active life-style in about 6 to 8 weeks.[10,11]

There is no conclusive evidence that physical conditioning during the postinfarction period exerts a beneficial effect on the course of the disease.[10,11] Physical conditioning does not appear to alter collateral development or the electrical stability of the heart, reduce the rate of subsequent myocardial infarctions, or increase the patient's life expectancy. However, a reduction in symptoms does occur, and many patients have an improved sense of well-being and improved function. These positive factors warrant an active conditioning program for the patient who has had an infarction.

DENTAL MANAGEMENT
MEDICAL CONSIDERATIONS

Patients who have the stable form of angina without a history of infarction generally have a much lower risk of complications occurring in the dental office than do patients who have unstable angina or a history of a recent myocardial infarction.

Patients who have had a recent myocardial infarction should not receive any routine dental care until 6 months after the infarction (possible complications decrease with time).[20] Even after 6 months the dentist should consult with the patient's physician before beginning dental treatment. The physician should be informed of the basic nature of the dental care to be rendered and the dental management plan based on what has been learned about the patient from the medical history and physical examination. Important medical points and medications should be confirmed, and information concerning the presence of other medical problems the patient may have and the patient's present status should be sought.

The dental management plan that is developed for the patient with a history of myocardial infarction should include the following considerations: First, what is the patient's current status in regard to presence of congestive heart failure, hypertension, and angina? Second, what medications is the patient taking?

Patients with a history of coronary atherosclerotic heart disease should be given short morning appointments and may be premedicated with 5 to 10 mg of diazepam (Valium) before the appointment in an attempt to reduce anxiety. Early morning appointments have been common practice for cardiac patients. However, recent clinical observations may force a reevaluation of this practice. The incidence of sudden death has been reported[13] to be highest in the early morning hours. Unpublished data from a study of patients receiving periodontal surgery showed a greater effect on blood pressure in patients treated in the morning than those treated in the afternoon. There is not enough evidence to stop using morning appointments, but it is suggested that during consultation with the patient's physician this issue be discussed.

The approach of the office staff and dentist should be one of openness so feelings of fear can be expressed by the patient and dealt with in a constructive way to reduce the patient's anxiety toward dental personnel and the process. Nitrous oxide–oxygen analgesia can be used, as long as hypoxia is avoided. An effective local anesthetic is a must for these patients. Epinephrine in the concentration of 1:100,000 can be used safely, even if the patient has hypertensive disease.[13] Patients with poorly controlled ischemic heart disease, with labile cardiac rhythms, or with a potentially life-threatening arrhythmia should not be given a local anesthetic with vasoconstrictors. Three percent mepivacaine or 4% prilocaine should be used in these cases.[13]

Usually no more than three cartridges of anesthetic with epinephrine should be given during any single appointment. This concentration of epinephrine can be tolerated quite well and should lead to no complications, unless injected intravascularly.

Therefore, aspiration for blood should be done before the anesthetic solution is deposited (slowly). Vasopressors must not be used to control local bleeding or used in gingival packing materials. The patient with an old infarction may still be receiving anticoagulation medication. If surgery or extensive scaling procedures are planned, the dosage of anticoagulation medication should be reduced by the patient's physician. A prothrombin time that is 1½ to 2½ times normal should be obtained on the day of the dental procedure for patients taking coumarin (Coumadin). For patients taking aspirin as an anticoagulant, a bleeding time 1½ times

TABLE 7–9
Dental Management of the Patient with Angina Pectoris

Schedule morning or early afternoon appointments
Keep appointments short
Reduce stress and anxiety
   Patient able to express fears
   Premedication—diazepam, 5 to 10 mg
   Nitrous oxide–oxygen; hypoxia must be avoided
Nitroglycerin tablets available
Local anesthetic with 1:100,000 epinephrine; aspirate, inject slowly, no more than three cartridges
Avoid use of vasopressors to control local bleeding
Avoid use of vasopressors in gingival packing material
If patient becomes fatigued or develops significant changes in pulse rate or rhythm during appointment, terminate appointment at that time

normal or less should be obtained on the day of the surgery[20] (Tables 7-9 and 7-10).

Patients who are receiving antihypertensive agents or digitalis may be prone to nausea and vomiting; thus excessive stimulation of the gag reflex should be avoided. Antisialagogues should not be used in patients with coronary atherosclerotic heart disease unless the patient's physician has been consulted, because these drugs tend to cause tachycardia. Antiarrhythmic agents such as quinidine and procainamide may cause nausea and vomiting, hypotension, and, on occasion, agranulocytosis. Any medication the patient is taking must be identified, and the *Physicians' Desk Reference*[24] must be checked for side effects and drug interactions.

If at any time during the dental appointment a patient with coronary atherosclerotic heart disease becomes fatigued or develops a significant change in pulse rate or rhythm, the appointment should be terminated. Thus it is important that the patient be told to inform the dentist if he or she becomes fatigued, notes a change in heart rate, or feels otherwise unable to continue at any time during the appointment.

Patients who have angina pectoris should bring their nitroglycerin medication with them

TABLE 7–10

Dental Management of the Patient with a
History of Myocardial Infarction

Consult physician concerning management
No routine dental care until at least 6 months
  postinfarction
Patients on anticoagulation therapy needing deep
  scaling or surgical procedures
  Check prothrombin time (coumarin [Coumadin])
    or bleeding time (aspirin)
  Have physician reduce prothrombin time to 2
    times normal or less; bleeding time reduced to
    1½ times normal
  Place on antibiotics following surgery to mini-
    mize possibility of postoperative infection
Schedule morning or early afternoon
  appointments; keep appointments short; reduce
  stress and anxiety; premedicate with diazepam
Use local anesthetic with 1:100,000 epinephrine
  three cartridges maximum, aspirate, inject slowly
Avoid use of vasopressors to control local blood
  loss
Avoid use of vasopressors in gingival packing
  material
If patient becomes fatigued or develops significant
  changes in pulse rate or rhythm during appointment, terminate appointment at that time

---

to every dental appointment. Prophylactic nitroglycerin may be considered for patients who
have frequent attacks. If pain develops during
the dental appointment in a patient with a
history of stable angina, all work should be
stopped and the patient should take a nitroglycerin tablet and be allowed to relax. If the pain
is not relieved within 1 to 2 minutes, a blood
pressure cuff should be placed on the patient's
arm and the blood pressure measured and pulse
rate and rhythm determined. If the patient is
stable but still having pain, then another nitroglycerin tablet should be taken. If the pain
continues after a 2-to-3-minute wait, a third
nitroglycerin tablet should be taken by the
patient. Thus up to three nitroglycerin tablets
can be given within a 15-minute period. If after
15 minutes the patient is free of pain and stable,
the dentist can consider completing the work
planned for the appointment. Patients who have
the stable form of angina pectoris with no
history of myocardial infarction can usually

tolerate continuation of a dental appointment
once they are free of pain and relaxed. If the
patient is pain-free but the vital signs are not
stable, arrangements should be made for transfer to the patient's physician's office or nearest
emergency facility (Table 7-11).

If the pain is not relieved in the patient with
a history of stable angina within 15 minutes after
nitroglycerin is taken, the possibility of a myocardial infarction must be considered and emergency steps taken. If the patient's pulse and
blood pressure are stable, the patient's physician should be called and immediate arrangements made for the patient to be seen. Appropriate transportation should be arranged for the
transfer. Patients who do not have a physician or
whose physician cannot be reached should be
taken to the nearest emergency facility or
physician's office, depending on the local circumstances.

If the patient's status becomes unstable before the transfer, appropriate emergency lifesaving procedures should be started. Regardless
of whether the patient is stable or not, the
dentist must accompany him or her during the
transfer[20] (Table 7-12).

Patients with unstable angina or a history of
myocardial infarction who develop chest pain
during a dental appointment would be managed
as above, except the vital signs would be
evaluated first and then up to 3 nitroglycerin
tablets would be given within a 15-minute
period. If the patient becomes pain-free and is
stable within the 15-minute period, the appointment should be terminated and the patient's
physician called to see if he or she would like to
see the patient, and then the patient should be
so informed (Table 7-12).

TREATMENT PLANNING
MODIFICATIONS

Patients who have a history of a myocardial
infarction within the last 6 months should not
receive any routine dental treatment. In general, it is also best that patients who have
unstable angina receive no routine dental treatment since they are high-risk patients for
myocardial infarction. The stress of the dental
appointment could be a precipitating factor for
infarction.

Patients who have the stable form of angina
or who have had a myocardial infarction that is

TABLE 7–11
Dental Management of the Patient with a History of Stable Angina Who Develops Chest Pain during the Dental Appointment

1. Stop dental procedure
2. Give patient nitroglycerin tablet under tongue (from patient's own medication if possible); wait 2 to 3 minutes
   a. If pain is relieved
      (1) Let patient rest and continue with appointment
      (2) Terminate appointment and reschedule for another day
      (3) If possible inform patient's physician of what happened
   b. If pain is not relieved
      (1) Take patient's blood pressure and pulse, repeat procedures as needed
      (2) If patient's condition is stable, give second nitroglycerin tablet; if pain is relieved in 2 to 3 minutes, manage as in 2a above
      (3) If patient's condition remains stable but pain continues, give third nitroglycerin tablet; if pain is relieved, manage as in 2a above
      (4) If pain is not relieved following 3 nitroglycerin tablets given within 15-minute period or if patient becomes unstable at any time
         (a) Provide immediate emergency care as needed
         (b) Call patient's physician and arrange for patient to be seen
         (c) Attend patient until in hands of his or her physician or is being managed by hospital emergency room personnel

TABLE 7–12
Dental Management of the Patient with a History of Unstable Angina or Myocardial Infarction Who Develops Chest Pain during the Dental Appointment

1. Stop dental procedure
2. Give patient nitroglycerin tablet under tongue (from patient's own medication if possible); measure blood pressure and pulse; wait 2 to 3 minutes
   a. If pain is relieved and patient is stable, terminate appointment and inform patient's physician of what happened
   b. If pain is not relieved
      (1) If patient's condition is stable, give second nitroglycerin tablet; if pain is relieved in 2 to 3 minutes, manage as in 2a above
      (2) If patient's condition remains stable but pain continues, give third nitroglycerin tablet; if pain is relieved, manage as in 2a above
      (3) If pain is not relieved following three nitroglycerin tablets within 15-minute period or if patient becomes unstable at any time
         (a) Provide immediate emergency care as needed
         (b) Call patient's physician and arrange for patient to be seen
         (c) Attend patient until in hands of his or her physician or is being managed by hospital emergency room personnel

at least 6 months old can receive any indicated dental treatment. Before dental treatment is begun, however, the patient's physician should be contacted whenever possible to confirm the dental management plan.

ORAL COMPLICATIONS

There are no lesions associated directly with coronary atherosclerotic heart disease. Drugs used in the treatment of this disease and its complications may result in oral changes. Some of these drugs may cause allergic or toxic reactions that can result in oral ulceration and infection. Patients receiving dicumarol may have significant bleeding problems following trauma or surgical procedures.

Patients with coronary atherosclerotic heart disease with brief pain may have the pain, in rare cases, referred to the lower jaw. The pattern of the onset of pain caused by physical activity and its disappearance with rest will usually serve as clues to its cardiac origin.

REFERENCES

1. Braunwald E, Cohn PF: Ischemic heart disease. In Peterdorf RG, et al, editors: *Harrison's Principles of internal medicine,* ed 10, New York, 1983, McGraw-Hill Book Co.
2. Burckhardt D, Hoffmann A, Kiowski W, et al: Effect of antiarrhythmic therapy on mortality after myocardial infarction, *J Cardiovasc Pharmacol* 17(suppl 6):S77-S81, 1991.
3. Chung EK: *Controversy in cardiology,* New York, 1976, Springer-Verlag.
4. Collen D, Bennett WF: Recombinant tissue-type plasminogen activator. *Biotechnology* 19:197-223, 1991.
5. Dawber RT, Kannel WB: Susceptibility to coronary heart disease, *Mod Conc Cardiovasc Dis* 30:671-676, 1961.
6. Felner JM: Techniques of echocardiography. In Hurst JW, editor: *The heart, arteries, and veins,* ed 5, New York, 1982, McGraw-Hill, pp 1773-1799.
7. Gordon R, Kannel WB: Premature mortality from coronary heart disease, the Framingham study, *JAMA* 215:1617, 1971.
8. Glueck CJ: Role of risk factor management in progression and regression of coronary and femoral artery atherosclerosis, *Am J Cardiol* 57:356-416, 1986.
9. Healy BP: Pathology of coronary atherosclerosis. In Hurst JW, editor, *The heart, arteries, and veins,* ed 7, New York, 1990, McGraw-Hill, pp 924-940.
10. Hurst JW, editor: *The heart, arteries, and veins,* ed 4, New York, 1978, McGraw-Hill.
11. Hurst JW: Atherosclerotic coronary heart disease: historical benchmarks, methods of study and clinical features, differential diagnosis, and clinical spectrum. In Hurst JW, editor: *The heart, arteries, and veins,* ed 7, New York, 1990, McGraw-Hill, pp 961-1001.
12. Hurst JW, King SB III, Walter PF: Atherosclerotic coronary heart disease: angina pectoris, myocardial infarction, and other manifestations of myocardial ischemia. In Hurst JW, editor: *The heart, arteries, and veins,* ed 5, New York, 1982, McGraw-Hill, pp 1009-1149.
13. Jastak JT, Yagiela JA: Vasoconstrictors and local anesthesia: a review and rationale for use, *J Am Dent Assoc* 107:623-630, 1983.
14. Kannel WB, Castelli WP, Gordon T, et al: Serum cholesterol, lipoproteins, and risk of coronary heart disease: the Framingham study, *Ann Intern Med* 74:1, 1971.
15. Kannel WB, Thom TJ: Incidence, prevalence, and mortality of cardiovascular disease. In Hurst JW, editor: *The heart, arteries, and veins,* ed 6, New York, 1986, McGraw-Hill, pp 557-565.
16. Kannel WB, Thom TJ: Incidence, prevalence, and mortality of cardiovascular disease. In Hurst JW, editor: *The heart, arteries, and veins,* ed 7, New York, 1990, McGraw-Hill, pp 627-638.
17. Lau KW, Sigwart U: Novel coronary interventional devices: an update, *Am Heart J* 123(2):497-506, 1992.
18. Levy RI: Changing perspectives in the prevention of coronary artery disease, *Am J Cardiol* 57:176-266, 1986.
19. Little WC, Downes TR, Applegate RJ: The underlying coronary lesion in myocardial infarction: implications for coronary angiography, *Clin Cardiol* 14(11):868-874, 1991.
20. Malamed SF: *Handbook of medical emergencies in the dental office,* ed 3, St Louis, 1987, CV Mosby, pp 328-363.
21. Nestel PJ: Overview: extending the indications for treating hypercholesterolemia, *Am J Cardiol* 57:36-46, 1986.
22. Paspa PA, Movahed A: Thrombolytic therapy in acute myocardial infarction, *Am Fam Physician* 43(2):640-648, 1992.
23. Pasternak RC, Braunwald E: Acute myocardial infarction. In Wilson JD, et al, editors: *Harrison's principles of internal medicine,* ed 12, New York, 1991, McGraw-Hill, pp 953-964.
24. *Physicians' desk reference,* ed 46, Oradell, NJ, 1992, Medical Economics.
25. Pitt B, et al: Myocardial infarction. In Harvey A, editor: *Osler's Principles and practice of medicine,* ed 19, New York, 1976, Appleton-Century-Crofts.
26. Ross R: Coronary heart disease, factors influencing atherogenesis. In Hurst JW, editor: *The heart, arteries, and veins,* ed 5, New York, 1982, McGraw-Hill, pp 935-950.
27. Ross R: Medical progress: the pathogenesis of atherosclerosis-an update, *N Engl J Med* 314:488-489, 1986.
28. Selwyn AP, Braunwald E: Ischemic heart disease. In Wilson JD, et al, editors: *Harrison's Principles of internal*

medicine, ed 12, New York, 1991, McGraw-Hill, pp 964-971.

29. Setaro JF, Cabin HS: Right ventricular infarction, *Cardiol Clin* 10(1):69-90, 1992.

30. Shepherd JT, Vanhoutte PM: Spasm of the coronary arteries: causes and consequences, *Mayo Clin Proc* 60:33-46, 1986.

31. Shub C, Vlietstra RE, McGoon MD: Selection of optimal drug therapy for the patient with angina pectoris, *Mayo Clin Proc* 60:539-548, 1985.

32. Silber EM, Katz LM: *Heart disease,* New York, 1975, Macmillan Publishing.

33. Syrota A, Jehenson P: Complementarity of magnetic resonance spectroscopy, positron emission tomography and single photon emission tomography for in vivo investigation of human cardiac metabolism and neurotransmission, *Eur J Nucl Med* 18(11):897-923, 1991.

34. Tiefenbrum AJ: Clinical benefits of thrombolytic therapy in acute myocardial infarction, *Am J Cardiol* 69(2):3A-11A, 1992.

35. Vlietstra RE, Kronmal RA, Oberman A, et al: Effect of cigarette smoking on survival of patients with angiographically documented coronary artery disease, *JAMA* 255:1023-1027, 1986.

36. Young JB, Luchi RJ: Coronary heart disease. In Rose LF, Kaye D, editors: *Internal medicine for dentistry,* St Louis, 1983, CV Mosby.

37. Zaret BL, Berger HJ: Techniques of nuclear cardiology. In Hurst JW, editor: *The heart, arteries, and veins,* ed 5, New York, 1982, McGraw-Hill, pp 1803-1843.

8

Cardiac Arrhythmias

Individuals seeking dental treatment may have various forms of cardiac arrhythmias. Many of these arrhythmias are of little concern to the patient or dentist; however, some can produce symptoms and a few can be life-threatening, including arrhythmias that occur secondary to anxiety (e.g., those associated with dental care). Patients with significant arrhythmias must be identified prior to having dental treatment rendered.

Cardiac arrhythmias may be found in normal healthy individuals, in patients on various medications, and in patients with certain systemic diseases. The arrhythmias may be asymptomatic, symptomatic, or even life threatening (Table 8-1).

The purpose of this chapter is to describe the various types of cardiac arrhythmias, the identifying characteristics of patients with various arrhythmias, and the importance of the more significant arrhythmias in the dental patient. The dental management of patients with a cardiac arrhythmia will be presented—with emphasis on (1) the identification of a patient who has an arrhythmia, (2) identifying the patient who is susceptible to developing an arrhythmia, and (3) the management of patients

TABLE 8–1
General Causes of Cardiac Arrhythmias

Primary cardiovascular disease
Pulmonary disorders
Autonomic disorders
Systemic diseases
Drug-related side effects
Electrolyte imbalances

with a life-threatening arrhythmia in the dental office.

GENERAL DESCRIPTION
INCIDENCE AND PREVALENCE

A cardiac arrhythmia is any variation in the normal rhythm of the heartbeat. Cardiac arrhythmias may be disturbances of rhythm, rate, or conduction of the heart. They may be found in healthy individuals as well as in those with various forms of cardiovascular disease (Table 8-2).

Various drugs also may cause cardiac arrhythmias.[1, 4, 5] Digitalis, morphine, and beta-blockers can induce sinus bradycardia. Atropine, epinephrine, nicotine, and caffeine can cause sinus tachycardia. Alcohol, tobacco, digitalis, or coffee may precipitate premature atrial beats in normal individuals. Digitalis, alcohol, epinephrine, and amphetamines may cause ventricular extrasystoles in healthy individuals. Digitalis, quinidine, procainamide, potassium, and sympathetic amines may induce ventricular tachycardia in patients with cardiovascular disease.

Cardiac arrhythmias may be associated with various systemic diseases (Table 8-3). Pathologic sinus bradycardia may be found in patients with febrile illnesses, myxedema, obstructive jaundice, increased cranial pressure, and myocardial infarction. Pathologic sinus tachycardia may be found in patients with fever, infection, hyperthyroidism, and anemia. Atrial extrasystoles may occur in patients with congestive heart failure, coronary insufficiency, and myocardial infarction. Supraventricular tachycardias have been reported[5] in about 6% of individuals with mitral valve prolapse and may be found in patients with pneumonia or acute myocardial

TABLE 8–2

Incidence of Cardiac Arrhythmias in Healthy Individuals

Type of arrhythmia	Population group	Number	Percentage
Sinus bradycardia	Healthy children 7 to 11 years	—	45
	1000 aviators 20 to 30 years	380	38
	6014 Air Force personnel	902 to 1683	15 to 28
Sinus tachycardia	1000 aviators 20 to 30 years	3	0.3
Paroxysmal atrial tachy-cardia	98 healthy 60 to 85 year olds	13	13.3
Atrial flutter	98 healthy 60 to 85 year olds	1	1.0
	67,000 Air Force personnel	1	0.001
Atrioventricular (A-V) block (first-degree)	19,000 air crew applicants	59	0.3
	67,000 Air Force personnel	350	0.5
Atrial and ventricular extrasystoles	300 middle-aged men		62
	10-to-13-year-old boys		13 to 26
	22-to-28-year-old women		54 to 64
	60 to 85 year olds		80
Ventricular tachycardia	67,000 Air Force personnel	1	0.001
	98 healthy 60 to 85 year olds	4	4.0

Based on Marriott H, Myerberg RJ. In Hurst JW, editor: *The heart, arteries, and veins,* ed 6, New York, 1986, McGraw-Hill, pp 433–475.

TABLE 8–3

Cardiac Arrhythmias Associated with Various Systemic Diseases

Arrhythmia	Systemic condition
Sinus bradycardia	Infectious diseases, hypothermia, myxedema, obstructive jaundice, increased cranial pressure, myocardial infarction
Atrial extrasystoles	Congestive heart failure, coronary insufficiency, myocardial infarction
Sinoatrial (S-A) block	Rheumatic heart disease, myocardial infarction, acute infections
Sinus tachycardia	Febrile illnesses, infections, anemia, hyperthyroidism
Atrial tachycardia	Obstructive lung disease, pneumonia, myocardial infarction
Atrial flutter	Ischemic heart disease, mitral stenosis, myocardial infarction, open heart surgery
Atrial fibrillation	Myocardial infarction, mitral stenosis, ischemic heart disease, thyrotoxicosis, hypertension
Atrioventricular (A-V) block	Rheumatic heart disease, ischemic heart disease, myocardial infarction, hyperthyroidism, Hodgkin's disease, myeloma, open heart surgery
Ventricular extrasystoles	Ischemic heart disease, congestive heart failure, mitral valve prolapse
Ventricular tachycardia	Mitral valve prolapse, myocardial infarction, coronary atherosclerotic heart disease
Ventricular fibrillation	Blunt cardiac trauma, mitral valve prolapse, anaphylaxis, cardiac surgery, rheumatic heart disease, cardiomyopathy of any kind, coronary atherosclerotic heart disease

infarction. Atrial flutter may be found in patients with ischemic heart disease and complicates 2% to 5% of myocardial infarction cases.[5] Atrial fibrillation may be found associated with rheumatic mitral disease, hypertension, ischemic heart disease, or thyrotoxicosis.[5]

Ventricular extrasystoles are the most common form of rhythm disturbance found in patients with various illnesses.[5] They occur in patients with ischemic heart disease and congestive heart failure. They also occur in about 45% of individuals with mitral valve prolapse.[5] Ventricular tachycardia is almost always associated with a diseased heart and has been reported in 6% of patients with mitral valve prolapse as well as in 28% to 46% of monitored patients with myocardial infarction.[5] Ventricular fibrillation is a terminal arrhythmia unless rapid and effective therapy is given. It may be precipitated by coronary atherosclerotic heart disease, cardiomyopathy of any origin, rheumatic heart disease, blunt cardiac trauma, mitral valve prolapse, cardiac surgery, and cardiac catheterization.[1,4,5]

ETIOLOGY

The primary pacemaker for the heart is the sinoatrial (S-A) node. Impulses generated by the S-A node result in a normal rhythm of 60 to 100 beats per minute. Secondary pacemakers are present and include atrial, atrioventricular (A-V), and ventricular escape pacemakers.[1,12]

The impulse generated by the S-A node is usually conducted in the following sequence: (1) S-A node, (2) A-V node, (3) bundle of His, (4) bundle branches, and (5) subendocardial Purkinje network (Fig. 8-1). The ECG is a record of the electrical activity of the heart. The basic deflections and physiologic events recorded are shown in Figures 8-2 and 8-3. Figure

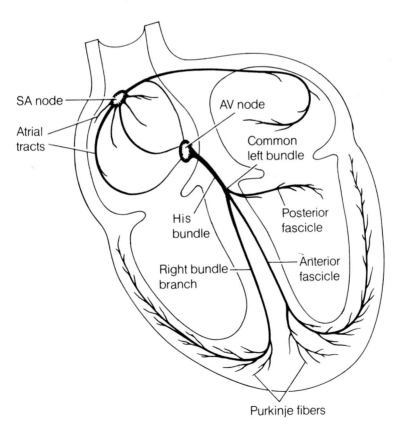

FIG. 8-1 The conduction system. (From Hurst C: *Dysrhythmia interpretation based on cardiac suppression and irritability,* Philadelphia, 1986, JB Lippincott, p 13.)

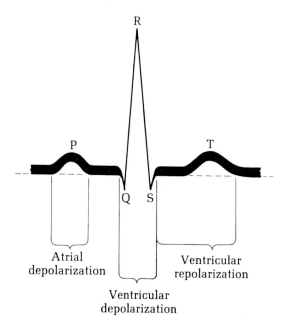

FIG. 8-2 Normal electrocardiographic deflections. The normal electrocardiogram consists of a P wave, a QRS complex, and a T wave. The P wave represents atrial depolarization; the QRS complex, ventricular depolarization; the T wave, rapid repolarization of the ventricles. (From Conover MB: *Understanding electrocardiography: arrhythmias and the 12-lead ECG,* ed 6, St Louis, 1992, Mosby–Year Book.)

8-4 demonstrates several methods of determining heart rate from an ECG tracing.

The A-V node serves as a gate preventing too many atrial impulses from entering the ventricle. It also slows the conduction rate of impulses generated in the S-A node.

Normal cardiac function depends on cellular automaticity (impulse formation), conductivity, excitability, and contractility. Disorders in automaticity and conductivity form the basis of the vast majority of cardiac arrhythmias. Under normal conditions the S-A node is responsible for impulse formation; however, other cells in the conduction system can generate impulses. Under abnormal conditions ectopic pacemakers can emerge outside the conduction system. After the generation of an impulse and its discharge the cells (S-A node) need time for recovery; this is termed *refractoriness.* Complete refractoriness will result in a block, and partial refractoriness in a delay, of conductivity.[1,4,8]

Disorders of conductivity (block or delay) can paradoxically lead to a rapid cardiac rhythm through the mechanisms of reentry. (For a more complete explanation of the mechanism of arrhythmias, see the chapter on arrhythmias in the seventeenth edition of the *Cecil Textbook of Medicine.*[1]

The type of arrhythmia may suggest the nature of its cause. For example, paroxysmal atrial tachycardia with block suggests digitalis toxicity.[1,8] However, many cardiac arrhythmias are not specific for a given cause. In these patients a careful search is made to identify the etiology of the arrhythmia. The most common

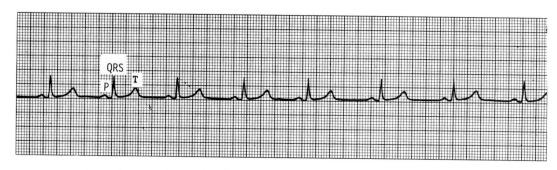

FIG. 8-3 Cardiac cycle. The basic P-QRS-T cycle repeats itself again and again. (From Goldberger AL, Goldberger E: *Clinical electrocardiography: a simplified approach,* ed 4, St Louis, 1990, Mosby–Year Book.)

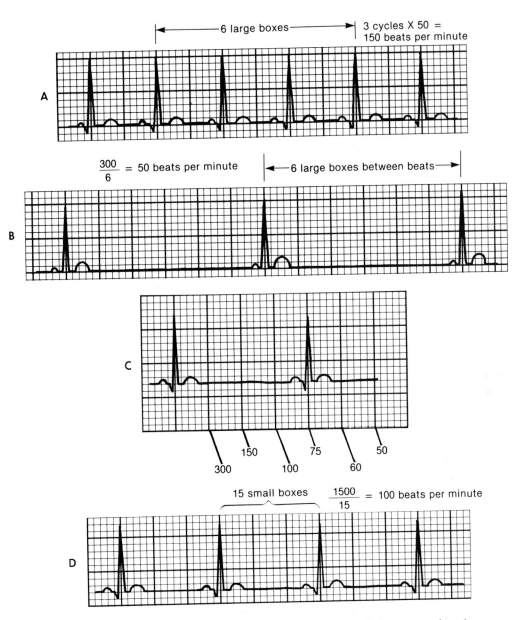

FIG. 8-4 Methods of determining heart rate. The rates shown (in beats per minute) are as follows: **A,** 150; **B,** 50; **C,** 75; **D,** 100. (From Johnson R, Swartz MH: *Simplified approach to electrocardiography,* Philadelphia, 1986, WB Saunders, p 19.)

TABLE 8-4
Cardiac Arrhythmias

Isolated ectopic beats

Premature atrial beats
Premature atrioventricular (A-V) beats
Premature ventricular beats

Bradycardias

Sinus bradycardia
Sinoatrial (S-A) heart block
A-V heart block

Tachycardias

Sinus tachycardia
Atrial tachycardia
Atrial flutter
Atrial fibrillation
Ventricular tachycardia

Preexcitation syndrome

Cardiac arrest

Ventricular fibrillation
Ventricular asystole
Agonal rhythm

causes include (1) primary cardiovascular disorders, (2) pulmonary disorders (embolism, hypoxia), (3) autonomic disorders, (4) systemic disorders (thyroid disease), (5) drug-related side effects, and (6) electrolyte imbalances (Table 8-1).

Arrhythmias can be classified into the following: isolated ectopic beats, bradycardias, tachycardias, preexcitation syndrome, and cardiac arrest (Table 8-4).

PATHOPHYSIOLOGY AND COMPLICATIONS

Arrhythmias may be asymptomatic and cause no hemodynamic changes. However, some can affect cardiac output[1,8] by (1) producing insufficient forward flow because of a slow cardiac rate, (2) reducing forward flow because of insufficient diastolic filling time with a rapid cardiac rate, (3) decreasing flow because of poor sequence in A-V activation with direct effects on ventricular function.

The effect of an arrhythmia often is dependent on the physical condition of the patient. For example, a young healthy person with paroxysmal atrial tachycardia may have minimal symptoms whereas an elderly patient who has heart disease with the same arrhythmia may develop shock, congestive heart failure, or myocardial ischemia.[1,8]

Isolated ectopic beats
PREMATURE ATRIAL BEATS

Premature impulses arising from ectopic foci anywhere in the atrium may result in premature atrial beats. They are common in conditions associated with dysfunction of the atria such as congestive heart failure.

PREMATURE ATRIOVENTRICULAR BEATS

Premature A-V beats are less common than premature atrial or premature ventricular ectopic beats. Impulses can spread toward either the atria or the ventricles. When present, digitalis toxicity should be suspected.

PREMATURE VENTRICULAR BEATS

Premature ventricular beats are the most common form of arrhythmia with or without heart disease. In one study[5] over 50% of middle-aged men and up to 80% of persons 60 to 85 years of age were found to have premature ventricular beats. Eighty percent of myocardial infarction patients will have premature ventricular beats.[1] They also are common with digitalis excess and hypokalemia. Late premature ventricular beats can lead to ventricular tachycardia or fibrillation in the presence of ischemia (Fig. 8-5).

Bradycardias
SINUS BRADYCARDIA

A sinus rate of less than 60 beats per minute is defined as bradycardia.[1,4,5] It is a normal finding in young healthy adults and well-conditioned athletes. Bradycardia can occur secondary to medications. Medications with parasympathetic effects such as digoxin and phenothiazines may slow the heart rate. In addition, medications that suppress the excitability of the heart—such as beta–adrenergic blockers (propranolol, metoprolol)—may cause bradycardia.[14] A sinus bradycardia that persists in the presence of congestive heart failure, pain, or exercise and following atropine administration is considered abnormal. Sinus bradycardia

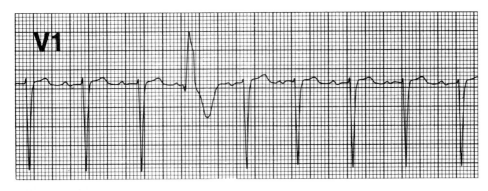

FIG. 8-5 Ventricular premature contraction. Note that this wide complex comes prematurely compared to the next sinus P wave. (From Johnson R, Swartz MH: *A simplified approach to electrocardiography,* Philadelphia, 1986, WB Saunders, p 19.)

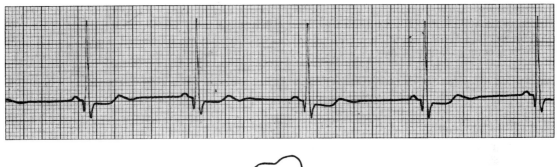

FIG. 8-6 Sinus bradycardia. In this tracing the sinus rate is 50 beats per minute. (From Conover MB: *Understanding electrocardiography: arrhythmias and the 12-lead ECG,* ed 6, St Louis, 1992, Mosby–Year Book.)

is a common finding early in myocardial infarction. It may also occur in infectious diseases, myxedema, and obstructive jaundice and in cases of hypothermia (Fig. 8-6).

SINOATRIAL HEART BLOCK

S-A heart block is relatively uncommon. Most cases are caused by rheumatic heart disease, myocardial infarction, acute infection, or drug toxicity (digitalis, atropine, salicylates, quinidine). The block may occur in stages or degrees:

(1) first-degree block—impulse takes undue time to enter the atrium, (2) second-degree block—one or some impulses fail to emerge from the S-A node, and (3) complete block—no impulses emerge from the S-A node.

ATRIOVENTRICULAR HEART BLOCK

Rheumatic fever, ischemic heart disease, myocardial infarction, hyperthyroidism, and drugs (digitalis, propranolol, potassium, quinidine) may cause A-V heart block. About 50% of the cases are associated with congenital heart disease.[3] A-V block also occurs in degrees: (1) first-degree block—slow impulses with increased conduction time, (2) second-degree block—some impulses fail to reach the ventricles, and (3) complete block—no impulses reach the ventricles. Sarcoidosis, Hodgkin's disease, myeloma, and open heart surgery (aortic valve, ventricular septal defects) also may result in complete heart block (Fig. 8-7).

Tachycardias

SINUS TACHYCARDIA

A sinus rate greater than 100 beats per minute is defined as sinus tachycardia.[1,4,5] It is most often caused by a physiologic response to exercise, anxiety, stress, and emotions. Pharma-cologic causes of sinus tachycardia include atropine, epinephrine, nicotine, and caffeine. Pathologic causes are fever, hypoxia, infections, anemia, and hyperthyroidism.

ATRIAL TACHYCARDIA

In atrial tachycardia ectopic impulses may result in atrial rates of 150 to 200 per minute.[1] Often there will be some degree of A-V block with ectopic atrial tachycardia. In about 75% of the cases digitalis toxicity or hypokalemia is present.[5] Atrial tachycardia is also seen in some cases of chronic obstructive lung disease, advanced pathology of the atria, acute myocardial infarction, pneumonia, and drug intoxications (alcohol, catechols)[1,4,5] (Fig. 8-8).

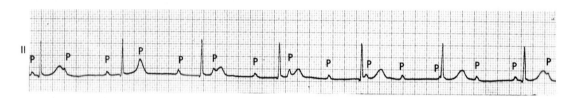

FIG. 8-7 Complete heart block is characterized by independent atrial *(P)* and ventricular *(QRS)* activity. The atrial rate is always faster than the ventricular rate. PR intervals are completely variable. Some P waves fall on the T wave, distorting the shape of the T wave. Others fall in the QRS complex and are "lost." Note that the QRS complexes are of normal width, indicating that the ventricles are being paced from the A-V junction. (From Goldberger AL, Goldberger E: *Clinical electrocardiography: a simplified approach,* ed 4, St Louis, 1990, Mosby–Year Book.)

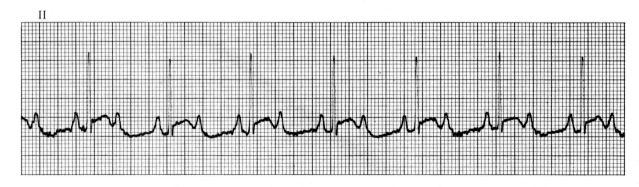

FIG. 8-8 Atrial tachycardia with 2:1 A-V conduction. (From Conover MB: *Understanding electrocardiography: arrhythmias and the 12-lead ECG,* ed 6, St Louis, 1992, Mosby–Year Book.)

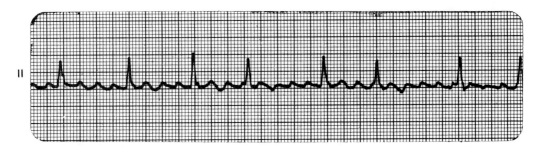

FIG. 8-9 Variable ventricular rate in a patient with atrial flutter. (From Goldberger AL, Goldberger E: *Clinical electrocardiography: a simplified approach,* ed 4, St Louis, 1990, Mosby–Year Book.)

ATRIAL FLUTTER

A very rapid, regular atrial rate of 220 to 360 beats per minute is defined as atrial flutter. Rare in healthy individuals,[1] atrial flutter is most often associated with ischemic heart disease in individuals over 40 years of age. It complicates about 2% to 5% of the cases of myocardial infarction and is a rare complication of digitalis intoxication.[5] Atrial flutter also is seen as a complication in patients with mitral stenosis or cor pulmonale and following open heart surgery. It may result when patients with atrial fibrillation have been treated with quinidine or procainamide (Fig. 8-9).

ATRIAL FIBRILLATION

Atrial fibrillation is characterized by a very, very rapid atrial rate of 400 to 650 per minute with no discrete P waves on the ECG tracing.[1] Ventricular response is irregularly irregular. Atrial fibrillation may be found in healthy individuals although it usually is associated with rheumatic heart disease, hypertension, ischemic heart disease, or thyrotoxicosis. It is more common than the other forms of atrial tachyarrhythmias and occurs in 7% to 16% of patients with myocardial infarction. It is also found in about 90% of persons with mitral stenosis who have had peripheral emboli.[5]

Two major hemodynamic events occur with atrial fibrillation: (1) poor atrial transport of blood and (2) generation of impulses that excite rapid and irregular ventricular response. A secondary complication of poor atrial transport of blood is peripheral or pulmonary emboli. Thirty percent of individuals with long-standing atrial fibrillation experience at least one embolic episode. Atrial fibrillation can precipitate congestive heart failure in patients with a history of heart disease[1,4,5] (Fig. 8-10).

VENTRICULAR TACHYCARDIA

Three or more ectopic ventricular beats occurring at a rate of 100 or more per minute is defined as ventricular tachycardia. This arrhythmia almost always occurs in diseased hearts. Certain drugs—such as digitalis, sympathetic amines, potassium, quinidine, and procainamide—may induce ventricular tachycardia. On rare occasion it may be found in young healthy adults. When ventricular tachycardia occurs, it may be either nonsustained or sustained or it may degenerate into ventricular fibrillation (Fig. 8-11).

Preexcitation syndrome (WPW)

Three events appear to be involved in the Wolfe-Parkinson-White (WPW) preexcitation syndrome: First, an accessory A-V pathway is present that allows for the normal conduction systems to be bypassed. Second, this accessory pathway allows for rapid conduction and short refractoriness, with impulses being passed rapidly from atrium to ventricle. Third, the parallel conduction system provides a route for reentrant tachyarrhythmias. This pattern constitutes a syndrome when patients become symptomatic from paroxysmal supraventricular tachycardia. Paroxysmal atrial fibrillation and flutter also may occur, leading to ventricular fibrillation and death.[1,4,5,12]

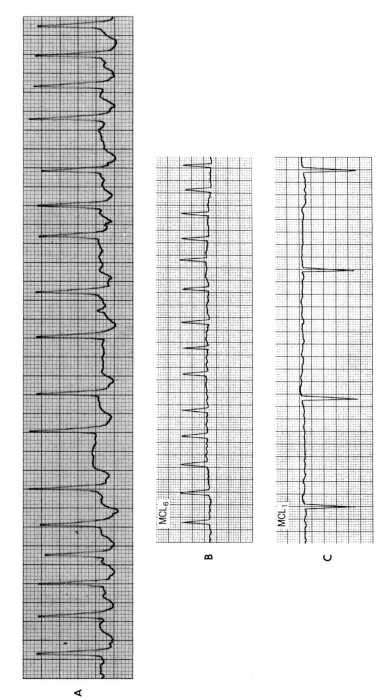

FIG. 8-10 **A,** Atrial fibrillation with an uncontrolled ventricular response and a fine fibrillatory line. **B,** Atrial fibrillation with a rapid ventricular response. **C,** Atrial fibrillation with a slow ventricular response. Chaotic atrial activity is demonstrated by the undulating baseline. (**A** from Conover, MB: *Understanding electrocardiography: arrhythmias and the 12-lead ECG*, ed 6, St Louis, 1992, Mosby–Year Book; **B** and **C** from Guzzetta CE, Dossey BM: *Cardiovascular nursing: holistic practice*, ed 2, St Louis, 1992, Mosby–Year Book.)

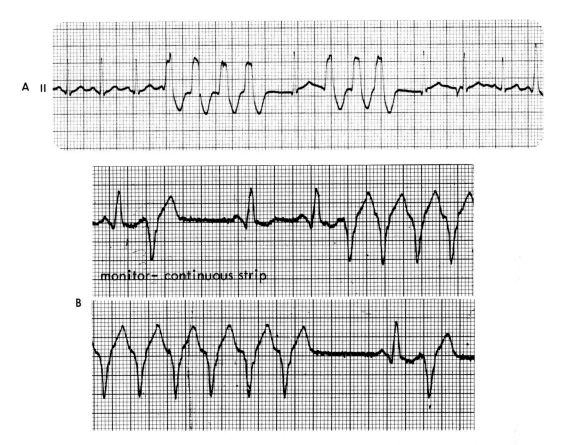

FIG. 8-11 **A,** Two short bursts of ventricular tachycardia, defined as three or more consecutive PVCs. **B,** The monitor lead shows bursts of ventricular tachycardia. (**A** and **B** from Goldberger AL, Goldberger E: *Clinical electrocardiography,* ed 4, St Louis, 1990, Mosby–Year Book.)

Continued.

Cardiac arrest

Ventricular fibrillation, ventricular asystole, and agonal rhythm are all lethal arrhythmias that require immediate therapy for survival. (See Table 8-6.)

VENTRICULAR FIBRILLATION

Ventricular fibrillation is represented as chaotic activity on the ECG, with the ventricles contracting very rapidly but ineffectively. This is usually a terminal arrhythmia unless therapy is rapidly administered. Coronary atherosclerosis is the most common form of heart disease predisposing to ventricular fibrillation. Other causes of this arrhythmia include rheumatic heart disease, anaphylaxis, blunt cardiac trauma, mitral valve prolapse, cardiac surgery, digitalis intoxication, and cardiac catheterization. Ventricular fibrillation in young healthy adults is rare[1,4,5] (Fig. 8-12).

VENTRICULAR ASYSTOLE

In ventricular asystole, cardiac standstill occurs when no impulses are being conducted to the ventricles and no muscular activity is taking place. The conditions causing ventricular fibrillation can also lead to ventricular asystole (Fig. 8-13).

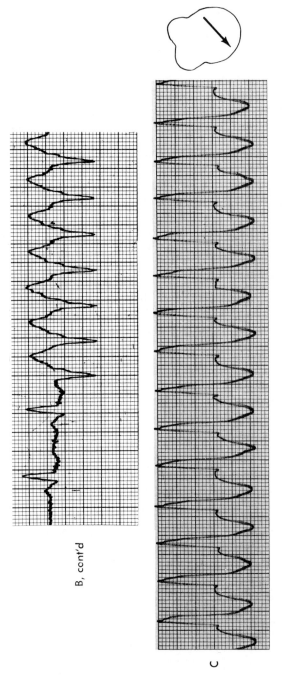

B, cont'd

C

FIG. 8-11, cont'd   **C**, Ventricular tachycardia. (C from Conover MB: *Understanding electrocardiography: arrhythmias and the 12-lead ECG*, ed 6, St Louis, 1992, Mosby–Year Book.)

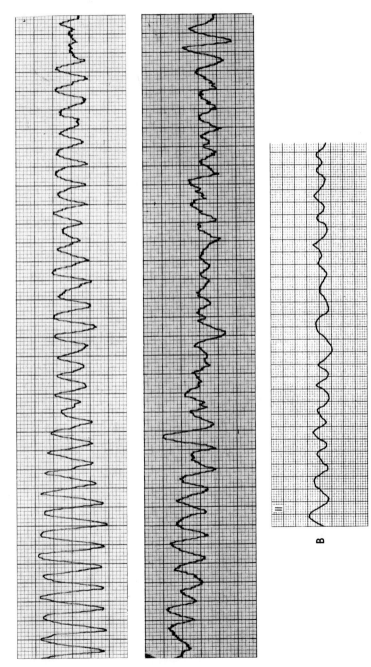

FIG. 8-12 **A,** Ventricular flutter deteriorating into ventricular fibrillation (continuous strip). **B,** Ventricular fibrillation. (A from Conover MB: *Understanding electrocardiography: arrhythmias and the 12-lead ECG,* ed 6, St Louis, 1992, Mosby–Year Book; **B** from Guzzetta CE, Dossey BM: *Cardiovascular nursing: holistic practice,* ed 2, St Louis, 1992, Mosby–Year Book.)

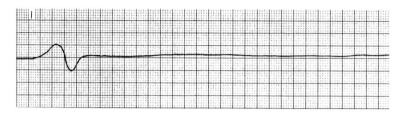

FIG. 8-13   Ventricular standstill. Note the agonal beat at the beginning of the strip. (From Guzzetta CE, Dossey BM: *Cardiovascular nursing: holistic practice,* ed 2, St Louis, 1992, Mosby–Year Book.)

AGONAL RHYTHM

Again, in agonal rhythm, effective ventricular contraction ceases. Although impulse conduction is taking place, the ECG shows wide distorted complexes, with no mechanical activity in the ventricles.[5]

CLINICAL PRESENTATION
SIGNS AND SYMPTOMS

Cardiac arrhythmias may be asymptomatic but detected because of a change in the rate and/or rhythm of the pulse. A slow pulse may indicate a form of bradycardia, and a fast pulse may indicate a tachyarrhythmia. Electrocardiographic monitoring is needed to identify the true nature of many cardiac arrhythmias.[1,12]

The impact of an arrhythmia on the circulation is more important than the arrhythmia itself. Symptoms that may indicate the presence of an arrhythmia include fatigue, dizziness, syncope, congestive heart failure, angina, and cardiac arrest. The patient may complain of heart palpitations occurring on a regular or irregular basis[1,4,5,8] (Table 8-5).

TABLE 8–5
Signs and Symptoms of Cardiac Arrhythmias

Signs	Symptoms
Slow heart rate (less than 60 beats per minute)	Palpitations Fatigue Dizziness
Fast heart rate (greater than 100 beats per minute)	Syncope Congestive heart failure Angina
Irregular heart rate	Cardiac arrest

LABORATORY TESTS

The ECG is very helpful in the identification and diagnosis of cardiac arrhythmias. Electrode catheter techniques now allow for intracavitary recordings of the specialized conducting systems, which aids greatly in diagnosing arrhythmias. (See the chapter on cardiac arrhythmias in the seventeenth edition of the *Cecil Textbook of Medicine*[1] for a more complete explanation of the above techniques in arrhythmia identification and diagnosis.)

MEDICAL MANAGEMENT

The management of cardiac arrhythmias involves medication, a pacemaker, surgery, or cardioversion. Asymptomatic arrhythmias usually require no therapy. Symptomatic arrhythmias, in general, are treated first with medications. Those that do not respond to medications are then treated by a pacemaker. If both medications and pacing fail to control the arrhythmia, then surgery may be attempted. Cardioversion is indicated for any tachyarrhythmias that compromise hemodynamics and/or life. Cardiac arrest also is treated by cardioversion.[1,4,8,13]

ANTIARRHYTHMIC DRUGS

With many antiarrhythmic drugs the toxic/therapeutic ratio is very narrow; therefore dosage for a given patient must be individualized. Measurement of plasma levels of the medication is often an important part of therapy. The following medications are used for control of arrhythmias[1,4,8,13] (Table 8-6):

1. *Digoxin.* Digoxin improves the mechanical efficiency of the myocardium by slowing conduction in the A-V node, prolonging refractoriness in the A-V node, and de-

TABLE 8–6
Drugs Used in the Management of Cardiac Arrhythmias

Drug	Usual dosage (maintenance)
Digoxin	PO 0.125 to 0.5 mg per day
Digitoxin / Digitalis	PO 0.1 mg per day
Quinidine	PO 200 to 600 mg every 6 hours
Procainamide	PO 250 to 750 mg every 3 to 4 hours
Disopyramide	PO 100 to 300 mg every 6 hours
Lidocaine	IV 20 to 50 mg/min to total dose of 5 mg/kg
Propranolol	PO 20 to 80 mg every 6 hours
Verapamil	PO 200 to 400 mg every 6 hours

creasing the refractoriness of atrial tissue. These effects are useful in treatment of supraventricular tachycardias—atrial flutter and atrial fibrillation. *Digitoxin* and *digitalis* are also used as antiarrhythmic agents.

2. *Quinidine.* Quinidine depresses automaticity arising from abnormal or ectopic locations. It also increases the threshold of excitability of the atrium and ventricle, slows conduction (except in the A-V node, where it increases conduction), and prolongs refractoriness. It is often effective in the treatment of a variety of supraventricular and ventricular arrhythmias—including atrial and ventricular premature beats, atrial flutter, and atrial fibrillation. Patients are usually given digitalis before starting quinidine therapy. Quinidine is generally not used in patients with second-degree or complete A-V block or in those with congestive heart failure. Adverse effects of quinidine include diarrhea, nausea, vomiting, tinnitus, hearing loss, vertigo, and thrombocytopenia; on occasion, it may precipitate ventricular tachycardia or fibrillation.

3. *Procainamide.* The indications for procainamide are the same as for quinidine, except that procainamide is more effective in the treatment of ventricular than of atrial arrhythmias. Toxic effects include nausea, vomiting, rarely diarrhea, and in about 20% to 25% of patients a systemic lupus erythematosus–like syndrome that spares the brain and kidney.

4. *Disopyramide.* The actions of disopyramide are similar to those of quinidine; however, prominent anticholinergic side effects—such as dry mouth, blurred vision, constipation, and urinary hesitancy—have been reportedly associated with the use of disopyramide. It must be used with caution in patients who have prostatic hypertrophy or congestive heart failure and in older patients with significant myocardial ischemia. Disopyramide is contraindicated in patients with glaucoma.

5. *Lidocaine.* Lidocaine is used primarily in the emergency management of patients with a serious ventricular arrhythmia. It is effective in abolishing ventricular reentry impulses and has minimal effect on atrial tissues. Side effects include dizziness, paresthesias, confusion, muscle tremors, and seizures.

6. *Propranolol.* Propranolol slows conduction and prolongs refractoriness in the A-V node; hence it is useful for a variety of supraventricular arrhythmias. Its effect also is mediated by blockage of the beta–adrenergic stimulating action of catecholamines on the heart. Propranolol is used with digoxin to slow ventricular response in patients with atrial fibrillation. It is also used for arrhythmias associated with hyperthyroidism, exercise, and mitral valve prolapse. Propranolol may lead to severe hypotension in some patients and cause pulmonary vasoconstriction in patients with asthma or obstructive lung disease. Sudden withdrawal of the drug should be avoided in patients with ischemic heart disease, such as angina and myocardial infarction, since severe arrhythmias may be precipitated.

7. *Verapamil.* Verapamil is an antiarrhythmic agent that acts by interfering with the movement of calcium through the so-called slow channel. It is the drug of choice for paroxysmal A-V junction tachycardias. Verapamil is not used with propranolol, disopyramide, or quinidine. It can cause heart block in patients with underlying abnormalities in the A-V node.

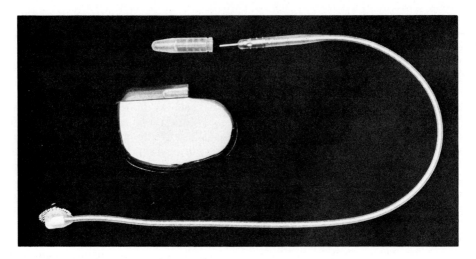

FIG. 8-14   One type of implantable pacemaker (pulse generator). This device is usually implanted subcutaneously in the right anterior chest below the clavicle. (From Phipps WJ, et al: *Medical-surgical nursing,* ed 4, St Louis, 1991, Mosby–Year Book.)

PACEMAKERS

In 1984 about 500,000 persons in the United States had permanent pacemakers. About 100,000 new implants are performed each year. Today's pacemakers are smaller, lighter, and more reliable, and last longer, than those available 10 to 15 years ago.[7,10]

A pacing system consists of a generator that will produce an electric impulse that is transmitted by a lead to an electrode that is in contact with endocardial or myocardial tissue. A variety of pacing systems is available. For example, the atrium and/or ventricle may be paced; transvenous or transmediastinal leads may be used; demand, asynchronous, or programmable pulse generators (Fig. 8-14) are available; and active or passive electrodes can be placed[7,10] (Table 8-7).

Pacemakers are useful in the management of several conduction system abnormalities: symptomatic sinus bradycardia, symptomatic A-V block, and tachyarrhythmias refractory to drug therapy.

The most common pacing system in use today is the demand ventricular pacemaker with a lithium-powered generator and transvenous leads.[10] This pacemaker has a sensing circuit that can detect the patient's natural heartbeat and avoid competitive pacemaker firing. In addition, there are dual-chambered pacemakers capable of sensing and pacing both atria and ventricles. The newer units contain pacing circuits that allow for programming, memory, and telemetry.[1,7,10]

A classification code for modes of pacing has been developed[8] (Table 8-8). The code shows the chamber that is paced, the chamber that is sensed, and the mode of response. It also shows programmable functions (e.g., rate modification) and the system used for tachyarrhythmias found in the more complex pacemakers.[8] The most common pacemaker in use today has a code of VVI. This means it paces the ventricle, senses the ventricle, and is inhibited by the patient's own ventricular activity.[8]

A piezoelectric crystal bonded to the inner surface of the pulse generator is used to detect patient movement. Increased activity causes increased pacing.[8] Some side effects can result from pacemakers. Infection at the generator site

TABLE 8–7
Component Parts of a Pacemaker

Generator – demand, asynchronous
Lead – transvenous, transmediastinal
Electrode – active, passive

TABLE 8–8
Pacemaker Code*

Code positions†				
I Chamber(s) paced	**II** Chamber(s) sensed	**III** Response to sensing	**IV** Programmable functions	**V** Antitachyarrhythmic functions
V, Ventricle	V, Ventricle	T, Triggers pacing	P, Programmability (rate and/or output)	P, Antitachyar- rhythmia
A, Atrium	A, Atrium	I, Inhibits pacing	M, Multiprogramma- bility (rate, output, sensitivity, etc.)	S, Shock
D, Double	D, Double	D, Triggers and inhibits pacing	C, Communication (telemetry)	D, Dual (P + S)
			R, Rate modulation	
0, None	0, None	0, None	0, None	

*This code, first suggested in the 1970s by the Inter-Society Commission for Heart Disease Resources, was modified in 1980 and 1987.
†Positions *I* to *III* are used exclusively for antibradyarrhythmic pacing.
From Mond HG, Sloman JG. In Hurst JW, editor: *The heart, arteries, and veins,* ed 7, New York, 1990, McGraw-Hill, p 570.

and thrombosis on the leads or electrodes are uncommon but do occur. Skeletal muscle may be stimulated if insulation is lost around the lead or the generator rotates. In rare cases myocardial burning can occur.[8,9] Some patients become depressed, and suicide attempts have been reported.[8,9]

Electromagnetic interference from noncardiac electrical signals may interfere temporarily with the function of a pacemaker. This occurs by a mimicking of the frequency of spontaneous heartbeats, which causes inappropriate pacemaker inhibition. Examples would be transmission from high-powered television sets, radio and radar transmitters, or arc welders. Other forms of electrical signals can cause revision of the pacemaker mode to a fixed rate of transmission. These would include microwave ovens, Cavitrons, certain pulp testers, diathermy and electrocautery units, defibrillators, any electric motor, and direct-contact pulse generators in boat or automobile motors[10] (Table 8-9).

Internal shielding has been increased on the newer generators to minimize the adverse effects of electromagnetic interference. These units are now protected against adverse effects from microwave oven signals. However, problems still occur, particularly with dual-chamber pacemakers.[10]

Certain patients with ventricular fibrillation or unstable ventricular tachycardias are candidates for an automatic implantable cardioverter-defibrillator (AICD). The AICD is a self-contained diagnostic-therapeutic system that monitors the heart and, when it detects fibrillation or tachycardia of the ventricle, sends a correcting electric shock to restore normal

TABLE 8–9
Sources for Electromagnetic Interference With Pacemaker Function

Television set
Radio transmitter
Radar transmitter
Arc welder
Microwave oven
Diathermy unit
Electrocautery unit
Boat or automobile motor
Any electric motor
Cavitron
Electric pulp tester

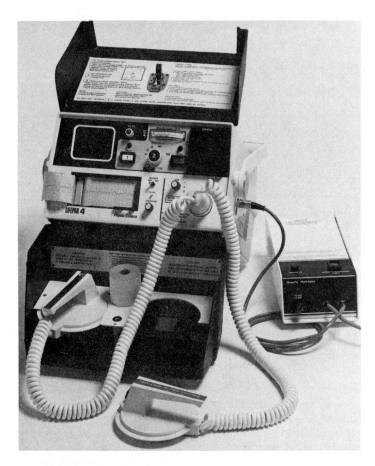

FIG. 8-15   Portable battery-powered monitor-defibrillator unit suitable for emergency use at the scene, during transport, or in hospital. The charger *(right)* can be disconnected. (Courtesy Physio-Control, Redmond Wash. From Burrell LO, Burrell ZL Jr: *Critical care,* ed 4, St Louis, 1982, CV Mosby.)

rhythm.[6] By 1987 over 2500 patients worldwide had had an AICD surgically implanted. (See Chapter 5.)

The AICD is 99% reliable in detecting ventricular fibrillation and 98% reliable in detecting ventricular tachycardias. Its conversion effectiveness is excellent. Usually one 25-joule (J) discharge converts the arrhythmia.[6] The surgical implantation of an AICD is covered in Chapter 5. The AHA does not recommend antibiotic prophylaxis for patients with either a cardiac pacemaker or an AICD.[7]

CARDIOVERSION

Direct-current cardioversion to convert atrial and ventricular arrhythmias was first described in 1962.[1] Cardioversion can be effective for treatment of reentrant arrhythmias—such as atrial flutter, atrial fibrillation, ventricular tachycardia, and ventricular fibrillation. Tachyarrhythmias that result in hemodynamic collapse, prolonged angina pectoris, or pulmonary edema should be treated promptly with direct-current cardioversion. The countershock simultaneously depolarizes the entire myocardium, allowing for synchronous repolarization and the resumption of sinus rhythm.[1,7,8,13]

A defibrillator is an electrical device that sends a pulse of current through the heart to arrest several types of arrhythmias (Figs. 8-15 and 8-16). The pulse is applied to electrodes placed on the thorax. One electrode is placed on

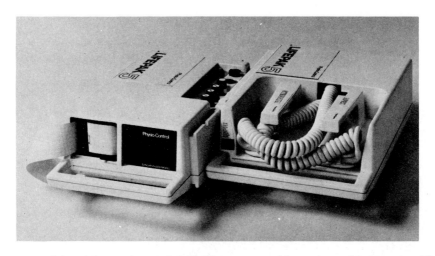

FIG. 8-16 Lightweight monitor and defibrillator powered by rechargeable batteries. Their light weight makes these devices ideal for field use. The monitor and defibrillator are detachable, so either unit can be operated independently. (Courtesy Physio-Control, Redmond Wash. From Burrell LL, Burrell ZL Jr: *Critical care,* ed 4, St Louis, 1982, CV Mosby.)

the left chest over the region of the apex, and the other on the right chest just to the right of the sternum and below the clavicle (Fig. 8-17). Usually a damped sine wave defibrillator is used that can store 400 J of energy and deliver about 350 J into a 50-ohm resistor. Either multiple low-energy shocks (2 J/kg) or a single high-energy first shock (4 J/kg) is employed. It is important to develop a dose concept, so the strength of the shock required is related to the size of the subject's heart. The practice of turning the output control to maximum and delivering a full "jolt" to all adults can be dangerous. Defibrillation is usually instantaneous, and cardiac pumping resumes within a few seconds. If defibrillation is unsuccessful (regular heartbeat does not occur), it may have to be repeated. Cardiopulmonary resuscitation (CPR) must be used until defibrillation has been successful. When defibrillation is attempted, all rescue personnel must stand clear of the patient except the individual who is holding the electrodes.

DENTAL MANAGEMENT
MEDICAL CONSIDERATIONS

Stress associated with dental treatment or excessive amounts of epinephrine may produce life-threatening cardiac arrhythmias in susceptible dental patients. Patients with an existing arrhythmia(s) are at risk in the dental environment. In addition, patients who are at risk for developing an arrhythmia also may be in danger in the dental office if they are not identified and measures taken to minimize stressful situations that could precipitate an arrhythmia. Other patients may have their arrhythmia under control by drugs or a pacemaker but will require special considerations when receiving dental treatment. The key to the dental management of patients prone to developing a cardiac arrhythmia and those with an existing arrhythmia is identification and prevention. Even under the best of circumstances, however, a patient may develop a cardiac arrhythmia that will require immediate emergency measures.

PREVENTION OF MEDICAL COMPLICATIONS

Identification of patients with an existing arrhythmia and those prone to developing an arrhythmia is most important. The dentist must obtain a medical history and evaluate the vital signs (pulse [rate and rhythm], blood pressure, respiratory rate) for all patients desiring dental treatment.

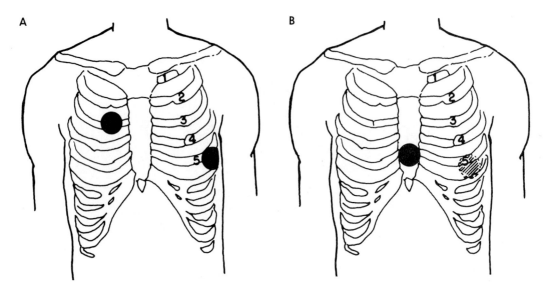

FIG. 8-17 Positioning of paddles for defibrillation or cardioversion with direct current shock. **A,** One paddle is placed to the right of the sternum, over the second and third interspaces. The other is placed on the left anterior axillary line, just below the apex of the heart, so electric current will pass through the heart. **B,** Anteroposterior view. Note that one paddle is over the sternum at the level of the heart apex and the second is under the left interscapular area. (From Goldberger E: *Treatment of cardiac emergencies,* ed 5, St Louis, 1990, Mosby–Year Book.)

TABLE 8–10
Dental Management of the Patient with a
Cardiac Arrhythmia—Medical Consultation

---

1. Refer for diagnosis and management any patient identified as having signs and symptoms suggesting presence of cardiac arrhythmia
2. Establish current status for patient with arrhythmia under medical treatment, also nature and severity of arrhythmia
3. Patient with pacemaker—attempt to establish
   a. Type of pacemaker being used
   b. Nature of arrhythmia being treated
   c. Need for prophylactic antibiotics
   d. Degree of shielding provided for generator and types of electrical equipment that should be avoided
4. Establish whether patient with atrial fibrillation is being treated with coumarin (Coumadin) to prevent atrial thrombosis and how dosage should be altered by physician
5. Establish presence and current status of underlying condition that may be cause of arrhythmia

---

Patients with a history of palpitations, dizziness, angina, dyspnea, and/or syncope may have a cardiac arrhythmia and should be evaluated by a physician before dental treatment is performed. Patients who have an irregular cardiac rhythm with or without symptoms should be referred for medical evaluation. Elderly patients with a regular heart rate that varies in intensity with respiration should be referred for evaluation of a possible sinus arrhythmias and sinus node disease[11,14] (Table 8-10).

Patients with a history of significant heart disease, thyroid disease, or chronic pulmonary disease must be detected and medical consultation obtained regarding their current status and risk for developing a cardiac arrhythmia. In addition, patients taking antiarrhythmic medication and those with a pacemaker must be identified through their medical history and, again, their current status established by medical consultation (Table 8-11).

Several recent studies[2,3] have reported the use

TABLE 8–11
Dental Management of the Patient with a
Cardiac Arrhythmia—Patient Identification

1. Undetected arrhythmia
   a. Rapid or slow pulse rate
   b. Irregular pulse rhythm
   c. Associated symptoms
      (1) Palpitations
      (2) Dizziness
      (3) Syncope
      (4) Angina
      (5) Dyspnea
2. Susceptible to development of arrhythmia
   during dental treatment
   a. History of ischemic heart disease
   b. History of valvular heart disease
   c. History of thyroid disease
   d. History of obstructive pulmonary disease
3. Under medical treatment for arrhythmia
   a. Taking antiarrhythmic medication
   b. With implanted pacemaker

of a 3-lead ECG unit, ViTel III,* to screen
dental patients for arrhythmias. The system
consists of a portable ECG unit (ViTel III) that
utilizes leads I, II, and III (the standard limb
leads of a 12-lead electrocardiogram). Electrode placement is standard—on the right
forearm, left forearm, and right or left leg. The
use of these three electrode sites allows testing
without the patient's needing to disrobe.

The ViTel III can record either a single-
channel 60-second ECG or a triple-channel 60-
second ECG (with three 20-second intervals);
each provides a distinct vector (angle) for view-
ing the electrical function of the heart. Three-
lead ECG monitoring has been used for a number of years and, when compared with the
standard 12-lead EKG system, is more than 90%
accurate.

Prior to the ECG recording, each patient is
asked to complete a cardiac screening questionnaire (CSQ) (Fig. 8-18). One or more positive
answers are interpreted as indicating increased
risk for an arrhythmia. Once the ECG is
recorded, it is transmitted by telephone to a
scanning service located in EquiMed's control
office in Plymouth, Minnesota. The transmitted

* EquiMed Corporation, Plymouth MN, 55447.

ECG is interpreted by a registered nurse or
technician trained in evaluating cardiac recordings, with a cardiologist available for consultation. The reading of the ECG strip includes
numerical data for heart rate, pulse rate, QRS
width, and QT interval and the classification of
any arrhythmia noted according to its origin or
nature. The interpretations of arrhythmias are
grouped into one of three classifications (Fig.
8-19): *Column I* consists of those considered to
be nonserious and in need of no follow-up
unless the patient is symptomatic. *Column II*
consists of those that could be serious and
require additional evaluation. *Column III* consists of those that are serious and could be
life-threatening. This information is communi-
cated to the transitting dentist and is followed by
a written report mailed to the dentist for
inclusion in the patient's dental record.

Based on the screening of over 10,000 patients,[2] about 4% were found to have column II
or III arrhythmias. This is a rather high yield
and would suggest a role for screening in the
dental office. Dental patients appeared to be
receptive to this activity.[3] Arrhythmias were
more common in patients with a positive CSQ,
in patients 60 years of age or older, and in males
generally.[2] Patients found to have a significant
arrhythmia are referred for medical evaluation.

The dentist can prevent many cardiac
arrhythmia–related medical emergencies by being aware of who are the high-risk patients
(Table 8-12) and by taking appropriate precautions during dental treatment (Table 8-13).
These precautions include the following:

1. *Reduce patient anxiety.* Any increases in sympathetic tone can precipitate an arrhythmia.
   Premedication with diazepam (Valium) 5 mg on
   the night before the appointment and 5 mg
   before the appointment may be utilized. Nitrous oxide inhalation can be initiated. An
   open, honest approach with the patient, explaining what will happen is most important.
2. *Minimize stressful situations.* Patients with coronary atherosclerotic heart disease, ischemic
   heart disease, or congestive heart failure
   should be managed to prevent or minimize
   acute exacerbation of these conditions that
   might trigger significant arrhythmias (Chapters
   7 and 9).
3. *Avoid excessive amounts of vasoconstrictive
   agents.* At the same time, however, vasoconstrictors in appropriate concentration in the local

Name _____ ID# _____ Age _____ Sex _____ Date _____

	Y	N			Y	N

1. Have you ever had any of the following?
   Episodes of passing out ___ ___
   Unusual shortness of breath ___ ___
   Unexplained fatigue ___ ___
   Frequent dizziness or light-headedness ___ ___

2. Do you ever experience chest tightness, heaviness, pressure, or pain? ___ ___

3. Are you currently taking any of the following medications? (please circle)

   Antianginals (nitroglycerin [Nitro-Bid], [Nitro-Patch], isosorbide dinitrate [Isordil]) ___ ___

   Calcium channel blockers (diltiazem [Cardizem], verapamil [Isoptin], [Calan], nifedipine [Procardia], [Adalat]) ___ ___

   Beta blockers (nadolol [Corgard], metoprolol [Lopressor], propranolol [Inderal], pindolol [Visken], timolol [Blocadren], [Timolide], atenolol [Tenormin]) ___ ___

   Antiarrhythmics (quinidine [Quinaglute], disopyramide [Norpace], procainamide [Procan SR], [Pronestyl], flecainide [Tambocor], amiodarone [Cordarone], mexiletine [Mexitil], tocainide [Tonocard], encainide [Encaid]) ___ ___

   Digitalis (digoxin [Lanoxin]) ___ ___

   Diuretics (water pills) (furosemide [Lasix], hydrochlorothiazide [Oretic], [Esidrix], spironolactone [Aldactone]) ___ ___

   Antihypertensives (blood pressure pills) (captopril [Capoten], hydralazine [Apresoline], prazosin [Minipress], triamterene [Maxzide], hydrochlorothiazide-triamterene [Dyazide], enalaprilat [Vasotec], minoxidil [Loniten], indapamide [Lozol], methyldopa [Aldomet], clonidine [Catapres]) ___ ___

4. Have you ever had palpitations, an irregular or slow heartbeat, or skipped beats? ___ ___

5. Do you have a family history of cardiac sudden death? (brothers, sisters, parents, grandparents, children) ___ ___

6. Are you a heart patient currently under the care of a doctor? ___ ___

7. Do you have a history of rheumatic fever? ___ ___

8. Do you have mitral valve prolapse? ___ ___

9. Do you have a history of heart murmurs? ___ ___

10. Are you over 70? ___ ___

11. Do you have high blood pressure? ___ ___

12. Do you have a pacemaker? ___ ___
    Type: _____ Rate: _____

13. Have you ever had a heart attack? ___ ___
    If so, when _____

14. Do you have chronic lung disease, bronchitis, emphysema, wheezing, or asthma? ___ ___

15. Have you ever had heart surgery? ___ ___

16. Have you ever had an abnormal exercise test? (eg. treadmill) ___ ___

17. Have you had an abnormal ECG? ___ ___

18. Do you have a history of any of the following?
    High cholesterol ___ ___
    Smoking more than one pack of cigarettes per day ___ ___
    Diabetes ___ ___
    High blood pressure ___ ___
    Family history of heart attacks ___ ___
    Being more than 30 lb overweight ___ ___

FIG. 8-18 Cardiac screening questionnaire used to select patients for ECG screening in the dental office.

Acct. #_____ Patient name _____ID #_____

Date _____ Age _____ Sex _____ Previous results _____

Medical history _____

CSQ results _____

Medication _____

_____

_____

Report # _____ EquiMed technician _____

Heart rate _____ PR interval _____ QRS width _____ QT interval _____

    (Normal 50 to 100)   (Normal 0.12 to 0.20)   (Normal 0.04 to 0.10)   (Normal 0.30 to 0.46 variable)

_____ Normal sinus rhythm _____ Sinus dysrhythmia _____ Other (below)

Comments

COLUMN I	COLUMN II	COLUMN III
Atrial arrhythmia		
___ Sinus pause, < 2 sec	___ Supraventricular extrasystoles, > 6/min (PJC, PAC)	___ Paroxysmal supraventricular tachycardia, > 10 sec
___ Sinus tachycardia, > 100 bpm	___ Paroxysmal supraventricular tachycardia, < 10 sec	___ Sinus pause, > 2 sec
___ Sinus bradycardia, < 50 bpm	___ Atrial fibrillation/flutter, controlled rate, < 120 bpm	___ Atrial fibrillation/flutter, ≥ 120
___ Wandering atrial pacemaker	___ Nonconducted PAC, ≥ 6/min	
___ Supraventricular extrasystoles, ≤ 6/min (PJC, PAC)	___ Junctional rhythm	
___ Nonconducted PAC, <6/min		

FIG. 8-19 Form used to report results of ECG screening by EquiMed Corp. *Column I* arrhythmias are the least serious and do not require immediate medical follow-up. *Column II* arrhythmias are more serious, and the patient should be referred for medical evaluation. *Column III* are the most serious and require immediate medical evaluation.

COLUMN I	COLUMN II	COLUMN III
CONDUCTION DISTURBANCE		
___ First-degree A-V block	___ Second-degree A-V block, Mobitz type I	___ High-degree A-V block
	___ Second-degree A-V block, Mobitz type II	___ Third-degree (complete) A-V block
	___ Bundle branch block, IVCD	
	___ BBB & first-degree A-V block	
Ventricular arrhythmia		
___ Ventricular extrasystoles, ≤ 6/ min	___ Ventricular extrasystoles, > 6/min	___ Sustained idioventricular rhythm
	___ Ventricular couplets	___ Sustained ventricular tachycardia
	___ Ventricular bigeminy	___ Ventricular fibrillation/flutter
Pacemaker	___ Nonsustained ventricular tachycardia	___ Ventricular standstill
___ Normal pacemaker function	___ Nonsustained idioventricular rhythm	___ Pacemaker malfunction
		Failure to sense ___
Other		Failure to pace ___ Other___
_____	___ S-T deviations, < 2 mm Elevation___ Depression___	___ S-T deviations, > 2 mm Elevation ___ Depression___
_____	___ Abnormally prolonged QT	
_____		

NOTE: The ECG interpretation has been made from a random 3-channel, 60-second rhythm strip and is based only on the rate and rhythm present at that time. It should not be considered a substitute for continuous ECG monitoring, 12-lead resting ECG monitoring, or cardiac stress testing. Any patient evaluation made must necessarily include appropriate consideration of the patient's medical history, vital signs, and complaints, as well as the 3-lead ECG, as false negatives can occur.

TABLE 8–12
Degree of Risk Involved in the Patient with Various Types of Cardiac Arrhythmias*

1. Low risk—no medications, infrequent symptoms
   a. Atrial arrhythmias
   b. Premature ventricular beats
   c. Young active individuals with sinus bradycardia
2. Moderate risk—chronic medication, asymptomatic
   a. Atrial arrhythmias
   b. Ventricular arrhythmias
   c. Medications known to affect function of sinus node
   d. Pacemaker
3. High risk
   a. Symptomatic patient
   b. Pulse greater than 100 or less than 60 with another type of arrhythmia
   c. Irregular pulse rhythm
   d. Irregular pulse and bradycardia
   e. Bradycardia with cardiac pacemaker

*Medical consultation is recommended to help establish the risk for each patient.

TABLE 8–13
Dental Management of the Patient at Risk for a Cardiac Arrhythmia—Precautions to be Taken

1. Reduce anxiety
   a. Premedication
   b. Open and honest communication
   c. Morning appointments
   d. Short appointments
   e. Nitrous oxide–oxygen inhalation
2. Avoid excessive amounts of epinephrine
   a. Use 1:100,000 in local anesthetic, except for patients with severe arrhythmias
   b. Use long-acting local anesthetic without epinephrine for patients with severe arrhythmias; confirm by medical consultation
   c. Use no more than three cartridges of anesthetic
   d. Do not use epinephrine in gingival packing
   e. Do not use epinephrine to control local bleeding
3. Avoid general anesthesia
4. Avoid use of electrical equipment that may interfere with function of pacemaker
5. Manage underlying problem—such as rheumatic heart disease—as indicated (i.e., antibiotic prophylaxis for endocarditis prevention, etc.)
6. Establish need for antibiotic prophylaxis by medical consultation for patients with cardiac pacemaker

anesthetic are indicated. The need to achieve profound local anesthesia and hemostasis far outweighs the very slight risk of using these agents in small amounts (e.g., 1:100,000 epinephrine). However, the use of more than three cartridges (1.8 cc) of anesthetic is not advised for any given appointment. In patients with severe arrhythmias it may be best to use a local anesthetic without epinephrine. Vasoconstrictors must not be used in gingival packing material for crown impressions or to control local bleeding.

4. *Avoid general anesthesia.* Patients susceptible to developing significant cardiac arrhythmias should not be given general anesthesia in the dental office.
5. *Be careful in use of electrical equipment.* During the medical consultation for patients with a pacemaker the risk for electromagnetic interference from electrical equipment used in the dental office should be established. Patients with a new, well-shielded generator are at low risk. However, patients with poor shielding may be at high risk for complications in pacing because of electromagnetic interference. Pulp testers, motorized dental chairs, belt-driven handpieces, and Cavitrons all may be capable of causing pacemaker malfunction in a patient with poor shielding in the pacemaker generator. Electrosurgery units can be of risk to all pacemaker patients, and their use in these patients is contraindicated.

6. *Consider the type of disorder.* Patients with underlying cardiac disease must be managed as indicated by the nature of the cardiac problem (e.g., those susceptible to endocarditis).[11,14]
7. *Minimize prophylactic antibiotics.* Although patients with a pacemaker are potentially susceptible to infective endocarditis, the incidence of this is extremely low; therefore antibiotic prophylaxis is not generally indicated. However, it may be discussed with the patient's physician.

In the rare case when a life-threatening cardiac arrhythmia occurs during dental treatment, the dentist and staff must be prepared to take immediate action (Table 8-14).

TABLE 8–14

Dental Management of the Patient with a Life-Threatening Arrhythmia in the Dental Office

---

Stop procedure

Evaluate vital signs: pulse rate and rhythm, blood pressure, also mental alertness of patient

Call for medical assistance if indicated

Administer oxygen

Place patient in Trendelenburg position (reduces hypotension)

Give nitroglycerin if indicated (chest pain)

Perform vagal maneuver (carotid massage) in cases of hypotension with tachycardia

Initiate cardiopulmonary resuscitation (CPR) as indicated for cardiac arrest

Patient with cardiac arrest will require cardioversion as soon as possible along with other advanced life-support measures; these in most cases will be provided as medical assistance becomes available or when patient has been transported to hospital

---

TREATMENT PLANNING CONSIDERATIONS

Once the patient who is susceptible to cardiac arrhythmias has been identified and the steps described above have been taken, these patients can receive virtually any indicated dental procedure. Complex dental procedures should be spread out over several appointments to avoid overstressing the patient. Some physicians want prophylactic antibiotics used to protect all patients with a pacemaker from infection secondary to transient dental bacteremias. In general, however, little evidence has been found to support the need for prophylactic antibiotics in these cases.[5,6] Patients with atrial fibrillation often are taking coumarin (Coumadin) to prevent atrial thrombosis. Minor surgical procedures can be done in these patients if the prothrombin time is 1½ to 2½ times normal, but each case must be evaluated prior to having dental procedures performed that will cause bleeding. This involves medical consultation, possible modification of coumarin dosage by the physician, and a prothrombin time test to verify that anticoagulation is in an acceptable range.

The dentist and staff must be prepared to deal with a life-threatening cardiac arrhythmia at any time and with any patient.

TABLE 8–15

Oral Complications of Antiarrhythmic Drugs*

Drug	Complication
Procainamide	Mucosal ulcerations
	Drug-induced lupus erythematosus
Propranolol	Mucosal ulcerations
	Petechiae
Disopyramide	Xerostomia
Quinidine	Mucosal ulcerations

*When findings are noted, the patient's physician should be contacted and informed.

ORAL COMPLICATIONS

The only significant oral complications found in patients with an arrhythmia are those occurring as side effects to the medication used to control the arrhythmia. Procainamide can cause agranulocytosis secondary to drug toxicity affecting the bone marrow. Mucosal ulcerations may occur in the mouth from agranulocytosis. Patients on procainamide who develop oral ulcerations should be evaluated for possible bone marrow suppression. Procainamide also has been reported to produce a lupus-like syndrome in some patients. Quinidine can cause a similar reaction leading to oral ulceration. Disopyramide, because of its anticholinergic effect, may cause xerostomia. If the xerostomia becomes severe, medical consultation is indicated to see if another antiarrhythmic agent could be used in place of the disopyramide. Propranolol may produce bone marrow suppression resulting in agranulocytosis and/or thrombocytopenia. In these patients, oral ulcers and/or petechiae may be found[11,14] (Table 8-15). (See Appendix B for treatment regimens to manage these oral lesions.)

REFERENCES

1. Gallagher JJ: Cardiac arrhythmias. In Wyngaardin JB, Smith LH, editors: *Cecil textbook of medicine,* ed 17, Philadelphia, 1985, WB Saunders Co.
2. Little JW, Kunik RL, Merry JW, et al: Evaluation of an EKG system for the dental office, *Gen Dent* 38(4):278-282, 1990.
3. Little JW, Simmons MS, Rhodus NL, et al: Dental patient reaction to EKG screening, *Oral Surg* 70:433-439, 1990.
4. Luck JC, Engel TR: Cardiac arrhythmias. In Rose LF,

Kaye D, editors: *Internal medicine for dentistry,* ed 2, St Louis, 1990, Mosby–Year Book.

5. Marriott HJ, Myerberg RJ: Recognition of arrhythmias and conduction abnormalities. In Hurst JW, editor: *The heart, arteries, and veins,* ed 6, New York, 1986, McGraw-Hill, pp 433-475.

6. Mirowski M: The implantable cardioverter-defibrillator. In Hurst JW, editor: *The heart, arteries, and veins,* ed 7, New York, 1990, McGraw-Hill, pp 2110-2113.

7. Mond HG, Sloman JG: Artificial cardiac pacemakers. In Hurst JW, editor: *The heart, arteries, and veins,* ed 6, New York, 1986, McGraw-Hill.

8. Mond HG, Sloman JG: The indications for and types of artificial cardiac pacemakers. In Hurst JW, editor: *The heart, arteries, and veins,* ed 7, New York, 1990, McGraw-Hill, pp 561-580.

9. Mond HG, Strathmore NF: The technique of using cardiac pacemakers: implantation, testing, and surveillance. In Hurst JW, editor: *The heart, arteries, and veins,* ed 7, New York, 1990, McGraw Hill, pp 2100-2110.

10. Riegel B, Purcell JA, Brest AN, Dreifus LS, editors: *Dreifus pacemaker therapy: an interprofessional approach,* Philadelphia, 1986, FA Davis.

11. Rose LF, Godfrey P, Steinberg BJ: Dental correlations; arrhythmia. In Rose LF, Kaye D, editors: *Internal medicine for dentistry,* St Louis, 1983, CV Mosby, pp 584-585.

12. Smith MB, Gallagher JJ: Mechanisms of arrhythymias and conduction abnormalities. In Hurst JW, editor: *The heart, arteries, and veins,* ed 6, New York, 1986, McGraw-Hill, pp 406-432.

13. Smith MB, Wallace AG: Management of arrhythmias and conduction abnormalities. In Hurst JW, editor: *The heart, arteries, and veins,* ed 6, New York, 1986, McGraw-Hill, pp 475-486.

14. Sonis ST, Frazio RC, Fang L, editors: *Principles and practice of oral medicine,* Philadelphia, 1984, WB Saunders.

9

Congestive Heart Failure

Over 2 million Americans have congestive heart failure. About 400,000 new cases occur each year. Once overt signs and symptoms appear, 50% of the patients will die within 5 years. Hypertension precedes congestive heart failure in about 75% of the cases, coronary artery disease with hypertension in about 39% of the cases, and rheumatic heart disease in about 21% of the cases.[5,7]

Congestive heart failure is one of the most common causes of death in the United States.[5,7,11] The 1-year survival rate for patients with severe congestive heart failure is 40% to 60%. Sudden death accounts for 30% to 50% of the deaths. About 50% of the patients with severe congestive heart failure develop ventricular tachycardias.[13] Patients who have untreated or poorly managed heart failure are at high risk for complications during dental treatment—such as infection, cardiac arrest, excessive bleeding, cerebrovascular accident, and myocardial infarction—that can occur in the dental office. The purpose of this chapter is to present the basic pathophysiology, clinical findings, medical management, and dental management for patients with congestive heart failure. The emphasis is on the role of the dentist in detecting these patients based on history and clinical findings, referring the patient for medical diagnosis and management, and working closely with the physician to develop a dental management plan that will be effective and safe for the patient.

GENERAL DESCRIPTION
INCIDENCE AND PREVALENCE

Congestive heart failure is much like anemia in that it represents a symptom complex that can be caused by any number of specific disease processes (Table 9-1). The three most common causes are cardiac valvular disease, coronary atherosclerotic heart disease and its complications, and hypertensive disease. The dominant cause of congestive heart failure is hypertension, which precedes cardiac failure in 75% of the cases.[5] Other causes include thyrotoxicosis, rheumatic fever, congenital heart disease, severe anemia, chronic obstructive lung disease, and pulmonary hypertension.[2,5,13]

Congestive heart failure may involve failure of the left ventricle, right ventricle, or both ventricles. Most of the acquired disorders that lead to congestive heart failure result in failure of the left ventricle. This often is followed by failure of the right ventricle. Initial failure of the right side of the heart is much less common and

TABLE 9–1

Precipitating Causes of Congestive Heart Failure

Hypertension
Myocardial infarction
Rheumatic and other forms of myocarditis
Arrhythmias
Infective endocarditis
Anemia
Thyrotoxicosis
Pulmonary infection
Pulmonary embolism
Pregnancy
Physical or emotional stress

From Braunwald E. In Wilson JD, et al, editors: *Harrison's Principles of internal medicine*, ed 12, New York, 1991, McGraw-Hill, pp 890–900.

is associated with certain congenital heart defects or with emphysema (cor pulmonale). By the time most patients are seen for medical treatment, failure of both sides of the heart has usually occurred.

PATHOPHYSIOLOGY AND COMPLICATIONS

Heart failure appears when the heart no longer functions properly as a pump. Congestive heart failure is the end stage of a disproportion between the required hemodynamic load and the capacity of the heart to handle the load. This imbalance can occur with chronic increase in the load or damage to the myocardium. In most cases a combination of these two factors is involved. Chronic congestive heart failure usually evokes compensatory adjustments consisting of increased peripheral resistance, redistribution of blood flow to the heart and brain, and increased erythropoietic activity to increase the oxygen-carrying capacity of the blood.

Heart failure usually occurs in stages.[13] The first stage involves ventricular dysfunction, with the development of a gallop rhythm. The second stage consists of congestive failure, with dyspnea, pulmonary congestion, and peripheral edema. The third stage, termed *compensated heart failure,* is when medical therapy has been able to control or eliminate the clinical signs and symptoms of congestion.

Failure of the heart most often begins with left ventricular failure, brought on by either increased work load or disease of the heart muscle. The increased work load may result from a variety of entities, including aortic valve disease, anemia, and arterial hypertension. Direct effects on the myocardium may be a result of infections, rheumatic fever, or infarction. The outstanding symptom of left ventricular failure is dyspnea, which results from blood accumulation in the pulmonary vessels. Acute pulmonary edema is often associated with left ventricular failure. Left-side heart failure leads to pulmonary hypertension, which increases the work of the right ventricle, pumping against the increased pressure, and often leads to right-side heart failure as well. In fact, the most common cause of right-side heart failure is preceding failure of the left ventricle. An important feature of left ventricular failure is the retention of sodium and water and the insufficient emptying of the left ventricle during systole.[4,11]

Failure of the right side of the heart alone is uncommon. The most common cause of pure right-side heart failure is emphysema. The major results are systemic venous congestion and peripheral edema (Fig. 9-1).

Ventricular failure will lead to dilation and hypertrophy of the ventricle as it attempts to compensate for its inability to keep up with the work load. Venous pressure and myocardial

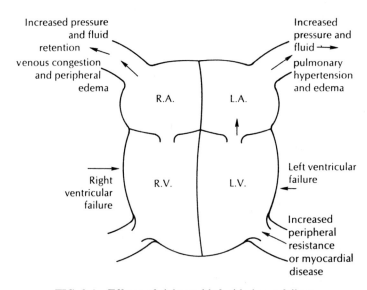

FIG. 9-1   Effects of right and left side heart failure.

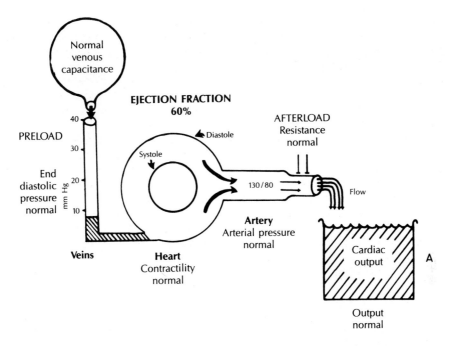

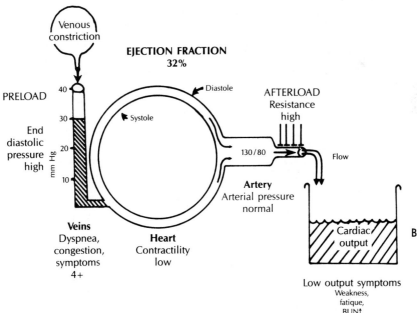

FIG. 9-2 **A,** Diagram of the normal heart and circulation. **B,** Diagram of the failing heart and circulation, showing the effects of Starling mechanisms (diastolic cardiac dilation causing increased force and volume of the subsequent systolic contraction and ejection), increased venous pressure, and increased peripheral resistance in the attempt to maintain central blood pressure and allocate limited cardiac output to vital areas such as the brain and heart. (From Spann JF: In Hurst JW, editor: *The heart, arteries, and veins,* ed 7, New York, 1990, McGraw-Hill, p 420.)

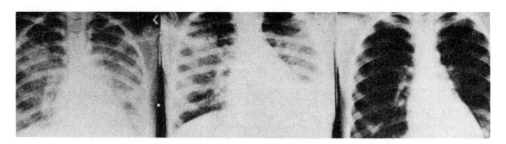

FIG. 9-3 Chest x-rays demonstrating the resolution of pulmonary edema (from *left* to *right*). (Courtesy J. Noonan, M.D., Lexington Ky.)

tone increase along with the increase in blood volume. The net effect is diastolic dilation, to increase the force and volume of the subsequent systolic contraction. This leads to dyspnea, orthopnea, and pulmonary edema.[13] Figure 9-2 denotes the circulation for both a normal and a failing heart.

An increased erythropoietic activity of the bone marrow in response to the need to increase the blood's oxygen-carrying capacity can lead to polycythemia, thrombocytopenia, and leukopenia. The clinical results of these changes are the same as those described in Chapter 4 that occur following the right-to-left shunting of blood that results from congenital heart lesions. These include (1) increased susceptibility to infection as a result of the decrease in circulating white blood cells and (2) excessive bleeding from trauma or surgical procedures brought on by the reduction in circulating platelets and coagulation factors (reduced because of thrombosis in the small vessels).

The natural history of severe congestive heart failure is to worsen and lead to death in 6 months to 5 years.[13] If the underlying cause can be treated, the prognosis is better. Patients who respond to the initial attempts of medical treatment have a better prognosis than those who do not. Sudden death due to ventricular fibrillation is common in patients with severe congestive heart failure.[2,13]

CLINICAL PRESENTATION
SIGNS

Patients with overt heart failure may demonstrate a gallop rhythm consisting of a ventricular, an atrial, or a summation gallop. The ventricular gallop occurs in the dilated heart during left ventricular filling. The atrial gallop results from the forceful presystolic distention of the ventricle by atrial contraction. The summation gallop consists of a triple rhythm that occurs during tachycardia because of the coincidence of atrial and ventricular gallops. A pulsus alternans — that is, the regular alternation of one strong beat with one weak beat — may be present.[4,11,13]

The circulation time is usually prolonged. The Decholin (dehydrocholic acid) time, a measurement of arm-to-tongue circulation time, is prolonged beyond normal (10 to 15 seconds). Radiographs of the chest may show enlargement of one or more heart chambers and the presence of pulmonary venous congestion and edema (Fig. 9-3).

Evidence of systemic venous congestion may be detected by the presence of distended neck

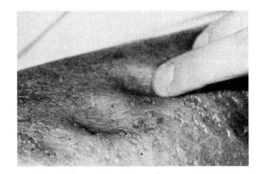

FIG. 9-4 Pitting pretibial edema in a patient with congestive heart failure. (Courtesy N. Wood, D.D.S., M.S., Ph.D., Chicago Ill.)

TABLE 9–2

Signs of Congestive Heart Failure

Gallop rhythm
Pulsus alternans
Prolonged circulation time
Cardiac enlargement shown on chest radiographs
Distended neck veins
Large tender liver
Jaundice
Peripheral edema
Ascites
Cyanosis
Sweating
Slight exophthalmos
Ruddy skin color
Polycythemia, thrombocytopenia, leukopenia
Weight gain, increased body girth

veins, a large tender liver, peripheral edema (Fig. 9-4), ascites (Fig. 9-5), and cyanosis. The retention of fluid will cause weight gain and may increase body girth. In addition, the patient may appear ruddy because of polycythemia and may show clubbing of the fingers (Fig. 9-6). (See Table 9-2.)

SYMPTOMS

Exertional dyspnea and fatigue in a patient suggest the possibility of beginning left-side heart failure. Symptoms of overt heart failure include orthopnea, paroxysmal nocturnal dyspnea (patient wakes gasping for breath), periodic breathing consisting of alternate periods of hyperventilation and apnea, and weakness. The patient may have a low-grade fever (Table 9-3).

LABORATORY FINDINGS

The laboratory findings of greatest importance to the dentist relate to the status of the red blood cells, white blood cells, platelets, and coagulation mechanism. Many patients with congestive heart failure will have polycythemia, thrombocytopenia, and leukopenia. In addition, the amounts of circulating coagulation factors may be depleted, possibly resulting in prolongation of the prothrombin time (PT) and partial thromboplastin time (PTT).

Urinalysis may show protein and an increase in specific gravity, indicating kidney involvement. Liver function tests may be abnormal, indicating liver involvement[13] (Table 9-4).

Special laboratory tests are utilized to diagnose congestive heart failure and its cause.

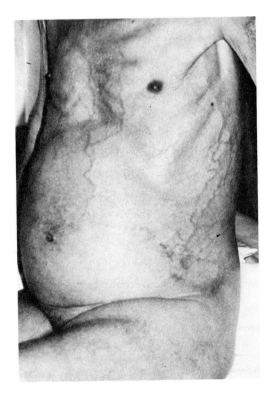

FIG. 9-5 Ascites. (Courtesy P. Akers, D.D.S., Evanston Ill.)

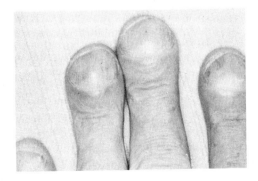

FIG. 9-6 Clubbing of the fingers in a patient with congestive heart failure.

TABLE 9–3
Symptoms of Congestive Heart Failure

Fatigue and weakness
Dyspnea (breathlessness)
Orthopnea (dyspnea in recumbent position)
Paroxysmal nocturnal dyspnea (dyspnea awakening
  patient from sleep)
Hyperventilation followed by apnea
Low-grade fever
Wheezing (cardiac asthma)
Anorexia, nausea, vomiting, constipation
Liver pain
Cough
Insomnia
History of weight gain
History of increased body girth
History of sweating
Dizziness, confusion

TABLE 9–4
Laboratory Findings in Congestive Heart
Failure*

Red blood cells
  Females—greater than 5,400,000/mm^3
  Males—greater than 6,200,000/mm^3
Hemoglobin
  Females—greater than 16 g/100 ml
  Males—greater than 18 g/100 ml
Hematocrit
  Females—greater than 47%
  Males—greater than 54%
Platelet count
  Less than 150,000/mm^3
White blood cell count
  Less than 5000/mm^3
Prothrombin time (PT)
  Greater than 14 seconds (depends on laboratory;
  must have control)
Partial thromboplastin time (PTT)
  Greater than 35 seconds (depends on laboratory;
  must have control)
Urinalysis
  Specific gravity—greater than 1.025
  Protein—usually indicates pathology
Liver function tests
  Aspartate aminotransaminase (AST)
    (serum glutamic-oxaloacetic transaminase
    [SGOT]) greater than 8 units per liter
  Alanine transaminase (ALT) (serum glutamic-
    pyruvic transaminase [SGPT]) greater than
    25 units per liter
  Alkaline phosphatase greater than 13 King-
    Armstrong units per 100 ml
  Lactic dehydrogenase (LDH) greater than 400
    units per liter
Total serum bilirubin greater than 1.5 mg/100 ml

*One or more of the above tests may show values that are
abnormal. The upper or lower range of normal is listed.

Swan-Ganz catheterization, radionuclide angiograms, and echocardiography may help in many cases.[13]

MEDICAL MANAGEMENT

Several factors relating to the prognosis for patients with congestive heart failure are important. The initial response to medical treatment is critical. A lack of response after several days of vigorous medical treatment usually indicates a poor prognosis for the patient.[4,11] The type of underlying cardiac disease also is important; for example, the patient with mitral stenosis has a much better prognosis than a patient with disease of the myocardium resulting from coronary atherosclerosis. The reason is that the diseased valve can be surgically opened or replaced whereas there is no way to replace the necrotic muscle that results from myocardial infarction other than by transplantation of a new heart. The presence of significant ventricular dilation is generally a poor sign.[2,13]

The classification of heart failure is shown in Table 9-5. The first indication of ventricular failure often is the development of a ventricular gallop rhythm. This occurs during ventricular filling from blood coming into a dilated chamber. Signs and symptoms of mild congestive failure may soon appear (Tables 9-2 and 9-3) and in time progress to intractable heart failure.[13]

The medical management of patients with mild, moderate, or severe congestive heart failure is shown in Tables 9-6 to 9-8. It is most important that the physician search for the causes of the congestive heart failure since medical or surgical treatment may be available to correct them. The management of congestive heart failure usually consists of attempting to increase cardiac output and decrease the work load on the heart, to improve myocardial

TABLE 9–5
Subsets of Heart Failure

Ventricular dysfunction
Ventricular gallop rhythm
No evidence of congestive failure

Congestive heart failure
Mild – moderate activity produces dyspnea
Moderate – mild activity produces dyspnea
Severe – dyspnea at rest

Compensated congestive heart failure
Treatment allows elimination of congestion

Intractable heart failure
Cannot be controlled by medical means

TABLE 9–6
Medical Management of the Patient with Mild
Heart Failure

Search for curable causes
Decrease slightly amount of physical activity
Give average loading dose of digitalis
Give average maintenance dose of digitalis
Omit salty foods, salt during cooking and eating

TABLE 9–7
Medical Management of the Patient with
Moderately Severe Heart Failure

1. Search for curable causes
2. Moderate decrease in physical activity
3. Loading dose of digitalis
4. Maintenance dose of digitalis
5. Thiazide diuretic 5 days per week
6. Potassium chloride, 1 g twice a day
7. If above therapy does not produce desired
   results
   a. Give thiazide diuretic (e.g., HydroDiuril)
      more often
   b. Change to another diuretic
      (1) Furosemide (Lasix)
      (2) Ethacrynic acid (Edecrin)
   c. Start venous vasodilator (if congestion
      continues)
      (1) Isosorbide dinitrate (Isordil)
   d. Start arterial vasodilator (if weakness occurs)
      (1) Hydralazine (Apresoline)
   e. Start angiotensin-converting enzyme (ACE)
      inhibitor if congestion and weakness both are
      present
      (1) Prazosin (Minipress)
      (2) Captopril (Capoten)

TABLE 9–8
Medical Management of the Patient with Severe
Chronic Congestive Heart Failure

1. Search for curable causes
2. Restrict physical activity but avoid bed rest if
   possible
3. Patients with severe nocturnal orthopnea – give
   topical nitroglycerin at bedtime
4. Loading dose and maintenance dose of digitalis
5. Furosemide, ethacrynic acid, or bumetanide
   should be given; if desired results not obtained
   a. First add potassium-sparing diuretic –
      triamterene
   b. Then add thiazide diuretic – hydrochlorothi-
      azide
6. If desired results not produced by above and
   a. Congestive symptoms predominate – use
      venous vasodilator
   b. Weakness predominates – use arterial vasodi-
      lator
   c. Congestion and weakness both present –
      use angiotensin-converting enzyme inhibitor
7. Surgical treatment when cause can be
   corrected – i.e., replacement of diseased
   heart valve

contractility, to mobilize excess tissue fluid, and, as stated above, to correct the cause whenever possible.[12,13]

Digitalis is an inotropic drug—i.e., one that increases the force of contractions in the failing heart and improves hemodynamics by increasing cardiac output. It also has antiarrhythmic effects on arterial and A-V nodal tissues.[6] Two forms, digoxin and digitoxin, were among the most commonly prescribed drugs in the 1980s.[6] Digitalis has a very narrow therapeutic index. The therapeutic/toxic ratios are similar for all digitalis preparations. The lethal dose for digitalis is only 5 to 10 times the dose that produces minimal therapeutic effects and is only two times the dose that results in minor toxic manifestations. The symptoms of digitalis intoxication are shown in Table 9-9.[2,6]

In a report on digitalis-induced arrhythmias in 926 patients,[6] the most common arrhythmias were ventricular (62%). Most of the ventricular arrhythmias were premature beats. However, 85 patients developed ventricular tachycardia. A-V block accounted for 34% of the arrhythmias, and atrial arrhythmias were found in 27% of the patients. A patient could have more than one arrhythmia.[6]

Diuretics that cause potassium loss increase the risk for digitalis toxicity. Quinidine decreases the renal clearance of digitalis and can lead to toxic blood levels. The retention of

TABLE 9–9
Clinical Manifestations of Digitalis Intoxication

CNS-stimulated anorexia, nausea, vomiting
Premature ventricular beats
A-V block
Nonparoxysmal atrial tachycardia
Vision changes—blurred, color
Fatigue, malaise, drowsiness
Headache
Ventricular tachycardias
Neuralgias
Weight loss
Gynecomastia
Delirium

From Braunwald E. In Wilson JD, et al, editors: *Harrison's Principles of internal medicine,* ed 12, New York, 1991, McGraw-Hill; and from Lathers CM. In Smith CM, Reynard AM, editors: *Textbook of pharmacology,* Philadelphia, 1992, WB Saunders.

digoxin is increased by verapamil, amiodarone, and spironolactone. Other agents—such as antacids, neomycin, and kaolin—can lead to digoxin toxicity by increasing the drug's absorption.[6]

When tachyarrhythmias occur due to digitalis intoxication, the drug must be withdrawn. Potassium, phenytoin, propranolol, or lidocaine can be given to control the arrhythmia. In severe cases electrical conversion or a pacemaker may be indicated.[2]

Sympathomimetic amines—epinephrine, isoproterenol, dopamine, and dobutamine—can be used to improve myocardial contractility. These agents are usually given by IV infusion, and a loss of responsiveness occurs in about 8 hours. Thus the sympathomimetic amines are used only in critical care settings.[2]

Drugs to treat congestive heart failure are shown in Table 9-10. Digoxin is the most commonly used agent to increase myocardial contractility. However, a new inotropic drug, amrinone, with a larger therapeutic index than digitalis, has been tested although it presently has only limited clinical use. Amrinone must be given IV and is used only in critical care settings for patients who do not respond to digitalis and diuretics. Clinical trials with oral amrinone[6] had to be stopped because of significant side effects that occurred. Diuretics are used in an attempt to decrease congestion by removing excess tissue fluid (reducing the cardiac preload). Venous vasodilators also are used to reduce the cardiac preload pressure. Arterial vasodilators are used to decrease the afterload and increase cardiac output. Prazosin (Minipress) is a drug with both arterial dilating and venous pooling effects that is used in patients with moderate to severe congestive failure. The last group of drugs used in treating congestive heart failure is the angiotension-converting enzyme (ACE) inhibitors.[4,13] Some of the complications caused by drugs used to treat congestive heart failure are shown in Table 9-11. Treatment with arterial vasodilators has been reported[13] to reduce the death rate in patients with severe congestive heart failure by 28%, and ACE inhibitors have reduced it by 27%.

Arrhythmias may develop as a complication of congestive heart failure. These arrhythmias are treated only if they cause symptoms or are hemodynamically significant. Reversible causes

TABLE 9–10

Drugs Used in the Medical Management of Chronic Congestive Heart Failure

1. To increase myocardial contractility
   a. Digoxin (Lanoxin) — loading dose, 1 mg; maintenance dose, 0.125 to 0.5 mg per day; given orally
   b. Amrinone — because of high rate (15%) of thrombocytopenia, not in general use
2. To decrease congestion by reducing preload
   a. Diuretics (taken orally)
      (1) Hydrochlorothiazide (HydroDiuril) — 50 to 150 mg per day
      (2) Ethacrynic acid (Edecrin) — 50 to 200 mg per day
      (3) Furosemide (Lasix) — 40 to 200 mg per day
      (4) Triamterene (Dyrenium) — 50 to 200 mg per day
      (5) Spironolactone (Aldactone) — 25 to 200 mg per day
   b. Venous vasodilators (taken orally)
      (1) Isosorbide dinitrate (Isordil) — 20 to 40 mg every 6 hours
3. To decrease afterload, increase cardiac output
   a. Hydralazine (Apresoline) — 50 to 70 mg every 6 hours, orally
4. With mixed arterial dilating and venous pooling effects and ACE inhibitor effects
   a. Prazosin (Minipress) — 2 to 7 mg every 6 hours, orally
   b. Captopril (Capoten) — 25 mg or less, every 6 hours, orally

TABLE 9–11

Complications of Drugs Commonly Used to Treat Congestive Heart Failure

Diuretics (thiazides, furosemide, ethacrynic acid)

Hypokalemia
Dehydration, xerostomia
Orthostatic hypotension
Hyperuricemia
Hyperglycemia
Allergic reactions

Cardiac glycosides overdose (digoxin)

Arrhythmias
Nausea, vomiting, anorexia
Blurred or yellow vision, headache, weakness
Gynecomastia

Vasodilators (prazosin, hydralazine)

Orthostatic hypotension
Dehydration, xerostomia
Nausea, headache, vomiting, diarrhea
Dizziness, weakness, drowsiness
Palpitations
Lichenoid skin and mucosal lesions

ACE inhibitors (captopril)

Neutropenia and agranulocytosis
Proteinurea, kidney damage
Thrombocytopenia, anemia
Pruritus, rash
Angioedema
Hypotension
Chest pain, tachycardia, palpitations

of arrhythmias — such as electrolyte imbalance, drug induced or ongoing ischemia — should be ruled out. Patients who are going to be placed on antiarrhythmic therapy should be hospitalized and monitored and the smallest effective dose established by using ECG results. Empirical treatment must be avoided.[10]

Patients who have severe dyspnea may be given 10 to 20 mg of morphine for 1 or 2 days to promote sleep and reduce the strenuous work of the respiratory muscles.[4,11,13] Barbiturates or tranquilizers may also be used for this purpose.

Patients who have acute pulmonary edema may require either an actual or a bloodless phlebotomy (the latter accomplished by placing a tourniquet on an extremity) to reduce the blood volume returning to the heart. Oxygen may be used, and at times thoracentesis may be indicated.

Pregnancy can be tolerated in some patients with congestive heart failure who are under good medical management. The greatest danger to the woman with congestive heart failure occurs in the seventh or eighth month of pregnancy, at which time previously undetected heart disease may manifest itself.[11]

The patient with congestive heart failure needs to be evaluated carefully to find the underlying cause of the problem. Once this has been accomplished, specific therapy for the

TABLE 9–12
Dental Management of the Patient with
Congestive Heart Failure

1. Consultation with physician
   a. Medications – confirm
   b. Present status – routine dental care if under good medical management and control
   c. Nature of underlying problem
      (1) Valvular disease
      (2) Hypertensive disease
      (3) Myocardial infarction
      (4) Hyperthyroidism
      (5) Emphysema
2. Receiving digitalis
   a. Prone to nausea and vomiting
   b. Avoid gagging
3. On diuretics, vasodilators, or ACE inhibitors
   a. Avoid excessive epinephrine (Chapter 6)
   b. Avoid orthostatic hypotension (Chapter 6)
   c. Look at complications listed in Table 9–11; refer patient for medical evaluation when present
4. Receiving dicumarol
   a. May have been bleeding problem
   b. Prothrombin time (PT) should be brought to less than 2½ times normal if any invasive procedures are planned.
   c. Adjustment of medication by physician
5. Polycythemia
   a. Thrombocytopenia and decreased fibrinogen levels may be present
   b. May have bleeding problem
   c. Avoid dehydration (thrombosis may occur)
   d. If white blood cell count is depressed, administer antibiotics to avoid postoperative infection
6. Place patient in upright position if pulmonary edema is present
7. In general, short morning appointments
8. Terminate appointment if patient becomes fatigued
9. Local anesthetic with 1:100,000 epinephrine can be used, except in patients with severe arrhythmias; nitrous oxide–oxygen inhalation sedation may be used, with caution

initiating problem should be rendered as appropriate.

DENTAL MANAGEMENT
MEDICAL CONSIDERATIONS

No patients with untreated congestive heart failure should undergo routine dental therapy until they have been referred for medical management.[1,8,12] Once the congestive heart failure is under control and the underlying cause has been identified, the patient should be encouraged to return for dental care. The dental management plan then must deal with the problems related to the congestive heart failure and its underlying medical problem (Table 9-12).

The patient who has congestive heart failure resulting from rheumatic heart disease may serve to demonstrate the problems involved and how they can be managed:

Consultation with the physician confirms that the patient, a 54-year-old man, is under good medical control and is being treated with digitalis (or digoxin), a thiazide diuretic, dicumarol, potassium supplementation, and 250 mg per day of oral penicillin to prevent recurrent attacks of rheumatic fever. He still has a significant degree of polycythemia, but his platelet count and white blood count are within normal ranges and his PT is being maintained at about 3 times normal value.

The following problems relate to all cases of congestive heart failure and its medical management:

1. Patients taking digitalis are prone to nausea and vomiting during dental treatment. Procedures that may cause gagging should be done with extra care in these patients, since gagging may trigger nausea and vomiting.
2. Patients who develop symptoms of digitalis intoxication (Table 9-9). The dentist needs to be aware of these signs and symptoms and, if they occur during a dental visit, refer the patient for immediate medical evaluation and treatment. If surgical procedures are planned or the patient develops an oral infection, dehydration must be prevented, since thrombosis may occur that could result in infarction of various organs (complication associated with the polycythemia).
3. Patients under good medical control may still have some degree of pulmonary edema. Thus if any evidence of pulmonary congestion develops with the patient in the supine chair position, he

or she should be raised to an upright position for the remaining dental treatment. In this patient the white cell count and platelet count are normal, and no special attention needs to be paid to preventing postoperative infection or bleeding related directly to these elements.

4. If a patient complains of weakness or fatigue developing during the dental appointment, the appointment should be terminated and the patient given an appointment on another day. In general, morning or early afternoon appointments are best for these patients. (See Table 9-12.)

Recent clinical observations, however, are beginning to question whether early morning appointments are best for the cardiac patient. The incidence of sudden death is greatest in the early morning hours. A recent study involving patients receiving periodontal surgery[9a] showed greater effects on blood pressure elevation in the morning than in the early afternoon. The dentist is best advised to discuss these factors with the patient's physician and to then select the best time for the dental appointment.

The problems that must be considered relative to the underlying cause in a case of heart failure, rheumatic heart disease, include the following: (1) The patient must be protected by prophylactic antibiotic coverage during and following all dental procedures to prevent infective endocarditis. (2) Because the patient is taking a low daily dose of oral penicillin, the oral flora may contain penicillin-resistant bacteria; thus erythromycin should be selected for the antibiotic coverage. (3) The physician should be consulted as to whether the patient needs to continue taking the oral penicillin during periods of erythromycin coverage. (See Chapter 2 for dosage, etc.) (4) If scaling or surgical procedures are planned, the physician should be asked to reduce the dicumarol dosage and the patient should be managed as described in Chapter 22.

Inhalation sedation with nitrous oxide–oxygen (oxygen levels greater than 27% to 30%) can be used for the cardiac patient. Hypoxia must be avoided in these patients, but with this level of oxygen the problem should not occur. Nitrous oxide–oxygen has been used in some European countries in the management of acute myocardial infarction.[9] The American Heart Association[3] has reported that nitrous oxide is a myocardial depressant (an effect that is reversible with calcium) and has recommended that it be used with care in cardiac patients. Current information suggests that, if used properly, nitrous oxide is safe in cardiac patients. If the dentist is planning on using nitrous oxide–oxygen inhalation sedation, these points should first be discussed with the patient's physician.

The dental management principles covered in Chapters 2, 6 to 8, 11, 12, 18, 22, and 23 may apply to certain cardiac patients, depending on the underlying cause of the congestive heart failure and the drugs used to treat it. The dentist must be prepared to recognize and deal with any of the serious medical emergencies that can arise during the dental visit in patients with a history of congestive heart failure.

TREATMENT PLANNING MODIFICATIONS

In general, patients with congestive heart failure who are under good medical management can receive any indicated dental treatment as long as the dental management plans deal effectively with the problems presented by the heart failure and its underlying cause.

ORAL COMPLICATIONS

There are usually no oral complications directly related to congestive heart failure — other than infection, spontaneous gingival bleeding, ecchymoses, and petechiae, which may result from the effects of the polycythemia (thrombocytopenia, leukopenia, thrombosis).[8]

REFERENCES

1. *Accepted dental therapeutics,* ed 39, Chicago, 1982, American Dental Association.
2. Braunwald E: Heart failure. In Wilson JD, et al, editors, *Harrison's Principles of internal medicine,* ed 12, New York, 1991, McGraw-Hill, pp 890-900.
3. *Cardiovascular disease in dental practice,* Publ. no. 71-0009, Dallas, 1991, American Heart Association, pp 27-30.
4. Fishman AP: Heart failure. In Wyngaarden JB, Smith LH, editors: *Cecil textbook of medicine,* ed 17, Philadelphia, 1985, WB Saunders.
5. Kannel WB, Thom TJ: Incidence, prevalence, and mortality of cardiovascular disease. In Hurst JW, editor: *The heart, arteries, and veins,* ed 7, New York, 1990, McGraw-Hill, pp 627-638.
6. Lathers CM: Treatment of congestive heart failure — digitalis glycosides. In Smith CM, Reynard AM, editors:

Textbook of pharmacology, Philadelphia, 1992, WB Saunders, pp 479-505.

7. Levy RI: Prevalence and epidemiology of cardiovascular disease. In Wyngaarden JB, Smith LH, editors: *Cecil textbook of medicine,* ed 17, Philadelphia, 1985, WB Saunders.

8. Lynch MA: Diseases of the cardiovascular system. In Lynch MA, editor: *Burket's Oral medicine, diagnosis and treatment,* ed 8, Philadelphia, 1984, JB Lippincott.

9. Malamed SF: *Handbook of medical emergencies in the dental office,* ed 3, St Louis, 1991, Mosby–Year Book, pp 328-366.

9a. Raab FJ II: Automatic ambulatory monitoring of circadian blood pressure and heart rate variations associated with periodontal therapy. Master's Thesis, University of Minnesota, pp 1-144, 1992.

10. Ravid S: Antiarrhythmic drug therapy in congestive heart failure: indications and complications, *Postgrad Med* 90(8):99-102, 1991.

11. Ross RS, et al: Management of the patient with congestive heart failure. In Harvey A, et al, editors: *The principles and practice of medicine,* ed 19, New York, 1976, Appleton-Century-Crofts.

12. Sonis ST, Fazio RC, Fang L: Congestive heart failure. In Sonis ST, Fazio RC, Fang L, editors: *Principles and practice of oral medicine,* Philadelphia, 1984, WB Saunders.

13. Spann JF, Hurst JW: The recognition and management of heart failure. In Hurst JW, editor: *The heart, arteries, and veins,* ed 7, New York, 1990, McGraw-Hill, pp 418-442.

14. William BO: The cardiovascular system. In Pathy MSJ, editor: *Principles and practice of geriatric medicine,* ed 2, New York, 1991, John Wiley, pp 573-625.

10

Pulmonary Disease

Many types of pulmonary disorders may compromise routine dental care and require special management of the patient. Some of the more commonly encountered pulmonary diseases—chronic obstructive pulmonary disease ([COPD], i.e., chronic bronchitis, emphysema), asthma, and tuberculosis—are discussed in this chapter.

Chronic obstructive pulmonary disease

GENERAL DESCRIPTION

COPD is a general term for pulmonary disorders characterized by the obstruction of airflow during respiratory efforts. The two most common diseases classified as COPD are chronic bronchitis and emphysema. Asthma is occasionally included in this list but will be presented in a separate following section. The basis for obstructed airflow in these two diseases is quite different. *Chronic bronchitis* is a condition associated with excessive tracheobronchial mucus production sufficient to cause cough with expectoration for at least 3 months of the year for more than 2 consecutive years. *Emphysema* is defined as distention of the air spaces distal to the terminal bronchioles with destruction of alveolar septa.[12] Although these diseases can be described as individual entities, it should be noted that they quite often coexist in a patient with overlapping symptoms, making differentiation difficult.

EPIDEMIOLOGY

COPD is an important health problem in the United States. It is the fifth leading cause of death and is estimated to affect 13.5 million people. In one large survey[5] 14% of males and 8% of females had COPD. Prevalence, incidence, and mortality rates increase with age and are highest in white men.[6,17] Emphysema, which can be definitively diagnosed only at autopsy, is found to some degree in two thirds of men and one fourth of women. Most of these affected individuals, however, have no recognized dysfunction.[12]

The most important etiologic factor in COPD is cigarette smoking, which accounts for 80% to 90% of COPD mortality in both men and women. The risk of COPD is dose related and increases as the number of cigarettes smoked per day increases and the duration of smoking increases.[18] In addition to cigarette smoking, it is felt that chronic exposure to occupational and environmental pollutants is of increasing etiologic importance.

PATHOPHYSIOLOGY

Although chronic bronchitis and emphysema both lead to obstruction of airflow, the pathophysiology of each is distinct.

In chronic bronchitis the pathologic changes consist of thickened bronchial walls with inflammatory cell infiltrate, an increase in size of the mucous glands, and goblet cell hyperplasia. Obstruction is caused by narrowing of small airways, mucus plugging, and collapse of peripheral airways from a loss of surfactant.[11] Obstruction is present on both inspiration and expiration.

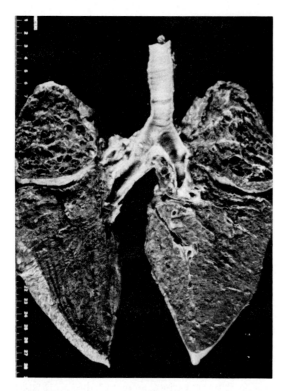

FIG. 10-1 Gross lung specimen from a patient with emphysema. (Courtesy Peggy Falace, M.D., Lexington Ky.)

In emphysema, by contrast, the pathologic changes consist of enlargement of air spaces distal to the terminal bronchioles with destruction of alveolar walls, which results in the loss of elastic recoil of the lungs. Obstruction is caused by the collapse of these unsupported and enlarged air spaces upon expiration (Fig. 10-1). There is no obstruction during inspiration.[11,12]

SEQUELAE AND COMPLICATIONS

COPD can lead to several serious complications that vary depending on the predominance of either chronic bronchitis or emphysema. With continued exposure to primary etiologic factors (cigarette smoking, environmental pollutants), COPD can result in progressive dyspnea and hypercapnia to the point of debilitation. Recurrent pulmonary infection with mucopurulent relapse is common, especially with bronchitis. Pulmonary hypertension frequently develops and can then lead to cor pulmonale (right-side heart failure). Thoracic bullae and pneumothorax are not uncommon. Patients with COPD also may have poor quality of sleep because of nocturnal hypoxemia. Emphysema is an irreversible process for which there is no cure. Avoidance of pulmonary irritants, however, can be of significant benefit in decreasing the morbidity and mortality of both diseases.

CLINICAL PRESENTATION
SIGNS AND SYMPTOMS

The clinical presentation of chronic bronchitis and emphysema is frequently indistinct since most patients have features of both. However, patients who have predominant chronic bronchitis often have a chronic cough with copious sputum production. Patients tend to be overweight and cyanotic, leading to the term "blue bloaters." Those in whom emphysema predominates may have severe exertional dyspnea with a minimal nonproductive cough. They are typically barrel-chested. Cyanosis is not usually seen, and these patients are labeled "pink puffers." Table 10-1 compares the predominant clinical features of these two diseases.

LABORATORY FINDINGS

Patients with predominant chronic bronchitis have an elevated Pco_2 and decreased Po_2, leading to erythrocytosis and an elevated hematocrit. The total lung capacity is usually normal with a moderate elevation of residual volume.

Patients with predominant emphysema have a relatively normal Pco_2 and a decreased Po_2, which maintains normal hemoglobin saturation, thus avoiding erythrocytosis. These patients also have a normal hematocrit. The total lung capacity and residual volume are markedly increased.

Chest radiographs in emphysema demonstrate a persistent and marked overdistention of the lungs with the presence of emphysematous bullae. In bronchitis, sputum examination may be helpful.

MEDICAL MANAGEMENT

The management of COPD is difficult in that there is no cure. However, much can be done to improve the quality of life for these patients and prevent progression of the disease.

TABLE 10-1
Predominant Clinical Features of Chronic
Bronchitis vs Emphysema

Chronic bronchitis	Emphysema
"Blue bloaters"	"Pink puffers"
Frequently overweight	Barrel chested
Chronic productive cough	Cough not prominent
Copious, mucopurulent sputum	Scanty sputum
Mild dyspnea	Severe dyspnea
Frequent respiratory infections	Few respiratory infections
Hypoxia, cyanosis, polycythemia	No hypoxia, cyanosis, or polycythemia

TABLE 10-2
Dental Management of the Patient with COPD

Upright chair position
Local anesthetic as usual, but avoid bilateral mandibular or palatal blocks
Avoid use of rubber dam in severe disease
Low-flow supplemental oxygen may be helpful
Avoid nitrous oxide–oxygen inhalation sedation
Low-dose oral diazepam acceptable
Avoid use of barbiturates, narcotics, antihistamines, and anticholinergics
If patient is taking steroids, may need supplementation
If patient is taking theophylline, avoid erythromycin
Outpatient general anesthesia contraindicated

The cornerstone of management is the elimination of smoking and exposure to environmental pollutants and irritants. This is probably the single most important aspect of treatment. There are other palliative measures that can be taken, including aggressive treatment of pulmonary infections, adequate hydration, and low-flow oxygen therapy. Bronchodilators are useful in many patients to relieve symptoms; they include methylxanthines, beta-adrenergic stimulators, and anticholinergics (Table 10-2). Corticosteroids are utilized in some patients; however, their use and effectiveness in COPD remains controversial. Encouragement of regular exercise commensurate with tolerance and good nutrition is thought to be of overall benefit to patients.

DENTAL MANAGEMENT
PREVENTION OF POTENTIAL PROBLEMS

Since patients with COPD already have compromised respiratory function, efforts must be directed toward the avoidance of anything that could further depress respiration (Table 10-3). Patients should be placed in an upright chair position for treatment, rather than the supine position, to avoid orthopnea and respiratory discomfort. There is no contraindication to the use of local anesthetic; however, bilateral mandibular blocks or bilateral palatal blocks are not recommended because of a possible unpleasant choking sensation or difficulty swallowing. With severe COPD, the use of a rubber dam is not advised, since this may result in a feeling of compromised air supply. A low flow of oxygen during dental procedures may be helpful.

If sedative medication is required, low-dose oral diazepam (Valium) may be used. Nitrous oxide–oxygen inhalation sedation is best avoided due to the possibility that high-flow oxygen will depress the respiratory drive. Narcotics and barbiturates are also to be avoided because of their respiratory depressant properties. Anticholinergics and antihistamines are contraindicated because of their drying properties and the resultant increase of mucus tenacity. Patients who are taking corticosteroids may require supplementation because of adrenal suppression. (See Chapter 18.) In patients taking theophylline, erythromycin should be avoided since the combination can retard the metabolism of theophylline. Outpatient general anesthesia is contraindicated for patients with COPD.

TREATMENT PLANNING MODIFICATIONS

No technical treatment planning modifications are required for patients with COPD.

ORAL COMPLICATIONS

There are no specific oral manifestations or complications of COPD.

Asthma

GENERAL DESCRIPTION
INCIDENCE, PREVALENCE, AND ETIOLOGY

Asthma is a syndrome consisting of dyspnea, cough, and wheezing caused by bronchospasm resulting from a hyperirritability of the tracheobronchial tree. Though it is a worldwide problem, its exact incidence is unclear. It may afflict as many as 5% of adults and 10% of children.[14] It is primarily a disease of children, however, affecting males more often than females, especially during the childhood age.

Asthma is a multifactorial disease whose exact etiology is not well-defined. Two types of asthma are classically described, allergic asthma (extrinsic) and idiosyncratic asthma (intrinsic); however, these classifications frequently overlap.

EPIDEMIOLOGY

Allergic or *extrinsic* asthma is the most common form of asthma and is usually seen in children and in young adults. There is generally an associated family history of allergic diseases in addition to positive skin testing to various allergens. Elevated serum levels of immunoglobulin E (IgE) are seen in affected individuals. Allergic asthma is often seasonal and may be associated with various grasses or pollen.[14] Approximately 50% of asthmatic children become asymptomatic by adulthood.[13]

The idiosyncratic or *intrinsic* type of asthma, by contrast, is seldom associated with a family history of allergy. Patients are usually nonresponsive to skin testing and demonstrate normal IgE levels. This form of asthma is generally seen in middle-aged adults, and its onset is frequently associated with an upper respiratory tract viral infection.[14]

Asthma may be precipitated by a number of substances or events.[14,19] Some of the more common are airborne substances (pollen, dust); aspirin and nonsteroidal antiinflammatory drugs (NSAIDs), especially in adults who have nasal polyps and recurrent rhinitis; sulfites; environmental pollutants (smoke, chemicals); respiratory infections (viruses); exercise, espe-

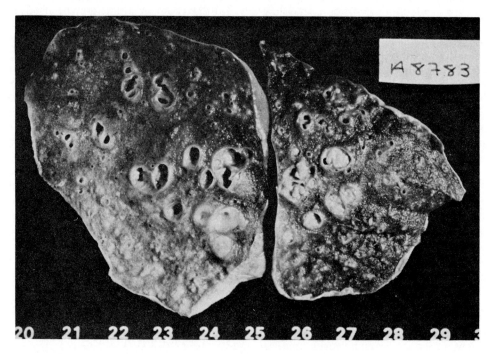

FIG. 10-2   Section of a lung with the bronchioles occluded by mucous plugs. (Courtesy A. Golden, M.D., Lexington Ky.)

cially in cold dry weather; and emotional stress (implicated in at least 50% of asthmatics).[14,19]

PATHOPHYSIOLOGY

The most striking macroscopic finding in the asthmatic lung is occlusion of the bronchi and bronchioles by thick, tenacious mucus plugs (Fig. 10-2). The characteristic histologic findings include (1) thickened basement membrane of the bronchial epithelium, (2) edema, (3) hypertrophy of the mucous glands, and (4) hypertrophy of the bronchial wall muscle.[11] All these changes result in decreased diameter of the airway.

SEQUELAE AND COMPLICATIONS

In terms of morbidity, asthma is relatively benign. Most patients can expect a reasonably good prognosis, especially those in whom disease develops during childhood. However, a small percentage of patients will develop status asthmaticus, the most serious manifestation of asthma. Status asthmaticus is a particularly severe and prolonged asthmatic attack that is refractory to usual therapy. It is often associated with a respiratory infection. Although death directly attributable to asthma is relatively uncommon, the disease has been estimated[13,14] to be associated with 5000 to 6000 deaths per year in the United States.

CLINICAL PRESENTATION
SIGNS AND SYMPTOMS

Asthma attacks often occur at night, for reasons that are unclear, but also may follow exposure to an allergen, exercise, respiratory infection, or emotional upset or excitement. The typical symptoms of asthma consist of paroxysms of dyspnea, cough, and wheezing. The onset is usually sudden, with a tightness in the chest and commonly a cough. Respirations become difficult and are accompanied by expiratory wheezing. Tachypnea and prolonged expiration are characteristic. The termination of an attack is commonly accompanied by a productive cough with thick, stringy mucus. Episodes usually are self-limiting, but severe episodes may require medical assistance.[13]

LABORATORY FINDINGS

Laboratory tests for asthma are nonspecific, and any one test alone is not diagnostic. Commonly ordered tests include chest radiographs (for hyperinflation), skin testing (for specific allergens), sputum smears (for eosinophilia), arterial blood gases, and spirometry (for pulmonary function).

MEDICAL MANAGEMENT

Avoidance or elimination of any known precipitating factor is the first step in preventing asthma attacks. For persons who have known allergies, desensitization injections may also be of some help.

The mainstay of asthma treatment is drug therapy. Drugs commonly used to treat asthma fall into five main categories. These are the beta-adrenergic agonists, methylxanthines, chromones, corticosteroids, and anticholinergic drugs (Table 10-3).

Inhalation of beta-adrenergic agonists is the preferred approach to management of an acute asthma attack and is usually accomplished by use of a metered-dose inhaler. Corticosteroids are also utilized, via the inhalation route or orally. The prophylaxis of chronic asthma is most commonly managed by oral theophylline preparations, oral chromones, or corticosteroids. Inhalation of beta-adrenergic agonists is also used.

DENTAL MANAGEMENT
PREVENTION OF POTENTIAL PROBLEMS

The goal of management for asthmatic dental patients must be to prevent an acute asthma attack (Table 10-4). The first step in achieving this goal is to identify asthmatics by history and to learn as much as possible about their problem and avoid precipitating factors.

Through a good history the dentist should be able to ascertain the type of asthma (allergic vs nonallergic), the precipitating substances, the frequency and severity of attacks, whether this is a current or past problem, how attacks are usually managed, and whether it has ever been necessary to receive emergency treatment of an acute attack. A past history of visits to an emergency facility for treatment of acute attacks signals more severe disease. For a severe asthmatic, consultation with the patient's physician is advised.

The patient should be instructed to bring his or her inhaler (bronchodilator) to each appoint-

TABLE 10-3
Drugs Used in the Outpatient Management of COPD and Asthma

Generic name	Product name	Route of administration
Bronchodilators, beta₂-adrenergic agonists		
Epinephrine	Primatene Mist, Bronkaid	Inhalation, parenteral
Ephedrine	Eted II	Oral, parenteral
Isoproterenol	Isuprel	Inhalation, oral, parenteral
Isoetharine	Bronkosol	Inhalation
Metaproterenol	Alupent	Inhalation, oral
*Terbutaline	Brethaire	Inhalation, oral, parenteral
*Albuterol	Proventil, Ventolin	Inhalation, oral, parenteral
*Bitolterol	Tornalate	Inhalation
*Pirbuterol	Maxair	Inhalation
Bronchodilators, xanthine derivatives		
Theophylline	Theo-Dur	Oral, inhalation, parenteral
Chromones		
Cromolyn	Intal	Inhalation
Corticosteroids		
Beclamethasone	Vanceril, Beclovent	Inhalation
Dexamethasone	Decadron	Inhalation
Flunisolide	Aerobid	Inhalation
Triamcinolone	Azmacort	Inhalation
Prednisone	Deltasone	Oral
Prednisolone	Delta-Cortef	Oral
Methylprednisolone	Solu-Medrol	Oral
Bronchodilators, anticholinergics		
Ipratropium	Atrovent	Inhalation

*Selective beta₂ stimulation.

ment and have it readily available for acute use. The inhalation of a selective beta₂ agonist is the preferred treatment for an acute asthma attack.

Since aspirin ingestion is associated with precipitating a small percentage of asthma attacks, it is advisable not to administer aspirin-containing medication or other NSAIDs to patients with asthma. Acetaminophen can safely be used for mild to moderate pain. Antihistamines should be used cautiously because of their drying effect. Patients taking theophylline preparations should not be given erythromycin, since this may result in a toxic blood level of theophylline.

Local anesthetic choice may require alteration. Seng and Gay[15] have suggested that acute asthma attacks may be precipitated by exposure to sulfites, which are used as preservatives in local anesthetic solutions containing epinephrine or levonordefrin. The precise threat of this occurring has not been determined; however, the use of local anesthetic without epinephrine or levonordefrin is advised. In 1987, the Food and Drug Administration[19] issued a warning for drugs containing sulfites as a cause of allergic-type reactions in susceptible individuals. Because data are limited concerning this problem, consultation with the physician is recom-

TABLE 10-4
Dental Management of the Patient with Asthma

1. Identification and assessment by history
   a. Type of asthma (allergic vs idiosyncratic)
   b. Precipitating factors
   c. Age at onset
   d. Frequency and severity of attacks
   e. How usually managed
   f. Medications being taken
   g. Necessity of emergency care
2. Avoidance of known precipitating factors
3. Medical consultation for severe, active asthmatic
4. Have patient bring medication inhaler to every appointment and keep it available
5. Drug considerations
   a. Avoid aspirin-containing medications (use acetaminophen)
   b. Avoid nonsteroidal antiinflammatory drugs (NSAIDs) (Table 15-3)
   c. Avoid barbiturates and narcotics
   d. Avoid erythromycin in patients taking theophylline
6. Local anesthetic considerations — may elect to avoid solutions containing epinephrine or levonordefrin because of sulfite preservative
7. Patients taking chronic corticosteroid medications may require supplementation (Chapter 18)
8. Provision of stress-free environment through establishment of rapport and openness
9. If sedation required, use nitrous oxide–oxygen inhalation sedation and/or small doses of oral diazepam

mended. Asthmatics who are chronically medicated with corticosteroids may require supplementation for dental procedures. (See Chapter 18.)

Since stress is implicated as a precipitating factor in asthma attacks, every effort should be made to identify those patients and to provide a stress-free environment through establishment of rapport and openness. Preoperative and intraoperative sedation may also be desirable. If sedation is required, nitrous oxide–oxygen inhalation is the approach of choice. Nitrous oxide is not a respiratory depressant, nor is it irritating to the tracheobronchial tree. Oral premedication also may be accomplished with small doses of diazepam. Outpatient general anesthesia is contraindicated for patients with asthma.

TREATMENT PLANNING MODIFICATIONS

No specific treatment planning modifications are required for the patient with asthma.

ORAL COMPLICATIONS

There are no specific oral complications of asthma. Oral candidiasis has been reported in patients using inhalation steroids; however, this is rare if a "spacer" or aerosol holding chamber is attached to the metered-dose inhaler and the mouth is rinsed with water after each use.[10]

Tuberculosis

Tuberculosis may be a cause for concern to the dentist from at least three standpoints. First, it is an infectious disease and as such is communicable in its active state. The dentist is in a high-risk population and may contract the disease from a patient, or patients may contract the disease from the dentist who might have an active case. Second, on rare occasions tuberculous lesions may be found in the oral cavity; thus the dentist must be alert to include tuberculosis in the differential diagnosis of oral lesions. Finally, the dentist may be the first person to discover that a patient has tuberculosis. The discovery may come about as a result of history, review of systems, or physical evaluation of the patient. Immediate referral to a physician may prove to be a great service to the patient and result in decreased morbidity and mortality.

GENERAL DESCRIPTION
INCIDENCE AND PREVALENCE

The occurrence of tuberculosis has decreased drastically in the last century. Around the turn of the century in the United States there were approximately 500 new cases of active tuberculosis per 100,000 population identified every year. In 1985 a rate of 9.3 per 100,000 population was reported to the Centers for Disease Control. In 1990 this figure had risen to 10.3, a 10% increase in a 5-year period.[5] This recent increase in occurrence is thought to be due to adverse social and economic factors, the AIDS epidemic, and the immigration of persons who have tuberculosis.

Although the present rate for the United

States as a whole is very low, minority residents of inner-city ghettos, the elderly urban poor, and persons with AIDS have occurrence rates several times the national average. As might be expected, tuberculosis is prevalent in areas of dense population and poor socioeconomic conditions and so remains a significant health problem in many areas of the world today. One author[7] estimates that 50% of the world's population has been infected with tuberculosis.

It is believed that the dramatic decrease in this century in the reported incidence of tuberculosis in the United States can be attributed to improved sanitation and hygiene measures more than to any other factor.

ETIOLOGY

In most cases of human tuberculosis the causative agent is *Mycobacterium tuberculosis,* an acid-fast nonmotile rod that is an obligate aerobe. Since it is an aerobe, it exists best in an atmosphere of high oxygen tension; therefore it most commonly infects the lung. Although *M. tuberculosis* is by far the most common causative agent in human infection, other species of mycobacteria are occasionally encountered— such as *M. bovis, M. avium,* and "atypical" mycobacteria.

The typical mode of transmission of the bacteria is by way of infected, airborne droplets of mucus or saliva that have been forcefully expelled from the lungs, most commonly by a cough but also by sneezing and talking. The quantity and size of the expelled droplets influence transmission. The smaller droplets evaporate readily, leaving the bacteria and other solid material as floating particles that are easily inhaled. The larger droplets quickly settle to the ground. Transmission by way of fomites rarely, if ever, occurs.[7,20] Transmission by ingestion also rarely occurs since the advent of pasteurized milk. A secondary mode of transmission, by ingestion, can occur when a patient coughs up infected sputum and inoculates oral tissues. It is through this mechanism that oral lesions of tuberculosis may be initiated.

PATHOPHYSIOLOGY

Tuberculosis can affect virtually any organ of the body; however, the lung is the most common site of infection. A typical infection of primary pulmonary tuberculosis begins with the inhala-

tion of infected droplets. The droplets are carried into the alveoli, where the bacteria settle out and begin to multiply. The infection progresses locally and may involve regional lymph nodes. If it is not controlled locally, distant dissemination through the bloodstream can occur; however, it is believed that the vast majority of disseminated bacteria are destroyed by natural host defenses. Approximately 2 to 8 weeks after infection, a hypersensitivity to the bacteria develops. This is manifested by conversion of the tuberculin skin test (purified protein derivative [PPD]) from negative to positive. Most infections of primary pulmonary tuberculosis are locally controlled, self-limited, and contained by natural host defenses. However, if they are not contained, the nidus of infection may become a productive tubercle with central necrosis and caseation. Cavitation may occur, resulting in the dumping of organisms into the airway for further dissemination either into other lung tissue or to the outside by means of forceful expulsion (Fig. 10-3).

The limitation and local containment of the infection may be due to a variety of factors— including host resistance, host immune capabilities, and the degree of virulence of the mycobacterium. Once the infection is successfully interrupted, the lesion heals spontaneously and then undergoes inspissation, hardening, encapsulation, and calcification. Even though the lesion is "healed," some bacteria may remain in a dormant state.

If the infection is not interrupted, dissemina-

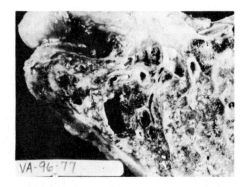

FIG. 10-3 Gross specimen of a tuberculous lung, demonstrating cavitation. (Courtesy R. Powell, M.D., Lexington Ky.)

tion of bacilli can occur through the lung parenchyma, resulting in extensive pulmonary lesions and lymphohematogenous spread. A widespread infection with multiple organ involvement is termed *miliary tuberculosis.*

Primary pulmonary tuberculosis is seen most often in infants and children; however, cavitation is rare in this age group. The majority of children produce no sputum, and, even if some bacilli are present in the bronchi, the child usually swallows the sputum.

The expression of the disease differs somewhat in teenagers and adults in that lymph node involvement and lymphohematogenous spread are not prominent features. However, cavitation commonly occurs. The usual form of disease found in adults is termed *secondary* or *reinfection tuberculosis.* This occurs with the reactivation of persistent dormant viable bacilli and probably represents a relapse of a previous infection. This form of the disease is usually confined to the lungs, and cavitation is common.

The reasons for relapse are inadequate or no treatment of the primary infection in addition to influences such as illness, immunosuppressive agents, and age. Acquired immune deficiency syndrome (AIDS) is responsible for a growing number of cases of reactivation tuberculosis.

SEQUELAE AND COMPLICATIONS

The manifestations of tuberculosis are extremely varied. Some of the more common sequelae include progressive primary tuberculosis, cavitary disease, pleurisy and pleural effusion, meningitis, and disseminated or miliary tuberculosis. Isolated organ involvement, other than of the lung, can occur and commonly affects the pericardium, peritoneum, kidneys, adrenal glands, and bone (especially the spine).[20] The tongue and other tissues of the oral cavity may also be involved, but this is infrequent.

Aside from complications associated with individual organ involvement, the ultimate complication is death. The decreased mortality rate from tuberculosis has paralleled the precipitous drop in its incidence in the United States; however, 5% to 10% of persons who develop tuberculosis die of it.[4] The advent of effective chemotherapy has undoubtedly been the most significant reason for the lower mortality rate of the disease.

CLINICAL PRESENTATION
SIGNS AND SYMPTOMS

A characteristic feature in most people who have tuberculosis is the relative lack of definitive signs and symptoms until the lesions have been extensive. The exceptions to this are a positive skin test or radiographic findings. Once symptoms become apparent, they are usually nonspecific and could be associated with any infectious disease. They include lassitude and malaise, anorexia, weight loss, night sweats, and fever. Temperature elevation commonly occurs in the evening or during the night and is accompanied by profuse sweating.

Specific local symptoms of the disease are dependent on the organ involved. Cough is associated with pulmonary tuberculosis, although it may be late in appearance. It is commonly seen with cavitary disease. The sputum produced is characteristically scanty and nonpurulent, and hemoptysis is common. Dyspnea is also seen in advanced pulmonary disease. Radiographic findings in pulmonary tuberculosis differ with the age of the patient. The radiographic findings of tuberculosis are not pathognomonic, and the diagnosis cannot be made from radiographs alone.

Manifestations of other organ involvement may include localized lymphadenopathy with development of sinus tracts, back pain over the affected spine, gastrointestinal disturbances (in intestinal tuberculosis), dysuria or hematuria (in renal involvement), heart failure, and neurologic deficits. Physical examination may be inconclusive.

LABORATORY FINDINGS

The tuberculin skin test (Mantoux) is the most useful and reliable method of determining when a person has been infected with *M. tuberculosis.* A positive test presumptively means that a person has been infected.[2,7] It does not mean that the person has clinical tuberculosis. This is determined by physical examination and culturing. Tuberculin is a standardized PPD of culture extract from *M. tuberculosis.* Specifically, PPD-S is used as the international testing standard. The test is administered by an intradermal injection of 0.1 ml of PPD containing 5 tuberculin units (TU) into the volar or dorsal surface of the forearm. The test is read 48 to 72 hours later, and evidence of induration is noted. A 5 mm or less area of induration is considered a negative result. An area of induration between 5 and 9 mm is considered inconclusive, and the test is usually repeated. If the result is still 5 to 9 mm of induration, it probably indicates infection with a mycobacterium other than *M. tuberculosis*. A 10 mm or greater area of induration is considered positive. A positive test necessitates a physical examination, radiographic evaluation, and, if necessary, sputum culture to rule out active disease. It is advisable for individuals at risk for tuberculosis, such as dentists, to obtain a tuberculin skin test annually.

Chest radiographs are extremely helpful in tuberculosis diagnosis. Multinodular infiltration in the apical posterior segments of upper lobes, cavitation, and infiltrates are common findings in active TB. Healed primary lesions leave a calcified peripheral nodule and a calcified hilar lymph node (Ghon complex).[7]

The definitive diagnosis of tuberculosis is based on the culture and identification of *M. tuberculosis* or other species from body fluids or tissues, usually sputum. A tentative diagnosis is frequently made from detection of acid-fast bacilli in smears; however, this must be verified by culture. Multiple specimens should be obtained for culturing to ensure positive results. It commonly takes several weeks for growth to occur.[20]

Other laboratory studies—such as sedimentation rate, complete blood count, and urinalysis—usually are not helpful in delineating the disease.

MEDICAL MANAGEMENT

With the initiation of chemotherapy, a cure is almost always assured provided proper selection of drugs is made and patient compliance is optimal. Effective chemotherapy of tuberculosis is dependent upon (1) patient compliance, (2) multiple drug utilization, and (3) continuance of drug administration for a sufficient time. In the past it was necessary to continue chemotherapy for 18 to 24 months, but now many treatment schedules include short courses of 9 to 12 months. Most relapses, however, follow the short courses of treatment. Table 10-5 lists the primary drugs used for the treatment of tuberculosis.

Following the initiation of chemotherapy, rapid reversal of infectiousness is achieved. Most patients become noninfectious within 2 weeks after the institution of appropriate chemotherapy from a decrease in the number of viable organisms and a decrease in coughing and sputum cultures. These will convert to negative within 3 to 6 months in up to 90% of patients.[1,3] Based on the early reversal of infectiousness, most patients are allowed to return to normal public contact within a few weeks provided they continue chemotherapy. Patients in whom sputum cultures have not converted to negative within 3 months should be evaluated for resistant bacteria.

The patient who has had a negative skin test and then, on retesting, converts to positive is considered infected with *M. tuberculosis*. Once it is established by physical examination and culturing that the disease is not active, the

TABLE 10-5
Primary Drugs for the Treatment of Tuberculosis

Drug	Product name	Dental management considerations
Isoniazid	INH, Laniazid, Nydrazid, Tubizid	Avoid acetaminophen (risk of hepatotoxicity)
Rifampin	Rifadin, Rimactane	Increased incidence of infection, delayed healing, gingival bleeding (due to leukopenia and thrombocytopenia), decreased metabolism of diazepam
Pyrazinamide	Generic	—
Ethambutol	Myambutol	—
Streptomycin	Generic	Avoid aspirin (risk of toxicity)

patient may be given a course of chemoprophylaxis to prevent clinical disease from developing. Not all patients with positive skin tests are placed on chemoprophylaxis. Those most likely to be include young persons, household contacts of patients with TB, and patients who have converted to positive within the past year as well as others considered to be at high risk for development of the disease (AIDS, immunosuppressed, renal failure). It must be recognized that many patients with infectious disease, including TB, cannot be clinically or historically identified; therefore all patients should be treated as though potentially infectious, and universal precautions for infection control strictly followed (Appendix A). Most commonly, chemoprophylaxis is provided by the oral administration of isoniazid (INH) daily for 6 to 12 months.[1] Even though this usually prevents active disease from occurring, the person retains hypersensitivity to the tuberculin test and will remain positive when skin-tested.

DENTAL MANAGEMENT
MEDICAL CONSIDERATIONS

Dental patients can be placed into one of four categories for management purposes: (1) patients with active tuberculosis, (2) patients with a past history of tuberculosis, (3) patients who have a positive tuberculin test, and (4) patients with signs or symptoms suggestive of tuberculosis. Each will be discussed in detail (Table 10-6).

Patients with clinically active sputum-positive tuberculosis

Patients with recently diagnosed tuberculosis and positive sputum cultures should not be treated on an outpatient basis. Treatment is best rendered in a hospital setting with appropriate isolation, sterilization (mask, gloves, gown), and special ventilation systems. Because of these precautions, it is best that treatment be limited to urgent care only.

After receiving chemotherapy for 2 to 3 weeks, a patient becomes noninfectious and can be treated on an outpatient basis in the same manner as any normally healthy individual. The physician should be consulted to verify that the patient is no longer infectious and to relate any complicating factors. If none are mentioned, no special precautions need be taken.

A child who has active tuberculosis and is receiving chemotherapy can usually be treated as an outpatient because bacilli are found only rarely in the sputum of young children. The child should be considered noninfectious unless a positive sputum culture has been obtained. This should be verified with the physician. The reasons that a child with tuberculosis is consid-

TABLE 10-6
Dental Management of the Patient with a History of Tuberculosis

1. Active sputum-positive tuberculosis
   a. Consult with physician before treatment
   b. Administer urgent care only (over age 6 years)
   c. Treat in hospital setting with isolation, sterilization (gloves, mask, gown), special ventilation
   d. Under age 6 years, treat as normal patient (noninfectious); consult physician
   e. When produces consistently negative sputum, treat as normal patient (noninfectious)
2. Past history of tuberculosis
   a. Approach with caution; obtain good history of disease and its treatment duration; appropriate review of systems is mandatory
   b. Patient should give history of periodic chest radiographs and physical examination, to rule out reactivation or relapse
   c. Consult with physician and postpone treatment if there is
      (1) Questionable history of adequate treatment time
      (2) Lack of appropriate medical follow-up since recovery
      (3) Signs or symptoms of relapse
   d. If present status is free of clinically active disease, treat as normal patient
3. Recent conversion to positive tuberculin skin test
   a. Should have been evaluated by physician to rule out active disease
   b. May receive isoniazid (INH) 6 months to 1 year for prophylaxis
   c. Treat as normal patient
4. Signs or symptoms suggestive of tuberculosis
   a. Refer to physician and postpone treatment
   b. If treatment necessary, treat as in 1 above

ered noninfectious are the rarity of cavitary disease in children and their inability to cough up sputum effectively. It is impossible to define exactly what age constitutes a "child" in this instance. As a general rule, children under the age of 6 years can be confidently treated. Over the age of 6, some degree of concern may exist. In any case the physician should be consulted before treatment is begun. Of greater concern in this case are the family contacts of the patient, since the disease was most likely contracted from an infected adult. On questioning, all family members who have had contact with the child should give a history of skin testing and chest radiograph to rule out the possibility of active disease. If such assurances are not obtained, then the physician or health department should be contacted to ensure that proper preventive action is taken.

Patients with a past history of tuberculosis

Fortunately, relapse is rare in patients who have received adequate treatment for the initial infection. However, this is not the case in patients who have not received adequate treatment. Regardless of what type of treatment the patient received, it is important to approach with initial caution any individual who has a past history of tuberculosis. The dentist should obtain a medical history—including diagnosis, dates of treatment, and type of treatment. Treatment duration of less than 18 months if treated in the past, or of 9 months if treated recently, would require consultation with the physician to determine the patient's status.

Patients should give a history of periodic physical examinations and chest radiographs to check for evidence of reactivation of the disease. Consultation with the physician is advisable to verify the current status. If the patient is found to be free of active disease, treatment may be rendered in the normal fashion with no special precautions.

A good review of systems is important with these patients, and referral to a physician is indicated if questionable signs or symptoms are present.

In summary, dental treatment should be postponed and consultation with a physician sought for patients who have any of the following:

1. Questionable history of proper treatment

2. Lack of appropriate medical evaluation following treatment
3. Signs or symptoms of tuberculosis suggesting relapse
4. Patients with a positive tuberculin test

A person who has a positive skin test for tuberculosis should be viewed as having been infected with tuberculosis. The patient should give a history of being evaluated for active disease by physical examination and chest radiograph. In the absence of clinically active disease, a regimen of prophylactic isoniazid may be started for 6 months to a year to prevent clinical disease. The patient is not infectious and can be treated in a normal manner. No special precautions are required.

Patients with signs or symptoms suggestive of tuberculosis

Any time a patient demonstrates unexplained, persistent signs or symptoms that may be suggestive of tuberculosis (dry nonproductive cough, pleuritic chest pain, fatigue, dyspnea, hemoptysis), no dental care should be rendered and the patient should be referred to a physician for evaluation.

DRUG ADMINISTRATION

Patients taking isoniazid should avoid acetaminophen-containing medications because of an increased potential for hepatotoxicity. If diazepam is administered during rifampin treatment, the clearance of diazepam is likely to be accelerated, thus requiring an adjustment of dosage. In addition, rifampin can cause leukopenia and thrombocytopenia—resulting in an increased incidence of infection, delayed healing, and gingival bleeding. Patients being administered streptomycin should not be given aspirin, because of the potential for increased ototoxicity.[9] Other than these possible effects, there are no apparent adverse interactions between the major antituberculous drugs and the drugs commonly used in dentistry.

TREATMENT PLANNING MODIFICATIONS

No treatment planning modifications are required for these patients.

ORAL COMPLICATIONS

Infrequently tuberculosis may be manifested by oral lesions. These are most commonly seen

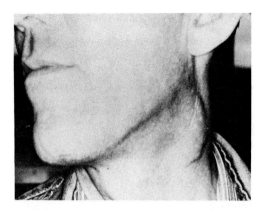

FIG. 10-4 Tuberculosis of the cervical lymph nodes.

as a painful deep ulcer on the dorsum of the tongue; however, other oral mucosal surfaces can be involved—including palate, lips, buccal mucosa, and gingiva.[8,16] Biopsy, in addition to culture, can be diagnostic if acid-fast bacilli are found. Treatment of the oral lesion is secondary to treatment of the tuberculosis. Pain can be managed symptomatically. (See Appendix B.)

The cervical and submandibular lymph nodes can become infected with tuberculosis, which is termed *scrofula*. The nodes are enlarged and painful, and abscesses may form and drain (Fig. 10-4). Usual treatment is the administration of antituberculous drugs.

REFERENCES

1. American Thoracic Society: Treatment of tuberculosis and tuberculosis infection in adults and children, *Am Rev Respir Dis* 134:355-363, 1986.
2. American Thoracic Society: The tuberculin skin test, *Am Rev Respir Dis* 124:356-363, 1981.
3. Centers for Disease Control: Bacteriologic conversion of sputum among tuberculosis patients—United States, *MMWR* 34:747-750, 1985.
4. Centers for Disease Control: Tuberculosis—United States, 1985, *MMWR* 35:699-703, 1986.
5. Centers for Disease Control: Summary of notifiable diseases, United States, 1990, *MMWR* 39(53):1, 1990.
6. Centers for Disease Control: Mortality patterns—United States, 1989, *MMWR* 41(7):121-125, 1992.
7. Daniel TM: Tuberculosis. In Wilson JD, et al, editors: *Harrison's Principles of internal medicine,* ed 12, New York, 1991, McGraw-Hill.
8. Dimitrakopoulos I, Zouloumis L, Lazaridis N, et al: Primary tuberculosis of the oral cavity, *Oral Surg* 72:712-715, 1991.
9. *Drug information for the health care professional,* ed 12, Rockville, Md, 1992, United States Pharmacopeial Convention.
10. Drugs for ambulatory asthma, *Med Lett Drugs Ther* 33(837):9-12, 1991.
11. Golden A, Powell DE, Jennings CD: *Pathology: understanding human disease,* ed 2, Baltimore, 1985, Williams & Wilkins.
12. Ingram RH Jr: Chronic bronchitis, emphysema, and airway obstruction. In Wilson JD, et al, editors: *Harrison's Principles of internal medicine,* ed 12, New York, 1991, McGraw-Hill.
13. Malamed SF: *Handbook of medical emergencies in the dental office,* ed 3, St Louis, 1986, CV Mosby.
14. McFadden ER Jr: Asthma. In Wilson JD, et al, editors: *Harrison's Principles of internal medicine,* ed 12, New York, 1991, McGraw-Hill.
15. Seng GF, Gay BJ: Dangers of sulfites in dental local anesthetic solutions: warning and recommendations, *J Am Dent Assoc* 113(5):769-770, 1986.
16. Shafer WG, Hine MK, Levy BM: *A textbook of oral pathology,* ed 4, Philadelphia, 1983, WB Saunders.
17. Snider GL: Chronic obstructive pulmonary disease. In Stein JH, editor: *Internal medicine,* Boston, 1990, Little, Brown.
18. US Department of Health and Human Services: *Chronic obstructive lung disease: the health consequences of smoking. A report of the Surgeon General,* Public Health Service Publ. no. 84-50205, 1984.
19. US Department of Health and Human Services: Warning on prescription drugs containing sulfites, *FDA Drug Bull* 17(1):2-3, 1987.
20. VonLichtenberg F: Infectious disease: viral, chlamydial, rickettsial, and bacterial diseases. In Cottran RS, Kumar V, Robbins S, editors: *Robbins' Pathologic basis of disease,* ed 4, Philadelphia, 1989, WB Saunders.

11

Chronic Renal Failure and Dialysis

There are 8 million people in the United States today with some form of kidney disease. Of these, some 60,000 die annually as a result of chronic, progressive, irreversible kidney failure (end-stage renal disease [ESRD]; chronic renal failure). Each year approximately 1.3 in 10,000 develop ESRD, and this is increasing by about 10% per year, most rapidly in patients over 65.[3]

The early phase of ESRD, which is usually asymptomatic except for some mild laboratory abnormalities, is called *renal insufficiency*. However, more damage occurs progressively, resulting in decreased ability of the kidney to perform its excretory, endocrine, and metabolic functions beyond compensatory mechanisms. The disease then becomes frank *renal failure*. This indicates inability of the kidneys to maintain normal homeostasis. The resulting syndrome — caused by kidney failure, retention of excretory products, and interference with endocrine and metabolic functions — is called *uremia*. The manifestations of uremia are seen in the cardiovascular, gastrointestinal, neuromuscular, hematologic, and dermatologic systems.

As the disease progresses, conservative medical management becomes inadequate and either artificial filtration of the blood by dialysis or transplantation of a kidney is required. Patients in both these categories pose significant management dilemmas for the dentist. This chapter will deal with the effects of renal failure and dialysis. Renal transplantation is covered in Chapter 26.

GENERAL DESCRIPTION
INCIDENCE AND PREVALENCE

ESRD is a bilateral, progressive, and chronic deterioration of nephrons that results in uremia and ultimately leads to death. The rate of destruction and the severity of disease depend on the underlying causative factors; however, in many cases the cause remains unknown. Some of the more common known causes of ESRD are diabetes, hypertension, glomerulonephritis, polycystic kidney disease, and systemic lupus erythematosus.

PATHOPHYSIOLOGY

Deterioration and destruction of functioning nephrons are the underlying pathologic processes of renal failure. The nephron includes the glomerulus, tubules, and vasculature. Various diseases affect different segments of the nephron at first, but the entire nephron is eventually affected. For example, hypertension affects the vasculature first whereas glomerulonephritis first affects the glomeruli.

Once lost, nephrons are not replaced. However, because of a compensatory hypertrophy of the remaining nephrons, normal renal function is maintained for a time. This is a period of relative renal insufficiency, during which time homeostasis is preserved. The patient remains asymptomatic and demonstrates only laboratory abnormalities that reflect a diminished glomerular filtration rate.[7]

Normal function is maintained until about 50% of the nephrons are destroyed.[3] At this point, compensatory mechanisms are overwhelmed and the signs and symptoms of uremia appear. Morphologically the end-stage kidney is markedly reduced in size and is scarred and nodular (Fig. 11-1).

SEQUELAE AND COMPLICATIONS

Although a patient with early renal failure may remain asymptomatic, physiologic changes invariably occur as the disease progresses.

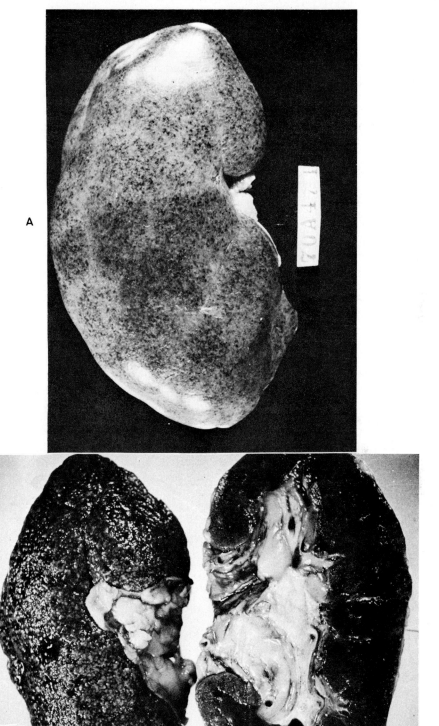

FIG. 11-1 Morphology of, **A,** a normal kidney and, **B,** a kidney in ESRD. (Courtesy A. Golden, M.D., Lexington Ky.)

These changes occur because of the loss of nephrons, which results in a loss of overall renal function. Because of tubular malfunction, the sodium pump loses its effectiveness and excretion of sodium occurs. Along with sodium, excess amounts of dilute urine also are excreted, which accounts for the polyuria that is commonly encountered.[2] The failing kidneys are unable to handle the sudden large intake of sodium or water, and sodium retention and fluid overload can become problems quickly.

With loss of the glomerular filtration function, there is a buildup of nonprotein nitrogen compounds in the blood, mainly in the form of urea. This is termed *azotemia.* In addition to nitrogenous waste products, other acids accumulate because of the tubular impairment. The combination of waste products results in acidosis, the major result of which is ammonia retention. In the later stages of renal failure, acidosis causes nausea, anorexia, and fatigue. Patients may tend to hyperventilate to attempt a respiratory compensation for the metabolic acidosis.

In the patient with acidosis of ESRD, adaptive mechanisms are already taxed beyond normal and any increase in demand can lead to serious consequences. For example, sepsis or a febrile illness can lead to a profound acidosis and be fatal.

As would be expected, there are severe electrolyte disturbances in renal failure. Sodium depletion has already been mentioned. With the progressive azotemia of later stages, hyperkalemia also may develop and becomes particularly evident as urine output falls.

Patients with ESRD demonstrate several hematologic abnormalities. Anemia is one of the most familiar manifestations of ESRD. It is due to decreased erythropoietin production by the kidney, inhibition of red blood cell (RBC) production by the effects of uremic serum on bone marrow, and RBC hemolysis; the last probably results from unidentified substances in the uremic plasma as well as other factors.[1,2]

There also are changes in the production and function of white blood cells (WBCs) that lead to alteration of the immune response, inflammation, and an enhanced susceptibility to infection.

Hemorrhagic diatheses, characterized by a tendency to abnormal bleeding and bruising, are common in patients with ESRD and are attributed primarily to abnormal platelet aggregation and adhesiveness, decreased platelet Factor III, and impaired prothrombin consumption.[2]

The cardiovascular system is affected by a tendency to develop congestive heart failure, pulmonary edema, or both. The most common complication, however, is arterial hypertension, which is due to fluid overload. Hypertrophy of the left ventricle also occurs and may compromise blood supply via the coronary vessels. This condition is worsened by anemia. There is also a tendency for accelerated atherosclerosis to develop in patients with ESRD, and pericarditis is common.[1,2]

A variety of bone disorders are seen in ESRD, commonly referred to as *renal osteodystrophy.* With decreasing nephron function there is decreased glomerular filtration, which results in an increased level of serum phosphate. Because phosphate is the driving force

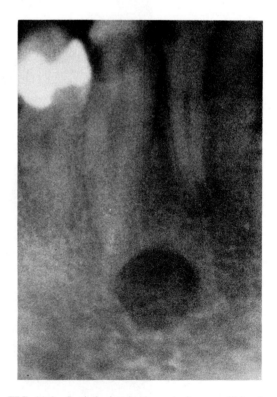

FIG. 11-2 Lytic lesion in the anterior mandible of a patient with hyperparathyroidism. (Courtesy L.R. Bean, D.D.S., Lexington Ky.)

of bone mineralization, the excess phosphate tends to cause serum calcium to be deposited in bone, leading to a decreased serum calcium level. In response to low serum calcium, the parathyroid glands are stimulated to secrete parathormone (PTH), which results in a secondary hyperparathyroidism. PTH (1) inhibits the tubular reabsorption of phosphate, (2) stimulates the renal production of vitamin D, which is necessary for calcium metabolism, and (3) enhances vitamin D absorption from the intestine. However, an additional defect in ESRD is the inability of the failing kidney to synthesize 1,25-dihydroxyvitamin D, the active metabolite of vitamin D. As a result there is a sustained high level of plasma PTH, which mobilizes calcium from the bones and promotes the excretion of phosphate. This leads to *osteomalacia* (increased unmineralized bone matrix), *osteitis fibrosa* (bone resorption and lytic lesions) (Fig. 11-2), and *osteosclerosis* (enhanced bone density) (Fig. 11-3) in varying degrees as well as to impaired bone growth in

children. With renal osteodystrophy there is also a tendency for spontaneous fractures with slow healing, myopathy, aseptic necrosis of the hip, and extraosseous calcifications.[1,2]

CLINICAL PRESENTATION
SIGNS AND SYMPTOMS

The signs and symptoms of uremia are manifested in a number of organ systems, several of which have already been mentioned.

Patients with renal failure (uremic syndrome) may demonstrate mental slowness or depression and become psychotic in later stages. They may also show muscular hyperactivity. Convulsion is a late finding that is directly correlated with the level of azotemia.

Patients with renal failure may also demonstrate a variety of gastrointestinal signs. Anorexia, nausea, and vomiting are common, as are a generalized gastroenteritis and peptic ulcer disease. Stomatitis, manifested by oral ulceration, and candidiasis can occur (Fig. 11-4). Parotitis may be seen, and there may be a urinelike odor to the breath. These patients commonly suffer from malnutrition and diarrhea.

Pallor of the skin and mucous membranes is most common and is due to anemia. Hyperpigmentation of the skin is seen and is characterized by a brownish yellow color caused by the retention of carotenelike pigments normally excreted by the kidney. These pigments also

Chronic Renal Failure

↓

Decreased Glomerular Function

↓

Increased Serum Phosphate

↓

Increased Calcium Depostion in Bone   ↓ 1,25 (OH)$_2$D$_3$

↓

Decreased Serum Calcium

↓

Increased PTH Secretion

↓

Increased Serum Calcium
Decreased Serum Phosphate

↓

"Renal Osteodystrophy"

(Osteomalacia, Osteitis Fibrosa Cystica, Osteosclerosia)

FIG. 11-3 Summary of changes that result in renal osteodystrophy.

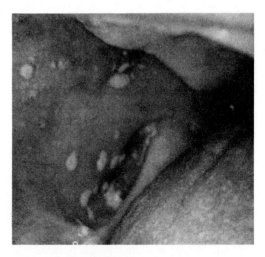

FIG. 11-4 Oral candidiasis in a patient with ESRD.

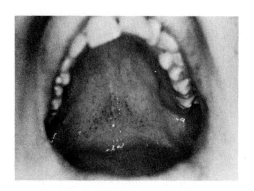

FIG. 11-5 Palatal petechiae in a patient with ESRD.

may cause a profound pruritus. An interesting occasional finding is a whitish coating on the skin of the trunk and arms produced by residual urea crystals left on the skin when perspiration evaporates (uremic frost).

Because of the bleeding diatheses that accompany ESRD, hemorrhagic episodes are not uncommon, especially in the gastrointestinal tract. In addition, ecchymoses or petechiae may be noted on the skin or mucous membranes (Fig. 11-5).

Cardiovascular manifestations of ESRD include hypertension, congestive heart failure (shortness of breath, orthopnea, dyspnea on exertion, peripheral edema), and pericarditis.

LABORATORY FINDINGS

There are several tests used to monitor the progress of ESRD—including urinalysis, urea nitrogen, serum creatinine, creatinine clearance, electrolyte measurements, and protein electrophoresis. However, the most basic test of kidney function is urinalysis, with special emphasis on the specific gravity and the presence of protein.

Creatinine is an excellent measure of glomerular filtration and tubular excretion and is commonly used as the index of clearance in a 24-hour urine collection. Serum creatinine is relatively constant, with a normal range of 0.6 to 1.20 mg. The blood urea nitrogen (BUN) is a common indicator of kidney function but is not as specific as the serum creatinine. Normal range for BUN is 8 to 18 mg/dl (3 to 6.5 mmol/L). Serum sodium ranges between 136 and 142 mmol/L, serum potassium between 3.8

and 5 mmol/L, serum chloride between 95 and 103 mmol/L, and total carbon dioxide between 22 and 26 mmol/L for venous blood.[9]

MEDICAL MANAGEMENT
CONSERVATIVE CARE

Once the diagnosis of ESRD is made, the goals of treatment are to retard the progress of disease and to preserve the quality of life. A conservative approach to treatment is the first step and may be adequate for prolonged periods.

Conservative care attempts to decrease the retention of nitrogenous waste products and to control fluids and electrolyte imbalances. This is accomplished by dietary modification with protein restriction and by closely monitoring fluid, sodium, and potassium intake. Calcium and vitamin D supplements are also important. Any treatable associated condition—such as hypertension, congestive heart failure, infection, volume depletion, urinary tract obstruction, hypercalcemia, and hyperuricemia—are corrected. Additionally, it is important to avoid nephrotoxic drugs or agents that are metabolized principally by the kidney.

The anemia that occurs in renal failure is generally refractive to conservative treatment but is well-tolerated by most patients.[8] No treatment is indicated unless the patient becomes severely symptomatic, develops an infection, or requires surgery. Even in that event, a hematocrit between 25 and 30 volumes per 100 ml is usually adequate. Infusion of packed RBCs is the treatment of choice if replacement becomes necessary.

DIALYSIS

As more and more nephrons are destroyed, attempts at medical management become inadequate to prevent or control azotemia. At this point, artificial filtration of the blood is required in the form of peritoneal dialysis or hemodialysis.

Peritoneal dialysis is accomplished by instilling a hypertonic solution into the peritoneal cavity. After a short time, the solution is drawn out. Dissolved solutes (e.g., urea) are also drawn out. The advantages of peritoneal dialysis are its relatively low cost and ease of performance. Disadvantages include the need for frequent sessions and its significantly lower effectiveness

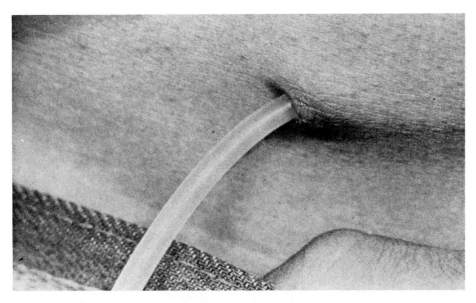

FIG. 11-6 Chronic ambulatory peritoneal dialysis catheter site in the abdominal wall. (Courtesy Dialysis Center, Lexington Ky.)

than hemodialysis. Its principal use is for patients who are in acute renal failure or require only occasional dialysis.

A newer method of peritoneal dialysis is the chronic ambulatory method. This is performed by the patient through a permanent peritoneal catheter (Fig. 11-6). Dialysate is instilled into the peritoneal cavity, the catheter is sealed, and then every 4 to 6 hours the dialysate is allowed to drain into a bag strapped to the patient and new dialysate is instilled. This method allows the patient more freedom than with the older method. A disadvantage is its high risk of peritonitis.

When dialysis must be used as a chronic treatment, hemodialysis is the method of choice. Most patients on dialysis are maintained by hemodialysis, approximately 72,000 currently in the United States.[1] Treatments are performed every 2 or 3 days depending on need. Usually 3 to 5 hours are required for each session (Fig. 11-7). Obviously, this consumes an enormous amount of the patient's time and is extremely confining; however, life-style between dialysis sessions is relatively normal.

The technique requires the surgical creation of a permanent arteriovenous fistula that is

readily accessible to cannulation with a large-gauge needle (Fig. 11-8). The patient is "plugged in" to the hemodialysis machine at the fistula site, and blood is passed through the machine, filtered, and returned to the patient. Heparin is administered during the procedure to prevent clotting.

Although hemodialysis is a lifesaving technique, there are complications associated with it. In addition to the problems attendant on ESRD, the risk of hepatitis B and C and AIDS is significant because these patients have usually had multiple blood exposures. It is estimated[5] that 3% to 10% of patients receiving chronic hemodialysis are carriers of hepatitis B (positive for hepatitis B surface antigen [HBsAg]) and thus constitute a reservoir of potential infection. The incidence of hepatitis C carrier state is unknown. A related concern is acquired immune deficiency syndrome (AIDS) infection in chronic hemodialysis patients. In a study of 520 dialysis patients,[6] however, only 0.8% were found to be truly reactive to enzyme immunoassay (EIA) and Western Blot tests. This incidence is much lower than in other high-risk groups but higher than in blood donors.

Infection of the arteriovenous fistula is an

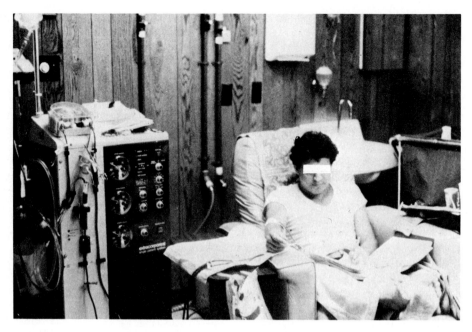

FIG. 11-7 Patient undergoing hemodialysis. (Courtesy Dialysis Center, Lexington Ky.)

ongoing concern and can result in septicemia, septic emboli, infective endarteritis, or endocarditis. However, the risk of fistula infection from surgical procedures (e.g., urogenital, oral surgical, or dental) is not precisely known but thought to be low.

As with all patients with ESRD, drugs that are metabolized primarily by the kidney or that are nephrotoxic must be avoided in patients receiving dialysis.

A final problem associated with dialysis is that of abnormal bleeding. As previously mentioned, patients with ESRD have bleeding tendencies because of altered platelet aggregation and decreased platelet Factor III. With hemodialysis there is the additional problem of platelet destruction by the procedure. One report[5] suggests that hemodialysis may also cause activation of prostaglandin I_2, which can reduce platelet aggregation. It is significant to note that because this compound has a half-life of 1 to 3 minutes its adverse effects may not be demonstrable by routine laboratory tests. An alternative to lifelong dialysis is renal transplantation. This has obvious advantages but is not without a significant number of problems. The reader is

referred to Chapter 26 for a discussion of organ transplantation.

DENTAL MANAGEMENT
PATIENT UNDER CONSERVATIVE CARE
Medical considerations

Consultation with the patient's physician is suggested before dental care is provided to patients under conservative care for ESRD. If the patient's disease is well-controlled, there is generally no problem in providing outpatient care. However, if the patient is in the advanced stages of failure, dental care may best be provided in a hospital setting. This decision should be made in concert with the physician and the patient (Table 11-1).

If it is decided to treat the patient as an outpatient, the blood pressure should be closely monitored before and during treatment. Any excessive readings should be reported to the physician. Because of the potential for bleeding problems, these patients should receive pretreatment screening for bleeding disorders — including bleeding time and platelet count. A hematocrit and a hemoglobin count should also

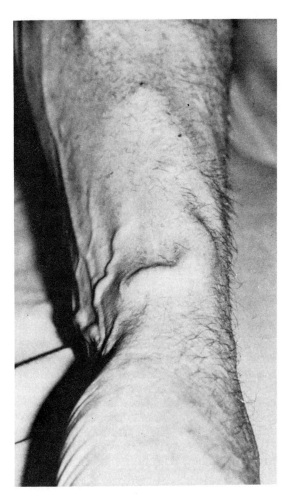

FIG. 11-8 Site of a surgically created arteriovenous fistula, with subsequent dilation and hypertrophy of the veins. (Courtesy Dialysis Center, Lexington Ky.)

TABLE 11-1
Dental Management of the Patient with End-Stage Renal Disease (Including Emergency Dental Care)

Under conservative care

Consultation with physician advised
Avoid dental treatment if disease is poorly controlled or advanced
Screen for bleeding disorder before surgery (bleeding time, platelet count, hematocrit, hemoglobin)
Monitor blood pressure closely
Pay meticulous attention to good surgical technique
Avoid nephrotoxic drugs (acetaminophen, acyclovir, aspirin, NSAIDs) (Table 15-3)
Adjust dosage of drugs metabolized by the kidney (Table 11-2)
Manage orofacial infections aggressively with culture and sensitivity test and antibiotics
Consider hospitalization for severe infection or major procedures

Receiving hemodialysis

Same as conservative care recommendations, plus
Consider antibiotic prophylaxis for dental work to prevent infective endarteritis or endocarditis
Avoid dental care on day of treatment (especially with first 4 hours afterward); best treated on day after
Screen for HBsAg before any treatment; treat as potential carrier

be obtained to assess the status of anemia. Any abnormal values should be discussed with the physician. Few problems are encountered if the hematocrit is above 25 volumes per 100 ml. If there is an orofacial infection, aggressive management is necessary using culture and sensitivity tests and appropriate antibiotics.

When surgical procedures are undertaken, meticulous attention to good surgical technique is necessary to decrease the risks of excessive bleeding and infection.

One of the major problems in treating a patient with ESRD is that of drug therapy. Of special concern are drugs that are primarily excreted by the kidney or that are nephrotoxic. Tetracycline, for example, is contraindicated in patients with renal dysfunction because it is excreted primarily by the kidney and is nephrotoxic. Drugs excreted by the kidney may not be metabolized normally and thus may reach toxic levels, and their dosage and timing of administration need to be altered. Nephrotoxic drugs should be avoided because of direct toxic effects on the kidney. Included in this group are acyclovir, acetaminophen, aspirin, and NSAIDs. An additional problem relates to certain drugs that are removed by hemodialysis and therefore require an additional dose to be administered

TABLE 11-2
Drug Therapy in Renal Disease

Drug	Route of elimination and metabolism	Normal dosage okay?	Method of dose adjustment	Require dosage supplementation following hemodialysis?
Lidocaine (Xylocaine)	Liver (kidney)	Yes		
Aspirin	Liver (kidney)	No	Increase interval between doses (avoid if possible)	Yes
Acetaminophen (Tylenol)	Liver	No	Increase interval between doses (avoid in severe failure)	Yes
Ibuprofen (Motrin)	Liver	No		Yes
Propoxyphene (Darvon)	Liver (kidney)	Yes		No
Codeine	Liver	Yes		No
Meperidine (Demerol)	Liver	Yes		No
Penicillin V	Kidney (liver)	No	Increase interval between doses	No
Erythromycin	Liver	Yes		
Cephalexin (Keflex)	Kidney	No	Increase interval between doses	Yes
Tetracycline (Doxycycline)	Kidney (liver)	No	Increase interval between doses	Yes
Diazepam (Valium)	Liver	Yes		No

Adapted from Bennett WM, et al: *Am J Kidney Dis* 3:155–176, 1983.

following hemodialysis. Table 11-2 provides a list of some of the more commonly used drugs in dental practice and recommendations for their use in patients with renal failure.

Treatment planning modifications

The goal of dental care for patients receiving conservative treatment for ESRD should be to restore the mouth to the healthiest condition possible and to eliminate possible sources of infection. Oral physiotherapy training is important for the maintenance of long-term oral health. Once an acceptable level of oral hygiene has been established, there is no contraindication to routine dental care. It is important to remember that ESRD is a progressive disease that will ultimately necessitate dialysis or transplant.

Oral complications

Several oral changes are seen with chronic renal failure. One of the most common is pallor of the oral mucosa secondary to anemia. There may also be diminished salivary flow, resulting in xerostomia and parotid infections. Patients frequently complain of a metallic taste, and the saliva may have a characteristic ammonia-like odor due to a high urea content. In severe failure a stomatitis may be present that can take two forms: an erythematopultaceous form (characterized by red, burning mucosa covered with a gray exudate) and an ulcerative form (characterized by frank ulceration).

Dental changes are also found to accompany chronic renal failure. Most classically described is the triad of loss of lamina dura, demineralized bone ("ground-glass"), and localized radiolucent jaw lesions. In the developing dentition a variety of manifestations have been described — including enamel hypoplasia, brown discoloration, and delayed or altered eruption. Tooth erosion can also be seen, resulting from persistent vomiting.

PATIENT RECEIVING HEMODIALYSIS
Medical complications

The recommendations for management of a patient receiving hemodialysis are the same as those for a patient under conservative care, with a few additional considerations (Table 11-1). Peritoneal dialysis really presents no additional problems, but this is not necessarily the case with hemodialysis. The surgically created arteriovenous fistula is potentially susceptible to infection (endarteritis) resulting from a dentally induced bacteremia and is a source of infectious emboli that can cause endocarditis. Both conditions are of low incidence. The threat of endarteritis to the hemodialysis patient is unknown, and data concerning emboli are scanty. The American Heart Association cites poor evidence and an apparent low risk for not making a recommendation to provide prophylactic antibiotics. Each case should be evaluated individually in concert with the managing physician.

Because hemodialysis tends to aggravate bleeding tendencies through physical destruction of platelets, it is important to determine the status of hemostasis before any surgery is performed. A battery of screening tests, including bleeding time and platelet count, should be ordered. Heparinization during dialysis will not produce significant residual bleeding tendencies because heparin's peak activity lasts only 3 to 4 hours after infusion. However, patients who have just had a hemodialysis session could have bleeding tendencies; therefore it is best to avoid dental care on the day of dialysis. If immediate care is necessary, protamine sulfate will block the anticoagulation effect of heparin. The best time for dental treatment is the day following hemodialysis.

All hemodialysis patients should have periodic testing for HBsAg, because a significant percentage of them are or will become carriers. However, even if the test has been negative in the past, all hemodialysis patients should be viewed as potential carriers because they may have acquired the disease since last tested or may be carriers of hepatitis C. (See Chapter 12.) All should be treated with universal infection control procedures.

Treatment planning modifications

No technical modifications are required for hemodialysis patients.

Oral complications

There are no additional oral manifestations peculiar to hemodialysis patients.

REFERENCES

1. Brenner BM, Lazarus JM: Chronic renal failure. In Wilson JD, et al, editors: *Harrison's Principles of internal medicine,* ed 12, New York, 1991, McGraw-Hill.
2. Centers for Disease Control: Recommendations for protection against viral hepatitis, *MMWR* 34:313-335, 1985.
3. Golden A, Powell DE, Jennings CD: *Pathology: understanding human disease*, ed 2, Baltimore, 1985, Williams & Wilkins.
4. Kuke RG: Dialysis. In Wyngaarden JB, Smith LH, Bennett JC, editors: *Cecil textbook of medicine,* ed 19, vol 1, Philadelphia, 1992, WB Saunders.
5. Milam SB, Cooper RL: Extensive bleeding following extraction in a patient undergoing chronic hemodialysis, *Oral Surg* 55:14-16, 1983.
6. Peterman TA, Lang GR, Mikos NJ, et al: HTLV-III/LAV infection in hemodialysis patients, *JAMA* 255:2324-2326, 1986.
7. Preuss HG, Podlasek SJ, Henry JB: Evaluation of renal function and water, electrolyte, and acid-base balance. In Henry JB, editor: *Clinical diagnosis and management of laboratory methods,* ed 18, Philadelphia, 1991, WB Saunders.
8. Sexauer CL, Matson JR: Anemia of chronic renal failure, *Ann Clin Lab Sci* 11:484-487, 1981.
9. Warnock DG: Chronic renal failure. In Wyngaarden JB, Smith LH, Bennett JC, editors: *Cecil textbook of medicine,* ed 19, vol 1, Philadelphia, 1992, WB Saunders.

12

Liver Disease

The dentist may encounter patients with one of many liver disorders. These patients are of significant interest because the liver plays such an important and vital role in metabolic functions. Impairment of liver function can lead to abnormalities of the metabolism of amino acids, ammonia, protein, carbohydrates, and lipids. In addition, many biochemical functions such as coagulation and drug metabolism may be adversely affected.

In considering the effects of liver disease on the provision of dental care, we have chosen two of the more common disorders for illustrative purposes: viral hepatitis and alcoholic liver disease.

Viral hepatitis

The term *hepatitis* is defined nonspecifically by *Dorland's Illustrated Medical Dictionary* as "inflammation of the liver." Hepatitis may result from a variety of causes. It may occur as a primary disease or secondarily to another disease. Examples of primary hepatitis are viral hepatitis, drug-induced hepatitis (e.g., caused by alcohol), and toxic hepatitis (e.g., caused by halothane). Examples of secondary hepatitis include that occurring with infectious mononucleosis, secondary syphilis, and tuberculosis. This discussion will be limited to viral hepatitis because of its special implications for dentistry.

GENERAL DESCRIPTION
ETIOLOGY

Acute viral hepatitis is caused by at least five distinct viruses—types A, B, delta, and non-A non-B (C and E). These viruses each have distinct antigenic properties, but their clinical expressions are similar. Type A hepatitis was formerly called *infectious hepatitis,* and type B hepatitis was formerly termed *serum hepatitis.* Delta hepatitis occurs only in association with hepatitis B. Non-A non-B (NANB) hepatitis occurs in at least two forms: a parenteral or community-acquired (sporadic) form called type C and a recently described enteric form (found in India, Southeast Asia, and Central America) termed type E. Table 12-1 shows the commonly used abbreviations in hepatitis terminology. Table 12-2 is a comparison of viral hepatitis types A, B, delta, and NANB. Delta hepatitis is not compared separately because it occurs only as a coinfection with type B or in a person who is a carrier of type B.

Hepatitis A

Type A hepatitis is caused by the hepatitis A virus (HAV), which is an RNA-type virus. Although this virus has been identified by electron microscopy, its properties are not completely understood. Serologic tests for HAV and its antibodies—anti-HAV, immunoglobulin M (IgM) anti-HAV (indicates recent infection), and immunoglobulin G (IgG)—are readily available.

Hepatitis B

Type B hepatitis is caused by the hepatitis B virus (HBV), which is a DNA-type virus. Electron microscopy has identified several virus-associated particles that are related to hepatitis B infection. The intact virus (HBV), or *Dane particle,* is composed of an outer shell and an inner core. The outer shell is the hepatitis B

TABLE 12-1
Hepatitis Terminology

Common Abbreviation	Term	Explanation
Hepatitis A		
HAV	Hepatitis A virus	Etiologic agent of hepatitis A
Anti-HAV	Hepatitis A antibody	Indicates past infection of hepatitis A; provides immunity
IgM anti-HAV	IgM class, hepatitis A antibody	Indicates recent infection of hepatitis A (4 to 6 months)
Hepatitis B		
HBV	Hepatitis B virus	Etiologic agent of hepatitis B
HBsAg	Hepatitis B surface antigen	Antigenic particle or antigen found on surface of virus; present during acute infection; persistence identifies carrier of hepatitis B
Anti-HBs	Antibody to hepatitis B s antigen	Indicates past infection of hepatitis B; appears after HBsAg disappears; provides immunity; denotes complete recovery
HBeAg	Hepatitis B e antigen	Antigenic particle whose presence is associated with increased infectivity in association with HBsAg
Anti-HBe	Antibody to hepatitis B e antigen	Presence is favorable sign in carriers; suggests low degree of infectiousness
HBcAg	Hepatitis B core antigen	No serologic test available
Anti-HBc	Antibody to hepatitis B core antigen	Indicates past or present infection of hepatitis B (more than 6 months)
IgM anti-HBc	IgM class antibody to hepatitis B core antigen	Indicates recent infection of hepatitis B (4 to 6 months)
Hepatitis D		
HDV	Hepatitis delta virus	Etiologic agent of delta hepatitis; requires HBV for coinfection
Anti-HD	Antibody to delta hepatitis	Indicates current or chronic infection
Hepatitis NANB		
HCV	Hepatitis C virus	Etiologic agent of parenteral and community-acquired (sporadic) NANB hepatitis
Anti-HCV	Hepatitis C antibody	Indicates past or present infection of hepatitis C and ineffective immunity
HEV	Hepatitis E virus	Etiologic agent of enterically acquired NANB hepatitis
Anti-HEV	Hepatitis E antibody	Indicates past or present infection of hepatitis E

TABLE 12-2

Comparison of Viral Hepatitides: Types A, B, Delta, and NANB

	Type A	Type B (delta*)	NANB (type C)	NANB (type E)
Etiologic agent	HAV	HBV (HDV)	HCV (similar to HBV)	HEV (similar to HAV)
Transmission	Predominantly fecal-oral	Predominantly parenteral	Predominantly parenteral; also sporadic	Fecal-oral
Incubation	2 to 5 weeks	1 to 6 months	1 to 6 months	2 weeks to 2 months
Age	Predominantly children and young adults	Any age; infrequent under 15 years	Any age; more common in adults	Young adults
Severity	Usually mild	Occasionally severe, especially delta coinfection	Occasionally severe	Usually mild
Complications	Rare	Yes	Yes; frequent	Rare
Immunity following infection	Probably lifetime	Probably lifetime	Very weak and ineffective	Probably lifetime
Immune serum globulin prophylaxis	Immune globulin (IG) usually effective	Hepatitis B IG (HBIG) usually effective	Effectiveness not established	Not known
Vaccine available	No	Yes	No	No
Carrier state	No	Yes; in 5% to 10% of patients	Probably; not yet defined	No

*Occurs as a coinfection or superinfection with B.

HAV, Hepatitis A virus; *HBV*, hepatitis B virus; *HBIG*, hepatitis B immunoglobulin.

surface antigen (HBsAg), and its antibody is anti-HBs. The inner core of the particle is the hepatitis B core antigen (HBcAg), with corresponding antibodies anti-HBc and IgM anti-HBc (indicate recent infection). A third particle is the hepatitis B e antigen (HBeAg), an antigenic component that is related to hepatitis B infectivity. Its corresponding antibody is anti-HBe. Serologic tests are available for all these antigen-antibody systems, except the HBcAg.

Delta hepatitis

Delta hepatitis is caused by a defective RNA-type virus that requires the presence of HBV for infection. It can occur as either a coinfection or a superinfection with hepatitis B.

The hepatitis delta virus (HDV) and its antibody anti-HD can be detected with serologic testing.

NANB hepatitis–type C

Non-A non-B hepatitis was originally a diagnosis of exclusion in posttransfusion hepatitis when serologic markers of types A and B were not present, a situation that was encountered in more than 90% of cases of post-transfusion hepatitis. Subsequently an antigenically distinct virus, the hepatitis C virus (HCV), was identified as the causative agent in most NANB hepatitides of parenteral and community-acquired (sporadic) origin. Serologic tests are now available for both the viral antigen (HCV) and its antibody (anti-HCV). The sensitivity and specificity of the antibody test are not well-defined, however.[13]

NANB hepatitis–type E

Another form of NANB hepatitis has been identified. This form is an enterically transmitted virus, similar to type A, and is called type E. Serologic tests for both antigen and antibody have recently become available.[15]

INCIDENCE AND PREVALENCE

Type A hepatitis occurrence declined for several years. In 1966 there were 32,859 cases reported in the United States whereas in 1983 there were 21,532 cases reported. Since then there has been a gradual steady increase in reported cases and in 1990 there were 31,441. The reasons for this increase are not immediately apparent. By contrast, the incidence of type B hepatitis has increased steadily, from 1497 reported cases in 1966 to 26,611 in 1985. From that year the occurrence has been gradually decreasing, and in 1990 there were 21,102 cases reported.[3,11] One can only speculate as to the reasons for the decrease; however, it seems likely to be associated with the increased emphasis on and awareness of infection control measures, including use of the vaccine against HIV infection, as a result of the AIDS epidemic. The occurrence of NANB remained stable from 1982 to 1990, averaging about 3000 cases per year. Nonspecified type reporting significantly decreased over this same time frame, from 11,000 to 1600.[11] This undoubtedly reflects improvements in serologic testing and type identification.

Because the means of transmission overlap and the clinical expression of the various forms of hepatitis are often indistinguishable, no absolute statements can be made regarding epidemiology. However, certain recurring patterns of disease are recognized for each type.

Hepatitis A

Type A hepatitis is transmitted almost exclusively by fecal contamination of food or water. Common sources include contaminated wells or water supplies, food sources (restaurants), and shellfish beds. Because the reservoir for infection is frequently a common food or water source, hepatitis A often occurs as an epidemic.

Transmission is also enhanced by poor personal hygiene. This may be especially apparent among school-age youngsters or food handlers. Hepatitis A is a common disease, with serologic evidence of infection in about 40% of urban populations in the United States.[15]

Persons of any age may be infected; however, the disease occurs primarily in children and young adults. In general, hepatitis A tends to be of mild severity. Of importance is the fact that no carrier state is known to exist for it. No vaccine is currently available, and recovery usually conveys immunity against reinfection.

Hepatitis B

Hepatitis B may be transmitted in a number of ways[6]—including (1) direct percutaneous inoculation of infected serum or plasma by needle or transfusion of infective blood or blood products, (2) indirect percutaneous introduction of infective serum or plasma, such as through minute skin cuts or abrasions, (3) absorption of infective serum or plasma, such as through mucosal surfaces of the mouth or eye, (4) absorption of other potentially infective secretions, such as saliva or semen through mucosal surfaces, as might occur following heterosexual or homosexual contact, and (5) transfer of infective serum or plasma via inanimate environmental surfaces or possibly vectors. Experimental data[5,10] indicate that fecal transmission of HBV does not occur and airborne spread is not epidemiologically important.

The role of saliva in HBV transmission, except by percutaneous or permucosal routes, does not appear to be significant. Observations reported to the Centers for Disease Control[4] suggest that transmission of hepatitis B to humans after surface oral contact with HBsAg-positive saliva is unlikely. Another study[38] reported that out of 19 dental professionals who had cutaneous contact with HBsAg- and HBeAg-positive saliva, none developed serologic evidence of hepatitis B. Transmission has been reported,[25] however, as a result of a human bite. Therefore it would appear that permucosal or percutaneous inoculation of infectious saliva is necessary for transmission of the disease.

The lifetime risk of hepatitis B occurrence among the general population is low; however, certain groups have a much higher risk. Included among these are health care workers

TABLE 12-3

Persons at Substantial Risk for Hepatitis B

Individuals with occupational risk
  Health-care workers
  Public-safety workers
Clients and staff of institutions for the developmentally disabled
Hemodialysis patients
Recipients of certain blood products
Household contacts and sex partners of HBV carriers
Adoptees from countries where HBV infection is endemic
International travelers
Illicit drug users
Sexually active homosexual and bisexual men
Sexually active heterosexual men and women
Inmates of long-term correctional facilities

From *MMWR* 40(RR-13):14–16, 1991.

(including dentists and dental personnel), refugees from Indochina and Haiti, residents of mental institutions and prisons, hemodialysis patients, users of illicit drugs, male homosexuals, heterosexuals with multiple partners, and recipients of blood transfusions (Table 12-3). The risk of infection is directly related to exposure to blood, resulting in a reported prevalence rate of past infection among general dentists ranging from 13% to 30%, whereas that among oral surgeons is as high as 38%.* A more recent report[14] cites the prevalence rate for general dentists at 8.89%. This reduction presumably reflects the effectiveness of prophylactic measures.

Of interest is the fact that, although hepatitis B can occur at any age, statistically it is unusual in persons under the age of 15. In fact, of the 21,102 cases of type B hepatitis reported to the Centers for Disease Control in the United States in 1990,[11] only 661 were in patients under age 15 years. This is an incidence rate of only 3.1%.

Compared with hepatitis A, hepatitis B tends to have greater associated morbidity and mortality, especially in older patients. One of the more significant features of hepatitis B is the existence of a chronic carrier state that can persist for variable periods after resolution of acute disease. A carrier is defined as an individual in whose serum the HBsAg persists and is detectable for longer than 6 months. A carrier state occurs in up to 10% of hepatitis B viral infections with or without symptoms.[13,15] It is estimated[9] that 0.1% to 0.5% of the general population in the United States is a carrier of hepatitis B whereas 5% to 15% of the populations of China, Southeast Asia, sub-Saharan Africa, most Pacific Islands, and the Amazon Basin are carriers. This marked difference reflects the endemicity of hepatitis B in these latter countries. The carrier rate of dentists in the United States has decreased, but the risk is still estimated[14] to be 3 to 10 times that of the general population. All carriers of hepatitis B should be considered potentially infectious; however, it has been shown[41] that not all carriers are equally infectious. There is a positive correlation between infectiousness and the simultaneous existence of HBsAg and HBeAg in the serum. Serum with HBeAg and HBsAg may be 10 times more infectious than serum with HBsAg alone.[41]

It is significant to note that most carriers are unaware that they have had hepatitis. An explanation for this is that many cases of hepatitis B are apparently mild, subclinical, and nonicteric. These cases may be essentially asymptomatic or may resemble a mild viral disease and therefore go undetected. Studies on dental school patients who were carriers of hepatitis B[18,39] found that up to 80% gave no history of hepatitis infection. This is indeed unfortunate, because these patients are not identifiable by medical history. It would require routine laboratory screening of every patient to identify these patients, which would not be practical.

Delta hepatitis

Delta hepatitis occurs only as a coinfection with acute hepatitis B or as a superinfection in carriers of hepatitis B and therefore is transmitted parenterally via infected blood or blood products. It is seen primarily in drug addicts and hemophiliacs and is frequently associated with more severe fulminant infections than is infection with hepatitis B alone.[8,13]

---

* References 1, 27, 28, 32, 37, 40.

NANB hepatitis—types C and E

As previously stated, two distinct forms of non-A non-B hepatitis have been confirmed. Type C hepatitis is similar to type B in behavior and characteristics. It is transmitted primarily parenterally and is the major etiologic agent of posttransfusion non-A non-B hepatitis, accounting for 80% to 90% of such cases.[36] Patients at risk for this disease include illicit drug users, health care workers exposed to blood, hemodialysis patients, and recipients of whole blood, blood cellular components, or plasma. Of interest, however, are the 40% of patients with hepatitis C that has occurred sporadically—in other words, with no identifiable risk factor for infection.[13] Heterosexual or homosexual contact has not been recognized as a significant factor in the transmission of hepatitis C, although this requires further study.

The enteric form of non-A non-B hepatitis, hepatitis E, resembles hepatitis A and is transmitted via fecal-oral contamination. The disease is endemic in India, Asia, Africa, and Central America.[15] It is not a significant factor in the United States at the present time.

PATHOPHYSIOLOGY

Although there is no single histopathologic lesion that is characteristic of viral hepatitis, the appearances of types A, B, delta, and NANB hepatitides are similar. Therefore they will be described together.

Commonly, acute viral hepatitis is characterized by degeneration and necrosis of liver cells with ballooning degeneration of the hepatocytes. The entire liver lobule is inflamed and consists of lymphocytes and mononuclear phagocytes.[19]

Icterus (jaundice) is commonly associated with hepatitis and is caused by an accumulation of bilirubin in the skin. Bilirubin is a degradation product of hemoglobin. It is one of the major constituents of bile and is yellowish in color. Bilirubin is normally transported to the liver by way of the plasma. In the liver it conjugates with glucuronic acid and is then excreted into the intestine, where it aids in the emulsification of fats and stimulates peristalsis. When liver disease is present, bilirubin tends to accumulate in the plasma because of decreased liver metabolism and transport.

Jaundice will usually become clinically apparent when the plasma level of bilirubin approaches 2.5 mg/100 ml (normal is less than 1 mg/100 ml).[15] If the plasma bilirubin does not reach this level, the patient is anicteric (without jaundice), thus explaining nonicteric hepatitis.

SEQUELAE AND COMPLICATIONS

Most cases of viral hepatitis, especially type A, resolve without any complications. However, occasional chronic problems do develop with hepatitis B, and a significant number of cases of type C result in chronic sequelae.

Approximately 3% to 5% of patients with acute hepatitis B and 40% to 50% with acute type C will develop chronic active hepatitis. This form of hepatitis is characterized by the persistence of signs and symptoms of chronic liver disease, persistent hepatic cellular necrosis, and biochemical abnormalities for longer than 6 months.[13,15] There also is a persistence of HBsAg in the serum with hepatitis B. It appears that patients who have HBeAg in their serum with the acute B infection have a greater chance than those who do not of developing this form of chronic hepatitis. The chronic liver destruction and resulting fibrosis can lead to cirrhosis in cases of chronic hepatitis.

The most serious complication of acute viral hepatitis is fulminant hepatitis, which sometimes occurs with hepatitis B and delta coinfection and with hepatitis C. This is, fortunately, a rare entity and is characterized by massive hepatocellular destruction. The mortality rate approaches 80%.

The complication of a persistent carrier state, which was previously discussed, is seen in 5% to 10% of cases of hepatitis B. There is noteworthy evidence that suggests a positive correlation between the chronic HBsAg carrier state and the development of hepatocellular carcinoma. This relationship is particularly strong in some selected Asian populations. Undoubtedly a carrier state is associated with type C, but this is not well-defined. There is, however, a positive correlation with chronic hepatitis C and hepatocellular carcinoma.

CLINICAL PRESENTATION
SIGNS AND SYMPTOMS

As previously indicated, it is frequently impossible to differentiate hepatitis type by clinical appearance; therefore it is appropriate to describe the clinical manifestations of acute viral hepatitis in general. Many of the signs and symptoms of acute viral hepatitis are common to viral diseases and may be described as flulike. This is especially true of the early, or prodromal, phase. There are classically three phases of acute viral hepatitis.

The prodromal *(preicteric)* phase usually precedes the onset of jaundice by 1 or 2 weeks and consists of anorexia, nausea, vomiting, fatigue, myalgia, malaise, and fever. With hepatitis B, 5% to 10% of patients will demonstrate serum sickness–like manifestations, including arthralgia or arthritis, rash, and angioedema.[15]

The *icteric* phase is heralded by the onset of clinical jaundice. Many of the nonspecific prodromal symptoms may subside, but gastrointestinal symptoms (e.g., anorexia, nausea, vomiting, and right upper quadrant pain) may increase, especially early in the phase. Hepatomegaly and splenomegaly are frequently seen. This phase usually lasts 6 to 8 weeks.[15]

During the convalescent or recovery *(posticteric)* phase the symptoms disappear, but hepatomegaly and abnormal liver function values may persist for a variable period. This phase can last for weeks or months, with recovery time for hepatitis types B and C generally being longer. The usual sequence is for recovery (clinical and biochemical) to be complete approximately 4 months after the onset of jaundice.[15]

LABORATORY FINDINGS

The laboratory studies most useful in making a diagnosis of acute viral hepatitis include the serum transaminases (aspartate aminotransferase [AST, SGOT] and alanine aminotransferase [ALT, SGPT]), serum bilirubin level, alkaline phosphatase level, WBC count, and prothrombin time. Antigen-antibody serologic tests also are of extreme importance.

The serum transaminase level will usually become elevated before elevation of the serum bilirubin occurs. The highest levels often correspond to the peak of the icteric phase and gradually subside during the convalescent phase. Jaundice will become clinically evident as the serum bilirubin level approaches 2.5 mg/100

ml. An elevated bilirubin level may persist after the transaminase level begins to fall. The serum alkaline phosphatase level may be mildly elevated or normal; however, this is a relatively nonspecific test.

There is usually an increase in the WBC count, with a relative lymphocytosis. Atypical lymphocytes are seen that are identical to those seen in infectious mononucleosis. It is important to monitor the prothrombin time because this may be elevated, especially in more extensive disease that results in hepatic cellular destruction. If the prothrombin time is severely elevated, abnormal hemostasis may be encountered.

Of particular interest in hepatitis B are antigen-antibody serologic tests and their relationship to the progress of the disease. Figure 12-1 demonstrates these serologic relationships. It should be recognized that the appearance of the antibody (anti-HBs) connotes recovery, and permanent immunity is usually conferred.

In type C the sensitivity and specificity of the currently available tests for anti-HCV are not well-defined. In posttransfusion cases the mean interval between date of transfusion and anti-HCV seroconversion is approximately 18 weeks but may be 6 to 12 months. The presence of anti-HCV is an indication of infectivity, not of recovery or immunity.[13,36]

MEDICAL MANAGEMENT

As is the case with most viral diseases, there is no specific treatment for acute viral hepatitis. Therapy is basically palliative and supportive. Bed rest may be prescribed, especially early in the course of the disease. A nutritious and high-calorie diet is advisable. Drugs metabolized by the liver are to be avoided. The effectiveness of corticosteroids is doubtful in treatment of acute viral hepatitis; they are usually reserved for fulminant hepatitis. Prophylaxis of viral hepatitis is the preferred form of treatment and is accomplished by administering either early postexposure immune globulins or preexposure or postexposure hepatitis B vaccine.

IG, also called *immune serum globulin,* is a pool of antibodies collected from human plasma that is free of HBsAg. This sterile solution contains antibodies against both hepatitis A and hepatitis B. Another type of IG is called

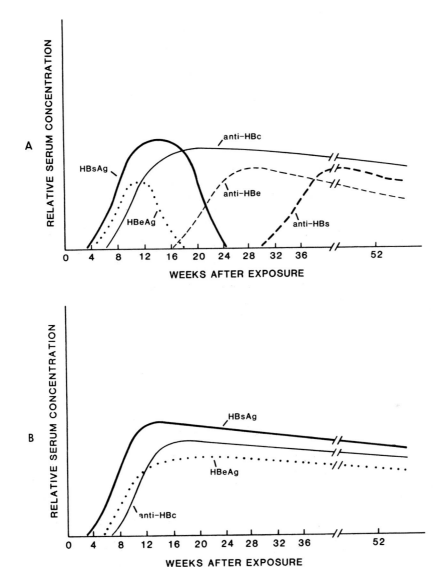

FIG. 12-1 Typical sequence of various HBV markers in, **A,** acute infection with recovery and, **B,** acute infection resulting in a chronic carrier state.

hepatitis B IG (HBIG) and is specially prepared from preselected plasma that is high in titers of anti-HBs. Administration of both IG and HBIG is safe and is not associated with transmission of the AIDS virus.[15]

In hepatitis A, IG given either before exposure or shortly after exposure is effective in preventing clinical infection. With hepatitis B,

however, IG is not recommended because of the low and unpredictable titers of antibodies to HBV. HBIG is the preparation of choice but is used only in certain postexposure instances.

Prophylaxis against hepatitis B is effectively accomplished by using the hepatitis B vaccine. Originally, the vaccine was derived from pooled donor plasma; however, this form is no longer available. Currently, two vaccines* are licensed for use, and both are produced by recombinant DNA technology. The vaccine is administered in three doses over a 6-month period and results in an effective antibody response in more than 90% of adults and 95% of infants, children, and adolescents.[12] This conversion rate is based upon injections given in the deltoid muscle, since injections administered in the buttocks resulted in only 81% of recipients' developing effective antibody titers.[9] Individuals who have received the vaccine in the buttocks should have serologic confirmation of their antibody titer status.

The duration of immunity and the need for booster doses remain somewhat uncertain. Current information is based on experience with the plasma-derived vaccine but results should be comparable to those with the recombinant vaccines. Long-term studies[12] indicate that immunity remains effective for at least 9 years and booster doses are not needed at this time. Further recommendations will be forthcoming as additional studies are completed.

In the past, considerable concern existed surrounding the possibility that plasma-derived hepatitis B vaccine could be a vehicle for transmission of AIDS. No evidence exists, however, linking the occurrence of AIDS with the plasma-derived vaccine. Based on extensive laboratory studies and epidemiologic monitoring,[7] the Centers for Disease Control concluded that there was no correlation between AIDS infection and the hepatitis B vaccine. It should be noted that, with the development of the recombinant DNA hepatitis B vaccine, this is no longer an issue.

The vaccine is intended for use not in mass inoculations but rather in selected target populations who are at high risk for contracting hepatitis B. Table 12-3 lists persons who are at substantial risk of contracting hepatitis B and should receive the vaccine. Note that health care workers (including dentists) are at the top of the list. It is strongly recommended that all dentists and dental personnel be inoculated with the vaccine.

If a vaccinated individual sustains a needle stick or puncture wound contaminated with blood from a patient known to be HBsAg

positive, it is recommended[12] that the vaccinated individual be tested for an adequate titer of anti-HBs, if unknown, and, if levels are inadequate, immediately receive an injection of HBIG and a vaccine booster dose. If the antibody titer is adequate, nothing further is required. If an unvaccinated individual sustains an inadvertent percutaneous or permucosal exposure to hepatitis B, immediate administration of HBIG and initiation of the vaccine are recommended.[12]

A question also arises concerning dentists who are carriers of HBsAg. As of this writing there have been nine reported outbreaks since 1974 of hepatitis B traceable to carrier dentists or oral surgeons. In each instance the practitioner was found to be seropositive for HBsAg and (if tested) HBeAg and did not use gloves during dental or surgical procedures. None of the practitioners were aware of their chronic infections. Two patients have died as a result of these infections.[20] It is interesting to note that almost all these reported outbreaks occurred before the increased awareness of transmission of blood-borne pathogens took place in the late 1980s.

Following the discovery of carrier state and documented transmission of disease, some dentists have ceased to practice permanently and others have faced lengthy periods of discontinuance. If a carrier dentist elects to continue practice, professional ethics and practice guidelines mandate aggressive efforts to prevent potential transmission by adherence to strict aseptic technique, periodic retesting of HBsAg, and informed consent from all patients.

DENTAL MANAGEMENT
MEDICAL CONSIDERATIONS

The dental management of patients with a history of hepatitis B begins with identification. The ideal goal is to identify potential or actual carriers of B, delta, or NANB hepatitis because they are potentially infectious. Unfortunately, this is not possible because in most instances carriers cannot be identified by history. The inability to identify potentially infectious patients extends to AIDS and other sexually transmitted diseases. Therefore it is necessary to manage all patients as though they are potentially infectious. The U.S. Public Health Service's Centers for Disease Control and the

---

* Recombivax HB and Engerix-B.

American Dental Association have published recommendations for infection control practice in dentistry that have become the standard of care to prevent crossinfection in dental practice. (See Appendix A.)

There are five categories of patients with a history of hepatitis that must be considered by the dentist. These are patients with active hepatitis, patients with a history of hepatitis, patients at a high risk for HBV infection, patients who are HBV carriers, and patients with signs or symptoms of hepatitis.

Patients with active hepatitis

Routine, elective dental care should not be performed for a patient with active hepatitis. If a patient is seen who has acute hepatitis, the physician should be contacted immediately. Unless the patient is clinically and biochemically recovered, no treatment should be rendered other than urgent care (Table 12-4).

Patients with a history of hepatitis

A primary concern of the dentist is to identify patients who are or could be carriers of type B, delta, or C hepatitis. As previously noted, however, the medical history will fail to identify up to 80% of carriers of hepatitis B and cannot be relied on for this purpose. In addition, it should be remembered that there is undoubt-

TABLE 12-4
Urgent Dental Care for the Patient with Hepatitis

Consult with physician to discuss patient's status and planned dental treatment

If surgery is necessary, obtain preoperative prothrombin time and bleeding time; discuss abnormal results with physician

Adhere to strict universal precautions (Appendix A)

Use isolated operatory

Minimize use of drugs metabolized by liver (Table 12-5)

Use rubber dam when possible to minimize contact with saliva and blood

Minimize aerosol production by using slow-speed handpiece when possible; use air syringe judiciously

Do only work that is absolutely necessary

---

edly a carrier state with hepatitis C though not well-defined as yet. Because it is estimated that there are between 750,000 and 1 million carriers of hepatitis B in the United States today, this means that there are 600,000 to 800,000 hepatitis B carriers who cannot be detected by history. Routine laboratory screening for all patients is economically impractical because of its low cost-effectiveness. Therefore the only practical method of protection from these individuals, and other patients with undetected infectious diseases, is to adopt a strict program of clinical asepsis for *all* patients (Appendix A). In addition, the availability and effectiveness of the hepatitis B vaccine can further decrease the threat of hepatitis B infection. Inoculation of all dental personnel with hepatitis B vaccine is strongly urged.

For those patients who provide a positive history of hepatitis, additional historical information will occasionally be of some help in determining the type of disease. For instance, if the infection occurred under age 15 years or was caused by contaminated food or water, this would suggest hepatitis A infection. Unfortunately, this approach will not reveal a person who has had infection with both type A and type B or C in which the B or C infection was subclinical or undiagnosed. This, again, supports the adoption of universal precautions for all patients and inoculation of dental personnel with hepatitis B vaccine.

An additional consideration in patients with a history of hepatitis of unknown type is to use the clinical laboratory to screen for the presence of HBsAg. This may be indicated even in patients who specifically indicate which type of hepatitis they have had, because studies[18] have shown that historically provided information of this type is unreliable 50% of the time. We do not currently recommend screening for anti-HCV due to the uncertain specificity and sensitivity of this test.

Patients at high risk for HBV infection

As indicated in Table 12-3, there are several groups of people who are at unusually high risk for HBV infection. Individuals who fit into one or more of these categories should routinely be screened for HBsAg before dental care is provided unless laboratory evidence exists for anti-HBs.

It may seem redundant to recommend screening patients for the presence of HBsAg, because all patients are to be managed in such a manner as to prevent the transmission of infection by following the Centers for Disease Control recommendations. Even if a patient is found to be a carrier, no modifications in treatment approach would theoretically be necessary. However, this information may still be of benefit in certain situations. If a patient is found to be a carrier, the information could be of extreme importance for the modification of life-style. In addition, the patient might have undetected chronic active hepatitis, which could lead to bleeding complications or drug metabolism problems. Finally, if an accidental needle stick or puncture wound occurs during treatment and the dentist is not vaccinated (or antibody titer status is unknown), it would be of extreme importance to know whether the patient was HBsAg positive, which would dictate the need for IG or HBIG vaccination.

Patients who are hepatitis carriers

If a patient is found to be a hepatitis B carrier (HBsAg positive) or to have a history of NANB hepatitis, the Centers for Disease Control recommendations (Appendix A) should be closely followed to avoid transmission of infection. In addition, some hepatitis carriers may have chronic active hepatitis, leading to compromised liver function and interfering with hemostasis and drug metabolism. Physician consultation or laboratory screening for liver function is advised.

Patients with signs or symptoms of hepatitis

Any patient who has signs or symptoms that suggest hepatitis should not be treated electively but referred immediately to a physician. If emergency care becomes necessary, it should be provided as for the patient with acute disease. (See Table 12-4.)

DRUG ADMINISTRATION

In a completely recovered patient there are no special drug considerations. However, if a patient has chronic active hepatitis or is a carrier of HBsAg and has impaired liver function, drugs metabolized by the liver should be avoided if possible, or the dosage decreased. As can be seen from Table 12-5, many drugs commonly

TABLE 12-5
Dental Drugs Metabolized Primarily by the Liver

Local Anesthetics

Lidocaine (Xylocaine)
Mepivacine (Carbocaine)
Prilocaine (Citinest)
Bupivicaine (Marcaine)

Analgesics

Aspirin
Acetaminophen (Tylenol, Datril)
Codeine
Meperidine (Demerol)
Ibuprofen (Motrin)

Sedatives

Diazepam (Valium)
Barbiturates

Antibiotics

Ampicillin
Tetracycline

used in dentistry are metabolized principally by the liver, but in other than the most severe cases of hepatic disease, these drugs can be used, although in limited amounts. For example, the maximum amount of lidocaine used should be limited empirically to approximately 120 mg (three cartridges of 2%).

TREATMENT PLANNING MODIFICATIONS

No treatment planning modifications are required for the patient who has recovered from hepatitis.

ORAL COMPLICATIONS

The only oral complication associated with hepatitis is the potential for abnormal bleeding in cases of significant liver damage. Before any surgery the prothrombin time should be checked to ensure that it is less than 2½ times normal (35 seconds). If it is greater than 35 seconds, the potential for severe postoperative bleeding exists. In this case, if surgery is necessary, an injection of vitamin K will usually correct the problem and should be discussed with the physician. It is also advisable to monitor the bleeding time to check platelet function, because liver damage can also result in decreased platelet count. The bleeding time should be less than 20 minutes. Values greater than this may require platelet replacement before surgery and should be discussed with the patient's physician.

Alcoholic liver disease

GENERAL DESCRIPTION
INCIDENCE, PREVALENCE, AND ETIOLOGY

Abuse of alcohol is a serious problem in the United States. It is estimated[33] that up to 90% of people drink alcohol, 40% to 50% of men have temporary alcohol-induced problems, and 10% of men and 3% to 5% of women develop pervasive and persistent alcoholism. In a recent survey[21] 9% of adults met the criteria for 1-year alcohol abuse and within this group there were three times as many men as women, although less of a difference in the younger age groups. Whereas problem drinking is primarily seen in adults, the prevalence among teenagers is rising alarmingly. One study[26] reported that an estimated 3.3 million youngsters aged 14 to 17 years could be classified as problem drinkers. Alcoholism among the elderly also is a significant problem as well, with prevalence estimates varying between 1% and 10%.[2]

The economic impact of alcohol abuse and dependence is staggering. In 1983 the cost was estimated at $116.9 billion. By 1990 this figure had increased to $136.3 billion, and it is projected to reach $150 billion by 1995.[35] In addition, alcohol has been implicated as the leading cause of accidental deaths in the United States. Motor vehicle accidents are the major cause of injury-related deaths, and alcohol is involved in at least half of them.

Alcohol abuse and dependence are not limited to any particular group. All ages and races, both sexes, and all socioeconomic levels are affected. The stereotypical picture of the skid row bum applies to only a small percentage of cases.

The chronic ingestion of large amounts of ethanol can result in a myriad of health problems[11,30]—including peripheral neuropathies, Wernicke's and Korsakoff's syndromes, cerebellar degeneration, dementia, esophagitis and gastritis, pancreatitis, malignancies, hematopoietic changes, and profound liver abnormalities leading to cirrhosis (the ninth leading cause of death among adults in the United States).

The quantity and duration of alcohol ingestion required to produce cirrhosis are not clear; however, the typical alcoholic with cirrhosis has a history of daily consumption of a pint or more of whiskey, several quarts of wine, or an equivalent amount of beer for at least 10 years.[30]

It has long been recognized that a relationship exists between excessive alcohol ingestion and liver dysfunction leading to cirrhosis. However, the exact effect of alcohol on the liver was not known until it was shown that alcohol is a direct hepatotoxic drug.[23] In light of this fact, it is curious that only 10% to 15% of heavy alcohol users ever develop cirrhosis.[30] This can probably be explained by hereditary factors and nutritional or biochemical differences among individuals.

PATHOPHYSIOLOGY

The pathologic effects of alcohol on the liver are expressed by one of three disease entities.[19,30] These conditions may exist alone but commonly appear in combination.

The earliest change seen in alcoholic liver disease is a *fatty infiltrate*. The hepatocytes become engorged with fatty lobules and distended, with enlargement of the entire liver. No other structural changes are usually noted. These changes may be seen after only moderate usage of alcohol for a brief time; however, they are considered completely reversible.

A second and more serious form of alcoholic liver disease is *alcoholic hepatitis*. This is a diffuse inflammatory condition of the liver characterized by destructive cellular changes, some of which may be irreversible. The irreversible changes can lead to necrosis. It is thought that nutritional factors may play a significant role in the progression of this disease. For the most part, alcoholic hepatitis is considered a reversible condition; however, it can be fatal if damage is widespread.

The third and most serious form of alcoholic

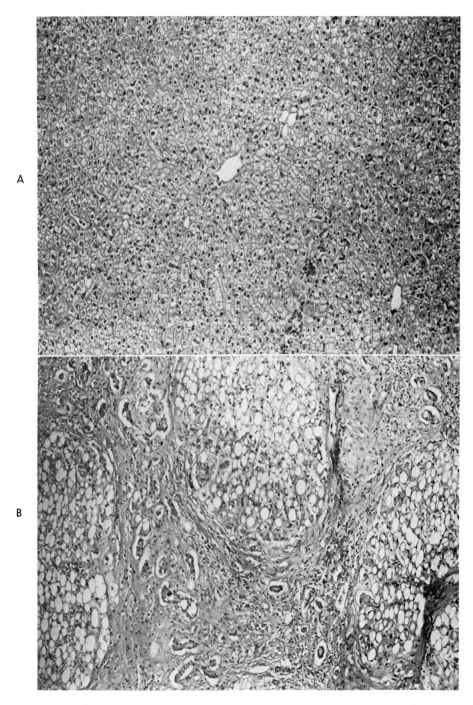

FIG. 12-2 Photomicrographs of, **A,** normal liver architecture and, **B,** liver architecture in alcoholic cirrhosis. (Courtesy A. Golden, M.D., Lexington Ky.)

liver disease is *cirrhosis,* which is generally considered an irreversible condition characterized by progressive fibrosis and abnormal regeneration of liver architecture in response to chronic injury or insult (Fig. 12-2). The insult, in this case, is prolonged and heavy use of ethanol.

Although cirrhosis is generally considered to be an end-stage condition, some evidence suggests that at least partial reversibility of the process is possible with complete and permanent removal of the offending agent.

SEQUELAE AND COMPLICATIONS

Cirrhosis results in the progressive deterioration of the metabolic and excretory functions of the liver and ultimately leads to hepatic failure. Hepatic failure is manifested by many abnormalities. Some of the more important of these are generalized malnutrition, weight loss, protein deficiency (including coagulation factors), impairment of urea synthesis and glucose metabolism, endocrine disturbances, encephalopathy, renal failure, portal hypertension, and jaundice. Accompanying portal hypertension is the development of ascites and esophageal varices[19,30] (Fig. 12-3).

Bleeding tendencies are a significant feature in advanced liver disease. The basis for this diathesis is in part a deficiency of coagulation factors, especially the prothrombin group (Factors II, VII, IX, and X). These all rely on vitamin K as a precursor for production. Vitamin K is absorbed from the large intestine and stored in the liver, where it is converted into an enzymatic cofactor for the carboxylation of prothrombin complex proteins. Widespread hepatocellular destruction as seen in cirrhosis decreases the liver's storage and conversion capacity of vitamin K, leading to deficiencies of the prothrombin-dependent coagulation factors. In addition to these deficiencies, thrombocytopenia may be caused by hypersplenism secondary to portal hypertension and to bone marrow depression. Anemia and leukocytosis may also be present, due to toxic effects of alcohol on the bone marrow as well as to nutritional deficiencies. Accelerated fibrinolysis is also seen.[22,23,29,30]

The combination of hemorrhagic tendencies and severe portal hypertension sets the stage for

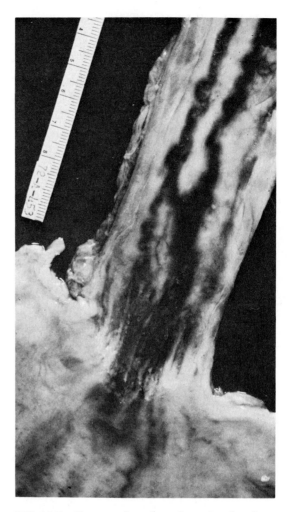

FIG. 12-3 Gross section of esophageal varices from an alcoholic patient. (Courtesy A. Golden, M.D., Lexington Ky.)

episodes of gastrointestinal bleeding, epistaxis, ecchymoses, or ruptured esophageal varices. In fact, most patients with advanced cirrhosis die of hepatic coma, often precipitated by massive hemorrhage from esophageal varices or intercurrent infection.[30]

A complication associated with abrupt alcohol withdrawal is delirium tremens (DTs)—characterized by hallucinations, disorientation, and extreme agitation.

CLINICAL PRESENTATION
SIGNS AND SYMPTOMS

With the possible exception of enlargement, there are no clinical manifestations of a fatty liver, and the diagnosis is usually made incidentally in conjunction with another illness.

The clinical presentation of alcoholic hepatitis is often nonspecific and may include features such as nausea, vomiting, anorexia, malaise, weight loss, and fever. More specific findings include hepatomegaly, splenomegaly, jaundice, ascites, ankle edema, and spider angiomas. With advancing disease, encephalopathy and hepatic coma may ensue, ending in death.

Alcoholic cirrhosis may remain asymptomatic for many years until there is sufficient destruction of the liver parenchyma to produce clinical evidence of hepatic failure. Ascites, spider angiomas (Fig. 12-4), ankle edema, or jaundice may be the earliest signs, but frequently hemorrhage from esophageal varices is the initial sign. The hemorrhagic episode may progress to hepatic encephalopathy, coma, and death. Some other, less specific, signs of alcoholic liver disease include purpura, ecchymoses, gingival bleeding, palmar erythema, nail changes, and parotid gland enlargement.

LABORATORY FINDINGS

The laboratory findings in alcoholic liver disease vary from minimal abnormalities caused by a fatty liver to the characteristic manifestations of alcoholic hepatitis and cirrhosis. These include elevations of bilirubin, alkaline phosphatase, aspartate aminotransferase (AST, SGOT) and alanine aminotransferase (ALT, SGPT). Deficiencies of clotting factors lead to elevations in the prothrombin time and partial thromboplastin time. Thrombocytopenia may be present, causing a decreased platelet count and increased bleeding time. Increased fibrinolytic activity may be evidenced by an increased bleeding time, prolonged thrombin time, or decreased euglobulin clot lysis time. Leukopenia (or leukocytosis) or anemia may also be present.[30]

MEDICAL MANAGEMENT

In all forms of alcoholic liver disease, the cornerstone of treatment is identification of the problem and then withdrawal and abstinence from alcohol. In addition, strict dietary modifications are required—including a high-protein, high calorie, and low-sodium diet. Fluid restriction as well as vitamin supplementation may be necessary. Anemia is corrected by iron replacement and folic acid supplementation. Infection or sepsis is treated appropriately. Steroids may be of some benefit, although this is controversial.

Hemorrhage from esophageal varices and hepatic encephalopathy require immediate treatment. Ascites mandates measures to control fluids and electrolytes.

DENTAL MANAGEMENT
MEDICAL CONSIDERATIONS
(Table 12-6)

There are two major treatment considerations in an alcoholic patient: (1) bleeding tendencies and (2) unpredictable metabolism of certain drugs. Correct dental management of these patients begins with detection, by history or clinical examination or both. Because alcohol abuse is frequently denied, the dentist must remain alert to the visible and obvious physical signs that may suggest alcoholic liver disease. These include spider angiomas of the skin, palmar erythema, white or banded nails, unexplained bruising, enlargement of the parotid glands (Fig. 12-5), swelling of the ankles, ascites, and jaundice (most evident in the sclerae and mucosa) (Table 12-7). In addition, the patient may admit to frequent use of alcohol, or its odor may be detectable on the breath. Family mem-

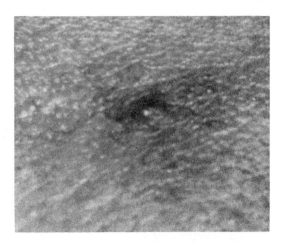

FIG. 12-4 Spider angioma.

TABLE 12-6
Dental Management of the Patient with
Alcoholic Liver Disease

1. Detection by
   a. History
   b. Clinical examination
   c. Alcohol odor on breath
   d. Information from family members or friends
2. Referral or consultation with physician to
   a. Verify history
   b. Check current status
   c. Check medications
   d. Check laboratory values
   e. Discuss suggestions for management
3. Laboratory screening (if otherwise not available
   from physician)
   a. CBC with differential
   b. AST, ALT
   c. Bleeding time
   d. Thrombin time
   e. Prothrombin time
4. Minimize drugs metabolized by liver
   (Table 12-5)
5. If screening tests abnormal, for surgical
   procedures consider using
   a. Antifibrinolytic agents
   b. Fresh frozen plasma
   c. Vitamin K
   d. Platelets

TABLE 12-7
Signs Suggestive of Advanced Alcoholic
Liver Disease

Spider angiomas
Jaundice (sclerae, mucosa)
Ankle edema
Ascites
Ecchymoses and petechiae
Parotid gland enlargement
Palmar erythema
White nails
Transverse pale bands on nails
Sweet, musty breath odor

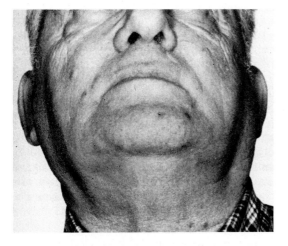

FIG. 12-5 Painless enlargement of the parotid glands associated with alcoholism. (Courtesy Valerie Murrah, D.M.D., San Antonio Tex.)

bers may also volunteer this information, in confidence. It should be kept in mind that alcoholism transcends the age, sex, and socio-economic spectrum.

If suggestive signs or symptoms are noted, the dentist should question the patient about alcohol use, including what is used, quantity on a daily or weekly basis, and how long the use has occurred. The questioning should be done in a nonjudgmental manner. Whether or not the patient admits to the heavy use of alcohol, a high index of suspicion should be followed by a series of laboratory tests for screening purposes. A complete blood count (CBC) with differential, AST and ALT, bleeding time, thrombin time, and prothrombin time are sufficient to screen for the most significant problems. Abnormal laboratory values, accompanied by abnormal clinical examination or positive history, are the basis for referral to a physician for positive diagnosis and treatment. A patient with untreated alcoholic liver disease is not a candidate for elective, outpatient dental care and should be referred to a physician. Once the patient is managed medically, dental care may be provided after consultation with the physician.

If a patient provides a history of alcoholic liver disease or alcohol abuse, the physician should be consulted to verify the patient's current status, medications, laboratory values, and contraindications for medications, surgery, or other treatment.

Bleeding diatheses, as reflected in abnormal laboratory tests, should be managed in conjunction with the physician and may entail using fresh frozen plasma, vitamin K, platelets, and antifibrinolytic agents. (See Chapter 22.)

If the patient has not been seen by a physician within the past several months, it would be wise to order screening laboratory tests—including CBC with differential, AST and ALT, bleeding time, thrombin time, and prothrombin time.

Another area of concern in patients with alcoholic liver disease is the unpredictable metabolism of drugs. The concern is twofold.

First, in mild to moderate alcoholic liver disease, significant enzyme induction is likely to have occurred, leading to an increased tolerance of sedative drugs, hypnotic drugs, and general anesthesia. Thus larger than normal doses of these medications may be required to obtain the desired effects.

Second, with more advanced liver destruction, drug metabolism may be markedly diminished and can lead to an increased or unexpected effect. For example, using acetaminophen in usual therapeutic doses in chronic alcoholics has been reported[34] to result in severe hepatocellular disease with a mortality rate of 20%. The dentist should use the drugs listed in Table 12-5 with caution when treating chronic alcoholics and should adjust their doses or avoid using them entirely when appropriate.

TREATMENT PLANNING MODIFICATIONS

There are no unique treatment planning modifications required in patients with alcoholic liver disease. However, cirrhotic patients tend to have more plaque, calculus, and gingival inflammation than do noncirrhotic patients. This seems to be the case in any patient who is a substance abuser and is related to oral neglect rather than to any inherent property of the abused substance. Based on the degree of neglect, caries, and periodontal disease, the prudent practitioner would be wise not to provide extensive care until the patient demonstrates an interest in and ability to care for his or her dentition.

ORAL COMPLICATIONS

Poor hygiene and neglect are prominent among the oral findings in chronic alcoholics. In addition, a variety of other abnormalities may be found[16,24] (Table 12-8). Nutritional deficiencies

TABLE 12-8
Oral Complications of Chronic Alcholism

Poor oral hygiene
Oral neglect
Glossitis
Angular or labial cheilosis
Candidiasis
Gingival bleeding
Oral cancer
Petechiae
Ecchymoses
Jaundiced mucosa
Parotid gland enlargement
Alcohol breath odor
Impaired healing
Bruxism
Dental attrition
Xerostomia

can result in glossitis and loss of tongue papillae along with angular or labial cheilosis, which is complicated by concomitant candidal infection. Vitamin K deficiency and disordered hemostasis can result in spontaneous gingival bleeding and mucosal ecchymoses and petechiae. In fact, in some instances, unexplained gingival bleeding has been the initial complaint of alcoholic patients.[17] Additionally, chronic alcoholics demonstrate impaired healing capabilities following surgery or trauma.

A bilateral, painless hypertrophy of the parotid glands is a frequent finding in patients with cirrhosis. The enlarged glands are soft and nontender and are not fixed to the overlying skin. The condition is reversible.[31] A sweet, musty odor to the breath may be associated with liver failure. Also, a finding of jaundiced mucosal tissue is not unusual.

Finally, it must be remembered that alcohol abuse and tobacco use are strong risk factors for the development of oral cancer, and the dentist must be aggressive (as with all patients) in the detection of unexplained or suspicious soft-tissue lesions in chronic alcoholics.

REFERENCES

1. Bass BD, Andors L, Pierri LK, et al: Quantitation of hepatitis B viral markers in a dental school population, *J Am Dent Assoc* 104(5):629-632, 1982.
2. Brody JA: Aging and alcohol abuse, *J Am Geriatr Soc* 30:123-126, 1982.

3. Centers for Disease Control: Hepatitis: United States, 1975-1976, *MMWR* 26:177, 1977.

4. Centers for Disease Control: Lack of transmission of hepatitis B to humans after oral exposure to hepatitis B surface antigen-positive saliva, *MMWR* 27:247, 1978.

5. Centers for Disease Control: Immune globulins for protection against viral hepatitis, *MMWR* 30:423-435, 1981.

6. Centers for Disease Control: Inactivated hepatitis B virus vaccine: Recommendations of the Immunization Practices Advisory Committee, *MMWR* 31:318-328, 1982.

7. Centers for Disease Control: Hepatitis B vaccine: evidence confirming lack of AIDS transmission, *MMWR* 33:685-686, 1984.

8. Centers for Disease Control: Hepatitis B among parenteral drug users — North Carolina, *MMWR* 35:481-482, 1986.

9. Centers for Disease Control: Recommended infection control practices for dentistry, *MMWR* 35:273, 1986.

10. Centers for Disease Control: Protection against viral hepatitis: recommendations of the Immunization Practices Advisory Committee (ACIP), *MMWR* 39:5-22, 1990.

11. Centers for Disease Control: Summary of notifiable diseases, United States, 1990, *MMWR* 39(53):1, 1990.

12. Centers for Disease Control: Hepatitis B virus: a comprehensive strategy for eliminating transmission in the United States through universal childhood vaccination: recommendations of the Immunization Practices Advisory Committee (ACIP), *MMWR* 40(RR-13):1-25, 1991.

13. Centers for Disease Control: Public Health Service inter-agency guidelines for screening disorders of blood, plasma, organs, tissues, and semen for evidence of hepatitis B and hepatitis C, *MMWR* 40(RR-4):6-17, 1991.

14. Cottone JA: Recent developments in hepatitis: new virus, vaccine, and dosage recommendations, *J Am Dent Assoc* 120(5):501-508, 1990.

15. Dienstag JL, Wands JR, Isselbacher KJ: Acute hepatitis. In Wilson JD, et al, editors: *Harrison's Principles of internal medicine,* ed 12, New York, 1991, McGraw-Hill.

16. Friedlander AH, Mills MJ, Gorelick DA: Alcoholism and dental management, *Oral Surg* 62:42-46, 1987.

17. Galili D, Kaufman E, Bodner L, Garfunkel AA: A modern approach to prevention and treatment of oral bleeding in patients with hepatocellular disease, *Oral Surg* 54:277-280, 1982.

18. Goebel WM: Reliability of the medical history in identifying patients likely to place dentists at an increased hepatitis risk, *J Am Dent Assoc* 98(6):907-913, 1979.

19. Golden A, Powell DE, Jennings CD: *Pathology: understanding human disease,* Baltimore, 1985, Williams & Wilkins.

20. Goodman RA, Soloman SL: Transmission of infectious diseases in outpatient health care settings, *JAMA* 265(18):2377-2381, 1991.

21. Grant BF, Harford TC, Chou P, et al: Prevalence of DSM-III-R alcohol abuse and dependence — United States, 1988, *Alcohol Health Research World* 15(1):91-96, 1991.

22. Kwann HC: Disorders of fibrinolysis, *Med Clin North Am* 56:163-176, 1982.

23. Lieber CS, Rubin E: Ethanol: a hepatotoxic drug, *Gastroenterology* 54:642-646, 1968.

24. Leonard RH: Alcohol, alcoholism and dental treatment, *Compendium* 12(4):274-283, 1991.

25. MacQuarrie MB, Forghani B, Wolochow DA: Hepatitis B transmitted by a human bite, *JAMA* 230:723-724, 1974.

26. McDonald RE: Substance abuse — can it be detected in your dental patient? (Editorial.) *Pediatr Dent* 20:120, 1984.

27. Reference deleted in proofs.

28. Mosley JW, Edwards VM, Casey G, et al: Hepatitis B viruses infection in dentists, *N Engl J Med* 293:729-734, 1975.

29. Pises P, Bick R, Siegel B: Hyperfibrinolysis in cirrhosis, *Am J Gastroenterol* 60:280-288, 1972.

30. Podolsky DK, Isselbacher KJ: Cirrhosis of the liver. In Wilson JD, et al, editors: *Harrison's Principles of internal medicine,* ed 12, New York, 1991, McGraw-Hill.

31. Rauch S, Gorlin RJ: Diseases of the salivary glands. In Gorlin RJ, Goldman HM, editors: *Thomas' Oral pathology,* ed 6, vol 2, St Louis, 1970, CV Mosby.

32. Schiff ER, DeMedina MD, Kline SN, et al: Veterans Administration cooperative study on hepatitis and dentistry, *J Am Dent Assoc* 113(3):390-396, 1986.

33. Schuckit JA: Alcohol and alcoholism. In Wilson JD, et al, editors: *Harrison's Principles of internal medicine,* ed 12, New York, 1991, McGraw-Hill.

34. Seeff LB, Cuccherini BA, Zimmerman HJ, et al: Acetaminophen hepatotoxicity in alcoholics: a therapeutic misadventure, *Ann Intern Med* 104:399-404, 1986.

35. *Seventh Special Report of the U.S. Congress on Alcohol and Health,* January 1990. Alcohol, Drug Abuse, and Mental Health Administration, Public Health Service, U.S. Department of Health and Human Services.

36. Smith DJ: Hepatitis C update. New answers, new questions, *Postgraduate Medicine* 90(8):199-206, 1991.

37. Smith JL, Maynard JE, Berquist KR, et al: From the Center for Disease Control: comparative risk of hepatitis B among physicians and dentists, *J Infect Dis* 13:705-706, 1976.

38. Sywassink JM, Lutwick LLI: Risk of hepatitis B in dental care providers: a contact study, *J Am Dent Assoc* 106(2):182-184, 1983.

39. Tullman MJ, Boozer CH, Villarejos VM, Feary TW: The threat of hepatitis B from dental school patients: a one year study, *Oral Surg* 49:214-216, 1980.

40. Weil RB, Lyman DO, Jackson RJ, et al: A hepatitis serosurvey of New York dentists, *NY State Dent J* 43:587-590, 1977.

41. Werner BG, Grady GF: Accidental hepatitis B surface antigen positive inoculations: use of e antigen to estimate infectivity, *Ann Intern Med* 97:367-369, 1982.

13

Sexually Transmitted Diseases

Sexually transmitted diseases (STDs) are a major health problem in the United States and the world and in many instances are on the increase. Included among this group of diseases are acquired immune deficiency syndrome (AIDS), gonorrhea, syphilis, chlamydia, genital herpes, hepatitis B, trichomoniasis, lymphogranuloma venereum, chancroid, genital warts, and pediculosis pubis. The morbidity and mortality of STDs vary from minor inconvenience or irritation to severe disability and death.

STDs have important implications for dentistry. First, many of them have oral manifestations that the dentist must be alert to identify so as to be able to refer patients for proper medical treatment. In addition, some STDs can be transmitted by direct contact with lesions, blood, or saliva, and because many patients may be asymptomatic the dentist much approach all patients as though disease transmission were possible and adhere to universal precautions.

Although the majority of STDs have the potential for oral infection and transmission, only gonorrhea, syphilis and genital herpes will be discussed because these entities are of special interest or importance to dental practice and will serve to illustrate basic principles. The reader is referred to Chapters 12 and 14 for information about hepatitis B and AIDS.

Gonorrhea

GENERAL DESCRIPTION
INCIDENCE AND PREVALENCE

Gonorrhea is the most commonly reported infectious disease in the United States, with over 690,000 cases recorded in 1990. This figure has declined, from its peak of over 1 million cases in 1979.[2] The decline is undoubtedly related to increased awareness of disease transmission due to the AIDS epidemic. However, it is believed that the number of cases reported represents only a small percentage of the actual number of cases.

Humans are the only natural host for this disease, and its occurrence is worldwide. The transmission of gonorrhea is almost exclusively via sexual contact—whether genital-genital, oral-genital, or rectal-genital. The primary sites of infection are the genitalia, anal canal, and pharynx.

Gonorrhea can occur at any age, though it is seen most commonly in the 20-to-24-year and 15-to-19-year age groups.[2] These groups include many single people who have a high potential for multiple sexual partners. Risk factors other than age include low education, low socioeconomic standing, being black, and being an urban dweller. Cases are reported more commonly in men than in women, at a ratio of 3:1. This difference is more apparent than real, however, because many women are asymptomatic and unaware that they have the disease.

ETIOLOGY

Gonorrhea is caused by *Neisseria gonorrhoeae,* which is a gram-negative diplococcus commonly found within polymorphonuclear leukocytes. *N. gonorrhoeae* is an aerobe that requires high humidity and specific temperature and pH for optimum growth. It is a fragile bacterium that is readily killed by drying, so it is not easily transmitted by fomites. It develops resistance to antibiotics rather easily, and many strains have become resistant to penicillin and tetracycline as well as to other antibiotics.

PATHOPHYSIOLOGY

The pathophysiology of gonorrhea is significant in that the type of host epithelium influences the invasiveness of the bacterium. Columnar epithelium (as found in the mucosal lining of the urethra and cervix) and transitional epithelium (as in the oropharynx and rectum) are highly susceptible to infection whereas stratified squamous epithelium (skin and mucosal lining of the oral cavity) is generally resistant to infection.[21] This explains the occurrence of rectal, pharyngeal, and tonsillar infection and the relative infrequency of oral infection. Another indication of the resistance of skin to gonococcal infection is the fact that there are no reported cases of gonorrhea of the fingers. Figure 13-1 demonstrates the areas of relative epithelial susceptibility to *N. gonorrhoeae* infection in the oral cavity and oropharynx.

Infection in men usually begins in the anterior urethra. The bacteria invade subepithelial tissues and produce a purulent exudate. The infection may remain localized or may extend to the posterior urethra, bladder, epididymis, prostate, or seminal vesicles. It is spread by means of lymphatics and blood vessels. Gonococcemia, although infrequent, may occur and results in dissemination of the disease to distant body sites.

Infection in women occurs most commonly in the cervix and urethra. The same subepithelial invasion with production of purulent exudate occurs. The infection tends to be less severe in women but may spread to the endometrium, fallopian tubes, ovaries, and pelvic peritoneum. Disseminated gonorrhea can also occur, with varying frequency. Many cases of pelvic inflammatory disease are a result of gonococcal infection.

In both sexes gonorrhea of the rectum may occur following anal-genital intercourse or by direct anal contamination from genital lesions. Infection of the pharynx and oral cavity is

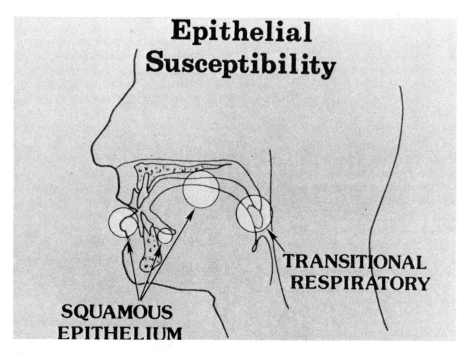

FIG. 13-1 Areas of relative epithelial susceptibility to infection by *Neisseria gonorrhoea* within the oral cavity.

predominantly seen in women and homosexual men following fellatio. It is also occasionally seen following cunnilingus.

Gonococcemia can lead to widespread dissemination and result in a variety of disorders — including migratory arthritis, skin and mucous membrane lesions, endocarditis, meningitis, and pericarditis.

CLINICAL PRESENTATION
SIGNS AND SYMPTOMS

In men, symptoms usually occur after an incubation period of 2 to 5 days. The most common findings include a mucopurulent urethral discharge, pain on urination, urgency, and frequency. Tenderness and swelling of the meatus may occur.

In women a significant percentage of cases may be asymptomatic or only minimally symptomatic. Women who have a symptomatic infection may demonstrate vaginal or urethral discharge and dysuria with frequency and urgency. Backache and abdominal pain may also be present.

Approximately 50% of women and 1% to 3% of men are asymptomatic or only mildly symptomatic.[10] This is unfortunate because these patients may not seek medical care for their problem and as a result constitute a large reservoir of infection.

Gonococcal infection of the anal canal is commonly less intense than genital infection, but similar symptoms can be noted including a copious purulent discharge and pain.

Within the oral cavity the pharynx is most commonly affected. Pharyngeal infection is found in 3% to 7% of heterosexual men, 10% to 20% of heterosexual women, and 10% to 25% of homosexual men.[10] It is usually seen as an asymptomatic infection with diffuse, nonspecific inflammation or as a mild sore throat. The likelihood of transmission of pharyngeal gonorrhea to the genitalia seems much less than that of genital-genital transmission.[6,13] Of significance, however, is the fact that *N. gonorrhoeae* has been cultured from the expectorated saliva of two thirds of patients with oropharyngeal gonorrhea.[11]

Gonococcal stomatitis or oral gonorrhea is thought to be uncommon, although several case reports[5,12,14,15,19] confirm its existence. It should be noted, however, that many of these reported

cases of oral gonorrhea lack definitive laboratory identification of *N. gonorrhoeae* and are based on presumptive evidence. Chue[4] has presented a review of the varied and nonspecific manifestations of oral gonorrhea. These include acute ulceration, diffuse erythema, necrosis of the interdental papillae, lingual edema, edematous tissues that bleed easily, vesiculations, and a pseudomembrane that is nonadherent and leaves a bleeding surface upon removal. Lesions may be solitary or widely disseminated. Symptoms include a burning or itching sensation, dryness, increased salivation, bad taste, fetid breath, fever, and submandibular lymphadenopathy. The lesions of oral gonorrhea may closely resemble the lesions of erythema multiforme, bullous or erosive lichen planus, or herpetic gingivostomatitis.

In a separate report Chue[3] describes an acute temporomandibular joint arthritis that was caused by disseminated gonococcal infection from a genital site.

LABORATORY FINDINGS

Laboratory diagnosis of *N. gonorrhoeae* infection can be made presumptively in a genital infection from finding gram-negative intracellular diplococci in a smear of purulent discharge (Fig. 13-2). Confirmation of the findings is made by culture. In suspected cases of oropharyngeal gonorrhea, however, because other species of *Neisseria* are normal inhabitants of the oral cavity, a smear and Gram stain are not as

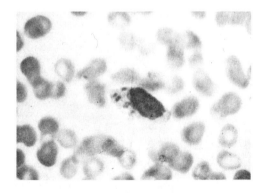

FIG. 13-2 Smear demonstrating gram-negative diplococci within a leukocyte. (Courtesy H.D. Wilson, M.D., Lexington Ky.)

helpful. Therefore culturing with selective media is necessary.

MEDICAL MANAGEMENT

Current recommendations for the treatment of uncomplicated urogenital or rectal infection include ceftriaxone and doxycycline. For patients who cannot take ceftriaxone, spectinomycin is the preferred alternative.[1] There is a very low treatment failure rate with ceftriaxone–doxycyline, and follow-up cultures are not considered essential. Following the institution of antibiotic therapy, infectiousness is rapidly diminished within a matter of hours.[8,17]

Syphilis

GENERAL DESCRIPTION
INCIDENCE AND PREVALENCE

Syphilis is the third most frequently reported infectious disease in the United States today, surpassed only by gonorrhea and chickenpox. In 1990 the record incidence of primary and secondary syphilis was 50,223 cases.[2] This represents a 27% increase from 1987 and occurred primarily among black men and women. As with gonorrhea, humans are the only known natural host for syphilis, although animal models have been experimentally infected.

The transmission of syphilis is predominantly sexual, including oral-genital and rectal-genital; however, transmission can also occur via nonsexual means such as kissing, blood transfusion, or accidental inoculation with a contaminated needle. Indirect transmission by fomites is possible but uncommon because the organism survives only a short time out of the body.[18] Congenital syphilis occurs when the fetus is infected in utero by an infected mother.

The primary site of syphilitic infection is usually the genitalia, although primary lesions also occur extragenitally at the lips, tongue, fingers, nipples, and anus.[18] Syphilis is most common in ages 20 through 40. The reported incidence is greater in males than females, by more than 2:1.[2]

ETIOLOGY

The etiologic agent of syphilis is *Treponema pallidum,* which is a slender fragile anaerobic spirochete. It is easily killed by heat, drying, disinfectants, and soap and water. The organism is difficult to stain, except with certain silver impregnation methods. Demonstration is best done using dark-field microscopy with a fresh specimen.

PATHOPHYSIOLOGY

It is believed the *T. pallidum* does not invade completely intact skin; however, it can invade intact mucosal epithelium as well as gain entry via minute abrasions or hair follicles.

Within a few hours after invasion, bacterial spread to the lymphatics and bloodstream occurs, resulting in early widespread dissemination of the disease. The early response to the bacterial invasion is an endarteritis and periarteritis.[18]

CLINICAL PRESENTATION
SIGNS AND SYMPTOMS

The manifestations and descriptions of syphilis are classically divided into stages of occurrence, with each stage having its own peculiar signs and symptoms that are related to time and antigen-antibody responses. The stages are primary, secondary, latent, tertiary, and congenital. Each will be briefly described.

Primary syphilis

The classic manifestation of primary syphilis is the *chancre,* which is a solitary granulomatous lesion. Accompanying the chancre are enlarged regional lymph nodes. The chancre usually occurs within 2 to 3 weeks after exposure (Fig. 13-3). Patients are infectious, however, before it appears. The lesion begins as a small papule and enlarges to form a surface erosion or ulceration that commonly is covered by a yellowish hemorrhagic crust and teems with *T. pallidum.* It is commonly painless. Associated with the chancre are enlarged, painless, hard regional lymph nodes. The chancre usually subsides in 3 to 6 weeks, leaving variable scarring in the form of a healed papule.[18,20] The genitalia, oral cavity, and anus are common sites for chancres. Figures 13-4 and 13-5 present examples of extragenital syphilitic chancres (lip and tongue).

Secondary syphilis

The manifestations of secondary syphilis appear 6 to 8 weeks after initial exposure. The

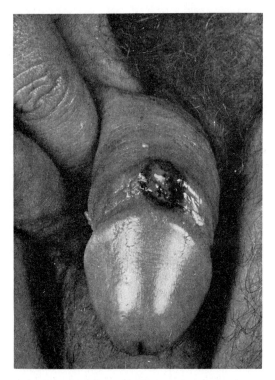

FIG. 13-3   Primary syphilis: chancre of the penis. (From Rudolph AW: In Top FH, Wehrle PF, editors: *Communicable and infectious diseases,* ed 8, St Louis, 1976, CV Mosby, p 674.)

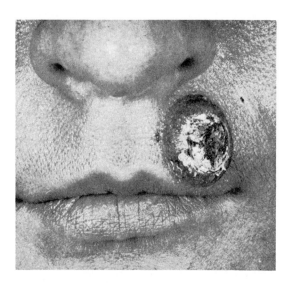

FIG. 13-4   Primary syphilis: extragenital chancre of the lip. (From Rudolph AW: In Top FH, Wehrle PF, editors: *Communicable and infectious diseases,* ed 8, St Louis, 1976, CV Mosby, p 674.)

chancre may or may not have completely resolved by this time. The symptoms and signs of secondary syphilis include fever, arthralgia and malaise, generalized lymphadenopathy, and generalized eruptions of the skin and mucous membranes. Oral manifestations of secondary syphilis include pharyngitis, papular lesions, erythematous or grayish white erosions (mucous patches) (Fig. 13-6), irregular linear erosions, and rarely parotid gland enlargement. The lesions of skin and mucous membranes are highly infectious.[18,20]

Latent syphilis

During the intermediate latent stage of syphilis, which follows untreated secondary syphilis, a person remains asymptomatic. The latent stage may last for many years or, in fact, for the remainder of the person's life. This stage follows the passing of secondary syphilis and is charac-

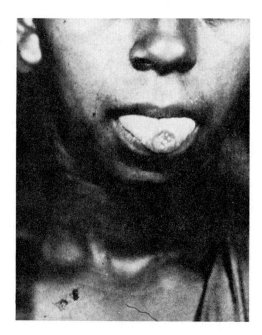

FIG. 13-5   Primary syphilis: extragenital chancre of the tongue.

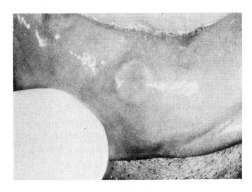

FIG. 13-6 Secondary syphilis: mucous patch of the lower lip.

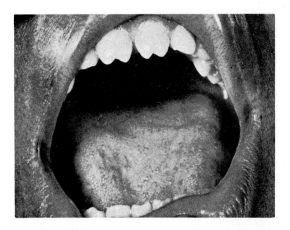

FIG. 13-7 Congenital syphilis: hutchinsonian teeth. (From Rudolph AW: In Top FH, Wehrle PF, editors: *Communicable and infectious diseases,* ed 8, St Louis, 1976, CV Mosby, p 681.)

terized by an asymptomatic period but with a persistently positive serologic test for syphilis. During the earlier phase of this stage (1 to 4 years) patients may have mucocutaneous relapses and are considered infectious. After 4 years relapses do not occur and patients are considered noninfectious (except for blood transfusions and pregnant women).[18]

Tertiary (late) syphilis

The tertiary (late) stage occurs as a result of untreated syphilis and is the destructive stage of the disease. Patients are noninfectious. Any organ of the body may be involved. Signs and symptoms of this stage do not occur until years after the initial infection.

The *gumma*—the classic localized lesion of tertiary syphilis—may involve the skin, mucous membranes, bone, nervous tissue, and/or viscera. It is believed to be the end result of a hypersensitivity reaction, basically an inflammatory granulomatous lesion with a central zone of necrosis. It is not infectious.

All the other manifestations of tertiary syphilis are essentially vascular in nature and result from an obliterative endarteritis. Cardiovascular syphilis is most commonly seen as an aneurysm of the ascending aorta. Neurosyphilis can result in a meningitis-like syndrome, Argyll Robertson pupils (which react to accommodation but not to light), altered tendon reflexes, general paresis, or tabes dorsalis (degeneration of dorsal columns of the spinal cord and sensory nerve trunks).

The oral lesions of tertiary syphilis are a diffuse interstitial glossitis and the gumma. The interstitial glossitis should be considered a premalignant condition. The tongue may appear lobulated and fissured with atrophic papillae, resulting in a bald and wrinkled surface. Leukoplakia is frequently present. The oral gumma is a rare lesion that most commonly involves the tongue and palate. It appears as a firm tissue mass with central necrosis. Palatal gummas may perforate into the nasal cavity or maxillary sinus.

Congenital syphilis

Syphilis or its sequelae will be present in the newborn if the mother is infected while carrying the child. The disease is transmitted to the fetus in utero, usually after the sixteenth week, since before this time the placenta prevents transmission of bacteria. Physical manifestations will vary depending on the time of infection. The sequelae of early infection include osteochondritis, periostitis, rhinitis, rash, and ectodermal changes. Syphilis contracted during late pregnancy can involve bones, teeth, eyes, cranial nerves, viscera, skin, and mucous membranes.

Oral manifestations or congenital syphilis include peg-shaped permanent central incisors with notching of the incisal edge (Hutchinson's incisors) (Fig. 13-7), defective molars with multiple supernumerary cusps (mulberry molars), and perioral rhagades (skin fissures).

LABORATORY FINDINGS

T. pallidum has never been cultured successfully on any kind of medium; therefore the definitive diagnosis of syphilis must be made from a positive dark-field microscopic examination. Dark-field examination is performed on fresh exudate from suspected lesions and is consistently positive only during primary and early secondary stages. Definitive diagnosis of oral lesions by this method is difficult since other *Treponema* species are indigenous to the oral cavity.

Although the dark-field examination is the only way to make a definitive diagnosis of syphilis, serologic tests for syphilis (STS) furnish presumptive evidence. These tests are of two basic types and are differentiated by the type of antibodies they investigate.

Nontreponemal tests

Nontreponemal tests are designed to detect the presence of an antibodylike substance called reagin that is produced when *T. pallidum* reacts with various body tissues. The Venereal Disease Research Laboratories (VDRL) slide test and the rapid plasma reagin (RPR) test are examples of these. A disadvantage of reaginic tests is the occasional biologic false-positive result that can occur.

Nontreponemal tests are consistently positive only 3 or 4 weeks after the appearance of the primary chancre. The highest titer (concentration) occurs during secondary syphilis. Positive results are variable during tertiary syphilis.

Treponemal tests

Treponemal tests are designed to detect the specific antibody produced against treponemes, which cause syphilis, yaws, and pinta.[18] They are more specific than the reaginic tests but less sensitive. The *Treponema pallidum* immobilization (TPI) test, fluorescent treponemal antibody (FTA) test, and fluorescent treponemal antibody absorption (FTA-ABS) test are examples. The test in most common use today is the FTA-ABS, which is considered the standard treponemal test in most laboratories. However, a newer instrument, the hemagglutination test, is less expensive and easier to perform and is replacing the FTA-ABS test in some laboratories.

In primary syphilis all serologic tests usually revert to negative within 12 months after successful treatment. In secondary syphilis up to 24 months may be required for the patient to become seronegative. Occasionally, a patient will remain seropositive for the rest of his or her life. With tertiary syphilis many patients remain seropositive for life.[1]

MEDICAL MANAGEMENT

The current medical management of syphilis includes the use of parenteral long-acting benzathine penicillins. Alternate drugs for patients allergic to penicillin include oral doxycycline and oral tetracycline.[1] Following treatment, patients should be periodically retested serologically to monitor their conversion to negative. This conversion will usually occur within a year. There is a low failure rate in the treatment of syphilis. An important aspect to note in the management of syphilis is that, as with gonorrhea, infectiousness is rapidly reversed, probably within a matter of hours upon the initiation of medical treatment.[17,18]

Genital herpes

GENERAL DESCRIPTION
INCIDENCE AND PREVALENCE

Genital herpes (herpes simplex type 2) is an important STD in the United States as well as the world. Its exact incidence is unknown, because it is not a reportable disease. The awareness and occurrence of genital herpes are rapidly increasing, however, as evidenced by coverage in the lay press and in the scientific literature. The Centers for Disease Control estimate that the number of patient consultations in the United States for genital herpes increased from 26,000 in 1966 to 423,000 in 1983. As with other STDs, this official estimate is probably grossly understated.

The herpes simplex virus (HSV) has been called the "virus of love," because the usual mode of transmission is by direct contact, usually kissing or sexual contact. Airborne droplet infection is not well-demonstrated, although it is possible.[16] Autoinoculation via face, fingers, eyes, and genitalia is a persistent clinical problem.

ETIOLOGY

HSV is a member of the herpesvirus group, which also includes cytomegalovirus, Epstein-Barr virus, and varicella-zoster virus. HSV is classified into two closely related types, 1 and 2 (HSV-1 and HSV-2).

HSV-1 is the causative agent of most herpetic infections that occur above the waist, especially on the mucosa of the mouth (herpetic gingivostomatitis, herpes labialis), nose, eyes, brain, and skin. Infection with HSV-1 is extremely common; most adults demonstrate antibodies to this virus. It is thought that many primary infections with HSV-1 are subclinical and thus are never known to the infected person. Transmission is usually by close contact, such as touching or kissing and transfer of infective saliva. HSV-1 is also transmitted via sexual contact.

HSV-2 is the causative agent of most herpes infections that occur below the waist, such as in or around the genitalia (genital herpes). HSV-2 is transmitted predominantly by sexual contact but may also be passed nonsexually. It can be transmitted to a newborn from an infected mother. There is a positive epidemiologic association with genital herpes and cervical carcinoma.

Although the primary site of occurrence of HSV-1 is above the waist and of HSV-2 below the waist, each infection may occur in either site and in fact can be inoculated from one site to the other[9] (Fig. 13-8). Furthermore, type cannot be differentiated clinically.

PATHOPHYSIOLOGY

The pathologic process of herpesvirus infections of HSV-1 and HSV-2 are essentially identical, and as such the lesions of skin and mucous membranes are identical. The infection arises from intimate contact with a lesion or infective fluid (e.g., saliva). Cells are invaded, and viral replication occurs. Characteristic cellular changes include ballooning degeneration intranuclear inclusion bodies, and the formation

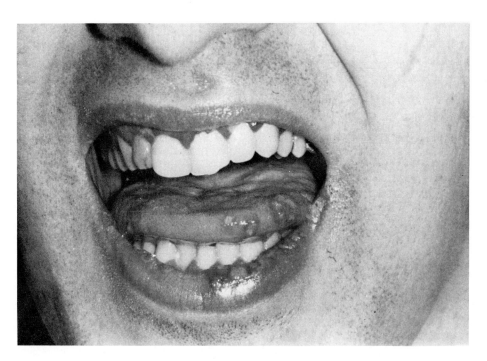

FIG. 13-8 Primary type II herpes simplex occurring in the oral cavity documented by laboratory testing. (Courtesy R.C. Noble, M.D., Lexington Ky.)

of multinucleated giant cells. With cellular destruction come inflammation and increasing edema, which result in a papular formation that progresses to fluid-filled vesicles. The vesicles rupture, leaving an ulcerated or crusted surface. Lymphadenopathy and viremia are prominent features. In normal individuals the infection is contained by usual host defenses; however, in an immunosuppressed person or infant an infection of this type may become systemic, widespread, and fatal.

When the infection has run its course, usually in 10 to 20 days, the viruses enter the ends of local peripheral neurons and migrate up the axonal sheath to the regional ganglion (HSV-1 in the trigeminal, HSV-2 in the sacral), where they reside. Then upon stimulation such as trauma, sunlight, menses, or intercourse the virus becomes reactivated, migrates down the axon, and produces a recurrent infection with lesions similar to the primary. However, the lesions of recurrent infection are generally of a less severe nature and tend to be more localized.

CLINICAL PRESENTATION
SIGNS AND SYMPTOMS

After an incubation period of 2 to 7 days, the lesions of primary genital herpes appear. In women both internal and external genitalia may be involved, as may the perineal region and skin of the thighs and buttocks. In men the external genitalia may be involved, as may the skin of the inguinal area. Lesions in moist areas tend to ulcerate early and are painful. Lesions on exposed dry areas tend to remain pustular or vesicular and then to crust over (Fig. 13-9). Painful regional lymphadenopathy accompanies the infection, along with headache, malaise, and symptoms of fever. These subside in about 2 weeks, with healing in 3 to 5 weeks.[9]

As previously stated, recurrent genital herpes is generally a less severe infection that is frequently precipitated by menses or intercourse. A prodrome of localized itching, tingling, pain, and burning may be noted and is followed by a vesicular eruption. Healing occurs in 10 to 14 days. Constitutional symptoms are generally absent.

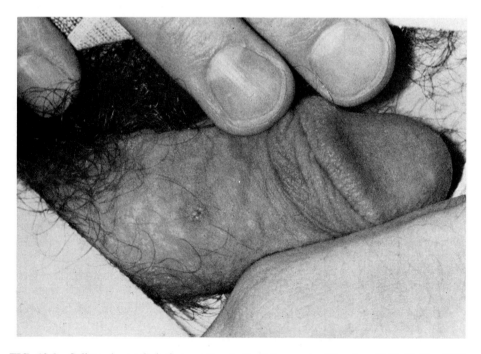

FIG. 13-9 Solitary herpetic lesion on the shaft of the penis. (Courtesy R.C. Noble, M.D., Lexington Ky.)

Whether the virus is HSV-1 or HSV-2, the lesions are highly infectious and therefore can be transmitted to other individuals or to other sites on the patient. The infectious period of herpetic lesions is of uncertain length but positive viral cultures can be obtained from every stage.[7] Therefore one should assume that all herpetic lesions are infectious, regardless of stage (papular, vesicular, pustular, ulcerative, or crusted).

LABORATORY FINDINGS

Cytologic examination of a smear taken from the base of a herpetic lesion will reveal typical features—including ballooning degeneration of cells, intranuclear inclusion bodies, and multinucleated giant cells.

Viral typing can be performed by using tissue cultures, isolation of viruses, and then specific type identification by a number of methods—restriction endonuclease, immunofluorescence, or immunoperoxidase.[7]

MEDICAL MANAGEMENT

The management of primary and recurrent genital herpes continues to be of a symptomatic and palliative nature, because no definitive treatment or cure yet exists. Many forms of therapy, both topical and systemic, have been tried. These include iododeoxyuridine (idoxuridine, IDU), photodynamic inactivation with viral dyes, adenine arabinoside (vidarabine), lysine, bacillus Calmette-Guérin (BCG) vaccine, smallpox vaccine, and herpes vaccines. All these approaches have proven to be of minimal or no value.

The first, and as yet only, drug that has been effective against HSV is acyclovir (Zovirax), which does not provide a cure but is effective in decreasing viral shedding, duration of lesions, and symptoms. The drug is available for oral, topical, and intravenous administration. The effectiveness of acyclovir is greatest when treatment is begun early in the infection, whether primary or recurrent. The following treatment recommendations[1] are for genital herpes only, although they may also be used for oral infections:

1. *Primary infection:* Oral acyclovir 200 mg, 5 times a day for 7 to 10 days
2. *Recurrent infection:* Oral acyclovir 200 mg, 5

times a day for 5 days, begun at the first signs or symptoms is appropriate

DENTAL MANAGEMENT
MEDICAL CONSIDERATIONS
(Table 13-1)

The dental management of patients with an STD necessarily begins with its identification. The obvious goal is to identify all individuals who have active disease, because many are potentially infectious. Unfortunately, this is not possible in every case because some persons will provide no history or may demonstrate no significant signs or symptoms suggestive of their disease. The inability to identify potentially infectious patients applies to other diseases—such as AIDS and viral hepatitis. Therefore it is necessary to manage all patients as though they were infectious. The U.S. Public Health Service, through its Centers for Disease Control, has published recommendations for universal precautions to be followed in controlling infection in dentistry that have become the standard for preventing cross-infection. (See Appendix A.) Strict adherence to these recommendations will, for all practical purposes, eliminate the danger of disease transmission between dentist and patient.

Even though these procedures are followed, some significant facts regarding STDs should be remembered.

Gonorrhea

The patient with gonorrhea poses little threat of disease transmission to the dentist. This is

TABLE 13-1

Dental Management of the Patient with a Sexually Transmitted Disease (STD)*

Gonorrhea—little threat of transmission to dentist; oral lesions possible

Syphilis—untreated primary and secondary lesions infectious; blood also potentially infectious

Genital herpes—little threat of transmission to dentist; oral lesions possible from auto-inoculation

*Because many patients with an active STD (as well as with other infectious diseases such as AIDS and hepatitis B) cannot be identified by the dentist, all patients should be considered potentially infectious and managed using universal precautions.

because of the specific requirements for transmission of the disease as well as the early reversal of infectiousness once antibiotics are administered. Therefore patients in this category can be provided whatever care is required.

Syphilis

The lesions of untreated primary and secondary syphilis are infectious, as is the patient's blood and saliva. Even after treatment is begun, absolute effectiveness of therapy cannot be determined except by conversion of the positive serologic test to negative; however, early reversal of infectiousness following the institution of antibiotics is to be expected. The time required for this conversion varies from a few months to over a year; therefore patients who are currently being treated or who have a positive STS following treatment should be viewed as potentially infectious. Still, any necessary dental care may be provided.

Genital herpes

The localized uncomplicated genital herpes infection poses no problem for the dentist. In the absence of oral lesions any necessary dental work may be provided. If oral lesions are present, elective treatment should be delayed to avoid inadvertent inoculation of adjacent sites.

PATIENTS WITH HISTORY OF AN STD

Patients who have had an STD should be approached with a measure of caution, because they are in a high-risk group for these diseases. This can include risk from the inadequate treatment of a previous infection or risk of a new infection. Special attention should be given to unexplained lesions of the oral, pharyngeal, or perioral tissues. Also a review of systems may reveal urogenital symptoms. Patients with a history of gonorrhea should give a history of antibiotic therapy. Patients treated for syphilis should receive a periodic STS for 1 year to monitor conversions from positive to negative. In the absence of medical follow-up care for these disorders, consultation and referral to a physician may be considered.

PATIENTS WITH SIGNS, SYMPTOMS, OR ORAL LESIONS SUGGESTIVE OF AN STD

Patients who have signs or symptoms suggesting an STD or who have unexplained oral or pharyngeal lesions should also be approached with caution. The index of suspicion should be even higher if the patient is between 15 and 24 years of age, black (male or female), an urban dweller, single, and from a lower socioeconomic group. Any patient who has these unexplained lesions should be questioned about possible relationships of the lesions with past sexual activity and advised to seek medical care. Herpetic lesions in or around the oral cavity, combined with a history of past involvement, should be recognizable. Patients with acute oral herpes lesions should not receive routine dental care but be given palliative treatment only. For a severe primary oral infection, the patient may require referral to a physician.

DRUG ADMINISTRATION

There are no adverse interactions between the usual antibiotics or drugs used to treat STDs and the drugs commonly used in dentistry. No drugs are contraindicated.

TREATMENT PLANNING MODIFICATIONS

No required modifications in the technical treatment plan are required for a patient with an STD.

ORAL COMPLICATIONS
Gonorrhea

As previously mentioned, the rare presentation of oral gonorrhea is nonspecific and varied and may range from slight erythema to severe ulceration with a pseudomembranous coating. The patient may be either asymptomatic or incapacitated with limitations of oral function (eating, drinking, talking). Definitive diagnosis of oral lesions should be attempted.

The initial step in treatment is to ensure that the patient is under the care of a physician and receiving proper chemotherapy. After this, treatment of the oral lesions is symptomatic. (See Appendix B.) The patient should be assured that the lesions will regress as the systemic infection resolves.

Syphilis

Syphilitic chancres and mucous patches are usually painless unless they become secondarily infected. These lesions are highly infectious. They regress spontaneously with or without

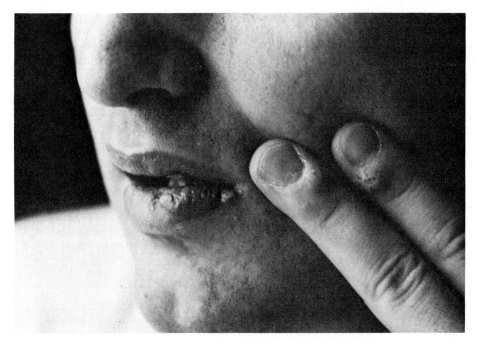

FIG. 13-10 Herpes simplex type I infection of the nailbeds (herpetic whitlow, herpetic paronychia) as a result of autoinoculation. (Courtesy R.C. Noble, M.D., Lexington Ky.)

antibiotic therapy, although chemotherapy is required to eradicate the systemic infection. As with gonorrhea, any oral treatment rendered is essentially symptomatic. The gumma is a painless lesion, but it may also become secondarily infected. It is noninfectious. Interstitial glossitis is viewed as a premalignant lesion.

Genital herpes

Since it is impossible to differentiate clinically between HSV-1 and HSV-2, all herpetic lesions of the oral cavity should be treated in the same way (Appendix B). All oral and perioral herpetic lesions should be considered infectious, regardless of stage (papular, vesicular, ulcerative, or crusted). It is recommended that elective dental treatment be delayed until the herpetic lesion is completely healed. This is because of (1) the danger of inoculation to a new site on the patient, (2) infection to the dentist (i.e., herpetic paronychia), and (3) aerosol or droplet inoculation of the conjunctivae of either patient or dental personnel.

A problem of particular concern to dentists is herpetic infection of the nail beds contracted by finger contact with a herpetic lesion of the lip or oral cavity of a patient (Fig. 13-10). The infection is called a herpetic whitlow or herpetic paronychia; it is serious, debilitating, and recurrent.

REFERENCES

1. Centers for Disease Control: 1989 Sexually transmitted diseases treatment guidelines, *MMWR* 38(S-8): 1, 1989.
2. Centers for Disease Control: Summary of notifiable diseases, United States, 1990, *MMWR* 39(53):1, 1990.
3. Chue PWY: Gonococcal arthritis of the temporomandibular joint, *Oral Surg* 39:572-577, 1975.
4. Chue PWY: Gonorrhea—its natural history, oral manifestations, diagnosis, treatment, and prevention, *J Am Dent Assoc* 90:1297-1301, 1975.
5. Escobar V, Farman AG, Arm RN: Oral gonococcal infection, *Int J Oral Surg* 13:549-554, 1984.
6. Feldman YM, Nikitas JA: Pharyngeal gonorrhea, *NY State J Med* 80:957-959, 1980.
7. Fife KH: Laboratory diagnosis of herpes simplex virus infections and the realm of rapid diagnostic tests. *Clinical update—herpes simplex: diagnosis and manage-*

ment, Research Triangle Park NC, 1986, Burroughs Wellcome.

8. Giunta JL, Fiuamara NJ: Facts about gonorrhea and dentistry, *Oral Surg* 62:529-531, 1986.

9. Goodman JL: Infections caused by herpes simplex viruses. In Hoeprich PD, Jordan MC, editors: Infectious diseases, ed 4, Philadelphia, 1989, JB Lippincott.

10. Hook EW, Handsfield HH: Gonococcal infections in the adult. In Holmes KK, et al, editors: Sexually transmitted diseases, ed 2, New York, 1990, McGraw-Hill Information Services.

11. Hutt DM, Judson FN: Epidemiology and treatment of oropharyngeal gonorrhea, *Ann Intern Med* 104:655-658, 1986.

12. Jamsky RJ, Christen AG: Oral gonococcal infections: report of two cases, *Oral Surg* 53:358-362, 1982.

13. Karus SJ: Incidence and therapy of gonococcal pharyngitis, *Sex Trans Dis* 6:143-147, 1979.

14. Kohn SR, Shaffer JF, Chomenko AG: Primary gonococcal stomatitis, *JAMA* 219:86, 1972.

15. Merchant HW, Schuster GS: Oral gonococcal infection, *J Am Dent Assoc* 95(4):807-809, 1977.

16. Nahmias AJ, Roizman B: Infection with herpes simplex viruses 1 and 2. III, *N Engl J Med* 289:781-789, 1973.

17. Noble RC: Personal communication, 1981.

18. Rudolph AH: Syphilis. In Hoeprich PD, Jordan MC, editors: *Infectious disease,* ed 4, Philadelphia, 1989, JB Lippincott.

19. Schmidt H, Hjorting-Hanssen E, Philipsen HP: Gonococcal stomatitis, *Acta Derm Venereol* 41:324-327, 1961.

20. Thin RN: Early syphilis in the adult. In Holmes KK, et al, editors: *Sexually transmitted diseases*, ed 2, New York, 1990, McGraw-Hill Information Services.

21. vonLichtenberg F: Infectious disease: viral, chlamydial, rickettsial, and bacterial diseases. In Cotran RS, Kumar V, Robbins SL, editors: *Robbins' Pathologic basis of disease*, ed 4, Philadelphia, 1989, WB Saunders.

14

AIDS and Related Conditions

The acquired immune deficiency syndrome (AIDS) is a recently recognized disease that was first reported in the United States in 1981. The initial report of the disease came from Los Angeles, where five "healthy" male homosexuals were diagnosed as suffering from an unusual type of pneumonia, caused by the protozoan *Pneumocystis carinii*. These individuals also were found to be immunosuppressed, for no obvious reason. From this seemingly innocuous beginning 11 years ago, over 200,000 cases of AIDS have been reported in the United States as of January, 1992, resulting in more than 120,000 deaths, and the number of cases continues to increase (Tables 14-1 and 14-2). The disease has been reported with increasing frequency in many European countries as well as elsewhere in the world. The mortality rate for individuals infected with AIDS is now thought to be virtually 100%.[1,19,23,75,84]

The AIDS epidemic continues unabated, with more than 3000 cases being reported to the Centers for Disease Control monthly.[12,75] These 3000 cases do not include those individuals with persistent generalized lymphadenopathy (PGL) or AIDS-related complex (ARC) or those who are asymptomatic antibody-positive carriers. All efforts in medicine have thus far led only to more unanswered questions. There is currently no vaccine or treatment, and only limited federal funding, for this nationwide epidemic. The best treatment approach for AIDS is preventive education and counseling for infected patients and their contacts (family, lover, friends, co-workers) plus the use of drugs to slow the progress of the disease. AIDS is an infectious disease that is transmitted predominantly by intimate sexual contact and by paren-

teral means. Unfortunately, because of its frequent association with homosexuality and IV drug abuse, the adverse social implications have caused AIDS to be viewed prejudicially and moralistically by many. However, it is becoming increasingly clear that all segments of society are potentially susceptible to this disease.

In 1982 a total of 24 papers on AIDS were published. Between 1982 and 1991 some 30,000 papers were published. In 1983 over 25% of the papers published concerned etiology, and by 1988 only 13% related to prevention. In 1990 only 3% of the published papers dealt with etiology and 12% with prevention. Based on these findings, clearly more emphasis needs to be placed on the etiology and prevention of AIDS in the 1990s.[26]

AIDS, as now defined by the Centers for Disease Control, consists of Kaposi's sarcoma, a *Pneumocystis carinii* pneumonia or other life-threatening opportunistic infection, the wasting syndrome, and/or CNS syndromes with dementia and associated immunosuppression. The predominant stipulation is that the complex cannot be accounted for by another disease or medication. From the time of diagnosis, most AIDS patients can be expected to live approximately 2 years. Death usually results from an opportunistic infection and in some cases from complications associated with the various malignancies seen with AIDS.

It is now estimated that all individuals infected with HIV will eventually develop AIDS and die. This will remain true until effective antiviral treatment agents become available. There may be as many as 330,000 to 405,000 cases of AIDS in the United States by the end of 1993. A few cases (52) of HIV-2 infection

TABLE 14-1
United States AIDS Cases by Age Group, Sex, and Exposure Category Reported to the Centers for Disease Control Through December 1991

	Men	Women	Children	Adult Total
Homosexual and bisexual	118,362 (65)*	–	–	118,362 (58)
IV drug use	5048 (19)	10,705 (50)	1430 (mothers)	45,753 (23)
Homosexual or bisexual and IV drug use	13,135 (7)	–	–	3135 (6)
Hemophilia or coagulation disorder	1671 (1)	42 (<1)	165 (5)	1713 (<1)
Mother with or at risk for AIDS or HIV	–	–	2936 (85)	–
Heterosexual contact	4687 (3)	7249 (34)	–	1936 (6)
Sex with IV drug user	1882	4407	606 (mothers)	
Sex with bisexual man	–	651	61 (mothers)	
Sex with hemophiliac	10	94	13 (mothers)	
Born in pattern-II country†	1805	718	244 (mothers)	
Sex with person from pattern II country†	98	76	14 (mothers)	
Sex with HIV-transfusion recipient	79	161	13 (mothers)	
Sex with HIV infected person	813	1065	144 (mothers)	
Other	–	–	414 (mothers)	
Transfusion recipient, blood component or tissue	2679 (1)	1668 (8)	289 (8)	4,347 (2)
Other and undetermined	6114 (3)	1561 (7)	83 (2)	7,675 (4)
Total	181,696 (100)	21,225 (100)	3,471 (100)	202,921 (100)

Total cases: Children + Adults and adolescents 206,392

*Figures given are the number of cases, with percent in parentheses.
†Country where HIV is spread by heterosexual contact (usually an underdeveloped country in Africa, etc.).
From Centers for Disease Control. *AIDS* 6(3):343–345, 1992.

TABLE 14-2
Number of Reported Cases of AIDS per Year in the United States

Year	Adults and Adolescents		Children less than 13 years old	
	Cases diagnosed	Deaths	Cases diagnosed	Deaths
Before 1981	79	30	6	1
1981	299	125	15	9
1982	1084	436	29	13
1983	2926	1447	75	29
1984	5938	3332	111	50
1985	11,132	6620	227	114
1986	18,171	11,469	323	157
1987	27,084	15,293	474	280
1988	33,016	19,585	574	297
1989	37,506	25,632	648	346
1990	37,633	26,961	647	350
1991	28,052	20,255	342	199
Totals	202,921	131,383	3,471	1850

From Centers for Disease Control. *AIDS* 6(3):343–345, 1992.

have been reported by the Centers for Disease Control,[11] all in individuals having immigrated from Africa.

By the end of 1991, AIDS was the leading cause of death in men 25 to 44 years of age—with some eight to ten million adults and one million children throughout the world infected. By the year 2000 an estimated 40 million individuals will be infected. In the last 5 years in the United States there has been a steady increase in the heterosexual transmission of AIDS whereas the cases of AIDS associated with blood and/or blood products has stabilized and is actually expected to start declining over the next few years. The largest proportionate increase in AIDS cases since 1989 has been among women (blacks, Hispanics, heterosexuals, and those living in the South). About half of these women have a history of IV-drug abuse.[12]

The impact and importance of AIDS on dentistry have been significant. The American Dental Association has established national guidelines and standards for infection control, identification of potential AIDS patients, and the management of these patients in the dental setting.

The remainder of this chapter will describe AIDS and related conditions, the dental implications of these conditions, and management concerns as they apply to patients and dental personnel.

GENERAL DESCRIPTION
INCIDENCE AND PREVALENCE

In the United States as of January, 1992, more than 120,000 people had died of AIDS. One to two million Americans have HIV antibodies[1,12,75] (Table 14-2). Prior to 1988 the majority of AIDS cases in the U.S. were found in four states—California, New York, Florida, and New Jersey—and cities reporting the largest numbers of AIDS cases were New York, San Francisco, Miami, Newark, and Los Angeles.[12,75] These cities continue to report new cases but not at the rate experienced during the period 1981 to 1988. By contrast, cities that are now in the early stages of the epidemic are reporting a doubling of the number of AIDS cases every 6 months to a year. Significant numbers of AIDS cases have occurred in all 50 states.

About 66% of AIDS cases are reported to involve homosexual or bisexual males, with approximately 7% of these homosexual IV drug users. The 66% figure has decreased from a high of 74% since late 1988. IV drug users (particularly those who share needles) now constitute some 22% of the AIDS cases, and this figure has increased sharply since 1988. Hemophiliacs with AIDS represent about 1% of all cases, and transfusion patients about 2%. AIDS found in heterosexuals (not included in the above groups) has increased from about 0.8% in 1985 to 6% of all cases reported by the end of 1991. There still remains a group of about 4% of the reported cases in which the method of transmission is unknown.* A reduction is now beginning to be seen in the number of AIDS cases in the transfusion and hemophiliac groups because of the testing (started in 1985) of donor blood for HIV antibodies and the heating of Factor VIII replacement preparations. (See Table 14-1).

Recent studies[21,80] have found the blood supply in the United States to be safe from transmission of the HIV virus. Nevertheless, there is still a (very small) risk of infection from individuals who become infected and donate blood just before seroconverting. This risk is estimated to be 1:153,000 for a single unit of blood and 1:28,000 for an average transfusion of 5.4 units of blood. Further reduction can be expected by attracting more women as donors, by obtaining more frequent donations from regular donors, and by constant improvement of the HIV screening test.[21] The mean time for AIDS to develop following blood transfusion transmission is 7 years.[21] The mean incubation period for individuals infected with HIV by blood transfusion is 1.97 years for children 1 to 4 years of age, 8.23 years for persons aged 5 to 59, and 5.5 years for individuals over 60 years of age.[70] In a study of hemophiliacs who had documented data of seroconversion,[37] AIDS was found to develop faster in the older patients. Older patients also had an earlier onset of low CD4 cell counts.

Children with AIDS are a true social and emotional concern. By the end of 1991 about 3300 cases had been reported. Eighty-four percent of these cases involved mothers with AIDS, mothers who were HIV-infected, or mothers who were at increased risk for developing HIV infection. About 9% of the children had received blood transfusions, and 5% were hemophiliac. The most common opportunistic infections in children are bacterial; Kaposi's sarcoma is rare.[1,60]

---

* References 1, 12, 23, 57, 75, 80.

The rate of HIV infection in the general population is not known. Seroprevalence studies of applicants for U.S. military service during the period 1985–1989 revealed a prevalence of about 0.34 per 1000. The rate was highest for blacks and lowest for whites.[8]

The 65 publicly funded HIV counseling and testing services reporting to the Centers for Disease Control (CDC) have stated that 3% (51,170 of 1,366,537) of the HIV antibody tests were positive during 1990. Based on CDC estimates, 3,250,000 individuals have been tested since 1985 through public services and 185,000 (5.69%) were positive for HIV antibodies. Only about half of the individuals with negative test results received post-test counseling, in contrast to about 75% of those with positive tests.[13]

By the end of 1991 some 20,000 women had been reported with AIDS. Fifty-one percent of these women were IV drug abusers, 34% were heterosexual contacts, 8% were transfusion recipients, and less than 1% were infected from blood products used to treat coagulation disorders. The cause in 8% was undetermined.[75]

No gender difference has been found in the rate of progression of HIV infection. A poorer survival rate for women has been found in several studies, but this appears to be related to less access to medical care. Pregnancy in HIV-infected women leads to infection in over 50% of the infants, although pregnancy itself does not appear to accelerate HIV infection. Women have an increased incidence of *Candida* esophagitis and HIV wasting syndrome over men.[7]

Approximately 10% of the patients with AIDS are over the age of 50 years. An estimated 1 million homosexual men are over 65. Many of these men engage in regular sexual activity into their 80s. Transfusion of infected blood, use of blood products, sexual activity, and IV drug abuse are the modes of transmission in the older population. Certain problems are unique to older patients with AIDS. HIV-related dementia may be diagnosed as Alzheimer's disease. Age changes in the immune system result in an increase in tumors and infections in non-HIV infected older individuals. Furthermore, the immune suppression found with HIV infection will only enhance the overall degree of immune suppression in older individuals. When dealing with neurologic, neoplastic, and infectious signs and symptoms in older patients, the dentist should consider possible HIV infection and investigate it.[70]

AIDS has been reported on five continents.[10,22,83] The majority of cases have been in the Americas, and the fewest in Asia. AIDS has also been reported in over 21 European countries, with the highest per capita rates appearing in Switzerland and France. The rate per million population for various countries up to October 1990 was as follows: Bermuda (2579), Bahamas (2003), Congo (1021), United States (589), Switzerland (225), Australia (118), Guyana (108), Japan (2.3), and China (0.003). It is now clear that the AIDS epidemic has the potential to be felt throughout the world.[10,22,83]

ETIOLOGY

In 1984 the etiologic agent for AIDS was identified independently by three laboratories. A French team from the Pasteur Institute identified a retrovirus termed *lymphadenopathy-associated virus* (LAV) and reported it as the causative agent for AIDS. In the United States a team from the National Institutes of Health isolated a retrovirus identified as *human T lymphotropic virus III* (HTLV-III) and labeled it the etiologic agent for AIDS. A team in San Francisco also isolated a retrovirus, *AIDS-related virus* (ARV), and designated it the causative agent for AIDS. All three viruses were similar retroviruses, with but minor differences in their amino acid sequences. The variations in disease patterns may be accounted for by the slight differences among the AIDS viruses — which also makes the production of a vaccine difficult.[62]

Since these early reports by the three groups, it has been established that they were essentially describing the same retrovirus, which can change its antigenicity, and most workers in the field up to 1986 referred to the virus as HTLV-III and considered it to be the causative agent for AIDS. In 1986 the World Health Organization recommended the AIDS virus be termed the *human immunodeficiency virus* (HIV) (Table 14-3).

What first appeared to be a single virus is now actually known to be a complex viral family composed of two subtypes (HIV-1 and HIV-2) with many different strains.[12] HIV can infect most human cells; however, the cells most commonly infected are those with CD4 receptors — including T-helper lymphocytes (CD4 cells) and

TABLE 14-3
Terminology for AIDS Viruses

LAV	Lymphadenopathy-associated virus
ARV	AIDS-related virus
HTLV-III	Human T lymphotropic virus III
HIV (HIV-1, HIV-2)	Human immunodeficiency virus

Current recommended terminology, World Health Organization Congress, 1986.

macrophages — and hence are the cells most involved with HIV infection.[53] Research[40] has suggested that a second receptor may be active in allowing the HIV to infect those human cells without CD4 receptors. Evidence has surfaced that HIV-antibody complexes may interact with Fc or a complement receptor, which then facilitates the entry of the virus into the cell. The action of certain viral cofactors in spreading HIV infection may be explained by activation of these second receptor sites.[49]

A small portion of the carboxy-terminal half of the viral envelope (GP-120), which represents less than 5% of the total genome, is associated with the most virulent features of HIV infection (Fig. 14-1). This segment of the GP-120 has been referred to as the V3 loop and may represent the best site for vaccine development.[49]

Recent studies[49] have indicated that a strong antiviral agent may be produced by suppressor lymphocytes (CD8 + cells). Long-term survivors of HIV infection have been found to have less virulent HIV strains, without the enhancing antibodies to HIV and with strong CD8 + cell antiviral activity.[49] When the viral regions responsible for neutralization enhancement are defined, it may be possible to develop *nef* proteins to block HIV replication. If researchers are able to develop a vaccine for the most virulent portion of HIV, to identify and produce the antiviral agent produced by CD8 + cells, or to develop *nef* proteins to block HIV replication, major steps will have been taken in the fight against this virus.[49]

PATHOPHYSIOLOGY AND COMPLICATIONS

The AIDS virus is transmitted by sexual means, through the exchange of body fluids (especially *infected semen* during intercourse),

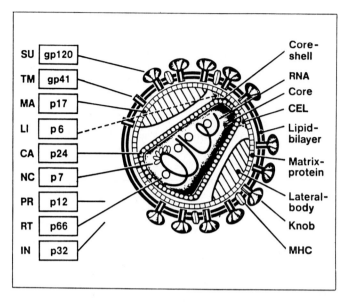

SU	gp120
TM	gp41
MA	p17
LI	p6
CA	p24
NC	p7
PR	p12
RT	p66
IN	p32

Core-shell
RNA
Core
CEL
Lipid-bilayer
Matrix-protein
Lateral-body
Knob
MHC

FIG. 14-1 HIV-1. (From Gelderblom H: *AIDS* 5:620, 1991. Used with permission.)

and by nonsexual means, via the parenteral transfer of *infected blood;* or it may be transmitted *vertically* (i.e., probably at birth or transplacentally[19a]) to infants born of infected mothers.

The most common method of sexual transmission is homosexual anal intercourse; however, heterosexual transmission has been documented from infected males to noninfected females. Transmission from infected females to noninfected males has also been reported.

Heterosexual transmission of HIV can occur through sexual contact of carriers who are heterosexual IV drug users, bisexual males, or blood recipients of either sex. HIV has been found in saliva, but transmission via saliva has been suggested in only one case as of this writing. HIV has also been isolated from tears, breast milk, cerebrospinal fluid, amniotic fluid, and urine. Only blood, semen, and vaginal secretions have been demonstrated to be associated with transmission of the virus, however.[11] Casual contact has not been demonstrated as a means of transmission.

Over 2 million Americans are estimated to have been exposed to the AIDS virus. Current data would suggest that most, if not all, of these individuals will develop AIDS as defined by the Centers for Disease Control. Antibody positivity

to HIV means that the person has been infected with the virus and can be viremic. Individuals who appear to be most susceptible to developing AIDS are those with repeated exposure to the virus and who also have an immune system that has been challenged by repeated exposure to various antigens (semen, hepatitis B, or blood products). Individuals infected with the virus will develop antibodies usually within 6 to 12 weeks. A few may take up to 6 months to seroconvert. In rare cases it may take as long as 35 months for seroconversion to occur.[11,12] The incubation period for AIDS appears to be lengthy[14]—*mean* 10 to 12 years. Ninety percent of individuals with AIDS are dead within 3 years of the diagnosis.[11,12]

Once HIV has gained access to the bloodstream, it selectively seeks out T lymphocytes (specifically T_4 or T-helper lymphocytes) for growth (Fig. 14-2). The virus is lymphotropic; hence the cells it selects for replication are soon destroyed. Once the virus has taken hold, it soon leads to a reduction in the total number of T helper cells and a marked shift in the ratio of T_4 to T_8 lymphocytes occurs. The normal ratio of T-helper to T-suppressor lymphocytes is about 2:1 (60% T-helper, 30% T-suppressor). In AIDS the T_4/T_8 ratio is reversed. The marked reduction in T-helper lymphocytes explains the

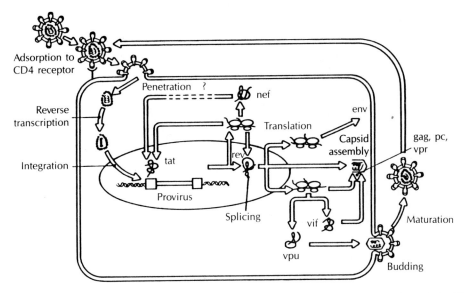

FIG. 14-2 The HIV replication cycle. (From Coffin JM: *AIDS 1990 Year Rev* 4(suppl):S1-S9, 1990. Used with permission.)

lack of immune response seen in AIDS patients and most likely is related to the increase in malignant disease found associated with AIDS: Kaposi's sarcoma, lymphoma, and carcinoma of the rectum.

The vast majority of individuals exposed to the virus at first do not develop evidence of immune suppression. These individuals respond by producing antibodies to HIV. The virus also may infect neurons or macrophages in the central nervous system, allowing the virus to be present within the body in latent form. These individuals may demonstrate a viremia on occasion and hence are considered carriers of the virus who have the potential to infect others. Of special concern is the fact that circulating antibodies fail to neutralize the virus because it has the capacity to alter its antigenicity. The alarming thing about these patients, in addition to having the potential to be infectious and to develop AIDS, is that about 50% will develop signs of dementia that can be rapidly progressive.[1,2,3] Following a long asymptomatic period, the infected individual may develop persistent generalized lymphadenopathy, symptoms such as fever, weight loss, diarrhea, night sweats, and malaise, and then eventually AIDS.

CLINICAL PRESENTATION
SIGNS AND SYMPTOMS

Following the initial infection with HIV, many patients will develop an acute flulike illness that may last 1 to 3 weeks. Others may not manifest this symptom complex. The severity of the initial acute infection with HIV is predictor of the course the infection will follow. In one study[36] 78% of the individuals with a long-lasting acute illness developed AIDS within 3 years; by contrast, only 10% of those individuals with no acute illness at seroconversion developed AIDS within 3 years.

Four groups of patients may be identified once exposure to the HIV virus has occurred. These groups are described here and summarized in Tables 14-4 and 14-5.

Group 1. Individuals who are antibody–positive to HIV but who are asymptomatic and show no other laboratory abnormalities

Group 2. Individuals who have minor laboratory changes in addition to being HIV antibody–positive and can also show clinical signs or symptoms—such as enlarged lymph nodes, night sweats, weight loss, etc. (persistent generalized lymphadenopathy [PGL])

Group 3. Individuals who have ARC, are HIV

TABLE 14-4
Categorization of HIV Exposures

Group 1	No symptoms, antibody-positive
Group 2	Minor symptoms, antibody-positive (persistent generalized lymphadenopathy, PGL)
Group 3	AIDS-related complex
Group 4	AIDS

TABLE 14-5
Signs and Symptoms of HIV Infection

Initial exposure or infection (seroconversion syndrome)
Flulike symptoms—fever, weakness, 10 to 14 days
Asymptomatic stage
Serologic evidence of infection
No signs or symptoms
Symptomatic stage
Serologic evidence of infection
T_4/T_8 ratio reduced to about 1
Persistent lymphadenopathy
Oral candidiasis
Constitutional symptoms—night sweats, diarrhea, weight loss, fever, malaise, weakness
Advanced symptomatic stage
Serologic evidence of infection
T_4/T_8 ratio suppressed to less than 0.5
HIV encephalopathy
HIV wasting syndrome
Major opportunistic infections
Neoplasms—Kaposi's sarcoma, lymphoma, carcinoma of rectum

antibody–positive, show an altered T-helper/T-suppressor ratio (usually less than 1), and can show lymphadenopathy with weight loss or complain of night sweats, fever, malaise, and diarrhea

Group 4. Individuals who have AIDS—including Kaposi's sarcoma, wasting syndrome, CNS symptoms with dementia and/or a life-threatening opportunistic infection, and an altered T-helper/T-suppressor ratio of 0.5 or less; they are HIV antibody–positive and can demonstrate generalized lymphadenopathy with severe weight loss, fatigue, chronic diarrhea, chronic fever, and night sweats (Fig. 14-1 and Table 14-5).

HIV can infect the CNS and often leads to a progressive form of dementia. Patients may become confused and disoriented or experience short-term memory deficits. Others can develop severe depression or paranoia and show suicidal tendencies.

LABORATORY FINDINGS

HIV can be isolated from the blood, semen, tears, and saliva of many patients with AIDS. Most patients exposed to the virus, with or without clinical evidence of disease, will show antibodies to the virus. Patients with ARC or AIDS will have an altered ratio of T_4/T_8 lymphocytes, a decrease in total number of lymphocytes, thrombocytopenia, anemia, a slight alteration in the humoral antibody system, and a decreased ability to show delayed allergic reactions to skin testing (cutaneous anergy).

In 1985 several screening tests became available for identification of antibodies to HIV. The enzyme-linked immunosorbent assay (ELISA) is sensitive but has a high rate of false-positive results. Current practice is to screen first with the ELISA. If the first results are positive, a second ELISA is performed. All positive results are then rescreened with a second test, the Western Blot Analysis. This combination of

screening tests is over 99% accurate. Positive ELISA and Western Blot tests indicate only that the individual has been exposed to the AIDS virus. They do not indicate whether AIDS, PGL, or ARC is present. Neither do they show if the patient is viremic, since for this special tests for the virus would have to be performed that are more expensive. However, patients with positive ELISA and Western Blot tests are considered potentially infectious.

An ELISA test developed by Wellcome has been found to be 98% sensitive in detecting antibodies to HIV in saliva. This test may have future application for general screening.[20]

A test to detect salivary secretory immunoglobulin A antibodies of nonmaternal origin in newborns of women at risk for HIV infection has been found accurate in detecting infected infants.[2]

MEDICAL MANAGEMENT

There is no effective treatment or cure for AIDS at present. Antiviral agents have been unsuccessful in killing the HIV virus. However, zidovudine (AZT) has been shown[73] to exert significant inhibitory effects on invitro replication cytopathogenicity of HIV. AZT has now been found to prolong life in both asymptomatic and symptomatic HIV-infected individuals,[31,48,79] although there is no evidence that it is effective in preventing infection once exposure to the virus has occurred.[71] Aerosol pentamide and oral sulfamethoxazole-trimethoprim have been shown to be effective prophylactic agents in preventing *Pneumocystis carinii* pneumonia. Ganciclovir, forcarnet, and acyclovir are used to treat opportunistic viral infections found in AIDS patients. Acyclovir also has been used[30] as a prophylactic treatment to prevent certain viral infections.

Attempts to improve the suppressed immune system are being investigated. Dithiocarb (Immuthiol) has shown promise. It appears to improve immune competence by modulating T-cell function.[30]

In addition, medical management consists of trying to protect the patient from exposure to infectious agents and to treat infections when they occur with isolation and high doses of antibiotics. Kaposi's sarcoma (epidemic form) associated with AIDS is a much more aggressive lesion than the classic form of this vascular tumor that is usually found in older men and may be difficult to manage using surgery or radiation techniques.

As the present time, treatment of the AIDS patient must be considered to be symptomatic in nature. At best, a vaccine is most likely several years away because of problems presented by the rapid change in antigenicity of the virus. Research efforts[1,23,49,57] indicate that agents may be found in the future that will kill the AIDS virus and others found that may help to restore the immune system to a more normal function.

Homosexual men are advised to reduce their risk of exposure to HIV by practicing safe sex through (1) reducing the number of sexual partners, (2) avoiding anonymous sexual partners, (3) modifying sexual practices to reduce the exchange of bodily secretions (including the use of condoms), (4) reducing the use of drugs such as volatile nitrites, alcohol, etc., and (5) adopting cleanliness procedures before and after the sex act. Heterosexuals are also advised to practice safe sex by reducing the number of sexual contacts and using a condom when having intercourse with anyone other than a long-standing partner.

The emotional and psychologic problems associated with AIDS are numerous and stressful. Psychosocial counseling intervention prior to testing, at the time of diagnosis, and during the course of the disease is extremely important. The emotional impact on a young adult faced with the trauma of a fatal disease can be severe. Patients must be helped to deal successfully with the fear of death, the liability of transmitting the disease, and the need to protect themselves from opportunistic infections; and they should be encouraged to communicate openly and honestly with lovers, friends, and family who serve as their support group. Psychosocial counseling intervention also can help to resolve problems such as how will patients support themselves, how will medical bills be paid, and how can group therapy be obtained. Psychosocial counseling intervention can help the patient obtain access to one of the various support groups for AIDS patients, provide education and literature about the infections and diseases, and serve as a liaison with community resources such as gay services agencies, cancer counseling, civil rights agencies, etc.[23] (Fig. 14-3).

DENTAL MANAGEMENT
MEDICAL CONSIDERATIONS

The major consideration for dentists providing care to AIDS patients is to minimize the possibility of transmission of HIV from an infected patient to themselves, their staff, or other patients. Although saliva has not been demonstrated to have transmitted the virus in a dental situation, the potential does exist.[5] Infected blood can transmit the AIDS virus. Dental procedures that result in soft tissue injury allow various amounts of blood to become mixed with saliva. Rubber (latex) gloves protect the hands of the operator from the mixture of blood and saliva in the mouth of an infected patient, but particles of blood and saliva could be splashed in the eye during various procedures. In addition, if an HIV-infected dentist cuts a finger through a glove, the potential to infect the patient also exists. Blood from the infected dentist could infect the patient through surgical wounds, ulcerations, or active periodontal disease. Current data[59,81] indicate that HIV can be transmitted by needle stick or an instrument wound. However, the frequency of

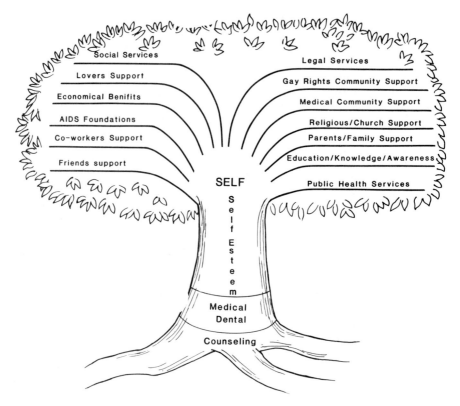

FIG. 14-3   Support tree needed to help a potential AIDS patient deal with the emotions and fears associated with AIDS, sources of educational information, and counseling services available.

such transfer is low. Needle stick surveillance studies performed by the Centers for Disease Control (CDC) have noted that 1948 health care workers (HCWs) with 2042 percutaneous exposures to blood from HIV-infected patients had a seroconversion rate of 0.29% and 668 with 1051 mucous membrane exposures had no seroconversions.[59] Nevertheless, although the problem of accidental instrument wounding remains a major concern in terms of potential transmission of HIV in the dental office, there is little the dentist can do to prevent it other than by being careful to avoid accidental injury. It should be pointed out that the possibility of developing hepatitis B from a single needle stick injury in a hepatitis B carrier is 6% to 30% whereas the possibility of developing HIV infection is 0.29%.[13,59]

As of March 31, 1991, a total of 168,913 cases

of AIDS in adults had been reported to the CDC. Occupational information was available for 80% of these: 6486 (4.8%) cases involved health care workers, and 171 (0.12%) dental health care workers (DHCWs). The majority (94%) of the 6486 cases had high-risk behavior for HIV infection. Four demonstrated seroconversion in a health care setting. Ten of the 171 DHCWs were classified as being at undetermined risk. Six of these were still being studied, and one was unavailable for study. The investigation has been completed for the remaining three (two dentists and one dental assistant), with no mode of transmission identified.

In two studies involving 5150 dental professionals,[16] three dentists were found to be HIV-infected. Two of the three had risk factors for HIV infection. No risk factors could be identified in the third infected dentist.

An observation study of 1307 general surgical procedures[35] showed a 1.7% rate of parenteral exposure to blood. The risk of exposure increased for procedures lasting longer than 3 hours and when patient blood loss was greater than 300 ml. Awareness of the surgical team to the patient's high risk or HIV infection status made no difference in the frequency of accidental wounds. Double gloving was found to prevent perforation of the inner glove. This study concluded that preoperative HIV testing would have had no beneficial effect on the frequency of accidental wounding in surgery.[35]

Through June 30, 1991, some 6800 AIDS cases had been reported in HCWs.[18] Three of these cases were determined to most likely have been infected from occupational exposure. (Included in this study were 46 surgeons and 190 DHCWs.[18])

In summary: The risk of exposure to HIV and seroconversion in the dental situation is present, but the probability of transmission to HCWs is low. However, when the added risks of hepatitis, herpes simplex, and syphilis are considered, the use of barrier techniques and universal precautions for *all* patients is well-justified.[1,18,52]

Until recently, the risk of transmitting HIV from an infected HCW to a patient has not been demonstrated. Various studies have looked for such transmission but could find no evidence it had occurred. This changed with the case of a Florida dentist who was found to have infected five of his patients. In look-back studies evaluating the patients treated by 60 HIV-infected HCWs, over 9000 cases have been studied. The only HCW found to have most likely transmitted infection to his patients was this Florida dentist,[14,15,18] who died of AIDS. A young woman patient of this dentist, who developed AIDS, came forward and was evaluated by the Florida Department of Health and the CDC. Following an extensive investigation, a total of four more patients were considered to have been infected by this Florida dentist. The young woman has since passed away, but before her death, she made a statement in strong support of mandatory HIV testing for all HCWs who perform invasive procedures. Over 700 of this dentist's former patients were tested for HIV antibodies. About 900 of his former patients elected not to be tested by the investigating personnel.[14,15]

It is now very clear that little risk is involved for the patient being treated by an HIV-infected surgeon or dentist. The possible risk of HIV infection resulting from such treatment is far smaller than the risk of an anesthesia-related death (100 per 1,000,000) or the risk of death from penicillin anaphylaxis (10 to 20 per 1,000,000). The risk in Minnesota for HIV transmission occurring during a surgical procedure has been estimated[56] to be between 1:2,100,000 and 1:21,000,000. This risk would be greater in urban areas in other parts of the United States. The available data clearly show a far greater risk for infection of HCWs by HIV-infected patients than vice-versa.[56]

Patients with severe immunosuppression associated with AIDS may be at risk for local or distant postoperative infections following invasive dental procedures that injure tissues and produce transient bacteremias. These patients may also be potential bleeders because of severe thrombocytopenia.

PREVENTION OF MEDICAL COMPLICATIONS

Patients who are identified as being carriers of HIV can be managed in the dental office using the protocol first developed for treating hepatitis B carriers but now recommended for all patients.[1,18,19,52] It has been estimated[13,61] that using laboratory screening tests for patients with a history of jaundice, hepatitis, or liver disease will pick up only 20% of the heptatitis B carriers. The other 80% are asymptomatic or have had nonspecific symptoms not identified with hepatitis and hence not picked up by history. The same is true of HIV exposed individuals; most are asymptomatic and not aware of their exposure. Hence, the history cannot be relied on for identification of infected individuals.[13,61]

In addition, pretreatment laboratory screening of all patients for HIV exposure is costly, impractical, and contrary to civil rights practices. Screening of all high-risk patients for HIV exposure is possible if these people are identified by history and clinical findings and will consent to screening. However, experience has shown that many individuals in the high-risk groups — homosexual males and IV drug users — are not willing to share that information and when identified are resistant to screening.

The American Dental Association[61] and the Centers for Disease Control[9] have recommended that all dental patients be considered as potentially infectious and universal precautions be used. These guidelines have been available since 1985. The Federal Government through the Occupational Safety and Health Administration (OSHA) has now set standards that describe how to prevent blood-borne pathogen transmission in the work place. These standards apply to dental offices with one or more employees.

The OSHA standard and the infection control procedures recommended by the ADA and the CDC are covered in detail in Appendix A. These recommendations should be used for all patients. If they are followed HIV-infected patients, other patients, and dental staff will be best protected from transmission of infectious agents.

PATIENT EVALUATION

The dentist can play an important role in detection of the patient with AIDS or a related condition. A health history should be taken and a head and neck examination performed as well as an intraoral soft tissue examination and a complete periodontal and dental examination on all new patients. History and/or clinical findings may indicate the patient who has AIDS or a related condition.

Patients with AIDS and those at high risk realize their lack of true privacy on questionnaires; in addition, there may be an AIDS-phobia or homophobia among members of the dental staff. Thus answers to certain questions may be less than factual. As a result, a patient's history should be obtained whenever possible via caring, understanding, verbal communication with a sharing of knowledge and facts through honesty, the avoidance of direct personal questions, and an openness with the patient. Because of the sensitive social and legal issues involved with AIDS, direct questions such as the following are not recommended for inclusion in the health history questionnaire: Are you homosexual or bisexual? Do you use IV drugs? We recommend that the questions listed below be included in some form on the health questionnaire and that the responses to these questions and various clinical findings serve as the foundation for leading into a discussion concerning lifestyle, etc. Questions suggestive of a high risk for AIDS or related conditions that can be included on the health questionnaire follow:

1. Have you had recurrent venereal infections such as syphilis or gonorrhea?
2. Have you had liver disease, jaundice, or hepatitis?
3. Do you use or have you used recreational drugs such as marijuana?
4. Have you had recent unexplained weight loss?
5. Do you have chronic unexplained fever?
6. Do you have chronic enlargement of lymph nodes?
7. Have you received multiple blood transfusions (1978 to 1985)?
8. Have you experienced malaise, fatigue, or weakness over an extended period?
9. Do you have a history of hemophilia?
10. Have you experienced unexplained night sweats, gastrointestinal discomfort, or diarrhea?
11. Are you under treatment for any form of cancer?
12. Do you have AIDS?
13. Are you HIV infected?
14. Are you at high risk for HIV infection?

Patients who, based on history and/or clinical findings, are found to be at high risk for AIDS or related conditions should be referred for HIV testing, medical evaluation, other appropriate diagnostic procedures, and psychosocial intervention. We do not recommend that the dentist undertake diagnostic laboratory screening but rather that the patient be referred to an appropriate medical facility.

This should follow a discussion concerning your findings and the possibility that AIDS or a related condition is present. At this time, sexual preference, IV drug use, etc. may be discussed and often will be mentioned by the patient. If not mentioned, the patient should still be strongly encouraged to seek diagnostic and supportive medical services. You should also encourage the utilization of professional support services—including those offered by social workers, gay rights groups, legal services, economic assistance, and civil rights groups—for counseling and support of the patient as well as the patient's own support group. The patient must be encouraged to allow the above types of activities to take place (Fig. 14-1).

High-risk AIDS patients who, for whatever reasons, fail to receive additional diagnostic testing and evaluation must be considered to have been exposed to the AIDS virus and to be potentially infectious. High-risk AIDS patients as well as diagnosed AIDS or HIV patients should be treated as any other with universal precautions. Attention should be directed to the handling of prosthetic procedures and fabrication of prostheses.[66] Biopsy specimens taken from patients also require special attention to processing.[1,66] (See Appendix A.)

All patients, regardless of their heptatis or AIDS status, must be treated using universal precautions and barrier techniques (Appendix A). This is strongly recommended because most HIV carriers and over 80% of the hepatitis B surface antigen (HBsAg) carriers cannot be identified on the basis of recommended clinical screening procedures.[1]

Several legal issues have been identified regarding the rights of dentists and a patient with AIDS.[1] The following guidelines have resulted as these issues were dealt with:

1. Dental treatment may not be withheld because the patient refuses testing for HIV exposure. We suggest the dentist assume that this type of patient is a potential carrier of HIV and treat him or her using barrier techniques.

2. An AIDS patient needing emergency dental treatment may not be refused care because the dentist does not want to treat AIDS patients.

3. An AIDS patient seeking routine dental care may be declined treatment by the new dentist regardless of the dentist's reason. However, the dentist should refer this patient to someone who would be willing to treat him.

4. A patient who has been under the care of a dentist and then develops AIDS or a related condition must be managed by that dentist or by a referral who is satisfactory to the patient.

5. The HIV-infected dentist does not need to inform patients that he (or she) is HIV-infected. The ADA recommends that infected dentists not perform invasive procedures. As demonstrated by public reaction to the case of the Florida dentist, a great deal of pressure for mandatory testing of dentists for their HIV status exists. Should a seropositive dentist be

allowed to practice is also a social as well as a professional question. These issues have not received sufficient public or professional attention as of this writing to demand testing or prohibit HIV-infected dentists from practicing, but this could change in the near future.

TREATMENT PLANNING CONSIDERATIONS

Patients who have been exposed to the AIDS virus but are asymptomatic may receive all indicated dental treatment. Patients who are symptomatic for ARC and early stages of AIDS can receive any dental care they may need and desire once the possibility of significant immunosuppression and thrombocytopenia has been ruled out. Complex treatment plans should not be undertaken before an honest and open discussion concerning the prognosis of the patient's medical condition.

Dental management of the HIV-infected asymptomatic patient is no different from that for any other patient in the practice. Universal precautions must be used for *all* patients. Any oral lesions found should be diagnosed and then managed by appropriate local and/or systemic treatment or should be referred for treatment. Lesions that are atypical or require special diagnostic procedures can be managed by the dentist who has experience with those procedures, or the patient can be referred for diagnosis and treatment.

Patients with lesions suggestive of HIV infection need to be evaluated for possible HIV infection. Patients with a history of IV drug abuse and infective endocarditis will require prophylaxis for invasive dental procedures. (See Chapter 3.) Patients with severe thrombocytopenia may require special measures before any surgical procedures (including scaling and curettage) are performed. Patients with advanced immunosuppression and neutropenia may require prophylaxis for invasive procedures (Table 14-6).

Acetaminophen should be used with caution in patient treated with zidovudine (AZT), because studies[36,69] have suggested that granulocytopenia and anemia, associated with zidovudine, may be intensified; also aspirin should be avoided in patients with thrombocytopenia.

Medical consultation is necessary for symp-

TABLE 14-6
Dental Management of the Patient with AIDS
or a Related Condition: General Procedures

Consult whenever possible with patient's physician
  to establish current status; if severe thrombocytopenia is present, platelet replacement may be
  needed before surgical procedures are performed
Determine if prophylactic antibiotics are needed to
  protect patient with severe immune suppression
  from postoperative infection
In general, render only more immediate treatment
  needs for patient with advanced AIDS
Dental procedures can be provided in most cases
  based on patient's wants and needs
All personnel working with AIDS patient must be
  informed of relative risks involved and how these
  can be minimized

tomatic HIV-infected patients before surgical procedures are performed. Current bleeding time and WBC count should be available. Patients with abnormal test results may require special management. All these matters need to be discussed in detail with the patient's physician.[36,69]

Any source of oral or dental infection should be eliminated in HIV-infected patients. They often require more frequent recall appointments for maintenance of periodontal health. Daily use of chlorhexidine mouth rinse is recommended. In patients with periodontal disease whose general health status is not clear, periodontal scaling can be done for several teeth to evaluate tissue response and bleeding. If no problems are noted, then the rest of the mouth can be treated. Root canal therapy may carry a slightly increased risk for postoperative infection in patients with advanced HIV disease. If infection occurs, it can be treated with local and systemic measures. Antibiotic prophylaxis is best avoided unless severe immune suppression and neutropenia are present.[36]

Antacids, phenytoin, cimetidine, and rifampin should be avoided in patients being treated with ketoconazole due to the possibility of altered absorption and metabolism.[38]

Individuals with severe symptoms of AIDS may be best managed by treatment of their more urgent dental needs to prevent pain and infection, with extensive restorative procedures not being provided. The main objectives of care are to avoid infection and to keep the patient free of dental or oral pain. Attention must be given to the prevention of infection and excessive bleeding in patients with severe immunosuppression and thrombocytopenia when planning invasive dental procedures. This may involve the use of prophylactic antibiotics. Platelet count or bleeding time should be ordered prior to any surgical procedure. If significant thrombocytopenia is present, platelet replacement may be needed. Medical consultation should precede any dental treatment (Table 14-6).

It is our strong recommendation that any dental practice can and should provide the needed dental care for patients with AIDS or related conditions. If the techniques described in this chapter are followed, the risk of HIV transmission to the dentist, staff, and other patients is very low, and the patient can be managed in a safe manner, with but minimum risk to others.

ORAL COMPLICATIONS

Clinical findings that suggest a high risk for AIDS or related conditions include candidiasis of the oral mucosa (Figs. 14-4 to 14-7), bluish purple or red lesion(s) that with biopsy are identified as Kaposi's sarcoma (Figs. 14-8 to 14-11), hairy leukoplakia of the lateral borders of the tongue (Figs. 14-12 and 14-13), and other oral lesions associated with HIV infection— including herpes simplex, herpes zoster, recurrent aphthous ulcerations, HIV gingivitis (Fig. 14-14), HIV periodontitis (Fig. 14-15), HIV necrotizing gingivitis, and necrotizing stomatitis. Other oral conditions that have been found in association with HIV infection are shown in Table 14-7.

The prevalence of six oral lesions reported to be associated with HIV infection was studied in a large number of homosexual and bisexual men (Tables 14-8 and 14-9).[29] The lesions investigated were hairy leukoplakia (HL), pseudomembranous candidiasis (PC), erythematous candidiasis (EC), angular cheilitis (AC), Kaposi's sarcoma (KS), and oral ulcers (OU). All were much more common in men with HIV infection. Seventy-one percent of the men with

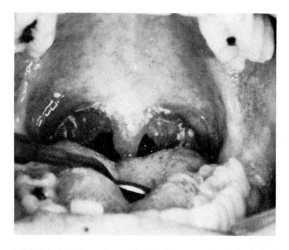

FIG. 14-4 Note the white lesions on the mucosa of the anterior and posterior tonsillar pillars. Cytologic study and culture established the diagnosis of candidiasis. The patient was found to have AIDS. (Courtesy Sol Silverman, D.D.S., San Francisco Calif.)

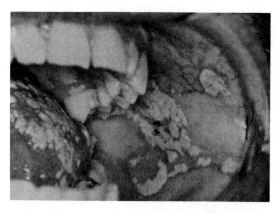

FIG. 14-5 Multiple, large white lesions in a patient with AIDS. The lesions could be removed with a tongue blade. The underlying mucosa was erythematous. Clinical and cytologic findings supported the diagnosis of pseudomembranesous candidasis. (Courtesy Eric Haus, D.D.S., Chicago Ill.)

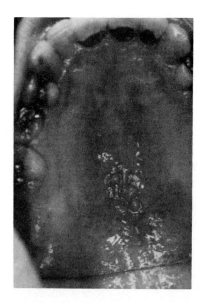

FIG. 14-6 Erythematous palatal lesion in an HIV antibody–positive patient. Smears taken from the lesion showed hyphae and spores consistent with *Candida*. The lesion healed following a 2-week course of antifungal medications. A diagnosis of erythematous candidiasis was made based on clinical and laboratory findings. (Courtesy Eric Haus, D.D.S., Chicago Ill.)

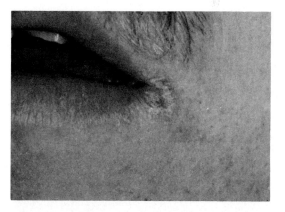

FIG. 14-7 AIDS patient with angular cheilitis. The lesion responded to antifungal medication. (Courtesy Eric Haus, D.D.S., Chicago Ill.)

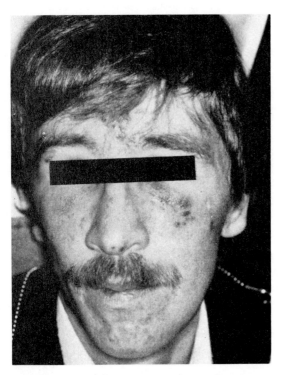

FIG. 14-8 Multiple erythematous lesions on the face of an AIDS patient. The lesions were established by biopsy as Kaposi's sarcoma. (Courtesy Sol Silverman, D.D.S., San Francisco Calif.)

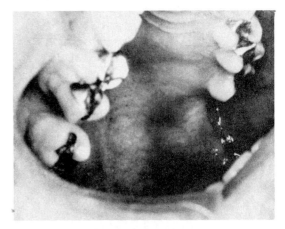

FIG. 14-9 Multiple large, flat, erythematous lesions involving the palatal mucosa. Biopsy revealed the lesions to be Kaposi's sarcoma, and the patient was eventually diagnosed as having AIDS. (Courtesy Sol Silverman, D.D.S., San Francisco Calif.)

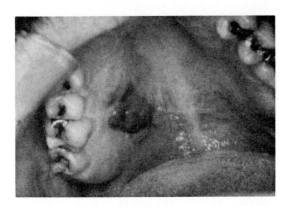

FIG. 14-10 A homosexual man with AIDS. Biopsy of the palatal lesion revealed Kaposi's sarcoma. (Courtesy Sol Silverman, D.D.S., San Francisco Calif.)

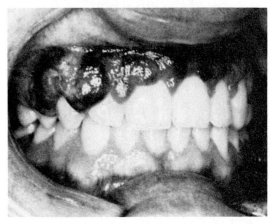

FIG. 14-11 Diffuse, elevated, erythematous lesion on the gingiva that biopsy revealed to be Kaposi's sarcoma. The patient was later diagnosed as having AIDS. (Courtesy Sol Silverman, D.D.S., San Francisco Calif.)

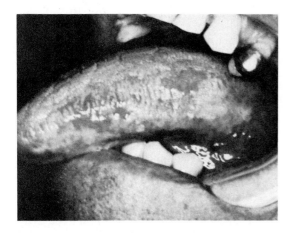

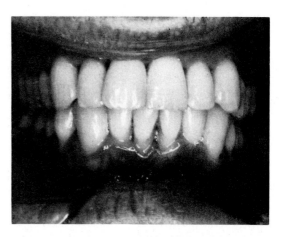

FIG. 14-12 Diffuse white lesion involving the tongue of a male homosexual. Biopsy supported the diagnosis of hairy leukoplakia. (Courtesy Sol Silverman, D.D.S., San Francisco Calif.)

FIG. 14-13 Diffuse white lesion involving the tongue of another male homosexual. Biopsy supported the diagnosis of hairy leukoplakia. (Courtesy Sol Silverman, D.D.S., San Francisco Calif.)

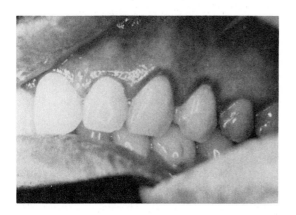

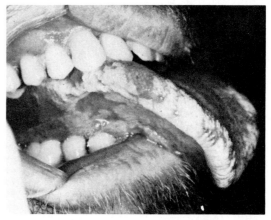

FIG. 14-14 HIV-gingivitis showing a linear band of erythema extending vestibularly from the gingival margin of the posterior teeth. (Courtesy James Winkler, D.D.S., San Francisco Calif.)

FIG. 14-15 HIV-periodontitis found in a young adult male. The diagnosis of AIDS was established following referral of the patient for medical evaluation. (Courtesy Sol Silverman, D.D.S., San Francisco Calif.)

hairy leukoplakia had a CD4 cell count below 200×10^6 per liter. HL, PC, KS, and AC were much more common in HIV-infected men with lower CD4 cell counts. HL was found in 20.4% of the HIV-infected men, and PC in 5.8%. The authors concluded that oral lesions can be used as an indirect marker for immune suppresion.[28]

In an interesting study[55] a strong relationship was found between an elevation of CD8+

lymphocytes before an oral examination and the appearance of oral lesions at the examination. This study involved asymptomatic HIV-infected individuals. It would suggest that both the CD8+ count (increased) and the CD4+ count (decreased) can be used in the management and

TABLE 14-7
Oral Manifestations of HIV Infections

Fungal infection

*Candidiasis
  Pseudomembranous
  Erythematous
  Hyperplastic
  Angular cheilitis
Histoplasmosis
Cryptococcosis
Geotrichosis

Bacterial infections

*HIV gingivitis
*HIV periodontitis
HIV necrotizing gingivitis
Necrotizing stomatitis
Mycobacterium avium intracellulare
Actinomycosis

Viral infections

*Herpes simplex
Herpes zoster-varicella
Cytomegalovirus
Human papillomavirus
  Oral warts
  Condyloma acuminatum
  Focal epithelial hyperplasia
Epstein-Barr virus
*Hairy leukoplakia

Neoplasms

*Kaposi's sarcoma
Non-Hodgkin's lymphoma

Others

Facial palsy
Trigeminal neuropathy
*Recurrent aphthous ulceration
  Minor
  Major
  Herpetiform
Immune thrombocytopenic purpura
Salivary gland enlargement
Xerostomia
Melanotic pigmentation

*More common oral lesions.
Based on Lemp GF, et al: *N Engl J Med* 321:1141–1148, 1989; Melnick SL: *Oral Surg* 68:37–43, 1989; Silverman S: *Dent Clin North Am* 35:259–267, 1991; Van Der Waal I, et al: *Int Dent J* 41:3–8, 1991.

TABLE 14-8
Oral Lesions in HIV-Infected and High-Risk Homosexual and Bisexual Men

Lesion	HIV-positive (n = 2235) (%)	HIV-negative (n = 2962) (%)
Hairy leukoplakia	18.7	0.3
Candidiasis	13	1.2
Pseudomembranous	6.6	0.1
Erythematous	2.1	0
Angular cheilitis	0.7	0.2
Kaposi's sarcoma	1.6	0
Oral ulcers	2	0.9

From Feigal DW, et al: *AIDS* 5:519–525, 1991.

evaluation of oral manifestations of HIV infection.[55]

In another study of 100 HIV-infected patients, which included 44 with AIDS,[78] 80% were found to have one or more of the HIV-associated oral lesions. In this study candidiasis was the most commonly found lesion—noted in 80.7% of the 44 AIDS patients and in 38% of the 56 HIV-infected individuals. In 6% of all the patients an oral lesion was the first clinical manifestation of HIV infection.[78]

Tables 14-10 and 14-11 summarize the frequency of oral lesions in high-risk and HIV-infected individuals. Seronegative high-risk patients had fewer lesions that did HIV-infected

TABLE 14-9
Prevalence of Oral Lesions by CD4 Lymphocyte Count on Baseline Examination of 737 HIV-Infected Subjects

Lesion	(n = 737) (%)	CD4 count (×10⁶/L)		
		Less than 200 (n = 126) (%)	200 to 499 (n = 335) (%)	Greater than 500 (n = 276) (%)
Hairy leukoplakia	150 (20.4)	43 (34.1)	74 (22.1)	33 (12)
Candidiasis				
Pseudomembranous	43 (5.8)	18 (14.3)	21 (6.3)	4 (1.5)
Erythematous	8 (1.1)	3 (2.4)	3 (0.9)	2 (0.7)
Angular cheilitis	9 (1.2)	5 (4)	2 (0.6)	2 (0.7)
Kaposi's sarcoma	11 (1.5)	8 (6.4)	2 (0.6)	1 (0.4)
Oral ulcers	14 (1.9)	0 (0)	10 (3)	4 (1.5)

From Feigal DW et al: *AIDS* 5:519–525, 1991.

TABLE 14-10
Specific Oral Lesions Related to Stage of HIV Infection: Percent of Patients with Lesions

Lesions	Seronegative high-risk (%)	Seropositive, but data not separated into clinical stages (%)	Asympto & PGL (%)	ARC (%)	AIDS (%)
Hairy leukoplakia	0.3 to 3	19	8 to 21	9 to 44	4 to 23
Candidiasis	0.8 to 10	11 to 31	5 to 17	11 to 85	29 to 87
Kaposi's sarcoma	0	0.3 to 3	1 to 2	0	35 to 38
Herpes simplex	0 to 0.5	0 to 1	0 to 5	11 to 29	0 to 9
Alphthous ulcerations	0 to 2	0 to 1	2 to 8	11 to 14	2 to 7
Veneral warts	0 to 0.7	0 to 1	0 to 1	0	0 to 1
ANUG	0 to 0.2		1 to 5	0	0 to 7
HIV gingivitis	0		0 to 1	0	51
HIV periodontitis	0		0 to 2	0 to 21	19

PGL, Persistent generalized lymphadenopathy; *ARC,* AIDS-related complex; *AIDS,* acquired immunodeficiency syndrome.
Based on Barone R, Ficarra G, Gaglioti D, et al: *Oral Surg* 69:169–173, 1990; Barr C, Croxson T, Dobles A, et al: *IADR* 1443, p 289, 1990; Feigal DW, Overby GL, Greenspan D, et al: *IADR* 65, p 190, 1989; Little JW, et al. Accepted for publication, *Gen Dent,* 1992; Melnick SL, Engel D, Truelove E, et al: *Oral Surg* 68:37–43, 1989; Roberts MW, Brahim JS, Rinne NF: *J Am Dent Assoc* 116(7):863–866, 1988; Silverman S Jr, Migliorati CA, Lozada-Nur, et al: *J Am Dent Assoc* 112(2):187–192, 1986.

TABLE 14-11
Association of Oral Lesions and Stage of HIV Infection: Percent of Patients with Lesions

	Patient HIV status		
	HIV-Infected		
Seronegative, high-risk (%)	Asymptomatic PGL (%)	ARC (%)	AIDS (%)
1 to 9	25 to 30	56 to 85	57 to 92

PGL, Persistent generalized lymphadenopathy; *ARC,* AIDS-related complex; *AIDS,* acquired immunodeficiency syndrome.
Based on Barone R, Ficarra G, Gaglioti D, et al: *Oral Surg* 69:169–173, 1990; Barr C, Croxson T, Dobles A, et al: *IADR* 1443, p 289, 1990; Feigal DW, Overby GL, Greenspan D, et al: *IADR* 65, p 190, 1989; Little JW, et al: (Accepted for publication, *Gen Dent,* 1992); Roberts MW, Brahim JS, Rinne NF: *J Am Dent Assoc* 116(7):863–866, 1988; Silverman S Jr, Migliorati CA, Lozada-Nur F, et al: *J Am Dent Assoc* 112(2):187–192, 1986.

patients, and asymptomatic HIV-infected individuals had an increased frequency of lesions though fewer than in the patients with ARC or AIDS. In a study of 106 patients with early HIV infection[51] 28% had a lesion reported to be associated with HIV infection (Table 14-12).

CANDIDIASIS

Worldwide, candidiasis is the most common oral manifestation of HIV infection.[24] Oral candidiasis, mentioned in the first report on

TABLE 14-12
Oral Lesions Found in 106 HIV-Infected Patients

	n (%)
Patients with at least one intraoral lesion	30 (28)
Candidasis	5 (5)
Recurrent herpes	6 (6)
Herpes zoster	0
Kaposi's sarcoma	0
HIV gingivitis	0
HIV periodontitis	2 (2)
Acute necrotizing ulcerative gingivitis	5 (5)
Oral warts	1 (1)
Ulcerations	8 (8)
Hairy leukoplakia	10 (9)

From Little JW, et al. (Accepted for publication, *Gen Dent,* 1992.)

AIDS in the United States,[65] occurs in about 45% of AIDS patients in the United States (Table 14-13). Its treatment is mandatory, to stop any spread to the esophagus. Oral candidiasis often occurs in multiple sites within the mouth. There is some evidence[65] to suggest that erythematous candidiasis precedes pseudomembranous candidiasis.

Oral lesions suspected of being candidiasis should be examined using cell study, culture, and/or biopsy techniques to confirm the clinical diagnosis. These are usually white lesions (pseudomembranous candidiasis) that can be scraped off, leaving small points of bleeding; however, some lesions are red (erythematous candidiasis). If the more common cause of oral candidiasis are absent—such as extended antibiotic usage, steroid therapy, radiation therapy, or diabetes mellitus—the dentist should suspect possible immunosuppression secondary to HIV infection.[37] The laboratory diagnosis, when used, should involve both Sabouraud and Pagano-Levin plates for primary isolation. The use of these culture media will allow identification of the various strains of *Candida*.[65]

Table 14-14 summarizes the topical and systemic antifungal medications used to treat oral candidiasis of HIV-infected individuals. Studies comparing the efficacies of ketoconazole and fluconazole in treating AIDS patients with oral candidiasis[65] have shown fluconazole to be superior. The yeasts may be developing resistance to the new systemic antifungals. Peridex, Listerine and hydrogen peroxide are

TABLE 14-13
Summary of Statistics Related to Oral Candidiasis in HIV-Infected Individuals Taken
From 17 Published Reports in the United States

Disease state	Papers	Prevalence frequences (%)		
		Range	Weighted mean*	Mean
Oral candidiasis	17	11 to 96	30.0	45.2
Erythematous	7	10 to 96	40.5	33.0
Pseudomembranous	6	6 to 69	22.2	25.6
Hyperplastic	6	2 to 20	3.8	3.8
Angular cheilitis	4	1 to 23	12.5	16.0

*Weighted by overall number of patients with oral candidiasis in each study.
From Samaranayake LP, Holmstrup P. *J Oral Pathol Med* 18:554–564, 1989.

TABLE 14-14
Antifungal Medications Used for Oral Candidiasis in HIV-Infected Individuals

Medication	Type	Frequency of dose	Dose	Duration* (days)
Chlortrimazole (topical)				
Mycelex	Oral troche	5 times daily	10 mg	7 to 14
Mycelex-G	Vaginal troche	1 time daily	100 or 500 mg	7 to 14
Nystatin (topical)				
Mycostatin	Vaginal tablets	1 tablet every 6 hours	100,000 units	10 to 14
Milstat	Vaginal tablets	1 tablet every 6 hours	100,000 units	10 to 14
Mycostatin	Oral Pastilles	1 tablet every 6 hours	200,000 units	10 to 14
Ketoconazole (systemic)				
Nizoral	Oral tablets	1 to 2 tablets (daily)	200 mg	10 to 14
Fluconazole (systemic)				
Diflucan	Oral tablets	1 tablet daily	100 mg	10 to 14

*Duration varies based on clinical response. Recurrence is common. Maintenance therapy can be considered using lower dose than treatment dose or every other day dosing with the systemic drugs.

mouth rinses that can be used for patients with candidiasis and other oral lesions associated with HIV infection.

Oral candidiasis found in patients with persistent generalized lymphadenopathy (PGL) may be of predictive value for the subsequent development of AIDS. In a study of 22 patients with PGL and oral candidiasis,[46] 13 (59%) developed AIDS within a median time of 3 months. By contrast, 20 patients with PGL without oral candidiasis were followed for a median time of 22 months and none of these patients developed AIDS.

The appearance of pseudomembranous candidiasis in HIV-infected individuals has been shown to be a strong indicator for the progression of infection to AIDS. A recent study[24] demonstrated that the erythematous form of candidiasis also indicates progression toward AIDS. In this study 169 HIV-infected patients with oral candidiasis were investigated. Ninety-two had pseudomembranous candidiasis, 37 had erythematous candidiasis, and 40 had both forms. Individuals in all three groups showed a rapid progression to AIDS (mean 25 months) and death (mean 43.8 months).[24]

KAPOSI'S SARCOMA

The classic lesion of Kaposi's sarcoma is a vascular neoplasm found in older men (over 50) of Jewish and Italian heritage. It is usually confined to the lower extremities and usually runs an indolent clinical course, with 10-to-15-year survivals occurring in over 37% of the cases. The variant of Kaposi's associated with AIDS has been termed *epidemic*. Epidemic Kaposi's sarcoma is most often disseminated throughout the body and runs a fulminant clinical course, with less than 20% survival at 2 years if associated with opportunistic infections.[23] In a study reported by Silverman,[71,83] Kaposi's sarcoma was found in the mouth as the first sign of AIDS in 22% of patients with HIV infection. Kaposi's sarcoma was found on the skin and in the mouth at the same time in another 45% of patients. Before December 1984, Kaposi's sarcoma was found in 21% of all AIDS patients. Since December 1984 only 13% of reported AIDS patients have had Kaposi's sarcoma.[76]

Kaposi's sarcoma is rare in children with AIDS and much less common in IV drug abusers, women, and hemophiliacs with AIDS than in homosexual men with AIDS.[22,60] Kaposi's sarcoma in patients with AIDS may be related to the release of HIV-induced growth factors by lymphocytes and macrophages. The growth factors stimulate angiogenesis and proliferation of fibroblasts and vascular (lymphatic) endothelium. In male homosexuals a sexually transmitted agent appears to play an important role in the development of this cancer.[6,71]

HAIRY LEUKOPLAKIA

Hairy leukoplakia is a virus-associated epithelial hyperplasia presenting as a corrugated white lesion on the mucosal surface of the mouth, usually involving the lateral borders of the tongue.[27,42,83] It has been reported[40,45,83] both in HIV-negative renal transplant patients and in a few HIV antibody–negative homosexual men. Lesions on the ventral surface of the tongue tend to consist of flat, white plaques whereas lesions on the lateral margins and dorsum of the tongue tend to be more corrugated. Hairy leukoplakia often is infected with *Candida* organisms, which makes the differential diagnosis from oral candidiasis important.[39-41,68]

Recent studies[17,42,44] have demonstrated that Epstein-Barr virus (EBV) replicates within the epithelial cells from hairy leukoplakia. The literature suggests that EBV is not associated with any other oral white lesions that must be differentiated from hairy leukoplakia. Thus hairy leukoplakia may be caused by a reactivation of EBV in the oral mucosa in association with HIV-induced immune deficiency.[67]

The diagnosis of hairy leukoplakia is based on the clinical appearance of the lesion, its lack of response to antifungal therapy, and histologic findings.[43] Researchers[17,38,43] have suggested that in the few cases of lesions found in HIV antibody–negative individuals, the EBV should be demonstrated for confirmation of the diagnosis. This can be done by immunocytochemistry, in situ hybridization, or electron microscopy. At the present time, techniques for the demonstration of EBV in lesions diagnosed by clinical and histologic findings are not available or practical for use by the general dentist, oral surgeon, or oral pathology services.

Patients with lesions diagnosed as hairy leukoplakia should be referred to a physician for

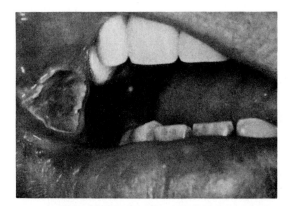

FIG. 14-16 Large aphthous ulcer (major type) found in a patient with AIDS. (Courtesy Eric Haus, D.D.S., Chicago Ill.)

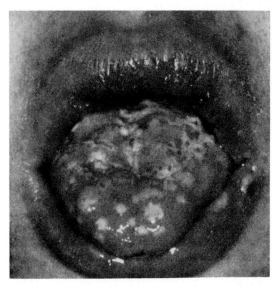

FIG. 14-17 Primary herpetic gingivostomatitis in a young patient with AIDS.

evaluation of their immune system and HIV antibody testing. Hairy leukoplakia is included in the 1986 Centers for Disease Control classification of HIV disease. The finding of hairy leukoplakia is also a predictive value for the subsequent development of AIDS. The probability of AIDS developing in an HIV-infected patient with hairy leukoplakia is 48% by 16 months and 83% by 30 months after the diagnosis of hairy leukoplakia.[22] The median time to death following the diagnosis of hairy leukoplakia is 41 months.[83]

APHTHOUS LESIONS

Three types of lesions are found in patients with recurrent aphthous ulcers. In non–HIV-infected subjects, minor aphthous ulcers are the most common lesions. In HIV-infected patients, herpetiform and major-type (Fig. 14-16) lesions appear to be most common. (Increased numbers of CD8+ cells are found at the base of ulcers in seronegative individuals.) The relative increase in CD8+ cells occurring in symptomatic HIV-infected individuals may, in part, explain the increased prevalence of herpetiform and major-type lesions seen in these people. Most HIV-infected patients with such lesions deny having had them as children.[53]

HIV PERIODONTAL DISEASE

HIV gingivitis and HIV periodontitis have been reported to be associated with HIV

infection (Fig. 14-17). Most studies include these conditions in patients with advanced HIV infection. The lesions appear to be related to alterations in the oral bacterial flora, to dysimmunoregulation, and decreased activity of polymorphonuclear leukocytes.[71] In a study of 97 individuals with early HIV infection (asymptomatic stage)[25] these lesions were rare. In fact, the overall periodontal health of these HIV-infected individuals was very good.

SALIVARY GLAND DISEASE

Several studies[68,78,84] have reported salivary gland enlargement in children and adults with HIV infection. The salivary gland enlargement may involve all the major salivary glands. These patients may have xerostomia. The HIV-associated salivary gland disease (HIV-sgd) is similar histologically to Sjögren's. However, autoantibodies are found in Sjögren's but are absent in HIV-sgd. Six percent of the patients seen at the Oral AIDS Center at the University of California–San Fracisco had HIV-sgd. No evidence has been found of direct invasion of the salivary glands by HIV-1.[68,78,84] Non-Hodgkin's lymphoma, Kaposi's sarcoma, benign lymphoepithelial cysts, and benign lymphoepithelial lesions have all been reported[74,84] in the major salivary glands of HIV-infected individuals.

Human salivary gland secretions have been found to contain a substance that inhibits HIV infection of human lymphocytes. Saliva from healthy women, men, and children was tested[33] and found to contain this factor—which, evidence suggests, may be a macromolecule (protein). In a recent study by Barr et al.[5] only 1% of 218 cultured whole saliva samples from HIV-infected homosexual or bisexual men contained cell-free HIV-1. These data support other studies showing that saliva is not important in the transmission of HIV-1.

An ELISA test developed by Wellcome has been found[20] to be 98% sensitive in detecting

TABLE 14-15
Treatment of the Oral Manifestations of HIV Infection

Condition	Regimen
Candidiasis	Topical and systemic antifungal agents
Hairy leukoplakia	Usually no treatment: acyclovir, 2.4 to 3 g orally per day for 2 weeks
Herpes simplex	Usually no treatment: acyclovir, 1 to 1.4 g, orally, per day for 7 to 10 days
Herpes zoster	Treat promptly to prevent scarring: acyclovir, 800 mg, orally, 5 times per day for 7 to 10 days
Recurrent aphthous ulceration	A small isolated lesion may not need treatment; other lesions can be treated by
	Topical fluocinonide ointment, 0.05%, mixed with Orabase; apply six times per day
	Dexamethasone elixir, 0.5 mg per 5 ml; rinse and expectorate two to three times per day
	A large atypical ulcer may require biopsy to rule out lymphoma or rare fungal infections
	Topical fluocinonide
	Metronidazole, orally, 250, mg, four times per day
Xerostomia	Sugarless gum, artificial saliva, topical fluorides; improve oral hygiene
Oral warts	CO_2 laser, surgical excision, cryosurgery, electrosurgery
Periodontal disease	
HIV gingivitis	Debridement, povidone-iodine, irrigation (Betadine 10%), Peridex (0.12% chlorhexidine gluconate mouth rinse, two times per day)
HIV periodontitis	Above plus scaling, root planning; for bone involve-
HIV necrotizing gingivitis	ment, metronidazole, 230 mg, four times per day, for 4 to 5 days
	Home irrigation with povidone-iodine; use of interproximal brushes
Kaposi's sarcoma	Debridement, dental prophylaxis, and scaling; intra-lesional vinblastine, CO_2 laser, surgical debulking, radiation
Oral lymphoma	Debridement, scaling, prophylaxis before treatment: radiation, chemotherapy

From Finberg J, Mills J. *Curr Sci* S209–S215, 1990; Fotos PG, Hellstein JW, Vincent SD. *Gen Dent* 422–433, 1991; Glick M. *Gent Dent* 418–424, 1990; Samaranayake LP, Holmstrup P. *J Oral Pathol Med* 18:554–564, 1989; Scully C, Porter SR, Luker J. *Br Dent J* 170:149–150, 1991; Silverman S. *Dent Clin North Am* 35:259–267, 1991; Stewart JS. *AIDS* 4(suppl):S217–S221, 1990; Workshop on oral healthcare in HIV disease, *Oral Surg* 73:138–142, 151–155, 1992; Zeitlen S, Shaha A. *J Surg Oncol* 47:230–232, 1991.

antibodies to HIV in saliva. This test may have application for population screening in the future. A test to detect salivary secretory immunoglobulin A antibodies of nonmaternal origin in newborns of women at risk for HIV infection has been found[2] to be accurate in detecting infected infants. One study[64] has shown that saliva might be an appropriate specimen for monitoring zidovudine (AZT) treatment in HIV-infected individuals.

LYMPHADENOPATHY

Lymphadenopathy, including cervical and submandibular locations, often is an early finding in patients infected with HIV. The lymphadenopathy is persistent and may be found in the absence of any current infection or medications known to cause lymph node enlargement. The nodes tend to be larger than 1 cm in diameter, and multiple sites of enlargement are found.

The dentist should perform a head and neck and intraoral soft tissue examination on all patients. White lesions in the mouth must be found and the patient managed in such a way that a diagnosis is established. This may involve cell study, culture, and/or biopsy by the dentist or referral to an oral surgeon. If red or purple lesions are found and cannot be explained by history (trauma—burn, chemical, physical) or proven by clinical observation (healing with in 7 to 10 days), they must be biopsied. Persistent lymphadenopathy must be investigated by referral for medical evaluation, diagnosis, and treatment.

Patients with AIDS or a related condition who have developed oral candidiasis can be treated as shown in Table 14-14. Treatment regimens for the various oral lesions associated with HIV infection are shown in Table 14-15 and can be found in Appendix B.

REFERENCES

1. American Association of Public Health Dentistry: The control of transmissible diseases in dental practice. (Position paper.) *J Public Health Dent* 46(1):13-22, 1986.
2. Archibald DW, Johnson JP, Nair P, et al: Detection of salivary immunoglobulin A antibodies to HIV-1 in infants and children, *AIDS* 4:417-420, 1990.
3. Barone R, Ficarra G, Gaglioti D, et al: Prevalence of oral lesions among HIV-infected intravenous drug abusers and other risk groups, *Oral Surg* 69:169-173, 1990.
4. Barr C, Croxson T, Dobles A, et al: HIV-associated oral lesions: immunologic and salivary parameters, *IADR 1443, 289, 1990.*
5. Barr CE, Miller LK, Lopez MR, et al: Recovery of infectious HIV-1 from whole saliva, *J Am Dent Assoc* 123(2):36-48, 1992.
6. Beral V, Peterman TA, Berkelman RL, Jaffe HW: Kaposi's sarcoma among persons with AIDS: a sexually transmitted infection? *Lancet* 335:123-127, 1990.
7. Brettle RP, Leen CLS: The natural history of HIV and AIDS in women, *AIDS* 5:1283-1292, 1991.
8. Burke DS, Brundage JF, Goldenbaum M, et al: Human immunodeficiency virus infections in teenagers: seroprevalence among applicants for US military service, *JAMA* 263:2074-2077, 1990.
9. Centers for Disease Control: Summary: recommendations for preventing transmission of infection with HTLV-III/Lav in the workplace, *MMWR* 34:45, 1985.
10. Centers for Disease Control: Update: AIDS—Europe, *MMWR* 35:2, 1986.
11. Centers for Disease Control: Surveillance for HIV-2 infection in blood donors—United States, *MMWR* 39:829-831, 1990.
12. Centers for Disease Control: The HIV/AIDS epidemic: the first 10 years, *MMWR* 40(22):357-363, 1991.
13. Centers for Disease Control: Publicly funded HIV counseling and testing—United States, 1990, *MMWR* 40(39):666-675, 1991.
14. Centers for Disease Control: Update: transmission of HIV infection during invasive dental procedures—Florida, *MMWR* 40(23):377-381, 1991.
15. Centers for Disease Control: Update: transmission of HIV infection during an invasive dental procedure—Florida, *MMWR* 40(2):21-27, 1991.
16. Ciesielksi C, Gooch B, Hammet T, Metler R: Dentists, allied professionals with AIDS, *J Am Dent Assoc* 122(9):42-44, 1991.
16a. Coffin JM: The virology of AIDS, *AIDS 1990 Year Rev* 4(suppl):S1-S9, 1990.
17. Corso B, Eversole LR, Hutt-Fletcher L: Hairy leukoplakia: Epstein-Barr virus receptors on oral keratinocyte plasma membranes, *Oral Surg* 67:416-21, 1987.
18. Cottone JA, Molinari JA: State-of-the-art infection control in dentistry, *J Am Dent Assoc* 122(9):33-40, 1991.
19. Council on Dental Therapeutics, American Dental Association: *Facts about AIDS for dental professionals,* Chicago, 1986, The Association.
19a. Cowan MJ, Hellman D, Chudwin DH, et al: Maternal transmission of acquired immunodeficiency syndrome, *Pediatrics* 73:382-386, 1984.
20. Crofts N, Nicholson S, Coghlan P, Gust ID: Testing of saliva for antibodies to HIV-1, *AIDS* 5:561-563, 1991.
21. Cumming PD, Wallace EL, Shore JB, Dodd RY: Exposure to patients to human immunodeficiency virus through the transfusion of blood components that test antibody-negative, *N Engl J Med* 321:941-946, 1989.
22. Curran JW, Morgan WM: AIDS—the beginning, the present, and the future. In Cole HM, Lundberg GD,

editors: *AIDS from the beginning,* Chicago, 1986, American Medical Association.

23. De Vita VT Jr, Hellman S, Rosenberg SA: *AIDS etiology, diagnosis, treatment, and prevention,* Philadelphia, 1985, JB Lippincott.

24. Dodd CL, Greenspan D, Katz MH, et al: Oral candidiasis in HIV infection: pseudomembranous and erythematous candidiasis show similar rates of progression to AIDS, *AIDS* 5:1339-1343, 1991.

25. Drinkard CR, Decher L, Little JW, et al: Periodontal status of individuals in early stages of human immunodeficiency virus infection, *Community Dent Oral Epidemiol* 19:281-285, 1991.

26. Elford J, Bor R, Summers P: Research into HIV and AIDS between 1981 and 1990: the epidemic curve, *AIDS* 5:1515-1519, 1991.

27. Eversole LR, Jacobsen P, Stone CE, Freckleton V: Oral condyloma planus (hairy leukoplakia) among homosexual men: a clinical pathologic study of thirty-six cases, *Oral Surg* 61:249-255, 1986.

28. Feigal DW, Katz MH, Greenspan D, et al: The prevalence of oral lesions in HIV-infected homosexual and bisexual men: three San Francisco epidemiological cohorts, *AIDS* 5:519-525, 1991.

29. Feigal DW, Overby GL, Greenspan D, et al: Oral lesions and immune function with and without HIV infection, *IADR* 65, 190, 1989.

30. Finberg J, Mills J: Treatment of opportunistic infections, *AIDS 1990 Year Rev* 4(suppl):S209-S216, 1990.

31. Fischl MA, Richman DD, Hansen N, et al: The safety and efficacy of zidovudine (AZT) in the treatment of subjects with mildly symptomatic human immunodeficiency virus type 1 (HIV) infection, *Ann Intern Med* 112:727-737, 1990.

32. Fotos PG, Hellstein JW, Vincent SD: Oral candidiasis revisited, *Gen Dent* 422-433, 1991.

33. Fox PC, Wolff A, Yeh CK, et al: Salivary inhibition of HIV-1 infectivity: functional properties and distribution in men, *J Am Dent Assoc* 118(6):709-711, 1989.

34. Garland FC, Lilienfeld AM, Garland CF: Incidence of human immunodeficiency virus seroconversion in US Navy and Marine Corps personnel, 1986 through 1988, *JAMA* 262:3161-3165, 1989.

35. Gerberding JL, Littel C, Tarkington A, et al: Risk of exposure of surgical personnel to patients' blood during surgery at San Francisco General Hospital, *N Engl J Med* 322:1788-1793, 1990.

36. Glick M: Clinical protocol for treating patients with HIV disease, *Gen Dent* 418-424, 1990.

37. Goedert JJ, Kessler CM, Aledort LM, et al: A prospective study of human immunodeficiency virus type 1 infection and the development of AIDS in subjects with hemophilia, *N Engl J Med* 321:1141-1148, 1989.

38. Greenspan D, Greenspan JS: Management of the oral lesions of HIV infection, *J Am Dent Assoc,* 122(9):26-32, 1991.

39. Greenspan D, Greenspan JS, Conant M, et al: Oral "hairy" leucoplakia in male homosexuals: evidence of association with both papillomavirus and a herpesgroup virus, *Lancet* 2:831-83, 1984.

40. Greenspan D, Greenspan JS, Hearst NG, et al: Relation of oral hairy leukoplakia to infections with the human immunodeficiency virus and the risk of developing AIDS, *J Infect Dis* 155:475-481, 1987.

41. Greenspan D, Greenspan JS, Pindborg JJ, Schiødt M, editors: *AIDS and the dental team,* Copenhagen, 1986, Munksgaard.

42. Greenspan JS, Greenspan D: Oral hairy leukoplakia: diagnosis and management, *Oral Surg* 67:396-403, 1989

43. Greenspan JS, Greenspan D, DeSouza Y, Freese UK: Diagnosis and investigation of hairy leukoplakia using noninvasive techniques, *J Dent Res* 66:184 (abstract 618), 1987.

44. Greenspan JS, Greenspan D, Lennette ET, et al: Replication of Epstein-Barr virus within the epithelial cells of oral "hairy" leukoplakia, an AIDS-associated lesion, *N Engl J Med* 313:1564-1571, 1985.

45. Itin P, Rufli T, Rüdlinger R, et al: Oral hairy leukoplakia in a HIV-negative renal transplant patient: a marker for immunosuppression? *Dermatologica* 177:126-128, 1988.

46. Klein RS, Harris CA, Small CB, et al: Oral candidiasis in high-risk patients as the initial manifestation of the acquired immunodeficiency syndrome. *N Engl J Med* 311:354-358, 1984.

47. Reference deleted in proofs.

48. Lemp GF, Payne SF, Neal D, et al: Survival trends for patients with AIDS, *JAMA* 263:402-406, 1990.

49. Levy JA: Changing concepts in HIV infection: challenges for the 1990s, *AIDS* 4:1051-1058, 1990.

50. Little JA: Differential diagnosis of white and red/purple lesions in HIV-infected individuals, *Compendium* 11(7):430-438, 1990.

51. Little JW, Melnick SL, Rhame FS, et al: Prevalence of oral lesions among individuals with asymptomatic human immunodeficiency virus infection and early AIDS-related complex. (Accepted for publication, *Gen Dent,* 1992.)

52. Lucatorto F: A comprehensive approach for the care of AIDS patients, *Am Acad Oral Med Newslett* 23:7, 1985.

53. MacPhail LA, Greenspan D, Feigal DW, et al: Recurrent aphthous ulcers in association with HIV infection: description of ulcer types and analysis of T-lymphocyte subsets, *Oral Surg* 71:678-683, 1991.

54. Melnick SL, Engel D, Truelove E, et al: Oral mucosal lesions: associations with the presence of antibodies to the human immunodeficiency virus, *Oral Surg* 68:37-43, 1989.

55. Melnick SL, Hannan P, Decher L, et al: Increasing CD8+ T lymphocytes predict subsequent development of intraoral lesions among individuals in the early stages of infection by the human immunodeficiency virus, *J Acquir Immune Defic Syndr* 4:1199-1207, 1991.

56. Minnesota Department of Health: *The Commissioner of Health's report and recommendations to the Gov-*

ernor on HIV infection and health care workers, October 1991.

57. Molinari JA, Merchant VA, Barrett ED: Acquired immunodeficiency syndrome (AIDS): clinical perspectives and considerations for dental patient treatment, *Compend Contin Educ Dent* 5(6):490-498, 1984.

58. Murrah VA, Scholtes GA: Antibody testing and counseling of dental patients at-risk for human immunodeficiency virus (HIV) infection and associated clinical findings, *Oral Surg* 66:432-439, 1988.

59. Neidle EA: A matter of policy, health groups face the AIDS crisis, *J Am Dent Assoc* 122(9):45-48, 1991.

60. Pahwa S, Kaplan M, Fikrig S, et al: Spectrum of human T-cell lymphotropic virus type III infection in children, *JAMA* 255:2299-2305, 1986.

61. Proceedings of the national symposium on hepatitis B and the dental profession, *J Am Dent Assoc* 110:614-650, 1985.

62. Robert-Guroff M, Gallo RC: A virological perspective on AIDS. In Cole HM, Lundberg GD, editors: *AIDS from the beginning*, Chicago, 1986, American Medical Association.

63. Roberts MW, Brahim JS, Rinne NF: Oral manifestations of AIDS: a study of 84 patients, *J Am Dent Assoc* 116(7):863-866, 1988.

64. Rolinski B, Wintergerst U, Matuschke A, et al: Evaluation of saliva as a specimen for monitoring Zidovudine therapy in HIV-infected patients, *AIDS* 5:885-888, 1991.

65. Samaranayake LP, Holmstrup P: Oral candidiasis and human immunodeficiency virus infection, *J Oral Pathol Med* 18:554-564, 1989.

66. Schaefer ME: Infection control in dental laboratory procedures, *CDA J* 13(10):81-84, 1985.

67. Schiødt M, Greenspan D, Greenspan JS: Can you recognize the oral manifestations of AIDS. *Resp Dis* 10:91-107, 1989.

68. Schiødt M, Greenspan D, Levy JA, et al: Does HIV cause salivary gland disease? *AIDS* 3:819-822, 1989.

69. Scully C, Porter SR, Luker J: An ABC of oral health care in patients with HIV infection, *Br Dent J* 170:149-150, 1991.

70. Ship JA, Wolff A: AIDS and HIV-1 infection: clinical entities in geriatric dentistry, *Gerodontology* 8:28-32, 1989.

71. Silverman S: AIDS update: oral manifestations and management, *Dent Clin North Am* 35:259-267, 1991.

72. Silverman S Jr, Migliorati CA, Lozada-Nur F, et al: Oral findings in people with or at high risk for AIDS: a study of 375 homosexual males, *J Am Dent Assoc* 112(2):187-192, 1986.

73. Simpson ML: Counseling and testing for human immunodeficiency virus, *Minn Med* 70:93-94, 1987.

74. Smith FB: Benign lymphoepithelial lesion and lymphoepithelial cyst of the parotid gland in HIV infection, *Arch Pathol Lab Med* 112:742-745, 1988.

75. Statistics from the Centers for Disease Control, *AIDS* 6:343-345, 1992.

76. Stewart JS: Current approaches to the treatment of HIV-related Kaposi's sarcoma and lymphoma by chemotherapy, *AIDS* 4(suppl 1):S217-S221, 1990.

77. Tsamtsouris A, Shein B, Rovero J: The periatric patient HIV infection: an overview for the pedodontist, *J Mass Dent Soc* 38(1):11-13, winter, 1991.

78. Van Der Waal I, Schulten EA, Pindborg JJ: Oral manifestations of AIDS: an overview, *Int Dent J* 41:3-8, 1991.

79. Volberding PA, Lagakos SW, Koch MA, et al: Zidovudine in asymptomatic human immunodeficiency virus infection: a controlled trial in persons with fewer than 500 CD_4 positive cell per cubic millimeter, *N Engl J Med* 322:941-949, 1990.

80. Ward JW, Bush TJ, Perkins HA, et al: The natural history of transfusion-associated infection with human immunodeficiency virus, *N Engl J Med* 321:947-952, 1989.

81. Weiss SH, Saxinger WC, Rechtman D, et al: HTLV-III infection among health care workers; association with needle-stick injuries, *JAMA* 254:2089-2093, 1985.

82. Winkler JR, Murray PA, Grassi M, Hammerle C: Diagnosis and management of HIV-associated periodontal lesions, *J Am Dent Assoc* (suppl) 25S-34S, November 1989.

83. Workshop on oral healthcare in HIV disease, *Oral Surg* 73:138-142, 151-155, 1992.

84. Zeitlen S, Shaha A: Parotid manifestations of HIV infection, *J Surg Oncol* 47:230-232, 1991.

15

Arthritis

Arthritis is a nonspecific term that means inflammation of the joints. It is one of the rheumatic diseases, a group of disorders that affect bones, joints, and muscles. The term *arthritis* is often used interchangeably by lay persons with the term *rheumatism;* the latter denotes aches, pains, and stiffness in the joints and muscles. There are over 100 arthritic diseases affecting different parts of the body. Some of the most common types include rheumatoid arthritis, osteoarthritis, systemic lupus erythematosus, juvenile arthritis, scleroderma, gout, ankylosing spondylitis, and psoriatic arthritis.

Arthritis is a serious disease with significant personal and economic impact. According to the Arthritis Foundation,[2] over 37 million Americans suffer from the various forms of arthritis, and over 7 million of these are disabled. In terms of its overall economic impact, arthritis costs the American economy more than $14 billion annually, with a loss of 26.6 million workdays per year.

Although arthritis is a large group of important diseases, this chapter is limited to a discussion of rheumatoid arthritis, osteoarthritis, and systemic lupus erythematosus, which are the most common forms encountered and can serve as models for the other forms.

Rheumatoid arthritis

GENERAL DESCRIPTION
INCIDENCE AND PREVALENCE

Rheumatoid arthritis (RA) is an autoimmune disease that is commonly mild and chronic but can be severe and crippling. It is estimated[7,14] that 4 to 6 million people in the United States have RA. Women are affected three times more frequently than men, with the age of onset usually between 35 and 50 years.[7,14]

The disease is characterized by symmetric inflammation of joints, especially the hands, feet, and knees. In addition, systemic involvement of the skin, muscles, eyes, lungs, blood vessels, and nerves is common.

ETIOLOGY

The cause of RA is not known, but a popular theory suggests a viral agent that perhaps alters the immune system in a genetically predisposed individual and leads to destruction of synovial tissues. Many persons who develop RA have a genetic predisposition in the form of a tissue marker called HLA-DR4; however, not everyone with this tissue type develops the disease. No evidence exists that any nutritional deficiency leads to rheumatoid arthritis or that certain foods or vitamins affect its outcome.[8,22]

PATHOPHYSIOLOGY

With RA, primary changes occur in the synovium—which is the inner lining of the joint capsule. There is edema of the synovium, followed by thickening and folding. This excessive tissue is called *pannus*. In addition, a marked infiltration of lymphocytes and plasma cells occurs into the capsule. Eventually granulation tissue covers the articular surfaces and destroys the cartilage and subchondral bone through enzymatic activity (Fig. 15-1). The process also extends to the capsule and ligaments. New bone or fibrous tissue is then deposited, and this results in fusion or loss of mobility.[5,8]

A likely sequence of events begins with a

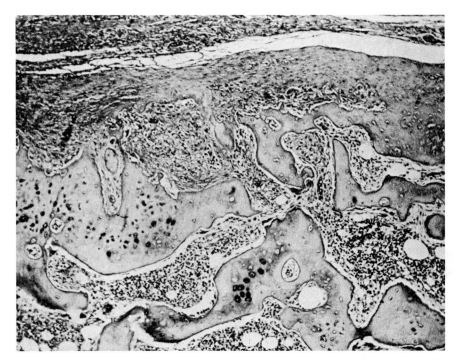

FIG. 15-1 The joint surface *(top)* has lost its cartilage and consists of granulation tissue with scar tissue. Subchondral bone shows degenerative changes and areas of necrosis. (Courtesy A. Golden, M.D., Lexington Ky.)

synovitis, perhaps of viral origin, that stimulates immunoglobulin G (IgG) antibodies. These antibodies form antigenic aggregates in the joint space and lead to the production of rheumatoid factor (autoantibodies). Rheumatoid factor then complexes with IgG complement and produces an inflammatory reaction that injures the joint space.[5]

An associated finding in 20% to 30% of patients with RA is subcutaneous nodules, usually found around the elbow.[14] These nodules are thought to arise from the same antigen-antibody complex that is found in the joint. A vasculitis confined to small- and medium-sized vessels also may occur and is probably caused by the same complexing.[5]

SEQUELAE AND COMPLICATIONS

The course and severity of RA are unpredictable but characterized by remissions and exacerbations. The most progressive period of the disease occurs during the first 6 years and thereafter slows. Approximately 15% of patients will undergo permanent remission within the first year whereas another 10% will experience relentless crippling, leading to nearly complete disability.[14] For the majority of patients, however, the disease is a sustained, lifelong problem that can be controlled or modified to allow a normal or nearly normal life.

The median life expectancy of persons with RA is shortened by 3 to 7 years. This increased mortality rate is usually associated with more severe disease and is attributed to infection and gastrointestinal bleeding.[14]

Many complications may accompany RA. Included among these are TMJ involvement, digital gangrene, skin ulcers, muscle atrophy, keratoconjunctivitis sicca (Sjögren's syndrome), pulmonary interstitial fibrosis, pericarditis, amyloidosis, anemia, thrombocytopenia, neutropenia, and splenomegaly (Felty's syndrome).[7,14]

TABLE 15-1
Comparison of Rheumatoid Arthritis and Osteoarthritis

Rheumatoid arthritis	Osteoarthritis
Multiple symmetric joint involvement	Usually one or two joints (or groups) involved
Significant joint inflammation	Joint pain without inflammation (usually)
Morning joint stiffness longer than 1 hour	Morning joint stiffness of less than 15 minutes
Symmetric spindle-shaped swelling of proximal interphalangeal (PIP) joints and volar subluxation of metacarpophalangeal (MCP) joints	Herberden's nodes of distal interphalangeal (DIP) joints and Bouchard's nodes of PIP joints
	No systemic involvement
Systemic manifestations (fatigue, weakness, malaise)	

CLINICAL PRESENTATION
SIGNS AND SYMPTOMS

The usual presentation of RA is as a process with an onset that is gradual and subtle (Table 15-1). It is commonly preceded by a prodromal phase of general fatigue and weakness with joint and muscle ache. Characteristically, these symptoms come and go over varying periods. Then painful joint swelling, especially of the hands and feet, occurs in several joints and progresses to other joints in a symmetric fashion. Joint involvement persists and gradually progresses to immobility, contractures, subluxation, deviation, and other deformities. Characteristic features include pain in the affected joints aggravated by movement, generalized joint stiffness after inactivity, and morning stiffness of greater than 1-hour duration.[14] The joints most commonly affected are fingers, wrists, feet, ankles, knees, and elbows. Multiple joint changes in the hands are seen and include a symmetric spindle-shaped swelling of the proximal interphalangeal (PIP) joints with dorsal swelling and characteristic volar subluxation of the metacarpophalangeal (MCP) joints[22] (Fig. 15-2). The TMJ is involved in up to 75% of patients.[9]

Rheumatoid nodules are seen in patients with RA and are most commonly found around the elbows, fingers, back of the head, and sacrum.[22]

The American Rheumatism Association[1] has developed revised criteria for the diagnosis and classification of RA (Table 15-2). These criteria have high specificity (89%) and sensitivity (91% to 94%) compared with controls when used to classify patients with RA. Four of seven of the criteria must be present for the diagnosis of RA to be made.[1]

LABORATORY FINDINGS

None of the laboratory tests are pathognomonic or diagnostic of RA although they may be used in conjunction with clinical findings to confirm the diagnosis.

Findings in RA include an increased erythrocyte sedimentation rate, positive rheumatoid factors (in two thirds of affected patients), normochromic and normocytic anemia, and the presence of C-reactive protein. In patients with Felty's syndrome (RA with splenomegaly) a marked neutropenia may be present.[14,22]

MEDICAL MANAGEMENT

The treatment of RA is, by necessity, palliative because there is no cure as yet for the disease. Treatment goals are to reduce joint swelling, relieve pain and stiffness, and facilitate and encourage normal function. These goals are accomplished by patient education, rest, physical therapy, and drug therapy (Table 15-3).

The nonsteroidal antiinflammatory drugs (NSAIDs), especially aspirin, constitute the cornerstone of treatment. Aspirin may be pre-

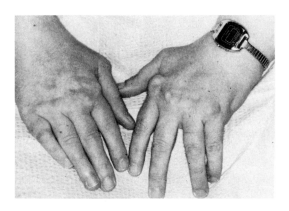

FIG. 15-2 Hands of a patient with rheumatoid arthritis who has undergone surgical replacement of deformed metacarpophalangeal joints of the right hand.

TABLE 15-2
Criteria for the Diagnosis of Rheumatoid Arthritis*

Morning stiffness
Arthritis of three or more joint areas
Arthritis of hand joints
Symmetric arthritis
Rheumatoid nodules
Serum rheumatoid factor
Radiographic changes

*At least four must be present to make a diagnosis of RA.
From Arnett FC, et al. *Arthritis Rheum* 31:315–324, 1988.

scribed in large doses on an individual basis. A common approach[13] is to start a patient on three 5-grain tablets four times a day and then adjust the dosage based on patient response. The most common sign of aspirin toxicity is tinnitus. Should this occur, dosage is decreased. In addition to aspirin, many NSAIDs are available. Some of the more common of these include ibuprofen (Motrin, Advil, Rufen, Nuprin), naproxen (Naprosyn), sulindac (Clinoril), tolmetin (Tolectin), fenoprofen (Nalfon), piroxicam (Feldene), dicloferac (Voltaren), flurbiprofen (Ansaid), diflunisal (Dolobid), etodolac (Lodine), and nabumetone (Relafen). All the NSAIDs can cause a qualitative platelet defect that may result in prolonged bleeding, especially in high doses. (See Chapter 22.)

In addition to NSAIDs, a variety of other drugs are used to treat RA. Many of these drugs can cause blood dyscrasias that lead to increased infections, delayed healing, and prolonged bleeding. Gold compounds may be effective in decreasing inflammation and retarding the progress of the disease; but the incidence of toxicity is high, and dermatitis with mucosal ulceration, proteinuria, neutropenia, and thrombocytopenia may result.[13] Antimalarial drugs (chloroquine, hydroxychloroquine) are used to treat RA usually in combination with aspirin or corticosteroids. Side effects include severe eye damage. A blue-black intraoral pigmentation may also be seen. Penicillamine is used in the treatment of RA. Both the antimalarials and penicillamine, however, are associated with significant toxicity, which limits their use.

Corticosteroids (prednisone, prednisolone) are frequently useful in controlling acute symptoms; however, because of multiple side effects, long-term usage is avoided if possible. One of the more potentially significant side effects is adrenal suppression. (See Chapter 18.)

In cases of recalcitrant disease, immunosuppressive therapy has been used successfully. Drug therapy includes cyclophosphamide, azathioprine, and methotrexate. These drugs are associated with significant side effects including severe oral ulcerations. In addition, lymphopheresis, plasmapheresis, and lymph node irradiation are used.[13,14]

Surgical management of severely deformed joints is common and may involve a variety of procedures—including arthroplasty, reconstruction, synovectomy, and total joint replacement. (See Chapter 22.)

DENTAL MANAGEMENT
MEDICAL CONSIDERATIONS

Since patients may have multiple joint involvement with varying degrees of pain and immobility, dental appointments should be kept as short as possible and the patient should be allowed to make frequent position changes. The patient also may be more comfortable in a sitting or semisupine position as opposed to a supine one. Physical supports, such as a pillow or rolled towel, may be needed to provide support for deformed limbs, joints, or neck (Table 15-4).

TABLE 15-3
Drugs Used in the Management of Rheumatoid Arthritis and Systemic
Lupus Erythematosus

Generic name	Trade name	Dental and oral considerations
Salicylates	Aspirin, Ascriptin, Bufferin, Anacin, Ectotrin, Empirin	Prolonged bleeding
Nonsteroidal antiinflammatory drugs		
Ibuprofen	Motrin	Prolonged bleeding, oral ulceration, stomatitis
Fenoprofen	Nalfon	
Indomethacin	Indocin	
Naproxen	Naprosyn	
Meclofenamate	Meclomen	
Piroxicam	Feldene	
Sulindac	Clinoril	
Tolmetin	Tolectin	
Dicloferac	Voltaren	
Flurbiprofen	Ansaid	
Diflunisal	Dolobid	
Etodolac	Lodine	
Nabumetone	Relafen	
Glucocorticoids		
Prednisone	Deltasone, Meticorten,	Adrenal suppression,
Prednisolone	Orasone, Articulose-50,	masking of oral infec-
Methylprednisolone	Delta-Cortef, Medrol	tion, impaired healing
Penicillamine	Cuprimine, Depen	Increased infections, delayed healing, prolonged bleeding, oral ulcerations
Gold compounds		
Gold sodium thiomalate	Myochrysine Ridaura	Increased infections, delayed healing,
Auranofin	Solganal	prolonged bleeding,
Aurothioglucose		glossitis, stomatitis
Antimalarials		
Hydroxychloroquine	Plaquenil	Increased infections,
Chloroquine	Aralen	delayed healing, prolonged bleeding, intraoral pigmentation
Sulfasalazine	Azulfidine	Increased infections, delayed healing, prolonged bleeding
Immunosuppressives		
Azathioprine	Imuran	Increased infections,
Cyclophosphamide	Cytoxan	delayed healing,
Methotrexate	Rheumatrex	prolonged bleeding, stomatitis

TABLE 15-4

Dental Management of the Patient with Arthritis

---

1. Short appointments
2. Ensure physical comfort
   a. Frequent position changes
   b. Comfortable chair position
   c. Physical supports as needed
3. Drug considerations
   a. Aspirin and other NSAIDs — pretreatment bleeding time (less than 20 minutes)
   b. Gold salts, penicillamine, and immuno-suppressives — complete blood count with differential; bleeding time
   c. Corticosteroids (systemic) — may have significant adrenal suppression after prolonged high doses

---

The most significant complications associated with RA are drug-related (Table 15-3). Aspirin and other NSAIDs can cause decreased platelet adhesiveness and result in abnormal bleeding. Because of this, patients taking these drugs should have a pretreatment bleeding time performed. Abnormal results should be discussed with the patient's physician. Even if the bleeding time is moderately prolonged (up to 20 minutes), patients can usually be treated, as long as curettage or surgery is performed conservatively in small segments and no other bleeding problem is present. (See Chapter 22.)

Patients taking gold salts, penicillamine, sulfasalazine, or immunosuppressives are susceptible to bone marrow suppression that may result in anemia, agranulocytosis, and thrombocytopenia. As a rule, these patients should be followed closely by their physician to detect this problem. If a patient has not had recent laboratory tests, it is advisable to order a complete blood count with differential and bleeding time. Abnormal results should be discussed with the physician.

If corticosteroids are used for prolonged periods, the potential for adrenal suppression exists. Management of this problem is discussed in Chapter 18.

TREATMENT PLANNING MODIFICATIONS

Treatment planning modifications are dictated by the patient's physical disabilities. An individual with marked disability or limited jaw function caused by TMJ involvement should not be subjected to prolonged extensive treatment, such as complicated crown and bridge procedures. If replacement of missing teeth is desired, consideration should be given to a removable prosthesis because of the decreased chair time needed for preparation and the easier cleansability of the appliance. If a fixed prosthesis is elected, ease of cleansability must be a significant factor in design. Progressive or abrupt occlusion changes are possible because of loss of condylar height. Therefore the dentist should take these potential occlusal changes into consideration when planning any significant reconstructive treatment.

The disabled patient may have significant difficulty cleaning his or her teeth. Cleaning aids such as floss holders, toothpicks, irrigating devices, and mechanical toothbrushes may be recommended. Manual toothbrushes can be modified by placing acrylic or a rubber ball on the handle to improve the grip.

It should be remembered that RA is a progressive disease that may ultimately lead to severe disability and crippling in some patients, which can make providing dental care difficult. Therefore the dentist should be aggressive in providing good preventive care and should attempt to identify and treat or eliminate potential problems before the disease progresses.

ORAL AND MAXILLOFACIAL COMPLICATIONS

The most significant complication of the oral and maxillofacial complex in RA is TMJ involvement. This may present as bilateral pain, tenderness, swelling, stiffness, and decreased mobility of the TMJs. There may be periods of remission and exacerbation as with other joint involvement. Bony ankylosis can occur. A particularly disturbing event is the development of an anterior open bite caused by destruction of the condyles and the loss of condylar height (Fig. 15-3). Although palliative treatment such as interocclusal splints, physical therapy, medication, and heat may prove to be helpful, surgical intervention may become necessary to decrease pain, improve the appearance, or restore function.

Another oral complication seen in patients with RA is a troublesome stomatitis that may be

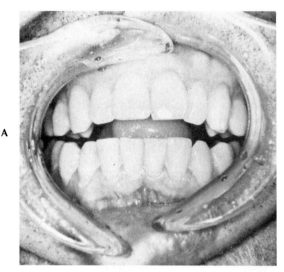

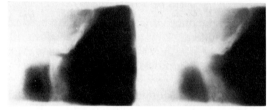

FIG. 15-3 A, Anterior open bite deformity in a patient with rheumatoid arthritis of the temporomandibular joints. Contact is present only on the second molars. **B,** Radiograph of the temporomandibular joints of this patient demonstrating extreme destruction and deformity of the condylar heads.

seen following the administration of gold compounds as well as with penicillamine and the immunosuppressives. This may be an indication of drug toxicity and should be reported to the physician. Palliative treatment may include bland mouth rinses, diphenhydramine elixir, or a topical emollient such as Orabase. (See Appendix B.)

Osteoarthritis

GENERAL DESCRIPTION
INCIDENCE AND PREVALENCE

Osteoarthritis (OA, degenerative joint disease) is another of the rheumatic diseases and is

the most common form of arthritis. Almost everyone past the age of 60 will have OA to some degree. Most people will be minimally symptomatic; however, it is estimated that 17 million people in the United States have OA to the extent that it results in pain, and it is the leading cause of disability among the elderly.[2,3]

OA is generally considered to be a regional disease and usually affects one or two joints at a time. It is more frequently found in stress-bearing or often-used joints such as hips, knees, feet, spine, and hands. The TMJ also is affected. Women are afflicted twice as often as men; however, men are afflicted at an earlier age. It is generally a disease of middle to older age, first appearing after the age of 40. There does not appear to be any racial or geographic predilection.

ETIOLOGY

The exact cause of OA is not known. It has been thought to be the end result of normal wear and tear on joints over a long period; however, other factors are now felt to be of significance. Preexisting structural joint abnormalities, intrinsic aging, metabolic factors, genetic predisposition, obesity leading to overloaded joints, and macro- or microtrauma are all considered causative or contributory factors in the origin of the disease.

PATHOPHYSIOLOGY

The initial change in the joint is a splitting of the articular cartilage, creating a fibrillated surface. This change is associated with the loss of proteoglycan. There is a progressive abrasion of cartilage down to the subchondral bone. The exposed bone becomes polished and sclerotic, resembling ivory (eburnation). There may be some resurfacing with cartilage if the disorder is arrested or stabilized. New bone forms at the margin of articular cartilage, in the non–weight-bearing part of the joint, creating osteophytes (or spurs), often covered by cartilage, that augment the degree of deformity.[5]

SEQUELAE AND COMPLICATIONS

OA, in contrast to RA, has a relatively favorable prognosis and less serious complications, depending on the joint(s) involved. The two most important complications with osteoarthritis are pain and disability. Conservative treatment can often retard the progress of the disease; however, surgery may be required to restore function and decrease pain.

CLINICAL PRESENTATION
SIGNS AND SYMPTOMS

The main symptom in OA is pain in one or two joints (Table 15-1). The pain is described as a dull ache and is accompanied by stiffness that is worse in the morning or after a period of inactivity. The pain and stiffness usually last 15 minutes or less.[3] Joint noises (crepitus) may variably be detected with movement. Redness and swelling are not usually features associated with OA.

The most common sign is a painless bony growth on the medial and lateral aspects of the distal interphalangeal (DIP) joints called Heberden's nodes. When these enlargements occur on the PIP joints, they are called Bouchard's nodes (Fig. 15-4). On occasion some pain may be associated with these nodes.

Depending upon which joint or group of joints is involved, patients may experience varying degrees of incapacitation. Hip and knee joints are particularly troublesome and can be a common source of disability.

A form of OA called primary generalized osteoarthritis is characterized by involvement of three or more joints or groups of joints, appears most often in women, and affects hands, knees, hip, and spine.[3]

Radiographic signs include narrowing of the joint space, articular surface irregularities and remodelings, and osteophytes or spurs. In addition, subchondral sclerosis (eburnation) and ankylosis may be seen.[3] It should be noted that

symptoms are often not well-correlated with radiographic signs.

LABORATORY FINDINGS

Laboratory findings in OA are essentially unremarkable. The erythrocyte sedimentation rate is usually normal, except for a mild elevation in primary generalized cases.

MEDICAL MANAGEMENT

The management of OA is palliative. Aspirin and the other NSAIDs (Table 15-3) form the cornerstone of drug treatment. Patient education, physical therapy, weight reduction, and joint protection are all aspects of management. Intraarticular steroid injections may be used intermittently to reduce acute pain and inflammation. Surgery is performed to improve function or for relief of pain.

DENTAL MANAGEMENT
MEDICAL CONSIDERATIONS

Depending upon which joints are involved, patients may not be comfortable supine in the dental chair for long periods. Consideration should be given to a more upright chair position, the use of neck, back, and leg supports, and the scheduling of short appointments (Table 15-4).

Altered platelet function caused by large doses of aspirin or other NSAIDs is a frequent finding, and patients should have a pretreatment bleeding time performed. Elevated results (up to 20 minutes) are not unusual but frequently are not clinically significant, as long as procedures that result in bleeding are kept to a minimum and other bleeding problems are not present. (See Chapter 22.) Grossly abnormal bleeding times should be discussed with the physician.

Adrenal suppression is generally not a concern with periodic intraarticular injections of steroids.

TREATMENT PLANNING
MODIFICATIONS

As for RA, actual modifications of dental treatment for OA are dictated by the patient's disabilities. For instance, severe disabilities of hip, knee, or other joint or TMJ involvement may prevent lengthy appointments, and therefore extensive treatment such as reconstruction or a long surgical procedure may not be appropriate.

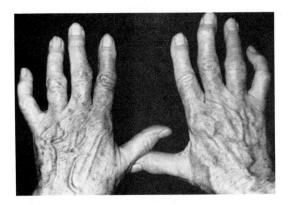

FIG. 15-4 Heberden's nodes and Bouchard's nodes in osteoarthritis.

Patients with hand disabilities may have difficulty cleaning their teeth, and aids such as floss holders or electric toothbrushes may be helpful. Modified toothbrush handles are also recommended to facilitate cleaning.

ORAL AND MAXILLOFACIAL COMPLICATIONS

The TMJ may be affected with OA and may constitute a problem for the patient. As would be expected, most people over the age of 40 show histologic changes in their TMJs, but most have no symptoms. TMJ pain caused by OA, however, is not uncommon.

The usual finding in patients with OA of the TMJ is an insidious onset of unilateral preauricular aching and pain with stiffness after a period of inactivity that decreases with mild activity. Severe pain may be elicited upon wide opening, and pain occurs with normal function and worsens during the day. Adjacent muscle splinting and spasm may occur. Crepitus is a common finding in the affected joint.[3] In most cases osteoarthritic pain in the TMJ will resolve within 8 months of onset.[10] Radiographic changes include altered joint space, remodeling, and osteophytes. Of significance is the lack of correlation of TMJ pain and symptoms with radiographic or histologic signs of osteoarthritis.[3] Treatment consists of aspirin or NSAIDs, muscle relaxants, limiting jaw function, physical therapy (heat, ultrasound, controlled exercise), and occlusal splints to unload the joint.[3] Conservative therapy is successful in many cases; however, should pain and/or dysfunction be severe and persistent, TMJ surgery may be necessary.

Lupus Erythematosus

There are two forms of lupus erythematosus: a form predominantly affecting the skin (discoid; DLE) and a more generalized form affecting many organ systems (systemic; SLE). The discoid form is characterized by chronic, erythematous, scaly plaques on the face, scalp, or ears. Most patients with DLE do not have systemic manifestations. The systemic form of the disease involves the skin as well as many other organ systems and is the more serious form. This chapter will focus on SLE.

GENERAL DESCRIPTION
INCIDENCE AND PREVALENCE

Systemic lupus erythematosus (SLE) is an autoimmune disease that predominantly affects women of childbearing age. Only 10% of cases are seen in men. The disease is more common and severe in blacks, Hispanics, and Asians than in whites.[2,6] The reasons for this distribution are not clear.

ETIOLOGY

The etiology of SLE is unknown although there is agreement that it is an autoimmune disease. Factors that may be involved in its pathogenesis include chronic viral infection, genetic predisposition, and environmental as well as hormonal influences.

PATHOPHYSIOLOGY

The production of pathogenic antibodies and immune complexes, coupled with the failure to suppress them, is the basic abnormality underlying SLE.[6] Thus antibodies are formed in response to some antigenic stimulus and the reaction between antigen and circulating antibodies forms antigen-antibody complexes. These complexes are then deposited in a variety of tissues and organs—including the kidney, skin, blood vessels, muscle and joints, heart, lung, brain, GI tract, lymphatics, and eye. The clinical expression of the disease reflects the organs or tissues involved and the extent of that involvement.

SEQUELAE AND COMPLICATIONS

Because of widespread organ involvement, multiple manifestations are seen. A migratory myalgia and arthritis are seen in most patients but with pain out of proportion to physical findings. Of significant concern is an avascular necrosis that is seen in up to 50% of patients and affects primarily weight-bearing joints such as the femoral head.[18]

Renal manifestations can be especially troublesome. Approximately 50% of patients with SLE have nephritis, which can lead to renal failure.[18] In patients with severe or more active lesions, renal failure is a major cause of death.[6]

Pulmonary abnormalities include pleuritis,

infection, pulmonary edema, pneumonitis, pulmonary hypertension, and diffusing abnormalities.[18] Cardiovascular abnormalities are seen frequently, with pericarditis being most common. Other manifestations include valvular insufficiency and myocardial infarction.

Myocarditis can also occur, resulting in arrhythmias and heart failure. Of particular significance are valvular abnormalities that are found in 50% of SLE patients at autopsy but that are frequently undetectable clinically. These lesions are known as nonbacterial thrombotic endocarditis (NBTE) and result from antigen-antibody complex deposition on the valvular endothelium. They can presumably become a nidus of infection and result in a verrucous endocarditis (Libman-Sacks endocarditis).[18]

Hematologic abnormalities in SLE are quite common and include anemia, leukopenia (which does not appear to predispose to infection), lymphocytopenia, and thrombocytopenia. In addition, 25% of patients with SLE possess an unusual antibody ("lupus anticoagulant") to clotting Factors VIII, IX, XI, XII, and XIII.[17] When it is found in the presence of thrombocytopenia, abnormal bleeding can occur.[12,20]

Vascular changes associated with SLE are thrombosis in capillaries and small vessels and a vasculitis (which can predispose to coronary artery disease). It is thought[6] that the lupus anticoagulant is responsible for this feature.

CLINICAL PRESENTATION
SIGNS AND SYMPTOMS

The classic picture of SLE is that of a young woman with polyarthritis and a butterfly-shaped rash across the nose and cheeks; however, presentation may vary, from mild to severe, and depends largely on the extent and selection of organ involvement. There are many signs and symptoms associated with SLE, none of which are pathognomonic. The diagnosis of SLE is based on criteria suggested by the American Rheumatism Association[21] (Table 15-5). The diagnosis of SLE is made if a patient demonstrates at least 4 of 11 of these criteria.

LABORATORY FINDINGS

The antinuclear antibody test is the best screening device for SLE. It is positive in virtually all patients with SLE.[6,18] Anti-DNA

TABLE 15-5

American Rheumatism Association Criteria for the Diagnosis of Systemic Lupus Erythematosus*

Malar rash	Renal disorder
Discoid rash	Neurologic disorder
Photosensitivity	Hematologic disorder
Oral ulcers	Immunologic disorder
Arthritis	Antinuclear antibody
Pleuritis and pericarditis	

*At least four must be present to make a diagnosis of SLE.

assays, double helix and single helix, also are elevated in 65% to 80% of patients with active untreated SLE.[23] Hematologic abnormalities include a normochromic normocytic anemia, leukopenia, lymphopenia, and thrombocytopenia. The Westergren sedimentation rate is often elevated. With active nephritis, proteinuria will be present as well as hematuria and cellular or granular casts. Other abnormalities include an increased partial thromboplastin time and false-positive serologic tests for syphilis.[6]

MEDICAL MANAGEMENT

There is no cure for SLE; thus all treatment is of a symptomatic or palliative nature. Many of the same drugs that are used in rheumatoid arthritis also are used in the management of SLE (Table 15-3). These include aspirin and nonsteroidal antiinflammatories for mild disease, antimalarials for dermatologic disease, glucocorticoids for more severe symptoms, and cytotoxic agents for symptoms unresponsive to other therapies or as adjuncts in severe disease. Several experimental approaches to therapy are under investigation—such as plasmapheresis, lymph node irradiation, cyclosporine injections, sex hormone therapy, and IV gamma globulin.

DENTAL MANAGEMENT
MEDICAL CONSIDERATIONS

As in rheumatoid arthritis, drug considerations and side effects in SLE are of major significance. Table 15-3 lists the dental and oral considerations with the use of these drugs. The leukopenia that is common in SLE is not associated with a significant increase in infection; however, when combined with chronic corticosteroids or cytotoxic drugs, the likelihood of infection is increased. Therefore, in patients taking corticosteroids or cytotoxins who also have leukopenia, the use of prophylactic antibiotics for periodontal and oral surgical procedures should be considered. Patients taking corticosteroids also may well develop significant adrenal suppression and could require supplementation, especially for extensive procedures or in cases of extreme anxiety. (See Chapter 18.)

Abnormal bleeding is a potential problem in SLE because of thrombocytopenia and abnormalities in some of the clotting factors. A coagulation profile should be obtained, especially noting the platelet count, bleeding time, and partial thromboplastin time. Bleeding times less than 20 minutes and a platelet count greater than 80,000 are indications of adequate platelet activity. Otherwise, abnormalities should be discussed with the physician.

Since cardiac valvular abnormalities are found in 50% of patients with SLE and are generally not clinically detectable, the potential for bacterial endocarditis resulting from dentally induced bacteremias exists. In a small retrospective study of endocarditis in patients with SLE,[15] the prevalence rate of bacterial endocarditis was found to be comparable to that in patients with prosthetic valves and was three times that in patients with rheumatic heart disease. Also, endocarditis is reported[18] to have been regularly observed in patients with SLE. Therefore, prudence suggests that patients with SLE should receive antibiotic prophylaxis for dental treatment likely to result in gingival bleeding. The current American Heart Association regimen for endocarditis prophylaxis is recommended.

Finally, patients with renal failure have the potential for drug interactions, hematologic disorders, and infection. (See Chapter 11 for management recommendations.)

TREATMENT PLANNING CONSIDERATIONS

No specific treatment planning modifications are required. Consideration, however, should be given to physical disabilities secondary to arthritis and myalgias. For patients with SLE the establishment and maintenance of optimum oral health are of paramount importance.

ORAL COMPLICATIONS

Oral lesions of the lip and mucous membranes has been reported to occur in up to 40% to 50% of patients with SLE as well as with DLE.[11,19] The lesions are rather nonspecific and may be erythematous with white spots or radiating peripheral lines and can also demonstrate painful ulcerations. They frequently resemble lichen planus or leukoplakia. When lesions occur on the lip, there may be a silvery scaly margin, similar to that seen on the skin.[11] Skin and lip lesions frequently occur following exposure to the sun. Treatment of these lesions is symptomatic. (See Appendix B.) One should always remain alert to oral eruptions and lesions secondary to any of a variety of the medications used to treat SLE, for they may be a sign of toxicity.

REFERENCES

1. Arnett FC, Edworthy SM, Bloch DA, et al: The American Rheumatism Association 1987 revised criteria for the classification of rheumatoid arthritis, *Arthritis Rheum* 31:315-324, 1988.
2. Arthritis Foundation: *Basic Facts,* Atlanta, 1990, The Foundation.
3. Brandt KD, Kavalov–St John K: Osteoarthritis. In Wilson JD, et al, editors: *Harrison's Principles of internal medicine,* ed 12, New York, 1991, McGraw-Hill.
4. Bulkley BH, Roberts WC: The heart in systemic lupus erythematosus and the changes induced in it by corticosteroid therapy, *Am J Med* 58:243-264, 1975.
5. Golden A, Powell DE, Jennings CD: *Pathology: understanding human disease,* ed 2, Baltimore, 1985, Williams & Wilkins.
6. Hahn BH: Systemic lupus erythematosus. In Wilson JD, et al, editors: *Harrison's Principles of internal medicine,* ed 12, New York, 1991, McGraw-Hill.
7. Harris ED: The clinical features of rheumatoid arthritis. In Kelly WN, et al, editors: *Textbook of rheumatology,* ed 3, Philadelphia, 1989, WB Saunders.
8. Harris ED: Pathogenesis of rheumatoid arthritis. In Kelly WN, et al, editors: *Textbook of rheumatology,* ed 3, Philadelphia, 1989, WB Saunders.
9. Kent JN, Carlton DM, Zide MF: Rheumatoid disease and related arthropathies. II. Surgical rehabilitation of the temporomandibular joint, *Oral Surg* 61:423-439, 1986.
10. Kreutziger KL, Mahan PE: Temporomandibular degenerative joint disease. I, Anatomy, pathophysiology and clinical description, *Oral Surg* 40:165-182, 1975.
11. Langlais RP, Miller CS: *Color atlas of common oral diseases,* Philadelphia, 1992, Lea & Febiger.
12. Laurence J, Nachman R: Hematologic aspects of systemic lupus erythematosis. In Lahita RG, editor:

Systemic lupus erythematosus, New York, 1986, Wiley & Sons.

13. Lightfoot RW: Treatment of rheumatoid arthritis. In McCarty DJ, editor: *Arthritis and allied conditions,* ed 10, Philadelphia, 1985, Lea & Febiger.

14. Lipsky PE: Rheumatoid arthritis. In Wilson JD, et al, editors: *Harrison's Principles of internal medicine,* ed 12, New York, 1991, McGraw-Hill.

15. Luce EB, Montgomery MT, Redding SW: The prevalence of cardiac valvular pathosis in patients with systemic lupus erythematosus, *Oral Surg* 70:590-592, 1990.

16. Mahan PE: The temporomandibular joint in function and pathofunction. In Solberg WK, Clark GT, editors: *Temporomandibular joint problems: biologic diagnosis and treatment,* Chicago, 1980, Quintessence Publishing.

17. Margolius A Jr, Jackson DP, Ratnoff OD: Circulating anticoagulants: a study of 40 cases and a review of the literature, *Medicine* 40:145-202, 1961.

18. Schur PH: Clinical features of SLE. In Kelly WN, et al, editors: *Textbook of rheumatology,* ed 3, Philadelphia, 1989, WB Saunders.

19. Shafer WG, Hine MK, Levy BM: *A textbook of oral pathology,* ed 4, Philadelphia, 1983, WB Saunders.

20. Shoenfeld Y, Schwartz RS: Hematologic manifestations. In Schur PH, editor: *The clinical management of systemic lupus erythematosus,* Orlando, Fla, 1983, Grune & Stratton.

21. Tan EM, Cohen AS, Fries JF, et al: The 1982 revised criteria for the classification of systemic lupus erythematosus, *Arthritis Rheum* 25:1271-1277, 1982.

22. Znaifler NJ: Etiology and pathogenesis of rheumatoid arthritis. In McCarty DJ, editor: *Arthritis and allied conditions,* ed 10, Philadelphia, 1985, Lea & Febiger.

23. Zweiman B, Lisak RP: Autoantibodies: autoimmunity and immune complexes. In Henry JB, editor: *Clinical diagnosis and management by laboratory methods,* ed 18, Philadelphia, 1991, WB Saunders.

16

Neurologic Disorders

Although there are many neurologic diseases, only two of the more common and significant, epilepsy and stroke, are discussed in this chapter. Alzheimer's disease, a closely related disorder, will be covered in Chapter 25.

Epilepsy

Epilepsy is a term that describes a group of disorders characterized by chronic, recurrent, paroxysmal changes in neurologic function (seizures) that are caused by abnormal electrical activity in the brain. Seizures may be either convulsive (i.e., accompanied by motor manifestations) or manifested by other changes in neurologic function (i.e., sensory, cognitive, emotional).[3] In the past much confusion existed about the nature and classification of epilepsy, but recent efforts have increased the understanding of these disorders.

In the 1800s Hughlings Jackson's discourse on epilepsy concluded that "a convulsion is but a symptom, and implies only that there is an occasional, an excessive, and a disorderly discharge of nerve tissue." This has proven accurate; however, it is too limited because there are many other forms of epilepsy besides the tonic-clonic generalized convulsion, many of which are focal, limited, and nonconvulsive. Therefore to redefine an expanded group of related seizure disorders, Sutherland and Eadie[16] proposed the following definition:

Epilepsy should be regarded as a symptom due to excessive temporary neuronal discharging which results from intracranial or extracranial causes. . . .

Epilepsy is characterized by discrete episodes, which tend to be recurrent [and] in which there is a disturbance of movement, sensation, behavior, perception, and/or consciousness.

Further help in understanding the spectrum of epilepsy is afforded by the International League Against Epilepsy,[1] which provided a revised classification of epilepsy in 1981 (Table 16-1). This classification is based on clinical behavior and electroencephalographic changes.

Partial seizures are limited in scope and clinical manifestations and involve motor, sensory, autonomic, or psychic abnormalities. Partial seizures are considered *simple* if consciousness is preserved and *complex* if consciousness is impaired. Generalized seizures—more global in scope and manifestation—involve an altered-consciousness state and frequently abnormal motor activity. Discussion in this section will be limited to generalized tonic-clonic seizures (idiopathic grand mal), since these represent the most severe expression of epilepsy that the dentist is likely to encounter.

GENERAL DESCRIPTION
INCIDENCE AND PREVALENCE

It is estimated[6] that 10% of the population will have at least one epileptic seizure in its lifetime and that the overall incidence rate is 0.5%. Seizures are most common during childhood, with as many as 4% of children having at least one seizure during the first 15 years of life. Fortunately, most children outgrow the disorder.[4]

The etiology of epilepsy is known in many patients. Common causes include head trauma, intracranial neoplasm, hypoglycemia, drug with-

TABLE 16-1
Classification of Epileptic Seizures

Partial (focal, local)

Simple partial seizures
Complex partial seizures
Partial seizures evolving to generalized
  tonic-clonic convulsions

Generalized (convulsive or nonconvulsive)

Absence seizures (petit mal)
Atypical absence seizures
Myclonic seizures
Clonic seizures
Tonic-clonic seizures (grand mal)
Tonic seizures
Atonic seizures
Unclassified epileptic seizures

From Commission on Classification and Terminology of the International League Against Epilepsy. *Epilepsia* 22: 489–501, 1981.

drawal, and febrile illness. Many patients, however, have epilepsy for which there is no known cause. This is termed *idiopathic epilepsy*.

Although the underlying cause of idiopathic generalized epilepsy is unknown, seizures can sometimes be evoked by a specific stimulus. Approximately 1 out of 15 patients reports that seizures follow exposure to a specific circumstance—such as flickering lights, monotonous sounds, music, or a loud noise. Of interest have been reports[2] of epileptic seizures in youngsters exposed to flickering lights and geometric patterns while playing video games.

PATHOPHYSIOLOGY

The basic event underlying an epileptic seizure is an excessive focal neuronal discharge that spreads to thalamic and brainstem nuclei. The cause of this abnormal electrical activity is not precisely known, although a number of theories have been proposed as explanations.[3,6,16] These include altered neuronal membrane potentials, altered synaptic transmission, diminution of inhibitory neurons, increased neuronal excitability, and decreased electrical threshold for epileptic activity.

A curious feature is that no specific type of brain lesion is absolutely correlated with epileptic seizures. In other words, the same lesion

in the same location of the brain may be epileptogenic in one patient but not in another. In fact, in many cases there is no identifiable lesion at all, which would seem to suggest an abnormality at the biochemical level.

SEQUELAE AND COMPLICATIONS

Approximately 60% to 80% of patients with epilepsy will achieve complete control over their seizures; the remainder will achieve only partial or poor control.[3,13]

A significant problem with epileptic patients is one of compliance (i.e., making sure that patients take their medication as directed). This problem is common to many chronic disorders, such as hypertension, because the patients may have to take medication for the rest of their lives even though they remain asymptomatic.

Another problem relating to anticonvulsant drugs is toxicity. Common examples are phenytoin-induced ataxia and phenobarbital-induced drowsiness. If a patient has frequent and severe seizures, there also may be altered mental function, resulting in dullness, confusion, or argumentativeness.

A common complication associated with phenytoin is gingival hyperplasia. This may occur in varying degrees and may become extensive enough to require surgical reduction. It is most common in children and adolescents.

The most serious acute complication of epilepsy (especially tonic-clonic) is the occurrence of repeated seizures over a short time without a recovery period. This is called status epilepticus, and it constitutes a medical emergency. Patients may become seriously hypoxic and acidotic during this event and suffer permanent brain damage or death.

CLINICAL PRESENTATION
SIGNS AND SYMPTOMS

The clinical manifestations of generalized tonic-clonic convulsions (grand mal seizure) are classic. The patient emits a sudden cry (caused by spasm of the diaphragmatic muscles) and immediately loses consciousness. The tonic phase consists of generalized muscle rigidity, followed by clonic activity that consists of uncoordinated beating movements of the limbs and head. Incontinence of urine or feces may occur. Movement ceases, and the person becomes comatose. Then, within a few minutes, there is a gradual return of consciousness, with stupor, headache, and confusion. Once the seizure has begun, the jaws and teeth are clamped tightly and cannot be pried apart. Jaw relaxation occurs only with termination of the seizure.

LABORATORY FINDINGS

Once the diagnosis of idiopathic epilepsy has been established, laboratory analysis is of little help. There are no characteristic findings associated with the disorder except for changes seen on the electroencephalogram (EEG). Each phase of the convulsion is associated with characteristic spike and wave patterns on the EEG. Even during intervals between seizures, many patients will demonstrate an abnormal EEG. It should be noted, however, that the EEG is not absolutely conclusive in making the diagnosis.

MEDICAL MANAGEMENT

The medical management of epilepsy is based on drug therapy. Phenytoin (Dilantin) is the anticonvulsant drug that is still most commonly used as a first line of treatment; however, there are several other drugs in common use. Table 16-2 is a list of the more commonly used drugs for control of generalized tonic-clonic epilepsy. Attempts are made to use single-drug therapy to

TABLE 16-2

Anticonvulsants Used in the Management of Generalized Tonic-Clonic (Grand Mal) Seizures

Generic name	Trade name	Usual daily adult dose (mg)	Drug interactions	Dental considerations
Phenytoin	Dilantin	300 to 400	—	Gingival hyperplasia, increased incidence of microbial infections, delayed healing, gingival bleeding (leukopenia)
Carbemazepine	Tegretol	600 to 1200	Propoxyphene, erythromycin	Xerostomia, increased incidence of microbial infection, delayed healing, gingival bleeding (leukopenia and thrombocytopenia)
Phenobarbital	Luminal	60 to 120	—	—
Valproic acid	Depakene	750 to 1250	Aspirin, NSAIDs	Excessive bleeding and petechiae, decreased platelet aggregation, increased incidence of microbial infection, delayed healing, gingival bleeding (leukopenia and thrombocytopenia)

avoid adverse drug interactions and facilitate compliance. Unfortunately, it is frequently necessary to use combination therapy.

DENTAL MANAGEMENT
MEDICAL CONSIDERATIONS

The first step in the management of an epileptic dental patient is identification. This is best accomplished by the medical history and discussion with the patient or family members. Once an epileptic patient is identified, it is important to learn as much as possible about the seizure history—including type of seizures, age at onset, cause if known, current medications, frequency of physician visits, degree of seizure

TABLE 16-3
Dental Management of the Epileptic Patient

1. Identification of patient by history
   a. Type of seizure
   b. Age at time of onset
   c. Cause of seizures (if known)
   d. Medications
   e. Frequency of physician visits (name and phone number)
   f. Degree of seizure control
   g. Frequency of seizures
   h. Date of last seizure
   i. Known precipitating factors
   j. History of seizure-related injuries
2. Provide normal care—well-controlled seizures pose no management problems
3. If questionable history or poorly controlled seizures, consult with physician before dental treatment—may require modification of medications
4. Be alert to adverse effects of anticonvulsants
   a. Drowsiness
   b. Slow mentation
   c. Dizziness
   d. Ataxia
   e. Gastrointestinal upset
   f. Allergic signs (rash, erythema multiforme)
5. Patients taking valproic acid (Depakene) may have bleeding tendencies because of platelet interference—order pretreatment bleeding time; if grossly abnormal, consult with physician
6. Be prepared to manage grand mal seizure
   a. Chair back in supported supine position
   b. Patient turned to side (to avoid aspiration)
   c. Do not attempt to use padded tongue blade

control, frequency of seizures, date of last seizure, and any known precipitating factors. In addition, a history of previous injuries associated with seizures and their treatment may be helpful (Table 16-3).

Fortunately, most epileptic patients are able to attain good control of their seizures with anticonvulsant drugs and are therefore able to receive normal routine dental care. In some instances, however, the history may reveal a degree of seizure activity that suggests noncompliance or a severe seizure disorder that does not respond to anticonvulsants. For these patients a consultation with the physician is advised before dental treatment is rendered. A patient with poorly controlled disease may require additional anticonvulsant or sedative medication, as directed by the physician.

Patients who are taking anticonvulsants may suffer from the toxic effects of these drugs, and the dentist must always be sensitive to their manifestations. Among the more common adverse effects are drowsiness, slow mentation, dizziness, ataxia, and gastrointestinal upset. Occasionally, allergy may be seen as a rash or an erythema multiforme–like reaction.

Phenytoin, carbemazepine, and valproic acid all can cause leukopenia and/or thrombocytopenia—resulting in an increased incidence of microbial infection, delayed healing, and gingival bleeding.[5] In addition, valproic acid can cause decreased platelet aggregation, lending to spontaneous hemorrhage and petechiae.[10]

Propoxyphene and erythromycin should not be administered to patients taking carbemazepine because of interference with metabolism of carbemazepine, which could lead to toxicity. Aspirin and nonsteroidal antiinflammatory drugs (NSAIDs) (Table 15-3) should not be administered to patients taking valproic acid; they can further decrease platelet aggregation, leading to hemorrhagic episodes.[5]

Seizure management

In spite of appropriate preventive measures taken by the dentist and patient, there is always the possibility that an epileptic patient may have a generalized tonic-clonic convulsion in the dental office. The dentist and staff should always anticipate this occurrence and be prepared to deal with it.

The primary task of management is to protect

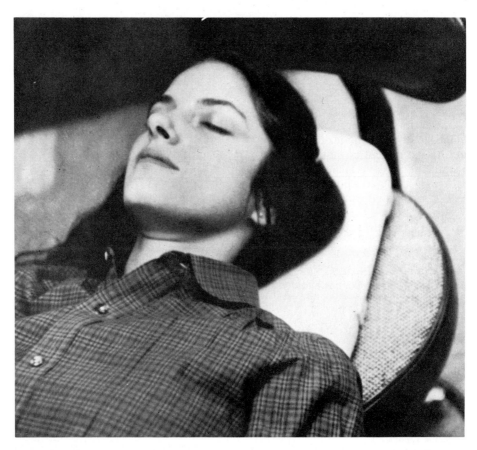

FIG. 16-1 Dental chair in the supine position with the back supported by the operator or the assistant's stool.

the patient and try to prevent injury. If the patient has a seizure while in the dental chair, no attempt should be made to move him or her to the floor. Instead, the chair should be placed in a supported supine position (Fig. 16-1) and the patient should, if possible, be turned to the side to control the airway and minimize aspiration of secretions. No attempt should be made to restrain or hold the patient down. Passive restraint should be used only to prevent injury from hitting nearby objects or from falling out of the chair.

One often is counseled to place a padded tongue blade between the teeth to prevent tongue biting. In reality, this is nearly an impossible task once the seizure has begun, and it may damage the teeth or oral soft tissue.

Therefore it is not advised. An exception to this would be if the patient senses a pending seizure and can cooperate. In this case a padded tongue blade or folded towel may be placed between the teeth before they are clenched.

Seizures generally do not last more than a few minutes. Afterwards the patient will fall into a deep sleep from which he or she cannot be aroused. Then in a few minutes the patient will gradually regain consciousness but may be confused, disoriented, and embarrassed. Headache is a prominent feature of this period.

No further treatment should be attempted, although any injuries sustained (e.g., lacerations or fractures) should receive immediate attention (Fig. 16-2). In the event of avulsed or fractured teeth or a fractured appliance, an

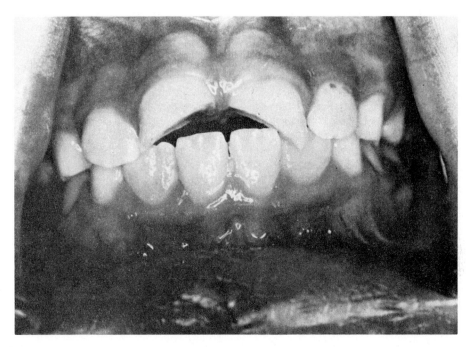

FIG. 16-2 Fractured teeth sustained during a grand mal seizure. (Courtesy G. Ferretti, D.M.D., Lexington Ky.)

attempt should be made to locate the tooth or fragments to rule out aspiration. A chest radiograph may be required to locate a missing fragment or tooth.

In the event a seizure becomes prolonged or is repeated (status epilepticus), intravenous diazepam, 10 mg, is effective in controlling it. However, measures for respiratory support should be available since respiratory function may be depressed postictally.

TREATMENT PLANNING CONSIDERATIONS

Because gingival hyperplasia is associated with phenytoin administration, every effort should be made to maintain a patient at an optimum level of oral hygiene. This may require frequent visits for monitoring progress.

If significant hyperplasia exists, surgical reduction will be necessary; however, this must be accomplished by an increased awareness of oral hygiene needs and a positive commitment by the patient to maintain oral cleanliness.

A missing tooth or teeth should be replaced if possible to prevent the tongue from being caught in the edentulous space during a seizure (as commonly happens). Generally, a fixed prosthesis is preferable to a removable one. The removable prosthesis is more easily dislodged. For fixed prostheses, all-metal units should be considered when possible to minimize the chance of fracture. When placing anterior castings, the dentist may wish to consider using three-quarter crowns or retentive acrylic facings in lieu of porcelain to facilitate repair if fracture occurs.

Removable prostheses are, nevertheless, sometimes constructed for epileptic patients. Metallic palates and bases are preferable to all-acrylic ones. If acrylic is used, it should be reinforced with a wire mesh.

ORAL COMPLICATIONS

The most significant oral complication seen in epileptic patients is gingival hyperplasia associated with phenytoin (Fig. 16-3). The incidence of this in epileptics is difficult to ascertain because of the variable criteria used in studies;

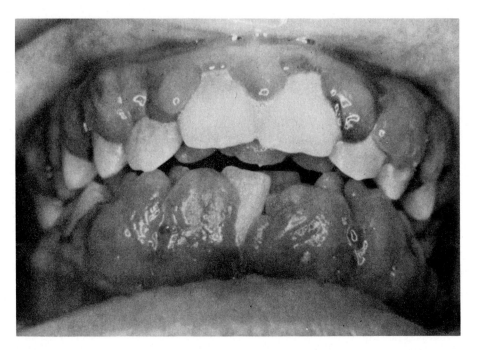

FIG. 16-3   Phenytoin-induced gingival hyperplasia. (Courtesy H. Abrams, D.D.S., Lexington Ky.)

reported incidences range from 0% to 100%, with an average of approximately 42%.[9] There seems to be a greater tendency for youngsters than for adults to develop hyperplasia. The anterior labial surfaces of the maxillary and mandibular gingivae are most commonly and severely affected.

Some disagreement exists in the literature as to the relationship between drug dosage and severity of hyperplasia, but the majority of studies do not support a statistically valid connection.

Another area of controversy is the effectiveness of oral hygiene in preventing gingival hyperplasia; however, the preponderance of evidence[7,9,15] suggests that meticulous oral hygiene will prevent or significantly decrease its severity. Good home care must always be combined with the removal of irritants—such as overhanging restorations and calculus. Frequently, hyperplastic tissues will become large enough to interfere with function or appearance, and surgical reduction will become necessary.

Stroke

A stroke (cerebrovascular accident, apoplexy, CVA) is a serious and often fatal event that is the end result of long-standing cerebrovascular disease. Even if a stroke is not fatal, the survivor is to some degree debilitated in motor function, speech, or mentation. The scope and gravity of stroke are reflected in the fact that stroke is the third most common cause of death in the United States (behind heart disease and cancer) and 5% of the population over age 65 has had one.[12]

GENERAL DESCRIPTION
INCIDENCE AND PREVALENCE

Stroke is a generic term used to refer to the acute development of neurologic deficit caused by cerebrovascular disease. A stroke results from the focal necrosis of brain tissue, which is due to interruption of the cerebral blood supply. There are many forms of cerebrovascular disease that can result in stroke, but the most common are atherosclerosis, hypertensive vascular disease, and cardiac pathosis (myocardial infarction, atrial fibrillation).[17] The actual interruption of blood supply is most commonly caused by thrombosis of a cerebral vessel. Other common causes of the interruption of cerebral blood flow include cerebral embolism and intracranial hemorrhage. Although the incidence of stroke has declined, it still remains as one of the most significant health problems in the United States today.

EPIDEMIOLOGY

Epidemiologic investigations have identified susceptible persons and associated risk factors that predispose to stroke. Included among these are the occurrence of transient ischemic attacks (TIAs) or a previous stroke. Also included are individuals with hypertension, cardiac abnormalities, atherosclerosis, diabetes mellitus, or elevated blood lipid levels and persons who smoke. Other, less well-documented, possible risk factors include physical inactivity and stress.

PATHOPHYSIOLOGY

The pathologic changes associated with stroke are infarction, intracerebral hemorrhage, and subarachnoid hemorrhage.

Cerebral infarctions are most commonly caused by either atherosclerotic thrombi or emboli of cardiac origin (Fig. 16-4). The extent of an infarction is determined by a number of factors—including site of the occlusion, size of the occluded vessel, duration of the occlusion, and collateral circulation.[14] Neurologic abnormalities depend on the artery involved and its area of supply.

The most common cause of intracerebral hemorrhage is hypertensive atherosclerosis, which results in microaneurysms of the arterioles. Rupture of these microaneurysms within brain tissue leads to extravasation of blood, which displaces brain tissue and causes increased intracranial volume until the resulting tissue compression halts bleeding[14] (Fig. 16-5).

The most common cause of subarachnoid hemorrhage is rupture of a saccular aneurysm at the bifurcation of a major cerebral artery.

SEQUELAE AND COMPLICATIONS

The most serious outcome of stroke is death, occurring in 47% of patients within a month of the event. Mortality rates are directly related to the type of stroke[17]—with 80% dying after an intracerebral hemorrhage, 50% after a subarachnoid hemorrhage, and 30% after occlusion of a major vessel by a thrombus. It should be noted that death from a stroke may not be immediate (sudden death) but rather may occur hours, days, or even weeks after the initial stroke episode.

If the victim survives, there is an excellent chance that a neurologic deficit or disability of varying degree and duration will remain. Of those surviving the stroke, 10% recover with no impairment, 40% have a mild residual disability, 40% are disabled and require special services, and 10% require institutionalization.[11] The deficit is directly dependent on the size and location of the infarct or hemorrhage. Deficits include unilateral paralysis, numbness, sensory impairment, dysphasia, blindness, diplopia, dizziness, and dysarthria.

Return of function is unpredictable and usually takes place slowly, over several months. Even with improvement, patients are frequently left with some permanent residual problem— such as difficulty in walking, using the hands, performing skilled acts, or speaking.

CLINICAL PRESENTATION
SIGNS AND SYMPTOMS

Familiarity with the warning signs and symptoms of stroke can lead to appropriate action that may be lifesaving. In many cases strokes are preceded by "minor strokes," or TIAs. These usually last less than 10 minutes and may be manifest dizziness, diplopia, hemiplegia, or speech disturbances. Most commonly a major stroke is preceded by one or two TIAs within a day to a week of the first attack.[17]

Warning signs of stroke include the following:
1. Sudden and temporary weakness or numbness of the face, arm, or leg on one side of the body
2. Temporary loss of speech or trouble in speaking or understanding speech
3. Temporary dimness or loss of vision, particularly in one eye (could be confused with migraine)
4. Unexplained dizziness, unsteadiness, or a sudden fall

Although these are classic manifestations of stroke, they are not pathognomonic. A differential diagnosis would include diabetes mellitus,

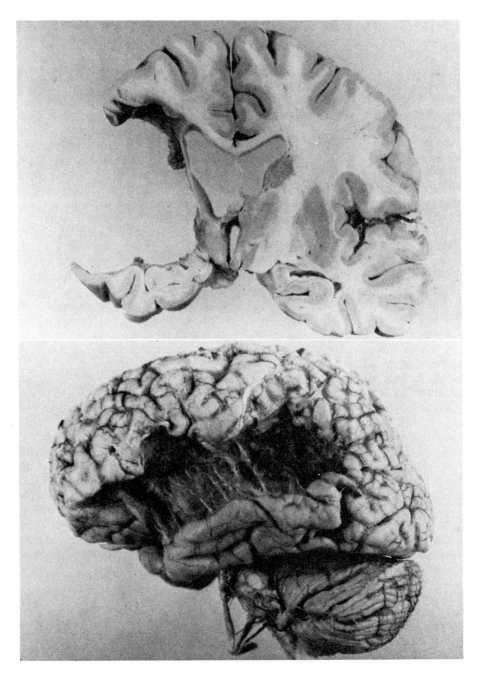

FIG. 16-4 Old cerebral infarction.

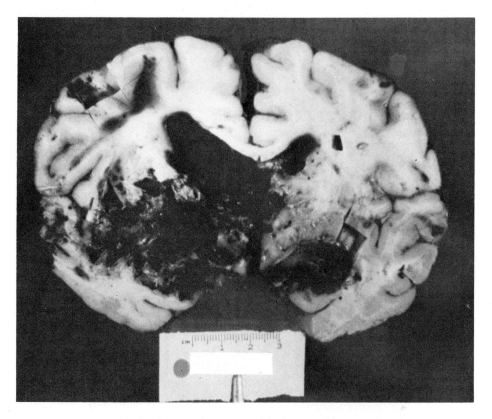

FIG. 16-5   Cerebral hemorrhage caused by hypertensive vascular disease.

uremia, abscess, tumor, acute alcoholism, drug poisoning, and extradural hemorrhage.[17] History and physical examination serve to make the correct diagnosis.

LABORATORY FINDINGS

Patients suspected of having had a stroke are usually submitted to a variety of laboratory tests—including urinalysis, blood sugar level, complete blood count, erythrocyte sedimentation rate, serologic tests for syphilis, blood cholesterol and lipid levels, chest radiographs, and electrocardiogram. Various abnormalities may be disclosed by these test results, depending on the type and severity of stroke as well as its causative factors. A lumbar puncture may also be ordered by the physician in an effort to check for blood or protein in the cerebrospinal fluid and for altered CSF pressure.[12,17]

A variety of neuroradiologic procedures may be performed—including arteriography, computed tomography (CT scan), and nuclear magnetic resonance (NMR) examination of the brain (Fig. 16-6).

MEDICAL MANAGEMENT

The first aspect of stroke management is prevention. This is accomplished by identifying risk factors in individuals (e.g., hypertension, diabetes, atherosclerosis, cigarette smoking) and then attempting to reduce or eliminate as many of these as possible. Antiplatelet therapy and carotid endarterectomy are methods of preventive treatment in some patients with a TIA.

If a patient has a stroke, treatment is generally threefold.

1. The immediate task is to sustain life during the period immediately following the

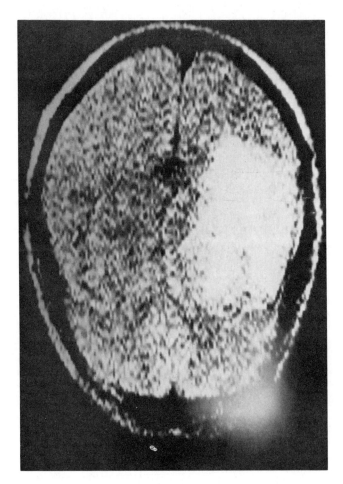

FIG. 16-6   NMR scan of the brain, demonstrating edema. (Courtesy L.R. Bean, D.D.S., Lexington Ky.)

stroke. This is done by means of life-support measures.

2. The second task is to prevent further thrombosis or hemorrhage. No therapy has been proven to reverse or restore damage already done; therefore treatment is by necessity of a prophylactic nature.

   a. Anticoagulant therapy is instituted in cases of thrombosis or embolism. Medications such as heparin, coumarin, aspirin, and dipyridamole (Persantine) are commonly used. Heparin is administered acutely whereas coumarin, dipyridamole, and aspirin are employed for prolonged periods.

   b. Corticosteroids may also be used acutely after a stroke to reduce the cerebral edema that accompanies cerebral infarction. This can markedly lessen complications.

   c. Surgical intervention may be indicated for removal of a superficial hematoma or management of a vascular obstruction. The latter is usually accomplished by thromboendarterectomy or by bypass grafts in the neck or thorax.

3. If the patient survives and prevention therapy is instituted, the third and final task is rehabilitation. This is generally accomplished by intense physical therapy

TABLE 16-4
Dental Management of the Stroke Patient

1. Identification of risk factors
   a. Hypertension
   b. Diabetes mellitus
   c. Coronary atherosclerosis
   d. Elevated blood cholesterol or lipid levels
   e. Cigarette smoking
   f. Transient ischemic attack (TIA) or previous stroke
2. Encouragement to control risk factors — refer to physician if appropriate
3. History of stroke
   a. Having had a stroke places patient at high risk for having another — caution
   b. Patient with TIAs — no elective care
   c. Anticoagulant drugs predispose to bleeding problems
      1. Aspirin or dipyridamole — pretreatment bleeding time less than 20 minutes
      2. Coumarin — pretreatment prothrombin time less than 35 seconds
   d. Short stress-free, morning appointments
   e. Monitor blood pressure
   f. Use minimum amount of anesthetic with vasoconstrictor
   g. No epinephrine in retraction cord

and (if indicated) speech therapy. Although marked improvement is common, many patients are left with some degree of permanent deficit.

DENTAL MANAGEMENT
MEDICAL CONSIDERATIONS

Some primary tasks of the dentist are stroke prevention and identification of the stroke-prone individual. Patients with a history of hypertension, diabetes mellitus, coronary atherosclerosis, elevated blood cholesterol or lipid levels, or cigarette smoking are predisposed to stroke as well as to myocardial infarction. The dentist should encourage these individuals to seek medical care and to eliminate or control all possible risk factors (Table 16-4).

A patient who has had a stroke or TIA is at greater risk for having another than a person who has not had one.[17] These individuals should be approached with a degree of caution. A patient suffering TIAs should not receive elective dental care. Medical consultation and referral to a physician are mandatory.

A patient taking coumarin or antiplatelet drugs is at risk for abnormal bleeding. The status of coumarin anticoagulation may be monitored by the prothrombin time. A level 2½ times normal or less (normal being 11 to 14 seconds) is acceptable for performing surgical procedures. If the prothrombin time is greater than 35 seconds, this may result in significantly abnormal hemostasis, and the physician should be consulted to decrease the dosage of the anticoagulant.

The effect of aspirin or dipyridamole on platelet aggregation is monitored by the bleeding time. Any BT greater than 10 minutes has the potential for a slightly increased risk of bleeding during the procedure; however, this risk does not become significant until the BT exceeds 20 minutes.[8] Abnormal results should be discussed with the physician.

Management of stroke-prone patients or patients with a history of stroke includes the use of short morning appointments that are as stress-free as possible. Blood pressure should be monitored to ensure good control. Pain control is important. Nitrous oxide may be given if good oxygenation is maintained at all times. A local anesthetic with 1:100,000 or 1:200,000 epinephrine may be used in judicious amounts (6 ml or less). Gingival retraction cord impregnated with epinephrine should not be used.

TREATMENT PLANNING MODIFICATIONS

Technical modifications may be required for patients with residual physical deficits that may make adequate oral hygiene difficult if not impossible. For these patients, extensive bridgework is not a good choice. All restorations should be placed with ease of cleansability in mind. Hygiene may be facilitated by an electric toothbrush, a large-handled toothbrush, or a water irrigation device. Flossing aids should also be prescribed. Frequent professional prophylaxis is advisable.

ORAL COMPLICATIONS

No specific oral findings are associated with stroke.

REFERENCES

1. Commission on Classification and Terminology of the International League Against Epilepsy: Proposal for revised clinical and electroencephalographic classification of epileptic seizures, *Epilepsia* 22:489-501, 1981.
2. Dalquist NR, Mellinger JF, Klass DW: Hazard of video games in patients with light-sensitive epilepsy, *JAMA* 249:776-777, 1983.
3. Dichter MA: The epilepsies and convulsive disorders. In Wilson JD, et al, editors: *Harrison's Principles of internal medicine,* ed 12, New York, 1991, McGraw-Hill, pp 1968-1977.
4. Dodson WE, Prensky AL, DeVivo DC, et al: Management of seizure disorders: selected aspects. I, *J Pediatr* 89:527-540, 1976.
5. *Drug information for the health care professional,* ed 11, Rockville Md, 1991, U.S. Pharmacopeial Convention.
6. Engel J: The epilepsies. In Wyngaarden JB, Smith LH, Bennett JC, editors: *Cecil textbook of medicine,* vol 2, ed 19, Philadelphia, 1992, WB Saunders.
7. Hall WB: Dilantin hyperplasia: a preventable lesion? *Compendium* (suppl) 14:5502-5505, 1990.
8. Handin RI: Bleeding and thrombosis. In Wilson JD, et al, editors: *Harrison's Principles of internal medicine,* ed 12, New York, 1991, McGraw-Hill.
9. Hassell TM: Epilepsy and the oral manifestations of phenytoin therapy. In Myers HM, editor: *Monographs in oral science,* vol 9, Basel, 1981, S Karger, pp 116-202.
10. Hassell TM, White GC II, Jewson LG, Peele LC III: Valproic acid: a new antiepileptic drug with potential side effects of dental concern, *J Am Dent Assoc* 99(6):983-987, 1979.
11. *1990 Heart and stroke facts.* Publ. no. 55-0376, Dallas, 1989, American Heart Association.
12. Kistler JP, Ropper AA, Martin JB: Cerebrovascular diseases. In Wilson JD, et al, editors: *Harrison's Principles of internal medicine,* ed 12, New York, 1991, McGraw-Hill.
13. Leppik IE: Antiepileptic medications, *Compendium* (suppl) 14:5490-5496, 1990.
14. Markesbery WR: The central nervous system. In Golden A, et al, editors: *Pathology. Understanding human disease,* ed 2, Baltimore, 1985, Williams & Wilkins.
15. Philstrom BL: Prevention and treatment of dilantin-associated gingival enlargement, *Compendium* (suppl) 14:5506-5510, 1990.
16. Sutherland JM, Eadie MJ: *The epilepsies: modern diagnosis and treatment,* ed 3, Edinburgh, 1980, Churchill Livingstone.
17. Toole JF: Vascular diseases. In Rowland LP, editor: *Merritt's Textbook of neurology,* ed 8, Philadelphia, 1989, Lea & Febiger.

17

Diabetes

Diabetes mellitus is a disease complex with metabolic and vascular components. The metabolic component involves the elevation of blood glucose associated with alterations in a lipid protein metabolism resulting from a relative or absolute lack of insulin. The vascular component includes an accelerated onset of nonspecific atherosclerosis and a more specific microangiopathy that particularly affects the eyes and kidneys.

In 1975 the American Diabetic Association classified diabetes as shown in Table 17-1. There were problems with this classification from several standpoints, however, primarily that it did not consider that juvenile or early-onset diabetes can be found in both children and adults and that adult or late-onset diabetes can be found in children.

In 1979 the National Diabetes Data Group[16] proposed a new classification for diabetes mellitus and related conditions. This classification, now in general use in the United States, is shown in Table 17-2. Its terminology will be used for this chapter.

Diabetes mellitus is of great importance to dentists because they are in a position, as members of the health care team, to detect new cases of diabetes. They must also be able to render dental care to patients who are already being treated for diabetes without endangering their lives.

The purpose of this chapter is to review the pathogenesis of diabetes, the detection of patients with undiagnosed diabetes, the referral of these patients to a physician for medical diagnosis and treatment, and the management of diabetic patients receiving dental treatment.

GENERAL DESCRIPTION
INCIDENCE AND PREVALENCE

There are over 200 million people in the world with diabetes mellitus. In the United States about 15 to 20 million persons have diabetes, which represents some 2% to 4% of the population. About half these people are unaware that they are diabetic. An estimated 11.2% of the general population in the United States has impaired glucose tolerance.[10] The cumulative incidence from birth to age 70 in a study of individuals in Rochester, Minnesota,[14] was 10.5 per 1000 for insulin-dependent diabetes mellitus (IDDM) and 100.3 per 1000 for non–insulin-dependent diabetes (NIDDM). In a span of 1 year, 6 to 25 individuals out of every 100,000 healthy persons developed diabetes and required insulin therapy. There were two peaks for the onset of IDDM found in the Rochester study; the first occurred at ages 10 to 19, and the second at ages 60 to 69.[14]

The incidence of IDDM has increased severalfold in children and teenagers during the past 30 years.[14] The distribution of NIDDM increases from 8 per 100,000 at age 15 to 163 per 100,000 at age 65. This rise in the distribution of NIDDM shows the powerful effect that age has on the disease.

Diabetes mellitus is the third leading cause of death in the United States and accounts for about 40,000 deaths per year. Twenty-five percent of all new cases of end-stage renal disease result from diabetes mellitus, and over 20,000 amputations per year are performed on patients with diabetes mellitus, which represents nearly 50% of all nontraumatic amputations.[18,26]

IDDM, or type I diabetes, rarely occurs

TABLE 17-1
Prior Classification of Diabetes by the American Diabetic Association, 1975

1. Hereditary, primary, or idiopathic diabetes
   a. Prediabetes
   b. Subclinical, latent, or stress diabetes
   c. Chemical diabetes
   d. Overt or clinical diabetes
      Juvenile or early-onset diabetes
      Maturity, adult, or late-onset diabetes
2. Nonhereditary, secondary diabetes
   a. Damage to or removal of pancreatic islet tissue
   b. Disorders of other endocrine glands
   c. Drugs or chemicals

From National Diabetes Data Group: *Diabetes* 28:1039–1057, 1979. Reproduced with permission of the American Diabetes Association Inc.

TABLE 17-2
Current Classification of Diabetes, National Diabetes Data Group, 1979

1. Diabetes mellitus
   a. Type I—insulin-dependent diabetes mellitus (IDDM)
   b. Type II—non–insulin-dependent diabetes mellitus (NIDDM)
   c. Type III—other types of diabetes
      Pancreatic disease
      Hormonal disease
      Drugs—thiazide diuretics, lithium salts
      Others
2. Impaired glucose tolerance (IGT)
   a. Nonobese IGT
   b. Obese IGT
   c. IGT associated with other conditions
      Pancreatic disease
      Hormonal disease
      Drugs
3. Gestational diabetes mellitus (GDM)
4. Previous abnormality of glucose tolerance (pre-AGT)
5. Potential abnormalities of glucose tolerance (pot-AGT)

From National Diabetes Data Group: *Diabetes* 28:1039–1057, 1979. Reproduced with permission of the American Diabetes Association Inc.

among the Chinese, Japanese, and Eskimos. The country with the highest prevalence is Finland (2.6 cases per 1000). The prevalence in the United States is about 1.89 cases per 1000 population. The incidence of IDDM in the United States has been increasing in the last 30 years.[8,10,26] NIDDM, or type II diabetes, is most common in the white population of North America, Europe, and Australia—with a prevalence of 10 to 100 per 1000 population. Since 1935 the incidence of NIDDM has been increasing in the United States.[8]

The number of cases of diabetes in the United States will continue to rise because (1) the population is increasing, (2) the life expectancy is increasing, (3) the number of people with obesity is increasing, and (4) persons with diabetes are living longer (because of better medical management) and are having more children who will pass on the disease.

A dental practice serving an adult population of 2000 can expect to encounter 40 to 80 persons with diabetes, about half of whom will be unaware of their condition.

ETIOLOGY

Diabetes mellitus may occur as a result of any of the following[3,10,14,20,27]: (1) a "genetic" disorder; (2) the primary destruction of islet cells by inflammation, cancer, or surgery; (3) an endocrine condition such as hyperpituitarism or hyperthyroidism; or (4) an iatrogenic disease following the administration of steroids. In this chapter the discussion will be limited to the "genetic" type of diabetes, which also has been termed *primary, hereditary,* or *essential diabetes* (Table 17-2).

There are two types of genetic diabetes: IDDM (type I) and NIDDM (type II). Both types appear to have a genetic component involved in their origin; however, the genetic role in NIDDM is much greater than in IDDM. In addition to a weak genetic role in IDDM, other environmental factors such as viral infections and autoimmune reactions appear to play important parts in its etiology. Studies of identical twins[18,26] have shown that if one twin has developed IDDM the other twin has only about a 50% chance of becoming diabetic, but if one identical twin develops NIDDM the other has a 100% chance of also developing it. Obesity plays an important but not well-understood part in the etiology of NIDDM.[18,26]

Diabetes mellitus appears to have multiple causes and several mechanisms of transmission. It can be thought of as a combination of diseases that share the cardinal clinical feature of glucose intolerance.[3,19,27]

It is estimated[18] that each year about 1% to 5% of individuals with impaired glucose tolerance (IGT) will develop clinical diabetes. Individuals with IGT have an increased risk for death secondary to atherosclerosis; however, they do not develop microvascular lesions in the retina or kidney as do individuals with overt diabetes mellitus.[18]

The onset of IGT or clinical diabetes during pregnancy is termed *gestational diabetes mellitus* (GDM). These patients usually return to "normal" following the birth of the child but have an increased risk of developing diabetes within 5 to 10 years. In addition, GDM carries an increased risk for loss of the fetus.

Several groups of patients fit into the classification *previous abnormality of glucose tolerance* (pre-AGT): patients who have had gestational diabetes, formerly obese individuals who have lost weight, patients with hyperglycemia following myocardial infarction, and patients with posttraumatic hyperglycemia.

Patients who have never had an abnormal glucose tolerance test but who are by genetic background at increased risk of developing diabetes mellitus fit into the *potential abnormalities of glucose tolerance* (pot-AGT) classification.

Patients with clinical signs and symptoms of diabetes mellitus may have IDDM, NIDDM, or type III diabetes. These individuals will show an elevation of the fasting blood glucose, abnormal glucose tolerance test, and microangiopathy.

Type I diabetes (IDDM) usually has a sudden onset of clinical symptoms and is usually found in individuals under 40 years of age; it may, however, occur at any age (Table 17-3). NIDDM generally occurs after the age of 40 in obese individuals. Its incidence increases with age, and insulin secretion may be low, normal, or high. Although most persons with NIDDM are able to secrete insulin, they have decreased numbers of insulin receptors in target cells and decreased postreceptor activity.[26]

The onset of diabetes mellitus in children is

TABLE 17-3

Hereditary Probability of Developing Type II Diabetes in Members of Families

Family member A	Family member B	Chance of developing diabetes mellitus (%)
Parent	Parent	85
Parent	Grandparent, aunt, uncle	60
Parent	First cousin	40
Parent		20
One grandparent		14
One first cousin		9

From Saadoun AP: *Periodont Abstr* 28:116–137, 1980.

usually preceded by a sudden growth spurt. These children have advanced height, bone age, and dental age at the time of onset of the disease compared with nondiabetic siblings. Puberty also appears earlier. In about 30% of patients with IDDM a short period of remission may occur but rarely exceeds 1 year.[3,18,26]

The etiology of IDDM has a weak genetic component. Studies[7,10] have shown that a person's susceptibility to IDDM is linked to the presence of certain genetically determined cell surface antigens found on lymphocytes. Major histocompatibility complex genes of the class II type appear to be involved in the etiology of type I diabetes. Ninety-five percent of whites with IDDM express HLA alleles DR3 or DR4 or the heterozygous DR3/DR4. There is now little doubt that the HLA-D region is somehow involved in the susceptibility to type I diabetes.[7,10]

Individuals who are HLA-identical to a sibling with type I diabetes have a 5% to 20% chance of developing the disease. This is somewhat less than the 50% chance for identical twins and would suggest that another gene outside the major histocompatibility complex contributes to diabetes susceptibility. HLA testing of the general population is not practical because of the low incidence of HLA-DR3, HLA-DR4, and HLA-DR3/DR4 individuals.[10,14]

Persons susceptible to type I diabetes may be triggered to develop the disease by an environmental event such as a viral infection. One established relationship in which a viral infection triggers IDDM is congenital rubella. Another is cytomegalovirus, which has been found in the beta cells of 20% of patients with type I diabetes. Other viral infections that have been implicated include mumps, hepatitis, and coxsackievirus.

As a result of viral infection or some other event, the susceptible individual appears to develop insulitis with lymphocytic infiltration of the pancreas. An alteration to the surface of the beta cells occurs in some way and they are converted from "self" to "non-self." An autoimmune destruction of the cells follows. Islet cell antibodies and insulin antibodies are found in circulation during this stage. However, overt diabetes may not develop for several years.

Immunofluoresence assay for cytoplasmic islet cell antibodies is positive in about 80% of the patients with new-onset type I diabetes. Less than 0.4% of the general population will show cytoplasmic islet cell antibodies. This increases to about 2% in first-degree relatives of individuals with type I diabetes.[7,10,14] In a study of 1590 individuals with IDDM,[22] 4015 nondiabetic relatives were investigated. Three percent (125) were found to have cytoplasmic islet cell antibodies. During the 10 years of this study, 40 relatives developed type I diabetes and 67% of these relatives had autoantibodies. The greatest risk for relatives of IDDM individuals to develop type I diabetes existed if they were 21 years of age or younger, had two or more diabetic relatives, and had cytoplasmic islet cell antibodies.[22]

Although little progress has been made in understanding the pathogenesis of NIDDM, it is known that there is a strong genetic influence in its etiology (Table 17-3). The modes of inheritance remain unknown except for one variant, maturity-onset diabetes of the young, which is transmitted as an autosomal dominant trait. Type II diabetes has no HLA association. Two processes underlie the development of NIDDM: increased insulin resistance and decreased insulin secretion. Obesity plays a major role in the onset of the disease. Sixty to eighty percent of individuals with type II diabetes are obese. Generally distributed obesity is related more to it than is uniformly distributed obesity.[7,10,14]

Just about all type II diabetics have some initial elevation of basal insulin levels. There often is a loss of the first-phase insulin release to a glucose load or meal. Most patients develop a glucose intolerance even with increased insulin levels. Insulin resistance may occur because of decreased receptors and decreased postreceptor activity. Decreased postreceptor activity is thought to account for the bulk of insulin resistance.[10,14]

There is an increase in the alpha cell/beta cell ratio in the pancreas. This leads to excess glucagon secretion relative to insulin secretion. Resistance to insulin can occur at several sites. Under normal conditions insulin binds to a receptor on the target cell. A transmembrane signal must then be generated by activation of receptor kinase. Postreceptor activation steps then occur within the cell. Defects with one or more of the above processes will result in insulin resistance. Insulin resistance appears to precede the loss of insulin secretion.[10]

PATHOPHYSIOLOGY

Glucose is the most important stimulus for insulin secretion. Insulin remains in circulation for only several minutes (half-life [or $T_{1/2}$] 4 to 8 minutes); then it interacts with target tissues and binds with cell surface insulin receptors. Secondary intracellular messengers are activated and interact with cellular effector systems, including enzymes and glucose transport proteins. Lack of insulin or insulin action allows glucose to accumulate in the tissue fluids and blood.[18]

The meal-stimulated secretion of insulin occurs in two phases. The first phase lasts only a few seconds and accounts for 3% to 5% of meal-stimulated insulin. The second phase lasts for about an hour and accounts for the majority of insulin secretion. A basal secretion of 0.5 to 1 unit of insulin per hour occurs during nonabsorptive states and accounts for some 40% of daily insulin secretion.

Insulin is needed for muscle, fat, and liver to utilize glucose from the blood; therefore, these tissues are described as being insulin-dependent. By contrast, the central nervous system and renal cortex can utilize glucose from the blood without insulin.[26]

As a meal is ingested, insulin is released from the islet cells of the pancreas. The four primary actions of insulin are as follows[26]: (1) to transfer glucose from blood to insulin-dependent tissues, (2) to stimulate transfer of amino acids from blood to cells, (3) to stimulate triglyceride synthesis from fatty acids, and (4) to inhibit breakdown of triglycerides for mobilization of fatty acids.

The current perception of IDDM[7,10,26] is that it represents a significant reduction in or absence of insulin secretion. NIDDM consists of low, normal, or high secretion levels of insulin but with reduced insulin receptors and postreceptor activity at target cells. In addition, the first phase of stimulated insulin secretion is missing in most NIDDM individuals. They have a delay in the second phase, with no peaks, and the second phase is prolonged.[7,10,26]

There appears to be a good correlation between the status of the beta cells and the clinical severity of the diabetes.[3,18,27] In the early stage of IDDM the islets of Langerhans may be enlarged and there is a lymphocytic infiltrate, which suggests the possibility of an autoimmune response. Later, the islets become smaller and essentially no insulin is produced. By contrast, most individuals with NIDDM are able to produce some insulin.[3,18,27]

The patient with uncontrolled diabetes is deprived of insulin or its action but will continue to use carbohydrates at the usual rates in the brain and nervous system because insulin is not required by these tissues. However, other tissues in the body are unable to take glucose into the cells or use it at a normal rate. Increased production of glucose may occur from glycogen and from protein; thus the rise in blood glucose in diabetic persons results from a combination of underutilization and overproduction.

Hyperglycemia leads to glucose excretion in the urine, which results in an increase in urinary volume. The increased fluid lost through urine may lead to dehydration and loss of electrolytes. In type II diabetics a prolonged hyperglycemia can lead to significant losses of fluid in the urine. When this type of severe dehydration occurs, the urinary output will drop and a hyperosmolar nonketotic coma can result. This condition is seen most often in eldery type II diabetics.[10]

The lack of glucose utilization by many of the cells of the body leads to cellular starvation. The patient will often increase the intake of food but in many cases still lose weight.

Cortisol secretion is often increased in the type I diabetic in response to the stress of the disease, leading to protein breakdown and difficulty incorporating amino acids into proteins. The result is conversion of amino acids to glucose and a loss of body nitrogen in the urine.

As the inability to utilize glucose progresses, the type I diabetic person shifts to fat metabolism. Body fat stores are mobilized, and the glycerol portion of the triglyceride is separated and converted to glucose. The fatty acids are metabolized through the Krebs cycle; but if excessive fat breakdown continues, the ability of the breakdown product, acetylcoenzyme A (acetyl-CoA), to be processed through the Krebs cycle fails. There is an excess of acetone and beta-hydroxybutyric acid, which build up in concentration in body fluids and are excreted in the urine.[3,18,27]

If these events continue to progress, the type I diabetic person will develop metabolic acidosis—resulting from the increased loss of electrolytes in the urine, the accumulation of acetoacetic acid and beta-hydroxybutyric acid in the body fluids, and an alteration of the bicarbonate and other buffer systems. For a time the body may be able to maintain the pH near normal levels; but as the buffer system and respiratory and renal regulators fail to compensate, the body fluids become more acidic (pH falls). Severe acidosis will lead to coma and death if it is not identified and treated. For unknown reasons, type II diabetics do not develop ketoacidosis. One possible explanation for this may be that the liver in these patients is resistant to glucagon, which allows malonyl-CoA levels to remain high and can inhibit fatty acid oxidation in the liver.[10]

The primary manifestations of diabetes—hyperglycemia, ketoacidosis, and vascular wall disease—contribute to the inability of uncontrolled diabetic patients to manage infections and heal wounds.[3,18,27] Hyperglycemia may reduce the phagocytic function of granulocytes and facilitate the growth of certain microorganisms. Ketoacidosis delays the migration of granulocytes in the area of injury and decreases phagocytic activity. The vascular wall changes lead to vascular insufficiency, which can result in decreased blood flow to an area of injury and could hamper granulocytic mobilization as well as reduce oxygen tension. The end results of

TABLE 17-4

Expected Years of Additional Life in Diabetic and Nondiabetic Individuals with Respect to Given-Age Cohorts

Attained age of diabetic individual	Expected years additional life of nondiabetic individual	Expected years additional life of diabetic individual	Years lost because of diabetes
10	61.5	44.3	17.2
20	51.9	36.1	13.8
30	42.5	30.1	12.4
40	33.3	23.7	9.6

these effects and others yet to be identified are to render the patient with uncontrolled diabetes much more susceptible to infection, to reduce the ability to deal with an infection once it is established, and to delay the healing of traumatic and surgical wounds.

COMPLICATIONS

A study of patients with IDDM conducted from 1939 to 1981[14] showed the significant effect of the disease on long-term survival. Few deaths occurred among these patients before the age of 30. By the age of 55 only 48% of the women and 34% of the men were still alive. When compared to the general population, diabetic women lived 22 years less than nondiabetic women and diabetic men 24 years less than nondiabetic men. In another study,[26] diabetes mellitus diagnosed at the age of 10 years was estimated to cause a loss of 17.2 years of life expectancy (Table 17-4). In addition to decreasing life expectancy, the complications of diabetes mellitus lead to significant signs and symptoms that affect the quality of life.

The complications of diabetes are associated with the vascular system and the peripheral nervous system (Table 17-5). The vascular complications result from two pathologic changes, microangiopathy and atherosclerosis. Some evidence[3,18,27] suggests that the microangiopathies seen in diabetic persons may be a basic part of the disease process and not a later complication. In any case, the vessel changes seen include thickening of the intima, endothelial proliferation, lipid deposition, and accumulation of para-aminosalicylic acid–positive material. These changes can be seen throughout the body but have particular clinical importance when they occur in the retina and small vessels of the kidney.[3,18,27]

Diabetic retinopathy consists of nonproliferative changes (microaneurysms, retinal hemorrhages, retinal edema, retinal exudates) and proliferative changes (neovascularization, glial proliferation, vitreoretinal traction). Diabetic retinopathy is the leading cause of blindness in the United States. The incidence of blindness in all diabetic persons is 0.2% per year but is 0.6% per year for diabetic individuals with retinopathy. Proliferative retinopathy is most common in IDDM, with a much lower incidence in NIDDM.[18,26] Cataracts occur at an earlier age and with greater frequency in diabetics.[21] The usual type of cataract, senile cataract, is found

TABLE 17-5

Complications of Diabetes Mellitus

Ketoacidosis (type I diabetes)
Hyperosmolar nonketotic coma (type II diabetes)
Diabetic retinopathy—blindness
Cataracts
Diabetic nephropathy—renal failure
Accelerated atherosclerosis
  Coronary heart disease
  Stroke
  Ulceration and gangrene of feet
Diabetic neuropathy
  Dysphagia
  Gastric distention
  Diarrhea
  Impotence
  Muscle weakness, cramps
  Numbness, tingling, deep burning pain
Early death

in 59% of diabetics 35 to 55 years of age but in only 12% of nondiabetics. Young diabetics are more prone to develop metabolic cataracts.[21]

Diabetic nephropathy leads to end-stage renal disease in 30% to 40% of individuals with IDDM. Renal failure occurs in only 5% of individuals with NIDDM. However, because NIDDM is much more common, the number of persons with renal failure is equal for the two types of diabetes.[6] Renal failure is the leading cause of death in patients with IDDM. Twenty-five percent of all patients using dialysis are diabetic. The microangiopathy in the kidney usually involves the capillaries of the glomerulus.[18]

Macrovascular disease (atherosclerosis) occurs earlier, and is more widespread and more severe, in diabetic than in nondiabetic persons. Atherosclerosis in IDDM seems to develop independent of microvascular disease (microangiopathy). Hyperglycemia appears to play a role in the evolution of atherosclerotic plaques. Uncontrolled diabetics have increased levels of low-density lipoprotein (LDL) cholesterol and reduced levels of high-density lipoprotein (HDL) cholesterol. Attainment of normal glycemia often will improve the LDL/HDL ratio. Atherosclerosis increases the risk of ulceration and gangrene of the feet (Fig. 17-1), hypertension, renal failure, coronary insufficiency, myocardial infarction, and stroke.[26]

The most common cause of death in patients with NIDDM is myocardial infarction. By the age of 55 years, a third of all diabetics die of complications from coronary heart disease. Coronary heart disease deaths in diabetics are rare before the age of 35. Death rate from

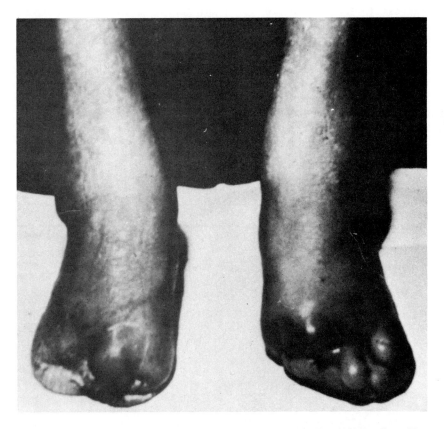

FIG. 17-1   Diabetic gangrene of the feet. (From Falace DA: In Wood NA, editor: *Treatment planning: a pragmatic approach,* St Louis, 1978, CV Mosby, p 63.)

coronary heart disease in the general population up to age 55 is about 8% for men and 4% for women. Diabetic women treated with insulin have greater risks for coronary heart disease than do non–insulin treated diabetic women. This is not true for insulin-treated diabetic men. A diabetic person also has less chance of surviving a myocardial infarction than a nondiabetic person has.[14]

From a clinical standpoint diabetics have more complaints concerning nerve disease than any other chronic complication, and there is growing evidence that hyperglycemia is a major factor in the onset and progression of diabetic neuropathy. Increased uptake of glucose by Schwann cells leads to the production of intracellular sorbitol, which attracts water into the cell and may cause cellular injury and nerve dysfunction. In the extremities diabetic neuropathy may lead to muscle weakness, muscle cramps, a deep burning pain, tingling sensations, and numbness. In addition, tendon reflexes, two-point discrimination, and position sense may be lost.[18,26] Some cases of oral paresthesia and burning tongue are caused by this complication.

Diabetic neuropathy also may involve the autonomic nervous system: esophageal dysfunction may cause dysphagia; stomach involvement may cause a loss of motility, with massive gastric distention; and involvement of the small intestine may result in nocturnal diabetic diarrhea. There may also be sexual impotence and bladder dysfunction. Diabetic neuropathy is common with both IDDM and NIDDM and may exist in over 50% of patients.[18,26]

Other complications found in diabetics are cataracts, skin rashes, and deposits of fat in the skin (xanthoma diabeticorum). In persons in whom diabetes has been diagnosed early and is well-controlled, these complications may not develop as quickly or to as great an extent as in those in whom the disease was detected late or was poorly managed.

CLINICAL PRESENTATION
SIGNS AND SYMPTOMS

With IDDM the onset of symptoms is sudden. The symptoms include polydipsia, polyuria, polyphagia, loss of weight, loss of strength, marked irritability, recurrence of bed wetting, drowsiness, and malaise. Patients with severe ketoacidosis may complain of vomiting, abdominal pain, nausea, tachypnea, paralysis, and loss of consciousness.[7,11] The onset of symptoms in NIDDM is usually slow, and the cardinal signs are less commonly seen. The signs and symptoms of IDDM and NIDDM are summarized in Tables 17-6 and 17-7.

Other signs and symptoms relating to the

TABLE 17-6
Clinical Pictures of IDDM and NIDDM

	IDDM	NIDDM
Frequency (percentage of diabetic persons)	5	85
Age at onset (years)	15	40 and over
Body build	Normal or thin	Obese
Severity	Extreme	Mild
Insulin	Almost all	25% to 30%
Plasma glucagon	High, suppressible	High, resistant
Oral hypoglycemic agents	Few respond	50% respond
Ketoacidosis	Common	Uncommon
Complications	90% in 20 years	Less common
Rate of clinical onset	Rapid	Slow
Stability	Unstable	Stable
Family history	Common	More common
Genetic locus	Chromosome 6	Chromosome 11(?)
HLA and abnormal autoimmune reactions	Present	Not present
Insulin receptor defects	Usually not found	Often found

complications of diabetes are skin lesions, cataracts, blindness, hypertension, chest pain, and anemia. The rapid onset of myopia in an adult is highly suggestive of diabetes mellitus.

LABORATORY FINDINGS

Two groups of patients should be screened for diabetes mellitus at periodic intervals[3,18,27]: (1) those individuals with signs and symptoms of diabetes or its complications and (2) those who have diabetic relatives, are obese, are over age 40, have delivered large babies, or have had spontaneous abortions or stillbirths.

The diagnosis of diabetes is established by the presence of a symptom complex consisting of microangiopathy involving the retina, abnormal glucose metabolism by clinical laboratory tests (which show glucose and acetone in the urine), a fasting blood glucose level at or above 140 mg/dl, a 2-hour postprandial blood glucose level

TABLE 17-7
Symptoms of Diabetes

1. IDDM
   a. Cardinal symptoms — common
      (1) Polydipsia
      (2) Polyuria
      (3) Polyphagia
      (4) Weight loss
      (5) Loss of strength
   b. Other symptoms
      (1) Recurrence of bed wetting
      (2) Repeated skin infections
      (3) Marked irritability
      (4) Headache
      (5) Drowsiness
      (6) Malaise
      (7) Dry mouth
2. NIDDM
   a. Cardinal symptoms much less common
   b. Usual symptoms
      (1) Slight weight loss or gain
      (2) Urination at night
      (3) Vulvar pruritus
      (4) Blurred vision
      (5) Decreased vision
      (6) Paresthesias
      (7) Loss of sensation
      (8) Impotence
      (9) Postural hypotension

at or above 200 mg/dl, and a lowered oral glucose tolerance level.

The use of laboratory tests for the diagnosis of diabetes mellitus has changed since 1979. Before that date the glucose tolerance test was considered to be *the* diagnostic laboratory test. Since then, the fasting glucose level and/or the 2-hour postprandial blood glucose level have become the standard laboratory tests.[6]

The use and interpretation of various clinical laboratory tests for evaluating and diagnosing diabetes will be described here in general terms.

Urinary glucose and acetone

The determination of urinary glucose and acetone is of limited value in detecting overt diabetes; and, in addition, finding glucose in the urine is not diagnostic of diabetes. A few people have a low renal threshold for glucose and may "spill" sugar into the urine on that basis. Other conditions may lead to glucose in the urine — such as renal disease and the administration of steroids. More important is the fact that failure to find glucose or acetone, or both, in the urine of a patient suspected of being diabetic does not rule out diabetes. Many studies have demonstrated that some persons with overt diabetes at times may not "spill" glucose into the urine and others may not show any evidence of acetone in the urine. Cases have been reported with blood glucose levels of 300 to 400 mg/dl without any evidence of urinary glucose. Except possibly for the patient who has the classic symptoms of diabetes, with glucose and acetone in the urine, most physicians depend on blood chemistry to establish the diagnosis of diabetes.

Blood glucose determination

When interpreting the blood glucose level, it is important to keep in mind that the source of blood, age of the patient, nature of the diet and physical activity of the patient will often affect the results. Also of great importance is the method used to measure the amount of sugar present in the blood sample.

Most clinical laboratories collect venous blood from the arm for analysis of blood gucose level. Venous glucose levels are lower than arterial glucose levels, with the greatest difference occurring about 1 hour after the ingestion of carbohydrates. Following an overnight fast, the arterial glucose levels are usually only 2 or

3 mg/dl higher than the venous glucose levels.

The capillary blood glucose values are closer to the arterial values than the venous levels are. However, methods that use capillary blood are subject to a greater variation in results because of the dilution of the blood sample with lymph. Normal fasting blood glucose levels range from 60 to 100 mg/dl for venous blood.

If the diet has been poor in carbohydrate for several days and the person is given 100 mg of glucose just before the blood glucose level is measured, it is possible to produce a condition termed *starvation hyperglycemia,* which could be misdiagnosed as diabetes mellitus. To prevent this from occurring, the diet should contain at least 250 to 300 g of carbohydrate on each of the 3 days before testing.

Physical activity tends to lower the blood glucose level. Excessive physical activity should be avoided by patients who are going to be tested for their blood glucose level.

The most accurate technique for determining blood glucose levels is one that measures only glucose. The Folin and Wu method gives higher results because it also measures other blood sugars (e.g., fructose and lactose). Methods that use glucose oxides give the lowest blood sugar value because they are specific for glucose. Most autoanalyzers use a ferricyanide method, which gives values a little higher than methods that use glucose oxides.

FASTING VENOUS BLOOD GLUCOSE

The 1979 international criteria for the diagnosis of diabetes mellitus[16] define diabetes as being present if the fasting blood glucose level is 140 mg/dl or greater on two or more occasions.

TWO-HOUR POSTPRANDIAL GLUCOSE

For the 2-hour postprandial glucose test the patient is given a 75 or 100 g glucose load after a night of fasting. The glucose can be given in the form of Glucola or in a meal containing about 100 g of carbohydrate. Glucola works well because it is a measured amount of glucose and can be given in the dental office. Blood glucose levels taken at 2 hours that are higher than 200 mg/dl on two or more occasions are diagnostic of diabetes mellitus.[18,26]

Oral glucose tolerance test

Glucose taken orally is absorbed from the small intestine, the maximum normal rate of absorption being 0.8 g/kg body weight/hour. The glucose tolerance test reflects the rate of absorption, uptake by tissues, and excretion in the urine of glucose. The glucose load can be given as Glucola, which contains 75 g of glucose in each 7 fl oz bottle. Some laboratories use a 75 g glucose load; others use a 100 g glucose load following a night of fasting. Venous blood samples are drawn from the arm just before and $\frac{1}{2}$, 1, 2, and 3 hours after the ingestion of glucose. Urine samples also are collected at each interval.

The most characteristic alterations seen in diabetes are an increased fasting blood glucose (above 140 mg/dl), an increased peak value (above 200 mg/dl) and/or a delayed return to normal at the 2- and 3-hour samples. Hypoglycemia may occur in the person with early, mild diabetes 3 to 5 hours after ingestion of glucose. For this reason some physicians will extend the glucose tolerance test to 5 hours for certain patients. The urine samples should not contain glucose at any point during the test.

As mentioned above, the glucose tolerance test is no longer the standard for diagnosing diabetes mellitus. This test is used to identify patients with impaired glucose absorption and gestational diabetes. Special tests can be performed to measure the release of insulin at various IV glucose infusion levels. However, they are basically for detection of special problems and are not part of the routine tests used to diagnose diabetes mellitus.[7,10]

Glycohemoglobin

The measurement of glycohemoglobin levels has been described as being of value in the detection and evaluation of diabetic patients (Table 17-8). It appears to reflect glucose levels in the blood over the 6 to 8 weeks preceding the

TABLE 17-8

Glycohemoglobin Measurement as a Laboratory Test for Evaluation of the Diabetic Patient

Glycohemoglobin level (% of total hemoglobin)	Clinical interpretation
4 to 8	Normal range in adults
Less than 7.5	Good control of diabetes
7.6 to 8.9	Fair control of diabetes
9 to 20	Poor control of diabetes

test. Patients do not have to fast before the test, and it can be useful in following the progress of the disease. However, at the present time this test is not generally used for the diagnosis of diabetes mellitus.[12]

MEDICAL MANAGEMENT

Diabetes mellitus is not a curable disease. Current evidence supports no precise relationship between hyperglycemia and the vascular complications of diabetes. However, the bulk of evidence weighs in favor of such a relationship; hence good control of glucose levels is a must. A key observation supporting the concept that good hyperglycemic control prevents complications in diabetics is to note what happens in transplanted kidneys. When a kidney is transplanted from a nondiabetic to a diabetic, it develops nephropathy within 3 to 5 years. However, if pancreatic transplantation is also performed, no nephropathy appears to develop.[10] Another example of how good hyperglycemic control can prevent diabetic complications from occurring is found in the eye. The rate of developing proliferative retinopathy is reduced with good diabetic control.[14]

Therapy must be a highly individual process and usually must continue for the rest of the patient's life. This need for lifelong compliance is a problem for many patients. The therapy and test results need to be reevaluated on a continuous basis, and patient education concerning the disease, its complications, and its management also is an ongoing process. The therapeutic goals for most patients are (1) to maintain as close to normal blood glucose levels as possible without repeated episodes of hypoglycemia, (2)

to strive to maintain normal body weight, and (3) to have a flexible treatment plan that does not dominate the patient's life any more than necessary.[26]

The patient with diabetes may be treated by control of diet and physical activity and the administration of oral hypoglycemic agents and/or insulin (Table 17-9). In many cases of NIDDM the disease can be controlled by weight loss, diet, and physical activity. Total calories must be balanced with physical activity and body weight, and a balanced diet is indicated (with rigid control of the total caloric content). Some physicians will start the diabetic patient on a diet that has a certain balance of carbohydrate, protein, and fat; others will allow the patient more freedom and will control only the total caloric content.[3,18,27]

If control of the diet and physical activity fails to affect the blood glucose level, hypoglycemic agents are used. Many patients with NIDDM can be managed with oral hypoglycemic agents. Certain oral hypoglycemics, specifically tolbutamide and related sulfonylurea drugs, were indicted in a report from the University Group Diabetes Program as being ineffective and tending to increase the risk of cardiovascular disease. Since that report there have been no further studies that would seem to support those conclusions.[3,18,27]

Although the fear of accelerated coronary heart disease has now been discounted, the oral hypoglycemics are still being used less for treatment of NIDDM. The reason for this is that currently the emphasis is on better hyperglycemia control. Thus a higher percentage of type II diabetics are being treated with insulin to prevent or slow the late complications of diabetes.[10]

In 1984 the second generation of oral hypoglycemic agents became available for use in the United States. The dosage of these new agents is about one hundredth that required for the first-generation oral hypoglycemics. The oral hypoglycemic agents available for treating NIDDM are shown in Table 17-10. Their mode of action is not completely understood; endogenous insulin must be present for these agents (sulfonylureas) to be effective. In some manner they appear to stimulate the secretion of insulin, increase the number of cell membrane insulin receptors, and improve insulin postreceptor activity. A number of patients with type II

TABLE 17-9
Treatment of Diabetes Mellitus

Type I diabetes (IDDM)
  Insulin
    Conventional
    Multiple injections
    Continuous infusion
    Pancreatic transplantation (Chapter 26)
Type II diabetes (NIDDM)
  Diet and physical activity
  Oral hypoglycemic agents
  Insulin plus oral hypoglycemic agents
  Insulin

TABLE 17-10
Metabolism, Potency, and Activity of the Hypoglycemic Agents Used for NIDDM

Agent	Maximum daily dose (mg per day)	Rate of metabolism	Duration activity known (hr)
Tolbutamide	3000	Rapid	6 to 8
Tolazamide	1000	Rapid	24
Acetohexamide	1500	Intermediate	12 to 18
Glyburide	20	Intermediate	24
Glipizide	45	Intermediate	24

diabetes are now being treated with a combination of insulin and oral hypoglycemic agents.[10,26]

Patients with type I diabetes, patients with type II diabetes who are pregnant, and patients who have renal disease or an acute illness should not be treated with oral hypoglycemic agents. If good patient selection is applied about 80% of the patients with type II diabetes will respond to sulfonylurea therapy for a variable time period. Five to ten percent per year of those treated with sulfonylureas will become nonresponsive to the medication. Three to five percent of the patients treated with sulfonylureas will experience adverse reactions—including nausea, vomiting, cholestasis, granulomatous hepatitis, blood dyscrasias, rashes, photosensitivity, water retention, and hypoglycemia.

Drug interactions with the sulfonylureas have been reported.[10,11,26] Barbiturates speed up the liver metabolism of sulfonylureas and can cause hyperglycemia. Sulfonamides compete with the sulfonylureas for metabolic pathways in the liver and can cause hypoglycemia. Warfarin, phenylbutazone, and aspirin also can affect the actions of oral hypoglycemic agents. Patients with IDDM require insulin to control their blood glucose level, although through diet control and adequate exercise the amount of insulin needed can be reduced.

Three types of insulin are available for the treatment of diabetes mellitus: human, pork, and beef. Pork insulin differs from human insulin in one amino acid and from beef insulin in three. The older animal insulin extracts contained a number of contaminants that caused significant adverse reactions. Allergic reactions at the site of injection were common; on occasion, serious systemic reactions occurred—including hives, angioedema, and anaphylaxis.

Another adverse reaction noted with the older animal insulin preparations was lipoatrophy, which consisted of a loss of subcutaneous fat at the injection site. Purified animal extracts of insulin are now available and have greatly reduced the frequency of these reactions in humans.[10,17]

Another form of insulin used in humans is derived by two processes. *Semisynthetic* insulin is produced by substituting alanine for threonine in pork insulin. *Biosynthetic* insulin is produced by recombinant DNA methodology in *Escherichia coli* (subtype K-12).[3a] There is little difference noted clinically between the uses of human insulin and purified pork insulin.[10,17]

Insulin therapy can be administered by using one of three methods: conventional therapy, multiple subcutaneous injections, and continuous subcutaneous infusion (Table 17-11). Conventional therapy is used most often and consists of one or two daily injections of insulin. The multiple injection method consists of injecting short-acting insulin prior to each meal and then a long-acting insulin injection in the evening. In continuous insulin infusion therapy a small battery-driven pump provides infusion pressure and sensors are used to detect the need for insulin, or the pump can be programmed to deliver insulin at certain times. Although the concept of continuous insulin infusion is attractive, many problems have yet to be solved.[10,17] Pancreas transplantation is used in selected diabetic patients to eliminate the need for exogenous insulin therapy. (See Chapter 26.)

Insulin is available in regular, neutral protamine Hagedorn (NPH), and lente preparation. Regular insulin is rapidly absorbed and is given first before meals. NPH and lente are intermediate-acting preparations and are usu-

TABLE 17-11
Types of Insulin Commonly Used in the United States

Type of insulin	Action	Buffer	Peak (hr)	Duration (hr)
Regular	Rapid	None	1 to 2	5 to 6
Neutral protamine Hagedorn (NPH)	Intermediate	Phosphate	2 to 8	24 to 28
Lente	Intermediate	Acetone	2 to 8	24 to 28
Protamine zinc	Long	Phosphate	8 to 12	36

ally given once a day in conventional therapy if less than total replacement is needed. A long-acting insulin preparation, potamine zinc, is available but is not used often[18,26] (Table 17-11).

In conventional therapy regular insulin can be mixed with either NPH or lente. By using a morning and an early evening injection of regular and NPH insulin, peak insulin levels will be available for breakfast, lunch, and dinner. A few patients may require a separate injection of long-acting insulin to prevent the dawn phenomenon (a rebound hypoglycemia that occurs in some patients at about 4 AM).[18,26]

Patients on conventional insulin therapy often use self–glucose monitoring to establish the effectiveness of their hyperglycemia control. These patients can alter their insulin dosage based on the results of the tests. The best results are obtained with a spring-driven lancet holder and an instrument to read the reagent strips that are used to measure the blood glucose levels. Two levels of control are sought using conventional therapy. *Acceptable* control is defined as maintaining the following blood glucose levels[10]: 60 to 130 mg/dl fasting and preprandial, less than 200 mg/dl postprandial, and greater than 65 mg/dl at 3:00 AM. *Ideal* control is defined for the following blood glucose levels: 70 to 100 mg/dl fasting and preprandial, less than 160 mg/dl postprandial, and greater than 65 mg/dl at 3:00 AM.[10]

Infection, emotional or physical stress, pregnancy, and surgical procedures will usually disturb the control of a patient's diabetes. This is particularly true in patients taking insulin, and additional control measures must be used during these periods. This often involves increasing the dosage of insulin or administering insulin for a short period to type II patients not being managed with insulin.

INSULIN SHOCK

It is important that patients being treated with insulin follow their diet closely. If they fail to eat in a normal pattern but continue to take their regular insulin injection, they may experience a hypoglycemic reaction caused by an excess of insulin (insulin shock). A hypoglycemic reaction can also be due to overdosage of insulin or an oral hypoglycemic agent. Reaction or shock caused by excessive insulin usually occurs in three well-defined stages, each more severe and dangerous than the preceding (Table 17-12).

TABLE 17-12
Signs and Symptoms of Insulin Reaction

Mild stage

Hunger
Weakness
Tachycardia
Pallor
Sweating
Paresthesias

Moderate stage

Incoherence
Uncooperativeness
Belligerence
Lack of judgment
Poor orientation

Severe stage

Unconsciousness
Tonic or clonic movements
Hypotension
Hypothermia
Rapid thready pulse

Mild stage

The mild stage is the most common and is characterized by hunger, weakness, trembling, tachycardia, pallor, and sweating; paresthesias may be noted on occasion. It occurs before meals, during exercise, or when food has been omitted or delayed.

Moderate stage

In the moderate stage the patient becomes incoherent, uncooperative and sometimes belligerent or resistive; judgment and orientation are defective. The chief danger during this stage is that patients may injure themselves or someone else if they are driving, etc.

Severe stage

Complete unconsciousness with or without tonic or clonic muscular movements occurs during the severe stage. Most of these reactions take place during sleep, after the first two stages have gone unrecognized. This stage may also occur after exercise or the ingestion of alcohol if earlier signs have been ignored. Sweating, pallor, rapid thready pulse, hypotension, and hypothermia may be present.

The reaction to excessive insulin can be corrected by giving the patient sweetened fruit juice or anything with sugar in it. Patients in the severe stage, unconsciousness, are best treated by giving a glucose solution IV; glucagon or epinephrine may be used for transient relief.

DENTAL MANAGEMENT
MEDICAL CONSIDERATIONS

Any dental patient who has the cardinal symptoms of diabetes (polydipsia, polyuria, polyphagia, weight loss, weakness) should be referred to a physician for diagnosis and treatment.

Patients with findings that may suggest diabetes (headache, dry mouth, marked irritability, repeated skin infection, blurred vision, paresthesias, progressive periodontal disease, multiple periodontal abscesses, loss of sensation) should be screened by the dentist for hyperglycemia or referred to a clinical laboratory or physician for screening tests (Table 17-13).

Patients who are obese, are over 40 years of age, or have close relatives who are diabetic should be screened once a year for any indication of hyperglycemia that may reveal the onset

TABLE 17-13
Detection of the Diabetic Patient

1. Known diabetic person
   a. Detection by history
      (1) Are you diabetic?
      (2) What medications are you taking?
      (3) Are you being treated by a physician?
   b. Establishing severity of disease and degree of "control"
      (1) When were you first diagnosed as diabetic?
      (2) What was the level of the last measurement of your blood glucose?
      (3) What is the usual level of blood glucose for you?
      (4) How are you being treated for your diabetes?
      (5) How often do you have insulin reactions?
      (6) How much insulin do you take with each injection and how often do you receive injections?
      (7) Do you test your urine for glucose?
      (8) When did you last visit your physician?
      (9) Do you have any symptoms of diabetes at the present time?
2. Undiagnosed diabetic person
   a. History of signs or symptoms of diabetes or its complications
   b. High risk for developing diabetes
      (1) Parents who are diabetic
      (2) Gave birth to one or more large babies
      (3) History of spontaneous abortions or stillbirths
      (4) Obese
      (5) Over 40 years of age
   c. Referral or screening test for diabetes

of diabetes. Women who have given birth to large babies (over 10 pounds) or who have had multiple spontaneous abortions or stillbirths also should be screened once a year for diabetes. These patients are best screened by their physician if they have one. Patients who do not have a physician can be screened in the dental office or referred to a clinical laboratory or physician for screening.

The dental office screening test for diabetes (hyperglycemia) is simple and inexpensive and, if done with care, is accurate in detecting patients with moderate to severe elevations of

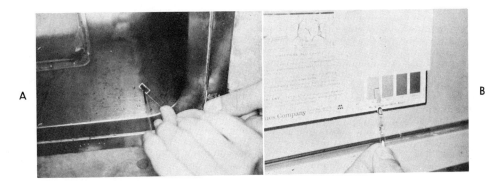

FIG. 17-2 Blood is transferred from the capillary tube to the reagent end of the Dextrostix, **A,** and the color of the activated end is matched with a color chart, **B.**

blood glucose. The procedures listed in Table 17-14 are suggested to screen the dental patient for hyperglycemia. The patient should be encouraged to eat a normal diet that contains about 250 to 300 g of carbohydrate per day for at least 3 days before screening. On the day of screening the patient should eat no breakfast and come into the dental office at about 8:30 to 9:00 AM. A fasting blood glucose test or a 2-hour postprandial blood glucose test can be performed. If the fasting blood glucose test is selected, blood is obtained when the patient comes into the office. If the 2-hour postprandial test is used, the patient is given a 75 g glucose load (in the form of Glucola, a convenient commercial product) before coming to the office.

When the 2-hour postprandial blood glucose test is utilized, blood is obtained 2 hours after ingestion of the Glucola. It is taken from the patient's finger, with a sterile lancet to produce the wound, and is collected in a capillary tube. A drop is expelled from the tube onto a Dextrostix (which contains a glucose oxide and a color indicator) (Fig. 17-2, *A*) and is washed from the Dextrostix after about a minute. The color of the reagent end is compared with a chart provided by the manufacturer to estimate the concentration of glucose (Fig. 17-2, *B*).

A patient with an estimated fasting blood glucose level of 140 mg/dl or higher should be

referred to a physician for medical evaluation and treatment if indicated. A patient with a 2-hour postprandial blood glucose level of 200 mg/dl or higher should also be referred.

All patients with diagnosed diabetes must be identified by history, and the type of medical treatment they are receiving must be established. The type of diabetes (IDDM, NIDDM, or type III) should be determined, and the presence of complications noted. Patients being treated with insulin should be asked how much insulin they use and how often they inject themselves each day. The frequency of insulin reactions and when the last one occurred should be determined. The frequency of visits to the physician should be established, as should whether or not the patient checks his or her urine for glucose. This information will provide the dentist with information concerning the severity and control of the diabetes (Table 17-14).

Patients with NIDDM who have no evidence of complications and whose disease is under good medical control will require little or no special attention when receiving dental treatment, unless they develop an acute dental or oral infection. By contrast, patients with complications such as renal disease or cardiovascular disease may need to be managed in special ways. Patients being treated with insulin or who are not under good medical management also will require special attention (Table 17-15).

Patients who have not seen their physician for a long time, who have had frequent episodes of

*Miles, Inc., Pharmaceutical Division, 400 Morgan Lane, West Haven, CT., 06516

TABLE 17-14
Screening for Diabetes in the Dental Office

1. Selection of patient
2. On each of 3 days before screening, patient's diet should contain 250 to 300 g of carbohydrate
3. Overnight fast before screening
4. Have patient come to dental office for 8:30 to 9:00 AM appointment on day of testing (no breakfast)
   a. Fasting blood glucose test
      (1) Make wound on finger pad with sterile blood lancet
      (2) Drop blood onto reagent end of Dextrostix
      (3) Wash blood off after 1 minute
      (4) Using color chart, estimate blood glucose level
   b. 2-hour postprandial blood glucose
      (1) Have patient ingest 75 g of glucose (Glucola)
      (2) 2 hours later, obtain blood sample and test as above
5. Refer patient to physician if
   a. Fasting blood glucose is 140 mg/100 ml or higher
   b. 2-hour postprandial blood glucose is 200 mg dl or higher

TABLE 17-15
Dental Management of the Diabetic Patient

1. Non–insulin-dependent patient
   a. All dental procedures can be performed
   b. No special precautions needed unless complications of diabetes present
2. Insulin-controlled patient
   a. Usually all dental procedures can be performed
   b. Morning appointments are usually best
   c. Advise patient to take usual insulin dosage and normal meals on day of dental appointment; confirm when patient comes for appointment
   d. Advise patient to inform you or your staff if symptoms of insulin reaction occur during dental visit
   e. Have source of glucose (orange juice, Glucola) available and give to patient if symptoms of insulin reaction occur
3. Extensive surgery needed
   a. Consult with physician concerning dietary needs during postoperaive period
   b. Consider prophylactic antibiotics for patient with brittle diabetes or one taking high doses of insulin to prevent postoperative infection
4. Special precautions may be needed for patient with complications of diabetes, renal disease, heart disease, etc

insulin shock, or who report signs and symptoms of diabetes may have disease that is out of control. These patients should be referred to their physician for evaluation, or the physician should be consulted to establish the patient's current status.

Some patients with IDDM who are being treated with large doses of insulin will have periods of extreme hyperglycemia and hypoglycemia (brittle diabetes), even with the best of medical management. These patients require close consultation with the physician before any dental treatment is started.

One major problem in the dental management of a diabetic patient being treated with insulin is to prevent insulin shock from occurring during the dental appointment. These patients should be told to take their usual insulin dosage and to eat their normal breakfast before the dental appointment, which is usually best scheduled in the morning. When the

patient comes for the appointment, the dentist should confirm that the patient has taken his or her insulin and eaten breakfast. In addition, patients should be instructed to tell the dentist if at any time during the appointment they feel symptoms of an insulin reaction occurring. A source of sugar, such as orange juice or Glucola, must be available in the dental office to give to the patient if symptoms of an insulin reaction occur (Table 17-15).

Any diabetic patient who is going to receive extensive periodontal or oral surgery procedures other than single simple extractions should be given special attention as regards dietary needs following surgery. It is important that the total caloric content and the protein/carbohydrate/fat ratio of the diet remain the same so control of the disease and proper blood glucose balance are maintained. The patient's

TABLE 17-16

Dental Management of the Diabetic Patient
with an Acute Oral Infection

1. Non–insulin-controlled patients—may require insulin; consult with physician
2. Insulin-controlled patients—usually will require increased dosage of insulin; consult with physician
3. Brittle diabetic or patient receiving high insulin dosage—should have culture(s) taken from infected area for antibiotic sensitivity testing
   a. Obtain culture, send for testing
   b. Initiate penicillin therapy
   c. In cases of poor chemical responses to penicillin, a more effective antibiotic can be selected based on sensitivity test results
4. Treat infection using standard methods
   a. Warm intraoral rinses
   b. Incision and drainage
   c. Pulpotomy, pulpectomy, extraction, etc.
   d. Antibiotics

physician should be consulted concerning diet recommendations for the postoperative period. One suggestion is to have the patient use a blender to prepare his or her usual diet so that it can be ingested with minimum discomfort; or special food supplements that are in a liquid form may be used.

Patients who have brittle diabetes or require a high dosage of insulin (IDDM diabetics) and are going to receive periodontal or oral surgery procedures may be placed on prophylactic antibiotic therapy during the postoperative period to avoid infection.

Patients with well-controlled diabetes can be given general anesthesia; however, in a dental office, management with local anesthetics is preferable.

Any diabetic patient with acute dental or oral infection presents an immediate problem in management (Table 17-16). This problem will be even more difficult for patients who take a high insulin dosage and those who have IDDM. The infection will often cause loss of control of the diabetic condition; as a result the infection is not handled by the body's defenses as well as it would be in the nondiabetic patient. Patients with brittle diabetes (difficult to control, high

dosage of insulin) may require hospitalization during the management of an infection. The patient's physician should be consulted and become a partner during this period.

The basic aim of treatment is to cure the oral infection and at the same time respond to the need to regain control of the diabetic condition. Patients receiving insulin usually will require additional insulin, which should be prescribed by their physician; non–insulin-controlled patients may need more aggressive medical management of their diabetes, which may include insulin during this period. The dentist must treat the infection by drainage extraction, pulpotomy, warm rinses, and/or antibiotics. Antibiotic sensitivity testing is recommended for patients with brittle diabetes or who require high insulin dosage for control. For these patients penicillin therapy can be initiated; and then, if the clinical response is poor, a more effective antibiotic can be selected based on the results of the antibiotic sensitivity testing. Attention also must be paid to the patient's electrolyte balance and fluid and dietary needs.

TREATMENT PLANNING MODIFICATIONS

The diabetic patient who is receiving good medical management without serious complications—such as renal disease, hypertension, or coronary atherosclerotic heart disease—can receive any indicated dental treatment. Those diabetic patients with serious medical complications may need to have an altered plan of dental treatment. (See Chapters 6, 7, and 11.)

ORAL COMPLICATIONS

The oral complications of uncontrolled diabetes mellitus may include xerostomia, infection, poor healing, increased incidence and severity of periodontal disease, and burning mouth syndrome. The oral findings in patients with uncontrolled diabetes most likely relate to the excessive loss of fluids through urination, the altered response to infection, the microvascular changes, and possibly the increased glucose concentrations in saliva.

The effects of hyperglycemia lead to increased amounts of urine, which depletes the extracellular fluids and reduces the secretion of saliva, and this results in the complaint of dry mouth. An increase in the rate of dental caries has been reported in young diabetic patients and would appear to be related to the reduced salivary flow.

The parotid saliva of persons with uncontrolled diabetes has been reported[4] to contain a slight increase in the amount of glucose. The glucose concentration in parotid saliva from nondiabetic individuals varies from 0.22 to 1.69 mg/dl whereas the glucose concentration in parotid saliva from persons with uncontrolled diabetes has been reported to range from 0.22 to 6.33 mg/dl. The effect of this slight increase (if any) on the incidence of dental caries and other oral conditions in diabetic patients remains to be established.

Several studies[1,2,9,16,23,25] have reported an increased incidence and severity of gingival inflammation, periodontal abscesses, and chronic periodontal disease in diabetic patients (Figs. 17-3 and 17-4). On the other hand, a well-controlled study by Shannon et al.[24] failed to demonstrate any difference in the amount or severity of periodontal disease in young diabetic and nondiabetic individuals.

The most impressive study showing an association of periodontal disease and diabetes[25] involved the Pima Indians in southwestern United States. This tribe has the highest incidence and prevalnce of type II diabetes in the world. In the study (of 3219 Pima Indians) 736 or 23% were found to have type II diabetes.[25] Fifty percent of the adults over 35 years were

diabetic. The dental status of 2878 of these persons in the study was determined. Periodontal disease was established by loss of epithelial attachment, and loss of crestal alveolar bone was estimated by clinical and radiographic techniques.[25] The prevalence of periodontal disease was significantly greater in those individuals with type II diabetes than in the nondiabetic individuals studied. Furthermore, periodontal disease was found to occur at an earlier age in diabetics.

Saadoun[23] reported small blood vessel changes in the gingival tissues of diabetic patients consisting of flattening of the endothelial cells, accumulation of periodic acid–Schiff positive material in the basement membrane, and a narrowing of the lumina. He also described an increase in the glucose level of the gingival fluids. The neutrophils appeared to be affected secondary to the hypoglycemia, showing decreased phagocytosis, diapedis, impaired adherence and impaired chemotaxis.

Saadoun[23] also reported that adults with uncontrolled diabetes who are prone to periodontal disease will have more severe manifestations of the disease than will nondiabetics prone to periodontal disease. This relationship is not clear in the patient with controlled diabetes. As a group, diabetic patients appear to have more severe periodontal disease than nondiabetic patients, but the differences are not great. Saadoun[22] also concluded that the glucose tolerance test results are not a reliable predictor of a patient's periodontal status. The time

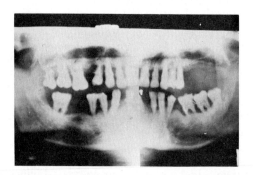

FIG. 17-3 Panoramic radiograph from a young adult with severe, progressive periodontitis. Following positive screening for diabetes, the patient was referred to physician and the diagnosis of diabetes mellitus was established. The patient required insulin treatment.

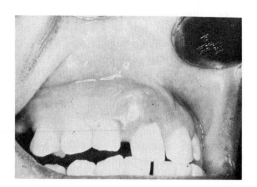

FIG. 17-4 Periodontal abscess in a patient with multiple abscesses. After evaluation by a physician the diagnosis of diabetes mellitus was estabished.

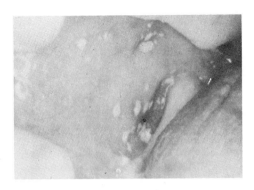

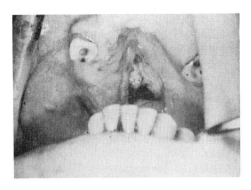

FIG. 17-5 Oral moniliasis in a diabetic patient. Note the multiple small white lesions on the buccal mucosa. The lesions could be scraped off. Cytologic study and cultures confirmed the clinical impression of infection by *Candidia albicans.*

FIG. 17-6 Lesion involving the palate in a diabetic patient. Cultures established the diagnosis of mucormycosis, a serious fungal infection that may occur in patients with systemic diseases such as diabetes or cancer. Treatment usually includes control of the diabetes, surgical excision of the lesion, and antibiotics and fungicides.

relationship between the diabetic state and periodontal disease is yet to be established. Cianciola et al.[5] evaluated the periodontal status of 263 patients with IDDM, 59 nondiabetic siblings and 149 nonrelated nondiabetic patients and concluded that periodontal disease is a complication of IDDM. The increased periodontal disease found in IDDM patients could not be explained by increased supragingival plaque accumulations. The periodontal disease found in these young patients (all less than 30 years of age) was usually asymptomatic and undetected.

In a recent unpublished study[19] the association between long-term control of diabetes mellitus and periodontitis was investigated. A total of 75 individuals with type I or type II diabetes were evaluated. Poor diabetic control and the presence of calculus increased the risk for periodontitis. Regular maintenance care, including patient motivation and instruction as well as professional calculus removal, was recommended for diabetic patients.

A study performed in Sweden involving children of diabetic mothers[7] showed a much higher frequency of enamel hypoplasia (28%) than in children of nondiabetic mothers (3%). The cause of this difference is not known, but it may be due to the effects of hyperglycemia on the formation and calcification of the enamel matrix.

Oral fungal infections may be found in the uncontrolled diabetic patient, including moniliasis and the more rare mucormycosis (Figs. 17-5 and 17-6). (See Appendix B for treatment regimens.) There appears to be general agreement that healing is delayed in individuals with uncontrolled diabetes and that they are more prone to various oral infections following surgical procedures. A recent report[1] suggested an association between diabetes mellitus and the atrophic-erosive form of lichen lanus. This association was not noticed for the reticular form of lichen planus.

Diabetic neuropathy may lead to oral symptoms of tingling, numbness, burning, or pain caused by pathologic changes involving nerves in the oral region. Early diagnosis and treatment of the diabetic state may allow for regression of these symptoms, but in long-standing cases the changes may be nonreversible.

Several studies have suggested that the status of patients thought to be "prediabetic" can be confirmed by gingival biopsy findings of thickened and hyalinized small vessels. However, at present this technique remains to be proven accurate and beneficial.

REFERENCES

1. Bagán-Sebastián JV, Milián-Masanet MA, Peñarrochia-Diago M, Jiménez Y: A clinical study of 205 patients

with oral lichen planus, *J Oral Maxiollofac Surg* 50(2):116-118, 1992.

2. Bartolucci EG, Parkes RB: Accelerated periodontal breakdown in uncontrolled diabetes: pathogenesis and treatment: *Oral Surg* 52:387-390, 1981.

3. Bennett PH, Seltzer HS: Diagnosis and epidemiology or diabetes mellitus. In Ellenbergy M, Refkin H, editors: *Diabetes mellitus: theory and practice*, New York, 1970, McGraw-Hill.

3a. Burrows W: *Textbook of microbiology*, ed 21 (Freeman BA, editor), Philadelphia, 1979, WB Saunders, p. 173.

4. Campbell MJ: Glucose in the saliva of the non-diabetic and the diabetic patient, *Arch Oral Biol* 10:197-205, 1965.

5. Cianciola LJ, Park B, Bruck E, et al: Prevalence of periodontal disease in insulin-dependent diabetes mellitus (juvenile diabetes), *J Am Dent Assoc* 104(5): 653-660, 1982.

6. DeFronzo RA: Diabetic nephropathy. In Becker KL, editor: *Principles and practice of endocrinology and metabolism*, Philadelphia, 1990, JB Lippincott, pp 1148-1158.

7. Eisenbath GS, Kahn CR: Etiology and pathogenesis of diabetes mellitus. In Becker KL, editor: *Principles and practice of endocrinology and metabolism*, Philadelphia, 1990, JB Lippincott, pp 1074-1084.

8. Ekoe JM: Recent trends in prevalence and incidence of diabetes mellitus syndrome in the world, *Diabetes Res Clin Pract* 1:249-264, 1986.

9. Faulconbridge AR, Bradshaw WC, Jenkins PA, Baum JD: The dental status of a group of diabetic children, *Br Dent J* 151:253-255, 1981.

10. Foster DW: Diabetes mellitus. In Wilson JD, et al, editors: *Harrison's Principles of internal medicine*, ed 12, New York, 1991, McGraw-Hill, pp 1739-1759.

11. Ganda OP, Weir GC: Oral hypoglycemic agents. In Becker KL, editor: *Principles and practice of endocrinology and metabolism*, Philadelphia, 1990, JB Lippincott, pp 1099-1102.

12. Goteiner DJ: Glycohemoglobin (GHb): a new test for the evaluation of the diabetic patient and its clinical importance, *J Am Dent Assoc* 102(1):57-58, 1981.

13. Grahnén H, Edlund K: Maternal diabetes and changes in the hard tissues of the primary teeth, *Odontol Rev* 18:157-162, 1967.

14. Krolewski AJ, Warram JH: Natural history of diabetes mellitus. In Becker KL, editor: *Principles and practice of endocrinology and metabolism*, Philadelphia, 1990, JB Lippincott, pp 1084-1087.

15. Napier JA: Field methods and response rates in Tecumseh community health study, *Am J Public Health* 52:208-216, 1962.

16. National Diabetes Data Group: Classfication and diagnosis of diabetes mellitus and other categories of glucose intolerance, *Diabetes* 28:1039-1057, 1979.

17. O'Hare JA, Weir GC: Insulin therapy: In Becker KL, editor: *Principles and practice of endocrinology and metabolism*, Phildelphia, 1990, JB Lippincott, pp 1102-1109.

18. Olefsky JM: Diabetes mellitus. In Wyngaarden JB, Smith LH, editors: *Cecil textbook of medicine*, ed 17, Philadelphia, 1985. WB Saunders.

19. Oliver R: Personal communication.

20. Owen OE, Shuman CR: Pathogenesis and diagnosis of diabetes mellitus. In Rose LF, Kaye D, editors: *Internal medicine for dentistry*, ed 2, St Louis, 1983, CV Mosby.

21. Rand LI: Diabetes and the eye. In Becker KL, editor: *Principles and practice of endocrinology and metabolism*, Philadelphia, 1990, JB Lippincott, pp 1158-1163.

22. Riley WJ, Maclaren NK, Krischer J, et al: A prospective study of the development of diabetes in relatives of patients with insulin-dependent diabetes, *N Engl J Med* 327(17):1167-1172, 1990.

23. Saadoun AP: Diabetes and periodontal disease: a review and update, *Periodont Abstr* 28:116-139, 1980.

24. Shannon IL, O'Leary TJ, Gibson WA, et al: Glucose tolerance responses in young adults of sharply contrasting periodontal status periodontal status, SAM-TR-66-9, *US Air Force Sch Aerospace Med*, 1-6, February 1966.

25. Shlossman M, Knowler WC, Pettitt DJ, Genco RJ: Type 2 diabetes mellitus and periodontal disease, *J Am Dent Assoc* 121(4):532-536, 1990.

26. Skillman TG: Diabetes mellitus. In Massaferri EL, editor: *Endocrinology*, ed 3, New York, 1986, Medical Examination Publishing.

27. Williams RH, Porte D Jr: The pancreas. In Williams RH, editor: *Textbook of endocrinology*, ed 5, Philadelphia, 1974, WB Saunders.

18

Adrenal Insufficiency

The adrenal glands are located bilaterally at the superior pole of each kidney. Each gland is actually a gland within a gland, the medulla contained within the cortex. The adrenal medulla functions as a sympathetic ganglion and secretes primarily epinephrine whereas the adrenal cortex secretes a variety of hormones with multiple actions (Table 18-1). This chapter will deal with hypofunction or insufficiency of the adrenal cortex and its hormones.

GENERAL DESCRIPTION
INCIDENCE AND PREVALENCE

The adrenal cortex manufactures three principal classes of adrenal steroids[6]: glucocorticoids, mineralocorticoids, and androgens. All are derived from cholesterol and share a common molecular nucleus.

Glucocorticoids

Cortisol, which is the primary glucocorticoid, is responsible for a wide variety of functions and effects. Some of the more important include regulation of carbohydrate, fat, and protein metabolism, maintenance of vascular reactivity, inhibition of inflammation, and maintenance of homeostasis during periods of physical or emotional stress.[12,13,19]

Regulation of cortisol secretion occurs via the hypothalamic-pituitary-adrenal (HPA) axis (Fig. 18-1). Central nervous system afferents mediating circadian rhythm and responses to stress stimulate the hypothalamus to release corticotropin releasing hormone (CRH), which stimulates the production and secretion of adrenocorticotropic hormone (ACTH) by the anterior pituitary. ACTH then stimulates the adrenal cortex to produce and secrete cortisol.

Plasma cortisol levels are increased within a few minutes following stimulation. Circulating levels of cortisol serve to inhibit the production of CRF and ACTH, thus completing a negative feedback loop.[12,13,19]

Cortisol secretion normally follows a diurnal pattern. Peak levels of plasma cortisol occur at about the time of awakening in the morning and are lowest in the afternoon and evening[13] (Fig. 18-2). This pattern is reversed in an individual who habitually works nights and sleeps during the day. The normal secretion rate of cortisol over a 24-hour period is approximatey 30 mg.[12,19] During periods of extreme stress this figure has been reported[9,14] to approach 300 mg. Anticipation of surgery or an athletic event is usually accompanied by only minimal increases in cortisol secretion, but surgery itself is one of the most potent activators of the HPA axis. The greatest response is found to occur in the immediate postoperative period, however, and

TABLE 18-1
Secretory Products of the Adrenal Glands

Adrenal cortex	Adrenal medulla
Glucocorticoids	Epinephrine*
Cortisol*	Norepinephrine
Corticosterone	Dopamine
Mineralocorticoids	
Aldosterone*	
Dexycorticosterone	
Sex hormones	
Dehydroepiandosterone*	
Androstenedone	

*Principal secretory products

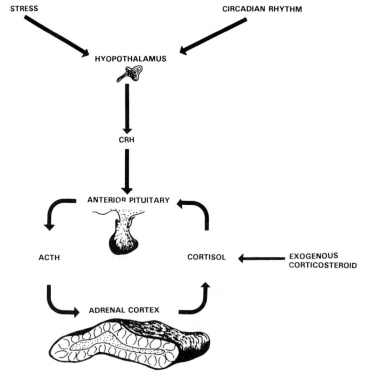

FIG. 18-1   Hypothalamic-pituitary-adrenal axis and the regulation of cortisol secretion.

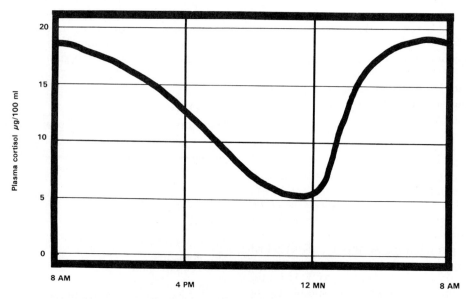

FIG. 18-2   Normal pattern of cortisol secretion over a 24-hour period.

TABLE 18-2
Glucocorticoid Preparations and Their Relative
Potency

Compound	Potency	Approximate equivalent dose (mg)
Short-acting (less than 12 hr)		
Cortisol	1	20
Cortisone	0.8	25
Intermediate-acting (12 to 36 hours)		
Prednisone	4	5
Prednisolone	4	5
Methylprednisolone	5	4
Triamcinolone	5	4
Long-acting (greater than 36 hours)		
Paramethasone	10	2
Betamethasone	25	0.75
Dexamethasone	25	0.75

Adapted from Haynes RC. In Gilman AG, et al, editors: *Goodman and Gilman's The pharmacological basis of therapeutics*, ed 8, New York, 1990, Pergamon Press, pp 1431–1462.

can be reduced by morphinelike analgesics or by local anesthesia.[13] This would seem to suggest a pain response mechanism.

Synthetic glucocorticoids are used in the treatment of many diseases — including rheumatoid arthritis, systemic lupus erythematosus, asthma, hepatitis, dermatoses, and mucositis. In addition, glucocorticoids are used during immunosuppressive therapy for organ transplantation. Many synthetic glucocorticoids are available and differ in potency relative to coritsol and in their duration of action (Table 18-2).

Mineralocorticoids

Aldosterone is the primary mineralocorticoid secreted by the adrenal cortex and is essential to sodium and potassium balance and to the maintenance of extracellular fluid (i.e., intravascular volume). Its actions are primarily on the distal tubule and collecting duct of the kidney. Aldosterone secretion is regulated by the renin-angiotensin system, ACTH, and plasma sodium and potassium levels — and is stimulated by a fall in renal blood pressure

resulting from a decrease in intravascular volume or a sodium imbalance.[6] The result is a release of renin, which activates angiotensin. Angiotensin causes aldosterone to be secreted, and this promotes sodium retention, potassium excretion, and fluid retention. Thus there is a negative feedback loop that ultimately inhibits the further production of aldosterone[6,19] (Fig. 18-3).

Androgens

Dehydroepiandrosterone is the principal androgen secreted by the adrenal cortex. The effects of adrenal androgens are the same as those of testicular androgens (i.e., masculinization and the promotion of protein anabolism and growth). The activity of the adrenal androgens, however, is only about 20% that of the testicular androgens and is of relatively minor importance.[6]

PATHOPHYSIOLOGY

Insufficiency of adrenocortical function may occur either primarily or secondarily.

Primary adrenocortical insufficiency is uncommon and is known as Addison's disease. It is due to a progressive destruction of the adrenal cortex, usually of an idiopathic nature (most likely autoimmune) but also resulting from infectious diseases (TB) or a malignancy. The signs and symptoms of the disease are the result of deficiencies of adrenocortical hormones.

The major hormones of the adrenal cortex are cortisol and aldosterone, and the presentation of Addison's disease is due primarily to insufficient quantities of these compounds. Lack of cortisol results in impaired glucose, fat, and protein metabolism, hypotension, increased ACTH secretion, impaired fluid excretion, excessive pigmentation, and an inability to tolerate stress. Aldosterone deficiency results in an inability to conserve sodium and eliminate potassium and hydrogen ions leading to hypovolemia, hyperkalemia, and acidosis.

Secondary adrenocortical insufficiency is a far more common problem and results from the administration of exogenous corticosteroids. The secretion of cortisol is directly dependent on the level of circulating ACTH. As the plasma cortisol level increases and demand is met, the production of ACTH decreases by virtue of negative feedback. With the administration of

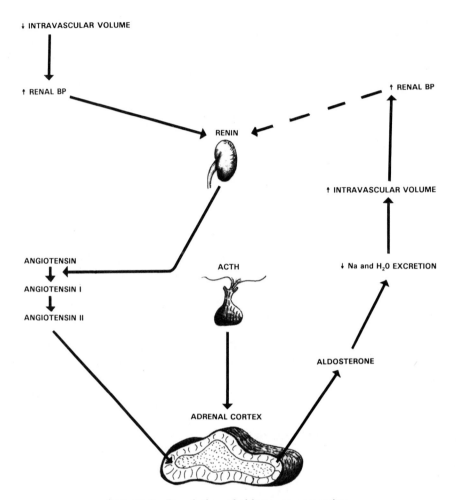

FIG. 18-3 Regulation of aldosterone secretion.

corticosteroids, the feedback system senses the elevated plasma steroid levels and inhibits ACTH production, which in turn suppresses the adrenal production of cortisol (Fig. 18-1). The result is a partial adrenal insufficiency. The production of aldosterone is not appreciably affected.

Although determination of adrenocortical suppression for a given patient is controversial, it is generally thought to depend on the dosage as well as the timing and duration of administration. Thus suppression is presumably more likely with supraphysiologic doses taken daily over an extended period. Prediction of suppression, however, based on the history of dosage or length of adminstration has been found[18] to be unreliable. Assessment of suppression is best accomplished by laboratory evaluation of the basal plasma cortisol and stimulation tests for functional cortisol production.

A common treatment modification of steroid therapy that attempts to minimize adrenal suppression is the alternate-day regimen[8,9,13] — i.e., steroids are given the morning of every other day instead of daily but a double dose is given to maintain an elevated serum level. The rationale for this is that the cortisol level normally is high in the morning, so a dose given at that time does not tend to suppress ACTH abnormally, whereas on the off-day the HPA axis can function normally and produce endogenous steroids. The result is less adrenal suppression than is seen with daily therapy. Unfortunately, however, this approach is not uniformly successful in controlling symptoms and many patients must return to daily therapy.

Topically applied corticosteroids also can induce adrenal suppression, by absorption through the skin or mucous membrane, although results are variable. Whereas the amount of topical steroid required to treat small noninflamed areas does not cause significant suppression, prolonged treatment of large inflamed areas may be a cause for concern, especially if occlusive dressings are used.[3,15] In this event one should assume that some adrenal suppression may have occurred. Similar comments can be made concerning the use of inhaled corticosteroids if given in frequent and high doses.[11]

Once corticosteroid administration ceases, the HPA axis regains its responsiveness and eventually normal ACTH and cortisol secretion resumes. The time required to regain normal adrenal responsiveness is thought to vary from days to months; however, studies from a large review[7] demonstrated a return to stress stimulation within 14 days of HPA function, in spite of supraphysiologic doses for a month or longer.

CLINICAL PRESENTATION
SIGNS AND SYMPTOMS

Primary adrenal insufficiency (Addison's disease) has signs and symptoms that relate to a deficiency of aldosterone and cortisol. The most common complaints are weakness, fatigue, and an abnormal pigmentation of the skin and mucous membranes (Fig. 18-4). In addition,

hypotension, anorexia, and weight loss are common findings. If a patient with Addison's disease is challenged by stress (e.g., illness, infection, or sugery), an adrenal crisis may be precipitated. This is a medical emergency manifested by a severe exacerbation of symptoms — including hypotension, nausea, vomiting, weakness, headache, dehydration, and hyperpyrexia. If not treated rapidly, the patient may die.[19]

Secondary adrenal insufficiency resulting from chronic corticosteroid administration is a partial insufficiency limited to glucocorticoids and usually does not present any symptoms unless the patient is stressed and does not have adequate circulating cortisol to cope with the stress. In that event, an adrenal crisis may be precipitated. It should be noted that an adrenal crisis in a patient with secondary adrenal suppression tends not to be as severe as that seen with primary adrenal insufficiency since aldosterone production is not altered.[13]

A patient who has been receiving long-term, high-dose corticosteroid therapy can begin to demonstrate the signs and symptoms of hyperadrenalism or Cushing's syndrome. A Cushingoid person may demonstrate weight gain, round or moon-shaped facies (Fig. 18-5) a "buffalo hump" on the back, abdominal striae, and acne. Other findings can include hypertension, heart failure, osteoporosis, diabetes mellitus, impaired healing, and mental depression or psychosis.[19]

LABORATORY FINDINGS

Since cortisol deficiency is of most concern from a dental management perspective, remarks

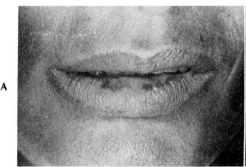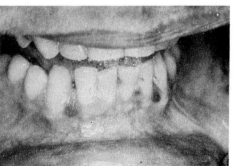

FIG. 18-4 Patient with Addison's disease. Note the bronzing of the skin with pigmentation of the lip, **A,** and oral mucosa, **B.**

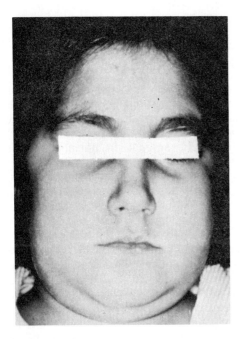

FIG. 18-5 Acquired Cushing's disease. (From Falace DA. In Wood NA, editor: *Treatment planning: a pragmatic approach,* St Louis, 1978, CV Mosby, p 56.)

will be limited to tests for the determination of cortisol secretion. These tests include basal plasma ACTH and cortisol, 24-hour urine excretion of 17-hydroxycorticosteroids (17-OHCS)and various stimulation tests. The usefulness of basal plasma testing and 24-hour urine testing is limited in that it measures cortisol production only at a given point or over a given period. These values can be altered by a variety of factors (circadian rhythm, diet and stress).

Normal plasma cortisol concentrations reflect a circadian rhythmicity. Values in the early morning range from 10 to 20 μg/dl whereas late afternoon values typicaly range from 3 to 10 μg/dl. Urinary excretion of 17-OHCS ranges from 3 to 8 mg per 24 hours.[13] All these values may be normal in adrenocortical hypofunction, and abnormality may become evident only with stimulation tests.

Stimulation tests of the HPA axis provide a much more accurate assessment of impairment. These tests include ACTH stimulation,

insulin-induced hypoglycemia, metyrapone, and corticotropin-releasing hormone. In cases of adrenal insufficiency, test results will be subnormal. Ironically, however, there is poor correlation between a subnormal stimulation test and the patient's clinical ability to respond to stress.[2]

MEDICAL MANAGEMENT

A patient with Addison's disease is treated by replacement of clinically significant hormones that are lacking. Glucocorticoid replacement is accomplished with 12.5 to 50 mg cortisone daily. Cortisol, 30 mg daily, or prednisone, 7.5 mg daily, is also given for substitution therapy. Current practice recommends giving two thirds of the dose in the morning and one third in the later afternoon, to reflect the normal diurnal cycle. Mineralocorticoid replacement is accomplished by the daily administration of fludrocortisone, 0.05 to 0.1 mg. Patients are also encouraged to ingest adequate sodium.[19]

Although patients with Addison's disease can lead essentially normal lives with appropriate treatment, the possible need for supplemental glucocorticoids during periods of illness or "stress" remains indefinitely. However, authorities differ on the need for and dosage of supplemental steroids.

For minor illness or minor surgery under local anesthesia, recommendations range from no supplementation to double or triple the normal dose.[2,10,13,19] Clinical experience, however, suggests most patients do not require any supplementation.[7]

For major surgery under general anesthesia or severe illness, there seems to be a consensus[2,13,19] that supplementation of approximately 200 mg of cortisol or its equivalent per day is required. These same recommendations are made for patients with secondary adrenal insufficiency.

Of interest is a recent review[7] of 200 cases in which surgery, both major and minor, was performed on patients who had been taking hydrocortisone at the equivalent of 20 to 320 mg/day for periods varying from 6 days to 20 years. The procedures were performed without supplemental corticosteroids, and no adverse sequelae were reported.

Acute adrenal insufficiency (adrenal crisis) may occur in spite of steroid supplementation. This requires immediate treatment—including injection of a glucocorticoid and fluid and electrolyte replacement. In addition, resolution of the event or condition that precipitated the crisis is required.

Patients taking corticosteroids for treatment of medical disorders can develop signs of hyperadrenalism, or Cushing's syndrome. If this occurs, the dosage or method of administration may require alteration.

DENTAL MANAGEMENT
MEDICAL CONSIDERATIONS

In developing recommendations for corticosteroid supplementation for dental patients taking steroids, the dentist must consider several issues. Predictions of adrenal suppression based on history of dosage or length of administration are not necessarily accurate. A recent study[18] investigating the cortisol stress response in patients taking a wide range of doses and types of corticosteroids over a wide range of time spans concluded that HPA axis function in patients receiving synthetic glucocorticoids cannot be appraised accurately on the basis of (history of) dose or duration alone. In addition, even if a patient has adrenocortical suppression as diagnosed by an abnormal stimulation test, this does not necessarily reflect how he or she will react clinically or, in fact, whether there will even be a reaction.[7]

One of the most important issues is determination of the normal adrenocortical response in response to various dental procedures. Some studies[1,13,16] have investigated the stress response to minor general and oral surgical procedures and have concluded that significant cortisol increases are not seen before or during the operation but are increased in the postoperative period. However, these postoperative cortisol increases are blunted by the use of analgesics, strongly suggesting a response to pain. A case report[17] of acute adrenal crisis in the postoperative period following dental extractions seems consistent with this observation. Until recently, no information was available about the response to other types of dental procedures.

In a recent study[5] of 42 healthy patients undergoing a variety of dental procedures performed by dental students, salivary cortisol (which directly reflects plasma cortisol) was measured pre-, intra-, and postoperatively. Procedures included routine examination, prophylaxis, endodontics, restorative treatment, and simple extractions. In all cases the procedures studied did not result in any significant increases in cortisol levels.

In a related study[4] salivary cortisol levels were measured in 39 dental students practicing local anesthetic techniques on each other. Samples were obtained before and following the injections. All students admitted to being a "little nervous" before the procedures. Thirty-six had no significant changes in cortisol levels. However, three had increases of 200% to 300%, and one of these had a syncopal episode. This demonstrates the potential role of anxiety in cortisol secretion.[4] Nevertheless, it would appear that most routine dental procedures, including extractions, are not associated with significant increases in cortisol secretion, except in cases of postoperative pain or extreme anxiety.

It should be recognized that there are not uniformly accepted guidelines; however, in light of current evidence and clinical experience, it appears that most patients who are taking corticosteroids and undergoing routine dental procedures with local anesthetic, including extractions, do not require supplemental steroids (Table 18-3). This, of course, assumes adequate pain and anxiety control. If it is decided that, because of the "stress" of a planned procedure or the extreme anxiety of a patient, supplementation would be appropriate, then doubling the normal daily dose on the day of the procedure should be adequate. If significant postoperative pain is anticipated, an additional day's supplementation may be provided.

When general anesthesia is planned, an acceptable approach is 100 mg of hydrocortisone on the morning of the procedure followed by 100 mg hydrocortisone 1 hour before the procedure. If postoperative pain is anticipated, doubling the maintenance dose on the next day is advised.

Once corticosteroid administration is discontinued, it may take weeks or months to regain normal adrenal function, and theoretically during this period patients are susceptible to adrenal crisis from the decreased adrenocortical response.[13,19] However, a large review of the literature[7] cited numerous references demonstrating that most patients regain an adequate

TABLE 18-3

Guidelines for Dental Management of the Patient Taking Corticosteroids

1. Routine dental procedures, including extractions, using local anesthetic:
   Patients currently taking corticosteroids — no additional supplementation generally required; be sure to obtain good local anesthesia and good postoperative pain control
   Patients with past history of regular corticosteroid usage — if less than 2 weeks, give normal daily maintenance dose on day of procedure; if more than 2 weeks, none generally required
   Patients using topical or inhalational steroids — generally no supplementation required
2. Extensive procedures or extreme patient anxiety, using local anesthetic:
   Patients currently taking corticosteroids — double normal daily dose on day of procedure; if postoperative pain is anticipated, double daily dose on first postoperative day
   Patients with past history of regular corticosteroid usage — if less than 2 weeks, give double daily maintenance dose on day of procedure; if more than 2 weeks, none generally required
3. General anesthesia:
   Should not be an outpatient procedure
   Supplementation recommended — 100 mg hydrocortisone on morning of procedure, then 100 mg hydrocortisone 1 hour before procedure; if postoperative pain is anticipated, double normal maintenance dose on following day.

clinical response to stress within 2 weeks after cessation of steroid administration, in spite of persistent subnormal plasma cortisol levels. If routine dental treatment is provided during this 2-week period, supplementation with physiologic doses on the day of the procedure would be advised.

Even though precautions are taken and patients are appropriately managed, the dentist should always remain alert to and anticipate the possibility of an acute adrenal crisis. Signs and symptoms of acute adrenal insufficiency include hypotension, weakness, nausea, vomiting, headache and frequently fever. Immediate treatment of this problem consists of 4 mg dexamethasone, IM, and immediate transportation to a medical facility.[13]

TREATMENT PLANNING MODIFICATIONS

No treatment planning modifications are required for the patient with Addison's disease.

ORAL COMPLICATIONS

In primary adrenal insufficiency, pigmentation of the oral mucous membranes is a common finding (Fig. 18-4). Patients with secondary adrenal insufficiency may be prone to delayed healing and have increased susceptibility of infection.

REFERENCES

1. Banks P: The adreno-cortical response to oral surgery, *Br J Oral Surg* 8:32-44, 1970.
2. Bethune JE: The diagnosis and treatment of adrenal insufficiency. In DeGroot LJ, et al, editors: *Endocrinology,* ed 2, vol 2, Philadelphia, 1989, WB Saunders, pp 1647-1659.
3. Coskey RJ: Adverse effects of corticosteroids. I. Topical and intralesional, *Clin Dermatol* 4(1):155-160, 1986.
4. Dembo JB, Falace DA: Salivary cortisol and the stress response in dental students. (Accepted for publication, *J Dent Educ.*)
5. Dembo JB, Miller CS, Falace DF: Adrenocortical response to dental treatment of varying stresses, *J Dent Res,* vol 71, Abstract 1583, 1992.
6. Ganong WF: *Review of medical physiology,* ed 15, Norwalk, Conn., 1991, Appleton & Lange, pp 334-359.
7. Glick M: Glucocorticosteroid replacement therapy: a literature review and suggested replacement therapy, *Oral Surg* 67:614-620, 1989.
8. Haynes RC: Adrenocorticotropic hormones; adrenocortical steroids and their synthetic analogs; inhibitors of the synthesis and actions of adrenocortical hormones. In Gilman AG, et al, editors: *Goodman and Gilman's The pharmacological basis of therapeutics,* ed 8, New York, 1990, Pergamon Press, pp 1431-1462.

9. Helfer EL, Roe LI: Corticosteroids and adrenal suppression; characterizing and avoiding the problem, *Drugs* 38(5):838-845, 1989.

10. Loriaux DL: Adrenal insufficiency. In Becker KL, editor, *Principles and practice of endocrinology and metabolism,* Philadelphia, 1990, JB Lippincott, pp 600-604.

11. Maxwell DL: Adverse effects of inhaled corticosteroids, *Biomed Pharmacother* 44:421-427, 1990.

12. Meikle AW: Secretion and metabolism of the corticosteroids and adrenal function and testing. In deGrott LJ, et al, editors: *Endocrinology,* ed 2, vol 2, Philadelphia, 1989, WB Saunders, pp 1610-1632.

13. Orth DN, Dovacs WJ, DeBold CR: The adrenal cortex. In Wilson JD, Foster DW, editors: *William's Textbook of endocrinology,* ed 8, Philadelphia, 1992, WB Saunders, pp 489-619.

14. Pescovitz OH, Cutler GB, Loriaux DL: Synthesis and secretion of corticosteroids. In Becker KL, editor: *Principles and practice of endocrinology and metabolism,* Philadelphia, 1990, JB Lippincott, pp 579-591.

15. Plemons JM, Rees TD, Zachariah NY: Absorption of a topical steroid and evaluation of adrenal suppression in patients with erosive lichen planus, *Oral Surg* 69:688-693, 190.

16. Plumpton FS, Besser GM, Cole PV: Corticosteroid treatment and surgery. 2. The management of steroid cover, *Anaesthesia* 24:12-18, 1969.

17. Scheitler LE, Tucker WM, Christian DG: Adrenal insufficiency: report of a case, *Spec Care Dent* 4(1):22-24, 1984.

18. Sclaghecke R, et al: The effect of long-term glucocorticoid therapy on pituitary-adrenal responses to exogenous corticotropin-releasing hormone, *N Engl J Med* 326:226-230, 1992.

19. Williams GH, Dluhy RG: Diseases of the adrenal cortex. In Wilson JD, et al, editors: *Harrison's Principles of internal medicine,* ed 2, New York, 1992, McGraw-Hill, pp 1713-1735.

19

Thyroid Disease

The patient with thyroid disease is of concern to the dentist from several aspects. The dentist may detect early signs and symptoms of thyroid disease and refer the patient for medical evaluation and treatment. In some cases this may be lifesaving whereas in others the quality of life can be improved and complications of certain thyroid disorders avoided.

Patients with untreated thyrotoxicosis may be in danger if surgical or operative procedures are performed by the dentist. Although uncommon, dental treatment may precipitate an acute medical emergency (thyrotoxic crisis or thyroid storm). Acute infections and trauma also may precipitate a thyrotoxic crisis in the untreated or inadequately treated patient.[2,5]

In this chapter the emphasis will be placed on disorders involving hyperfunction of the gland (thyrotoxicosis) and hypofunction of the gland (myxedema or cretinism). The standard abbreviations used for thyroid gland function and terminology are shown in Table 19-1.

GENERAL DESCRIPTION

The thyroid gland, located in the anterior portion of the neck just below and bilaterally to the thyroid cartilage, develops from the thyroglossal duct and portions of the ultimobranchial body. It consists of two lateral lobes connected by an isthmus. The right lobe is normally larger than the left,[8] and in some individuals a superior portion of glandular tissue can be identified, the pyramidal lobe. Thyroid tissue may be found anywhere along the path of the thyroglossal duct, from its origin (midline posterior portion of the tongue) to its termination (thyroid gland, in the neck). In rare cases the entire thyroid is found in the anterior mediastinal compartment; however, in most individuals the remnants of the duct atrophy and disappear. The thyroglossal duct, as it develops, is "divided" by the hyoid bone and remnants can become enclosed or surrounded by the bone.[8] Ectopic thyroid tissue may secrete thyroid hormones or become cystic or neoplastic; in a few individuals the only functional thyroid tissue is in these ectopic locations.

The thyroid gland secretes three hormones: thyroxine (T_4), triiodothyronine (T_3), and calcitonin. The tissue developing from the ultimobranchial bodies is thought to give rise to the parafollicular cells, which produce calcitonin. T_4 and T_3 are hormones that affect metabolic

TABLE 19-1

Standard Abbreviations Used for Thyroid Gland Function and Terminology

T_4	Thyroxine
T_3	Triiodothyronine
rT_3	Reverse triiodothyronine
TSH	Thyroid-stimulating hormone
TRH	Thyrotropin-releasing hormone
TT_4	Total thyroxine
TT_3	Total triiodothyronine
FT_3	Free triiodothyronine
FT_4	Free thyroxine
T_3U	Triiodothyronine uptake
FT_4I	Free thyroxine index
FT_3I	Free triiodothyronine index
TG	Thyroid globulin
TBG	Thyroid-binding globulin
TBPA	Thyroid-binding prealbumin
TBA	Thyroid-binding albumin

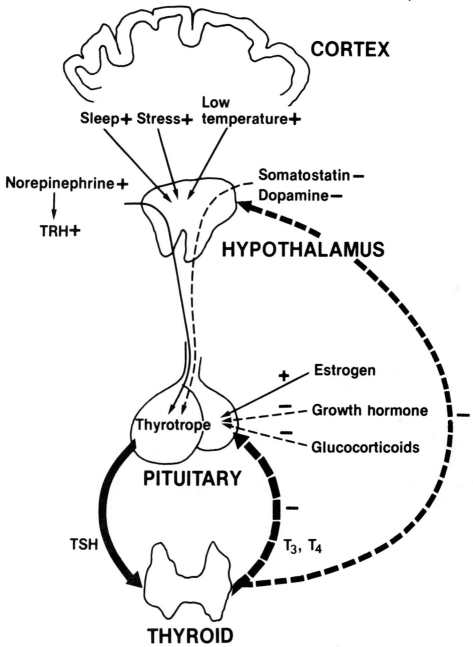

FIG. 19-1 Hypothalamic-pituitary-thyroid axis involved in the control of thyroid secretion. The secretion of thyrotropin (thyroid-stimulating hormone [TSH]) is regulated by interaction of a releasing factor (thyroid-releasing hormone [TRH]) and an inhibitory factor (somatostatin). Thyroid hormones (triiodothyronine [T_3] and throxine [T_4]) act directly on the pituitary to inhibit TSH secretion. Thyroid hormones also act at the hypothalamic level to stimulate somatostatin release. T_4 is converted to T_3 in the liver, kidney, and heart and in the pituitary and hypothalamus. T_3 is more potent T_4 at all sites. (From Mazzaferri EL: In Mazzaferri EL, editor: *Endocrinology,* ed 3, New York, 1986, Elsevier Science Publishing, p 152. With permission of the publisher.)

processes throughout the body and are involved with oxygen use.

Blood levels of T_4 and T_3 are controlled through a servofeedback mechanism mediated by the hypothalamic-pituitary-thyroid axis. Increased or decreased metabolic demand appears to be the main modifier of the system. Drugs, illness, thyroid disease, and pituitary disorders can affect the control of this balance. Recent findings[49,14] also show that age has some effect on the system (Fig. 19-1).

Under normal conditions thyrotropin-releasing hormone (TRH) is released by the hypothalamus in response to external stimuli (stress, illness, metabolic demand, and low levels of T_3 and to a lesser degree T_4). TRH stimulates the pituitary to release thyroid-stimulating hormone (TSH), which causes the thyroid gland to secrete T_4 and T_3.[4,9,14]

T_4 and T_3 also have a direct influence on the pituitary. High levels turn off the release of TSH and low levels turn it on. The effect of T_3 on the pituitary is greater than that of T_4.[4,9,14] T_4 is the main hormone secreted by the thyroid. The level of T_4 in the peripheral blood is 60 times that of T_3. T_4 is converted to T_3 peripherally by deiodination. T_3 is the more active hormone and is the main effector principle.[2] A small amount of an inactive form of T_3, called reverse T_3 (rT_3), is found in circulation.[14]

Goitrins are antithyroid agents that inhibit thyroid hormone synthesis. Foods such as cabbages, turnips, and rutabagas contain them. Thiocyanate, perchlorate, thiourea, methimazole, and prophylthiouracil are goitrins. Methimazole and propylthiouracil block both the iodination of tyrosine and the coupling of monoiodotyrosine (MIT) and diiodotyrosine (DIT) to form iodotyrosine.[9]

Under normal conditions, 10% to 20% of the circulating pool of T_3 comes from the thyroid gland and the rest comes from the monodeiodination of T_4. In cases of hyperthyroidism 30% to 40% of circulating T_3 comes from the thyroid.[8] The conversion of T_4 to T_3 can be inhibited by fasting, illness, steroids, and certain drugs (e.g., propylthiouracil).

Iodine must be available for the synthesis of T_4 and T_3. The inorganic form of iodine as used by the gland comes from the peripheral degradation and diodination of thyroid hormone and the diet. The minimum daily requirement of iodine is about 75 mg, and a typical 2800 calorie daily intake in the United States will contain some 700 mg of iodine. It is of interest to note that there has been a gradual increase in the dietary intake of iodine in the United States in recent years.[8] Iodine, which is stored in the thyroid gland, appears to be oxidized to a higher valence by a preoxidase, and then it combines with thyrosyl to form either MIT or DIT. These compounds then, by an oxidative coupling reaction, form either T_4 or T_3.

The thyroid hormones are stored in the colloid of the thyroid gland. A 3-to-4-month reserve is maintained. Thirty-five percent of the organic iodine content of the thyroid gland is stored as T_4, and about 5% to 8% as T_3. Phagocytosis of colloid droplets starts the secretion process. The colloid droplets are digested by proteases, and, once freed, thyroid globulin (TG), T_4, T_3, and small amounts of rT_3 are secreted into the blood.[9]

In the blood, T_4 and T_3 are almost entirely bound to plasma proteins. The binding plasma proteins are thyroid-binding globulin (TBG), thyroid-binding prealbumin (TBPA), and thyroid-binding albumin (TBA). TBPA binds only to T_4. TBA binds poorly to both T_4 and T_3. TBG binds both T_4 and T_3 but has less affinity for T_3. Therefore the free circulating level of T_3 (FT_3) is neary 10 times greater than the free level of T_4 (FT_4). Only 0.02 to 0.03% of FT_4 and about 0.3% of FT_3 are in plasma.[9]

Low T_4 and T_3 plasma levels are often found in ill and medicated older persons. Protein abnormalities can effect total T_4 and T_3 levels. Illness can reduce the conversion of T_4 to T_3 and increase rT_3. The free levels of T_4 and T_3 can also be affected by drugs and illness. The main age-related change seen in well older individuals is a fall in T_3 because of the reduced peripheral conversion of T_4 to T_3.[4]

The sites of action for thyroid hormones are the cell nucleus, mitochondria, cell membrane, adrenergic receptor pathway, and tyrosine metabolic pathway. The hormones stimulate mRNA synthesis and increase target cell protein synthesis through the cell nucleus. They also increase oxygen consumption, ATP generation, uncoupling of oxidative phosphorylation, and alpha-glycerophosphate dehydrogenase activity through the mitochondria. Finally, they stimulate the passage of Na^+ and K^+ across the cell membrane. In the adrenergic receptor pathway the thyroid hormones increase the number of receptors and amplify the beta-adrenergic signal. The tyrosine metabolic pathway is modified by the hormones to increase alternate adrenergic neurotransmitters.[9]

Calcitonin is involved, along with parathyroid hormone and vitamin D, in regulating serum calcium and phosphorous levels and skeletal remodeling. This hormone and its actions are considered in greater detail in Chapter 11.

INCIDENCE AND PREVALENCE

Worldwide, the most common thyroid disorder is iodine deficiency–related goiter with hyperthyroidism. There are few good studies demonstrating the prevalence of thyroid disorders. Studies in Great Britain have shown about 25 to 30 cases of hyperthyroidism per 10,000 women. The mean age at the time of diagnosis was 48 years. Some 2% of the women had established cases. The incidence of new cases was 3 per 1000 women per year. These studies showed that hyperthyroidism was 10 times more common in women than in men. The incidence of the disease in the United States has been reported[13] to be 3 cases per 10,000 women per year.

Hypothyroidism in Great Britain occurs at a rate of 3 cases per 1000 women per year. The number of established cases was reported to be 14 per 1000 women. The number of established cases in men was 1 per 1000. The mean age at diagnosis was 57 years. About a third of all cases resulted from surgical or radiation treatment for hyperthyroidism.[13]

In the United States hypothyroidism occurs in 3% to 4% of ill older patients admitted to hospital. It is 5 to 6 times more common than hyperthyroidism. Both hypothyroidism and hyperthyroidism are about 4 to 5 times more common in women in the United States.[4,13]

Asymptomatic autoimmune thyroiditis can lead to overt hypothyroidism. Thyroid antibodies are found in these patients, and with time about 5% per year will develop clinical hypothyroidism. Approximately 16% of women and 4% of men in the United States have circulating thyroid autoantibodies.[13] Six thyroid antibodies

have been reported. These are thyroglobulin, microsomal, colloid, antinuclear thyrotropin receptor, and thyrotropin-binding inhibitor antibodies.

Thyroglobulin and microsomal antibodies are the most commonly tested. Their frequency increases with age. They are found in 35% to 50% of patients with Graves' disease, 45% to 80% of patients with primary hypothyroidism, and 71% to 92% of patients with Hashimoto's thyroiditis.[9]

LABORATORY TESTS

The old protein-bound iodine test is not used any longer for detecting thyroid disease. It has been replaced by the radioimmunoassay for T_4 and T_3. The levels of free T_4 and T_3 can be measured, but these tests are time-consuming and expensive. Thyroid-binding globulin (TBG) can be measured. The T_3 uptake (T_3U) is another test that can be performed. It measures the number of unoccupied binding sites on TBG, TBA, and TBPA. Radioactive-labeled T_3 is added to the serum sample.[4,9,11]

The free thyroxine index (FT_4I) is the easiest and cheapest method to estimate the amount of free T_4. It is calculated by multiplying the T_4 by the T_3U. The FT_4I remains normal when the T_4 is elevated or decreased as a result of TBG changes. The FT_3I can be estimated in a similar way by using the T_3 level and T_3U.[4,9,11]

TSH levels are measured by using immuno-radiometric assay, enzyme immunoassay, or immunochemoluminometric assay. In some cases a TSH stimulation test is performed to measure the thyroid's ability to respond to TSH by increased output of T_4 and an increase in radioactive iodine uptake (RAIU) by the gland.[4,9,11]

Another test that can be used to evaluate thyroid function is T_3 suppression. In this test thyroid hormone is given to the patient and the effect on RAIU and T_4 concentration is evaluated. The RAIU and T_4 are measured before starting the test. Then daily dose of 75 to 100 µg of T_3 are given for 7 to 10 days. The RAIU and T_4 levels are measured again at the completion of the test. Under normal conditions the RAIU and T_4 levels should be decreased.[9]

Thyroid antibodies can be measured. The two that are tested for most commonly are thyroglobulin and microsomal antibodies. Patients with autoimmune thyroid disease will have elevated titers of these antibodies.

RAIU is used to evaluate thyroid function. It is not as useful a test now because other, newer, tests provide better data. RAIU uses either ^{131}I or [123]I. When available, ^{123}I is preferred because it gives off less radiation. The normal values for this test have decreased from 25% to 50% (20 years ago) to 10% to 25% now.[9]

A thyroid scan is a common test used to localize thyroid nodules and to locate functional ectopic thyroid tissue. [123]I or ^{99}Tc is injected and a scanner localizes areas of radioactive concentration. This technique allows for the identification of nodules 1 cm or larger. When a pinhole thyroid scan is used, 2 to 3 mm lesions can be detected.[9,10]

Ultrasonography is used to detect thyroid lesions. Nodules 1 to 2 mm in size can be identified. The technique is also used to distinguish solid from cystic lesions, measure the size of the gland, and guide needles for aspiration of cysts or biopsy of thyroid masses.[1,3,9]

Computed tomography has a limited role in evaluation of the thyroid gland. In general, it is an expensive procedure that adds little to the management of the patient. It is helpful in the postoperative management of patients with thyroid cancer. At present, magnetic resonance imaging plays no role in diagnosing thyroid disease.[3]

THYROTOXICOSIS (HYPERTHYROIDISM)
Etiology, pathophysiology, and complications

The term *thyrotoxicosis* refers to an excess of T_4 and T_3 in the bloodstream. This excess may be caused by ectopic thyroid tissue, Graves' disease, multinodular goiter, thyroid adenoma, or pituitary disease involving the anterior portion of the gland. In this section the signs and symptoms, laboratory tests, treatment, and dental considerations for the patient with Graves' disease will be considered in detail and will serve as the model for other conditions that can result in similar clinical manifestations. It should be emphasized that multinodular goiter, ectopic thyroid tissue, and neoplastic causes of hyperthyroidism are rare compared with toxic goiter (Graves' disease).

Patients with Graves' disease often have in

their serum an immunoglobulin G (IgG) called long-acting thyroid stimulator (LATS).[5,7,9,14] Lymphocytes from patients with Graves' disease stimulated with phytohemagglutinin to produce LATS have been found in the serum of about two thirds of patients with Graves' disease; however, the level of LATS does not correlate with the severity of symptoms of the disease. In addition, infants whose mothers have Graves' disease will show a transient period of goiter, ophthalmopathy, and clinical manifestations of Graves'. As the disease disappears the level of serum LATS diminishes.

Studies have shown that LATS is a seven-sulfur IgG produced by B lymphocytes. LATS will stimulate or induce thyroid hyperplasia and iodine accumulation in the thyroid gland, independent of the pituitary gland. A long-acting thyroid stimulator-protector (LATS-P) has been reported that prevents LATS from being neutralized. Graves' disease is now considered to be an autoimmune disease.[6,9,14]

In contrast to the preceding data, a familial tendency has been noted for the transmission of this disorder, with an increased incidence reported in monozygotic twins compared to other twins. In addition, ^{131}I uptake tests have been shown[5] to be increased in about 20% of the immediate relatives of patients with Graves' disease, particularly in sisters and daughters.

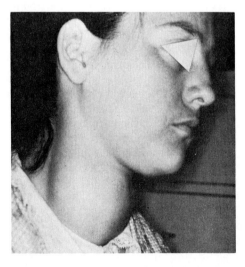

FIG. 19-2 Woman with toxic goiter (Graves' disease).

This disorder is much more common in women (7:1) and may manifest itself at puberty, pregnancy, or menopause (Fig. 19-2). Emotional stress—such as severe fright or separation from loved ones—has been reported associated with its onset. The disease may occur in a cyclic pattern and then "burn itself out" or continue in an active state.

Clinical presentation
SIGNS AND SYMPTOMS

The clinical picture in Graves' disease is due to direct and indirect effects of the excessive thyroid hormones.[2,5,9] The patient's skin will be warm and moist, the complexion rosy, and the patient may blush readily. Palmar erythema may be present, profuse sweating is common, and excessive melanin pigmentation of the skin occurs in many patients; however, pigmentation of the oral mucosa has not been reported. In addition, the patient's hair becomes fine and friable, and the nails soften.

Most patients will show eye changes: retraction of the upper lid, a bright-eyed stare (Fig. 19-3), lid lag, and jerky movements of the lids. The exophthalmos may be unilateral during initial phases of the disease but usually progresses to bilaterality. Corneal ulceration, optic neuritis, and ocular muscle weakness may develop as complications in these patients.

The increased metabolic activity caused by excessive hormone secretion increases circulatory demands, and an increased stroke volume and heart rate often develop in addition to widened pulse pressure, resulting in the patient's complaining of palpitations. Supraventricular cardiac dysrythmias develop in many patients. Congestive heart failure may occur and often is somewhat resistant to the effects of digitalis. Patients with untreated or incompletely treated thyrotoxicosis are highly sensitive to the actions of epinephrine or other pressor amines, and these agents must not be administered to them; however, once the patient is well-managed from a medical standpoint, these agents can be resumed.

Dyspnea not related to the effects of congestive heart failure may occur in some patients. The respiratory effect is caused by reduction in the vital capacity secondary to weakness of the respiratory muscles.

Weight loss even with an increased appetite is a common finding. Stools are poorly formed, and the frequency of bowel movements is increased. Anorexia, nausea, and vomiting are rare but, when they occur, may be the forerunners of thyroid storm. Gastric ulcers are rare in patients with thyrotoxicosis. Many of these patients have achlorhydria, and about 3% will develop pernicious anemia.

Thyrotoxic patients tend to be nervous and often show a great deal of emotional lability, losing their tempers easily and crying often; severe psychic reactions may occur. These patients cannot sit still and are always moving. A tremor of the hands and tongue, along with lightly closed eyelids, is often present; and a generalized muscle weakness may lead to the patient's complaining of easy fatigability (Tables 19-2 to 19-4).

The effect of the excessive thyroid hormones on mineral metabolism is complex and not well-understood. In addition, the role of calcitonin only complicates the problem; however, thyrotoxic patients have an increased excretion of calcium and phosphorus in their urine and stools, and radiographs demonstrate increased bone loss. Hypercalcemia occurs sometimes, but the serum levels of alkaline phosphatase are usually normal. The bone age of young individuals is advanced. (See Chapter 11.)

Infection or severe emotional trauma has been suggested[2] to act as a trigger for the onset of clinical manifestations of Graves' disease, but these relationships are unclear at present. The role of oral foci of infection as an etiologic factor in Graves' disease is also unclear; some evidence suggests that chronic oral infections may aggravate the symptoms.

The individual red blood cells in patients with

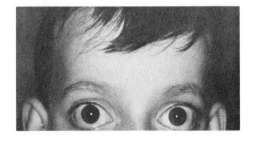

FIG. 19-3 Exophthalmos in a child with Graves' disease.

TABLE 19-2

Clinical Findings in the Patient with Thyrotoxicosis

Skeletal system
  Increased bone turnover
  Rate of resorption exceeds that of formation
  Osteoporosis (common in elderly)
Cardiovascular system
  Palpitations
  Tachycardia
  Arrhythmias (10% to 15% atrial fibrillation)
  Cardiomegaly, congestive heart failure
  Angina, myocardial infarction
Gastrointestinal system
  Weight loss—may have increased appetitite
  Decreased absorption of vitamin A
  Pernicious anemia (3%)
Central nervous system (CNS)
  Anxiety, restlessness, sleep disturbances
  Emotional lability
  Impaired concentration
  Weakness
  Tremors (hands, fingers, tongue)
Skin
  Erythema
  Hyperpigmentation
  Thin fine hair, areas of alopecia
  Soft nails—may lift from distal bed
Eyes
  Retraction of upper lid, exophthalmos
  Corneal ulceration, ocular muscle weakness
Others
  Increased risk for diabetes mellitus
  Decreased serum cholesterol level
  Increased risk for thrombocytopenia

TABLE 19-3

Frequency of Symptoms in 332 Thyrotoxic Patients

Symptom	Young and adult patients (%)	Elderly patients (%)
Nervousness	99	10
Heat intolerance	89	63
Palpitations	89	63
Tachycardia	82	58
Weight loss	85	75
Increased appetite	64	11
Angina	0	20
Tremor	0	55

From Mazzaferri EL. In Mazzaferri EL, editor: *Endocrinology,* ed 3, New York, 1986, Medical Examination Publishing. With permission of the publisher.

TABLE 19-4

Signs in 332 Thyrotoxic Patients

Sign	Young and adult patients (%)	Elderly patients (%)
Tachycardia	100	58
Goiter	100	63
Tremor	97	89
Eye signs	71	57
Atrial fibrillation	10	39
Muscle weakness	0	39

From Mazzaferri EL. In Mazzaferri EL, editor: *Endocrinology,* ed 3, New York, 1986, Medical Examination Publishing. With permission of the publisher.

thyrotoxicosis are usually normal; however, the red blood cell mass is enlarged to carry the additional oxygen needed for the increased metabolic activities. In addition to the increase in total numbers of circulating red blood cells, the bone marrow reveals an erythroid hyperplasia, and requirements for vitamin B_{12} and folic acid are increased. The white blood cell count may be decreased because of a reduction in the number of neutrophils whereas the absolute number of eosinophils may be increased. Enlargement of the spleen and lymph nodes occurs in some patients. The platelets and clotting mechanism are usually normal, but thrombocytopenia has been reported.[12]

The increased metabolic activities associated with thyrotoxicosis lead to increased secretion and breakdown of cortisol; however, serum levels remain within normal limits.

Laboratory findings

The T_4, T_3, TBG, and TSH tests are used to screen for hyperthyroidism. The normal values for these tests are shown in Table 19-5. The results found in hyperthyroidism are shown in

TABLE 19-5
Results for Thyroid Function Tests

Test	Normal range
T_4	5 to 12 μg/dl
T_3	80 to 200 ng/dl
rT_3	10 to 60 ng/dl
TBG	12 to 30 mg/l
TSH	Less than 5 mμ/l
FT_4	1.3 to 3.8 ng/dl
FT_3	260 to 480 png/dl
RAIU	10% to 25% per 24 hours

Based on Nickolai TF. In Rose LF, Kay D, editors: *Internal medicine for dentistry,* ed 2, St Louis, 1990, CV Mosby, pp 997–1019; Smallridge RC. In Becker KL, editor: *Principles and practice of endocrinology and metabolism,* Philadelphia, 1990, JB Lippincott, pp 278–284; Wartofsky L, Ingbar SH. In Wilson JD, et al, editors: *Harrison's Principles of internal medicine,* ed 12, New York, 1991, McGraw-Hill, pp 1692–1713.

TABLE 19-6
Thyroid Function Tests in Hyperthyroidism and Hypothyroidism

Test	Hyperthyroidism	Hypothyroidism
T_4*	Elevated	Decreased
T_3*	Elevated	Decreased
rT_3	Elevated	Decreased
FT_4	Elevated	Decreased
FT_3	Elevated	Decreased
T_3U	Increased	Decreased
FT_4I	Increased	Decreased
FT_3I	Increased	Decreased
RAIU	Increased	Decreased
TSH*	None or low	Elevated
TBG*	Increased	Decreased

*Tests that are used most frequently.

TABLE 19-7
Antithyroid Treatment Methods Used to Manage the Patient with Thyrotoxicosis

Acute stage of treatment	
Propylthiouracil	100 to 150 mg every 8 hours
Methimazole (Tapazole)	10 to 20 mg every 8 hours
Propranolol	20 to 40 mg every 6 hours
Dexamethasone	2 mg every 6 hours
Lithium (used with propylthiouracil)	800 to 1200 mg per day
Second stage of treatment	
Propylthiouracil	50 to 100 mg every 8 hours
Surgery	
Radioiodine ^{131}I	

Table 19-6. Other thyroid tests may be ordered depending on the clinical circumstances. These tests and their results in hyperthyroidism are also shown in Tables 19-5 and 19-6.

Medical management

Treatment of patients with thyrotoxicosis may involve antithyroid agents that block hormone synthesis, iodides, radioactive iodine, or subtotal thyroidectomy (Table 19-7). The most common antithyroid agents used are propylthiouracil and methimazole. Patients being treated with these antithyroid agents often will be given *United States Pharmacopeia* (USP) thyroid. The usual length of treatment is 18 to 24 months. Antithyroid agents may cause a mild leukopenia, but drug therapy is not stopped unless the white cell count is more severely depressed. If exophthalmos is present, it follows a course independent of the therapeutic metabolic response to antithyroid treatment modalities and is usually irreversible.

Management of thyrotoxic crisis

Patients with thyrotoxicosis who are untreated or incompletely treated may develop thyrotoxic crisis,[2,5] a serious but fortunately rare complication that may occur at any age and has an abrupt onset. Thyrotoxic crisis occurs in less than 1% of the patients hospitalized for thyrotoxicosis.[8] Most patients who develop thyrotoxic crisis have goiter, wide pulse pressure, eye signs, and long history of thyrotoxicosis.[8] Precipitating factors are infections, trauma, surgical emergencies, and operations. Early symptoms are extreme restlessness, nausea, vomiting, and abdominal pain; fever, profuse sweating, marked tachycardia, pulmonary edema, and congestive heart failure soon develop. The patient appears to be in a stupor, and coma may follow. Severe hypotension develops, and death may occur. These reactions appear to be associated, at least in part, with adrenocortical insufficiency.

Immediate treatment for the patient in a thyrotoxic crisis consists of large doses of antithyroid drugs (200 mg of propylthiouracil), potassium iodide, propranolol (to antagonize the adrenergic component), hydrocortisone (100 to 300 mg), IV glucose solution, vitamin B complex, wet packs, fans, and ice packs.[2,5] Start cardiopulmonary resuscitation if needed and seek immediate medical aid.

HYPOTHYROIDISM

Hypothyroidism is a rare condition—being responsible for only about one out of every 1500 hospital admissions. Acute hypothyroidism (myxedema) is five times more common in women and most common between the ages of 30 and 60 years. Childhood hypothyroidism is termed *cretinism.*[2,5]

Hypothyroidism can be congenital or acquired. Permanent hypothyroidism occurs about once in every 3500 to 4000 live births. Transient hypothyroidism occurs in 1% to 2% of newborns. Most infants with permanent congenital hypothyroidism have thyroid dysgenesis: ectopic, hypoplastic, or thyroid agenesis.[8] The acquired form may follow thyroid gland or pituitary gland failure. Radiation of the thyroid gland, surgical removal, and excessive antithy-roid drug therapy can cause hypothyroidism; however, some cases appear with no identifiable cause.

Neonatal cretinism is characterized by dwarfism, overweight, broad flat nose, wide-set eyes, thick lips, large protruding tongue, poor muscle tone, pale skin, stubby hands, retarded bone age, delayed eruption of teeth, malocclusions, a hoarse cry, umbilical hernia, and mental retardation that can be avoided with early detection and treatment (Fig. 19-4).

Hypothyroidism having its onset in older children and adults is characterized by a dull expression, puffy eyelids, alopecia of the outer

TABLE 19-8

Signs and Symptoms of Myxedema in 400 Patients

Clinical findings	Percent of patients
General	
Dry thick skin and/or dry hair	89
Fatigue	70
Edema, puffy hands, face, eyes	67
Cold intolerance	58
Hoarseness	48
Weight gain (15 lb or greater)	48
CNS	
Mental and physical slowness	57
Sleepiness	25
Headache	22
Gastrointestinal system	
Constipation	37
Anorexia	14
Nausea or vomiting	13
Musculoskeletal system	
Arthritis	15
Muscle cramps	10
Cardiovascular system	
Shortness of breath	19
Hypertension	18
Slow pulse	14
Genitourinary system	
Menstrual disturbances	17
Special senses	
Blurred vision	7
Tinnitus	7

From Mazzaferri EL. In Mazzaferri EL, editor: *Endocrinology,* ed 3, New York, 1986, Elsevier Science Publishing. (By permission.)

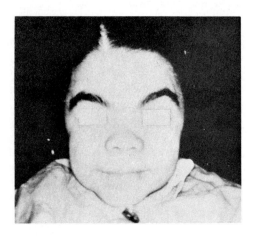

FIG. 19-4 Cretinism.

third of the eyebrows, palmar yellowing, dry rough skin, dry brittle and coarse hair, increased size of the tongue, slowing of physical and mental activity, slurred hoarse speech, anemia, constipation, increased sensitivity to cold, increased capillary fragility, muscle weakness, and deafness (Table 19-8).

The accumulation of subcutaneous fluid usually is not as pronounced in patients with pituitary myxedema as in those with primary (thyroid) myxedema. The serum cholesterol levels are closer to normal values in the patients with pituitary myxedema. Untreated patients with severe myxedema may develop hypothermic coma that is usually fatal.

The T_4, T_3, TBG, and TSH tests are used to screen for hypothyroidism. The normal values for those tests are shown in Table 19-5. The results found in hypothyroidism are shown in Table 19-6. Other thyroid tests can be ordered depending on the clinical circumstances. These tests and their results in hypothyroidism are also shown in Tables 19-5 and 19-6.

Patients with hypothyroidism are treated with thyroid extract or synthetic preparations containing sodium LT_4 (levothyroxin) (Table 19-9) or sodium LT_3 (liothyronine).[8] Patients with untreated hypothyroidism are sensitive to the actions of narcotics, barbiturates and tranquilizers, and these drugs must be used with caution. Stressful situations—such as cold, operations, infections, or trauma—may precipitate a hypothyroid (myxedema) coma, which is treated by parenteral T_3, steroids, and artificial respiration.

Myxedematous coma occurs most often in severely hypothyroid elderly patients.[2,5] It is more common during the winter months, has a high mortality rate, and is characterized by hypothermia, bradycardia, and severe hypotension; epileptic seizures may occur during the comatose state. Patients with hypothyroidism are treated with either synthetic thyroid hormone or thyroprotein derived from animal thyroid glands.

DENTAL MANAGEMENT
CLINICAL EXAMINATION

Examination of the thyroid gland should be part of a head and neck exam performed by the dentist. The anterior neck region can be scanned for indications of old surgical scars; the posterior dorsal region of the tongue should be examined for a nodule that could represent lingual thyroid tissue; and the area just superior and lateral to the thyroid cartilage should be palpated for the presence of a pyramidal lobe.

TABLE 19-9

Recommended Replacement Dosage of Sodium Levothyroxine (Synthetic Sodium LT_4) in Childhood and Adult Hypothyroidism

Age (yr)	Dose of sodium levothyroxine (μg/kg per day)
0 to 1	9
1 to 5	6
6 to 10	4
11 to 20	3
21 to 65	2.2
Over 65	1.8

From Mazzaferri EL. In Mazzaferri EL, editor: *Endocrinology,* ed 3, New York, 1986, Elsevier Science Publishing. (By permission.)

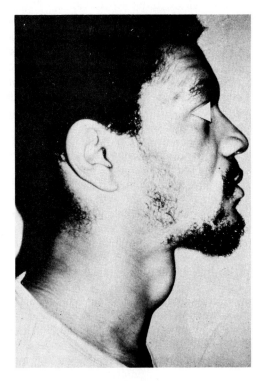

FIG. 19-5 Man with a thyroglossal duct cyst.

Although difficult to detect, the normal thyroid gland can be palpated in many patients.[2] It may feel rubbery and be more easily identified by having the patient swallow during the examination. As the patient swallows, the thyroid will rise and lumps in the neck that may be associated with it will also rise (move superiorly). Nodules in the midline area of the thyroglossal duct will move upward with protrusion of the patient's tongue (Fig. 19-5).

An enlarged thyroid gland caused by hyperplasia (goiter) will feel softer than the normal gland. Adenomas and carcinomas involving the gland will be firmer to palpation and usually be seen as isolated swellings. Patients with Hashimoto's disease or Riedel's thyroiditis will have a gland that is much firmer to palpation than the normal gland.

If a diffuse enlargement of the thyroid is detected, auscultation should be employed to examine for a systolic or continuous bruit that can be heard over the hyperactive gland of thyrotoxicosis or Graves' disease as a result of engorgement of the gland's vascular system.

MEDICAL CONSIDERATIONS
Thyrotoxicosis

The dentist should be aware of the clinical manifestations of thyrotoxicosis so undiagnosed or poorly treated disease can be detected and the patient referred for medical evaluation and treatment (Table 19-10). By doing this, dentists may be able to help reduce the morbidity and mortality rates associated with thyrotoxicosis.

Palpation and inspection of the thyroid gland should be part of the routine head and neck examination performed by the dentist. If a thyroid enlargement is noted, even though the patient appears euthyroid (normal thyroid function), a referral should be made for evaluation before dental treatment is rendered. A diffuse enlargement may be simple goiter or subacute thyroiditis. Isolated nodules may turn out to be an adenoma or carcinoma.

Patients with untreated or poorly treated thyrotoxicosis are susceptible to developing an acute medical emergency—thyrotoxic crisis, which is another important reason for detection and referral. Symptoms include restlessness, fever, tachycardia, pulmonary edema, tremor, sweating, stupor, and finally coma and death if treatment is not provided. Were a surgical

TABLE 19-10
Dental Management of the Thyrotoxic Patient

1. Detection of undiagnosed disease
   a. Symptoms
   b. Signs
   c. Referral for medical diagnosis and treatment
2. Patient with diagnosed disease
   a. Determination of original diagnosis
   b. Past therapy
   c. Present medication
   d. Assessment of clinical status (symptoms, signs, thyroid tests)
   e. Referral for reevaluation if signs and symptoms found
   f. Consultation prior to starting dental treatment
3. Avoidance of following in untreated or poorly treated patient:
   a. Surgical procedures
   b. Acute infection
   c. Epinephrine and other pressor amines (in local anesthetics, gingival retraction cords)
4. Recognition and management of initial therapy for thyrotoxic crisis
   a. Seeking of medical aid
   b. Wet packs, ice packs
   c. Hydrocortisone (100 to 300 mg)
   d. IV glucose solution
   e. Cardiopulmonary resuscitation
5. Patient under good medical treatment
   a. Avoidance of acute oral infections
   b. Treatment of all chronic oral infections
   c. Implementation of normal procedures and management

procedure to be performed on these patients, a crisis might be precipitated. In addition, an acute oral infection could precipitate a crisis. If a crisis occurs, the dentist should be able to recognize what is happening, begin emergency treatment, and seek immediate medical assistance. The patient can be cooled with cold towels, given an injection of hydrocortisone (100 to 300 mg), and started on an IV infusion of hypertonic glucose (if equipment is available). Vital signs must be monitored and cardiopulmonary resuscitation initiated if necessary. Immediate medical assistance should be sought; and, when available, other measures such as antithyroid drugs and potassium iodide can be started.

Although the role of chronic infection and thyrotoxicosis is unclear it is recommended that these sources be treated as in any other patient. Once the patient has been identified and referred for medical management, the treatment of oral foci of infection can be accomplished. Patients with extensive dental caries or periodontal disease, or both, can be treated after medical management of the thyroid problem has been effected.

The use of epinephrine or other pressor amines (in local anesthetics or gingival retraction cords, or to control bleeding) must be avoided in the untreated or poorly treated thyrotoxic patient. However, the well-treated thyrotoxic patient presents no problem in this regard and may be given normal concentrations of these vasoconstrictors.

Once the thyrotoxic patient is under good medical management, the dental treatment plan will be unaffected. If acute oral infection occurs however, consultation with the patient's physician is recommended as part of the management program.

Hypothyroidism

In general, the patient with mild symptoms of untreated hypothyroidism is not in danger when receiving dental therapy. Central nervous system (CNS) depressants, sedatives or narcotic analgesics, may cause an exaggerated response in patients with mild to severe hypothyroidism. These drugs must be avoided in all patients with severe hypothyroidism and used with care (reduced dosage) in patients with mild hypothyroidism; however, a few patients with untreated severe symptoms of hypothyroidism may be in danger if dental treatment is rendered. This is particularly true of elderly patients with myxedema. A myxedematous coma can be precipitated by CNS depressants, surgical procedures, and infections; thus, once again, the major goal of the dentist is to detect these patients and refer them for medical manage-

TABLE 19-11
Dental Management of the Hypothyroid Patient

1. Detection of undiagnosed disease
   a. Symptoms
   b. Signs
   c. Referral for medical diagnosis and treatment
2. Patient with diagnosed disease
   a. Determination of original diagnosis
   b. Past therapy
   c. Present medication
   d. Assessment of clinical status (symptoms, signs, thyroid tests)
   e. Referral for reevaluation if signs and symptoms of hyperthyroidism or hypothyroidism are found
3. Avoidance of following in untreated or poorly treated patient:
   a. Surgical procedures
   b. Oral infections
   c. CNS depressants (narcotics, barbiturates, etc)
4. Recognition and management of initial stages of myxedematous coma
   a. Seeking of immediate aid
   b. Hydrocortisone (100 to 300 mg)
   c. Artificial respiration
5. Patient under good medical management
   a. Avoidance of acute oral infections
   b. Implementation of normal procedures and management

TABLE 19-12
Medical Problems of Concern to the Dentist in a Patient with Undiagnosed or Poorly Controlled Thyroid Disease

Hyperthyroidism
  Adverse interaction with catecholamines (epinephrine)
  Life-threatening cardiac arrhythmias
  Congestive heart failure
  Complications of underlying cardiovascular pathologic conditions
  Thyrotoxic crisis can be precipitated by
    Infection
    Surgical procedures
Hypothyroidism
  Exaggerated response to CNS depressants
    Sedatives
    Narcotic analgesics
  Myxedematous coma can be precipitated by
    CNS depressants
    Infection
    Surgical procedures

ment before any dental treatment is rendered (Tables 19-11 and 19-12).

Patients with less severe forms of hypothyroidism also should be identified when possible, because the quality of their life can be greatly improved with medical treatment, and in young individuals permanent mental retardation can be avoided with early medical management. In addition, oral complications of delayed eruption of teeth, malocclusion, enlargement of the tongue, and skeletal retardation can be prevented with early detection and medical treatment.

Once the hypothyroid patient is under good medical care, no special problems are presented in terms of dental management, except for dealing with the malocclusion and enlarged tongue if present.

TREATMENT PLANNING MODIFICATIONS

No treatment planning modifications are required for the hypothyroid patient as long as the medical problems are well-controlled.

ORAL COMPLICATIONS
Thyrotoxicosis

Osteoporosis may be found involving the alveolar bone. Dental caries and periodontal disease appear more rapidly in these patients. The teeth and jaws develop more rapidly, and premature loss of the deciduous teeth with early eruption of the permanent teeth is common. Euthyroid infants of hyperthyroid mothers have been reported with erupted teeth at birth. A few patients with thyrotoxicosis have been found to have a lingual "thyroid" consisting of thyroid tissue below the area of the foramen cecum.

If the dentist detects a lingual tumor in a euthyroid patient, the patient should be evaluated by a physician for the presence of a normal thyroid gland before the mass is surgically removed. This is usually done with radioactive iodine scanning.

Hypothyroidism

Infants with cretinism may demonstrate thick lips, enlarged tongue, delayed eruption of teeth, and resulting malocclusion. The only specific oral change manifested by adults with acquired hypothyroidism is an enlarged tongue.

REFERENCES

1. Ahmann AJ, Wartofsky L: The thyroid nodule. In Becker KL, editor: *Principles and practice of endocrinology and metabolism,* Philadelphia, 1990, JB Lippincott, 312-319.
2. Barnes HV: The thyroid gland. In Harvey A, et al, editors: *The principles and practice of medicine,* ed 19, New York, 1976, Appleton-Century-Crofts.
3. Blum M: Thyroid sonography, computed tomography, and magnetic resonance imaging. In Becker KL, editor: *Principles and practice of endocrinology and metabolism,* Philadelphia, 1990, JB Lippincott, pp 289-293.
4. Green MF: The endocrine system. In Pathy MSJ, editor: *Principles and practice of geriatric medicine,* ed 2, New York, 1991, John Wiley & Sons, pp 1061-1122.
5. Ingbar SH, Woeber KA: The thyroid gland. In Williams RH, editor: *Textbook of endocrinology,* ed 5, Philadelphia, 1974, WB Saunders Co.
6. Ingbar SH, Woeber KA: Diseases of the thyroid. In Petersdorf RG, et al, editors: *Harrison's Principles of internal medicine,* ed 10, New York, 1983, McGraw-Hill.
7. Larsen PR: The thyroid. In Wyngaarden JB, Smith LH: *Cecil textbook of medicine,* ed 17, Philadelphia, 1985, WB Saunders.
8. Mazzaferri EL: The thyroid. In Mazzaferri EL, editor: *Endocrinology,* ed 3, New York, 1986, Medical Examination Publishing.
9. Nickolai TF: The thyroid gland. In Rose LF, Kaye D, editors: *Internal medicine for dentistry,* ed 2, St Louis, 1990, Mosby–Year Book, pp 997-1019.
10. Sarkar SD, Becker DV: Thyroid uptake and imaging. In Becker KL, editor: *Principles and practice of endocrinology and metabolism,* Philadelphia, 1990, JB Lippincott, pp 284-289.
11. Smallridge RC: Evaluation of thyroid function: blood tests. In Becker KL, editor: *Principles and practice of endocrinology and metabolism,* Philadelphia, 1990, JB Lippincott, pp 278-284.
12. Sonis ST, Fazio RC, Fang LF: *Principles and practice of oral medicine: thyroid disorders,* Philadelphia, 1984, WB Saunders.
13. Tunbridge WMG, Caldwell G: The epidemiology of thyroid diseases. In Braverman LE, Utiger RD, editors: *Werner and Ingbar's The thyroid,* ed 6, Phildelphia, 1991, JB Lippincott, pp 578-588.
14. Wartofsky L; Introduction of thyroid disease. In Becker KL, editor: *Principles and practice of endocrinology and metabolism,* Philadelphia, 1990, JB Lippincott, pp 264-267.
15. Wartofsky L, Ingbar SH: Diseases of the thyroid. In Wilson JD, et al, editors: *Harrison's Principles of internal medicine,* ed 12, New York, 1991, McGraw-Hill, pp 1692-1713.

20

Pregnancy and Breast-Feeding

A pregnant patient, although not "medically compromised" per se, poses a unique set of management considerations for the dentist. Therapeutic dental care must be rendered to the mother without adversely affecting the developing fetus. Although providing routine dental care to pregnant patients is generally safe, it must be recognized that the delivery of dental care involves some *potentially* harmful elements—including ionizing radiation and drug administration. Thus the prudent practitioner will minimize exposure of the patient to potentially harmful procedures or will avoid them altogether when possible.

Additional considerations arise during the postpartum period if the mother elects to breast-feed her infant. Although most drugs are only minimally transmitted from the maternal serum to the breast milk, so the infant's exposure is not significant, the dentist should avoid using any drug known to be harmful to the infant.

GENERAL DESCRIPTION
PHYSIOLOGY AND COMPLICATIONS

To define rational management guidelines, it is first necessary to review the normal processes of pregnancy and fetal development.

Endocrine changes are the most significant basic alterations that occur with pregnancy, and they result in most of the systemic alterations with which we are concerned. An increase occurs in the production of maternal hormones, and placental hormones begin to be produced.

Common neurologic findings in the first trimester include fatigue with nausea and/or vomiting. There is also a tendency for syncope and postural hypotension. During the second trimester, patients typically have a sense of well-being and relatively few symptoms. During the third trimester, increasing fatigue and mild depression may be seen.

Cardiovascular changes are varied. There is commonly a slight decrease in blood pressure, especially diastolic. Blood volume will increase 40% to 55%, and the cardiac output increases 30%.[15] Corresponding to these volume changes are tachycardia and heart murmurs. A systolic murmur will develop in 90% of pregnant women but disappears shortly after delivery.[9] A murmur of this type would be considered physiologic or functional; however, a murmur that preceded pregnancy or persisted after delivery would need further evaluation to determine its significance. There may also be dyspnea at rest that is aggravated by a supine position.

During late pregnancy a phenomenon known as supine hypotensive syndrome may occur—manifested by an abrupt fall in blood pressure, bradycardia, sweating, nausea, weakness, and air hunger when the patient is in a supine position.[4] The syndrome is due to impaired venous return to the heart resulting from compression of the inferior vena cava by the gravid uterus and leading to decreased blood pressure, decreased cardiac output, and impairment or loss of conciousness. The remedy for the problem is to roll the patient over onto her left side, which lifts the uterus off the vena cava. She should rapidly return to normal.

Blood changes in pregnancy include anemia and a decreased hematocrit. Because of the increased blood volume, there is a marked need for additional iron. It is not surprising that many pregnant women have some degree of iron deficiency, which is a problem that may be exaggerated after significant blood loss. There is also an increased white blood cell count due to a neutrophilia; however, changes in platelets are usually insignificant. Several blood clotting factors are increased, especially fibrinogen and Factors VII, VIII, IX, and X and fibrin split products.[15]

Pregnancy sometimes predisposes to an increased appetite and an appetite for unusual foods. As a result the diet may not be nutritious or balanced and may be high in sugars, which can adversely affect the dentition.

The general pattern of fetal development also should be understood when dental management plans are being formulated. Normal pregnancy lasts approximately 40 weeks. During the first trimester, formation of organs and systems occurs; thus the fetus is most susceptible to malformation during this period. After the first trimester the majority of formation has been completed and the remainder of fetal development is devoted primarily to growth and maturation. Thus the chances of malformation are markedly diminished after the first trimester. A notable exception to this is the fetal dentition, which is susceptible to dental staining caused by the administration of tetracycline during later pregnancy.

Another consideration relating to fetal growth is spontaneous abortion (miscarriage). Spontaneous abortion – the natural termination of pregnancy before the twentieth week of gestation – occurs in more than 15% of all pregnancies, the majority of which are caused by intrinsic fetal abnormalities.[21] Therefore it is most unlikely that any dental procedure would be implicated in spontaneous abortion. Febrile illnesses and sepsis, however, can precipitate a miscarriage; therefore prompt treatment of infection is advised.

Finally, it must be kept in mind that the fetus has a limited ability to metabolize drugs, because of its immature liver and immature enzyme system; therefore pharmacologic challenge of the fetus is to be avoided when possible.

DENTAL MANAGEMENT
MEDICAL CONSIDERATIONS

Management recommendations during pregnancy should be viewed as general guidelines, not as immutable rules. If possible, the first step in management is to contact the patient's obstetrician or physician to discuss the patient's medical status, her dental needs, and the proposed dental treatment. Not only is this beneficial from the standpoint of planning treatment, it also demonstrates to the patient a caring concern about her and her baby. It is interesting, however, to note that in a recent survey of obstetricians,[22] 91% of respondents indicated that they preferred not to be contacted in regard to "routine dental care." Nevertheless, 88% and 54% did want to be consulted prior to the dentist's prescribing, respectively, antibiotics and analgesics.

Pregnancy is a special event in a woman's life and, as such, is emotionally charged. Therefore establishment of a good patient-dentist relationship that encourages openness, honesty, and trust is an integral part of successful management. This kind of relationship greatly decreases stress and anxiety for both patient and dentist.

Preventive program

The most important objective in planning dental treatment for a pregnant patient is to establish a healthy oral environment and optimum oral hygiene level. This essentially consists of a plaque control program, which will minimize the exaggerated inflammatory response of the gingival tissues to local irritants that commonly accompanies the hormonal changes of pregnancy. The relationship of plaque and other local irritants, hormonal alterations, and periodontal disease is well-known and can be clearly explained to the patient. Acceptable oral hygiene techniques should be taught, reinforced, and monitored. Coronal scaling and polishing or root curettage may be performed whenever necessary. All these control measures should be stressed throughout pregnancy, including the first trimester.

The benefits of prenatal fluoride have been controversial, with little evidence that supported its use. However, two studies (by Glenn[12] and by Glenn et al.[13]) have suggested that when a daily 2.2 mg tablet of sodium fluoride was administered to mothers during the second and third trimester in combination with fluoridated water the offspring remained virtually free of caries for up to 10 years. In addition to the elimination of caries, the prematurity rate was significantly reduced and there was a slight increase in height and birth weight. There was no evidence of medical or dental defects (including fluorosis) in any of the children. Therefore it was concluded that fluoride tablet supplementation from the third through ninth month of pregnancy was safe and effective. These results are intriguing, but some authorities[14] suggest that adequate controls were not used and note that the studies have not been duplicated.

Treatment timing

Other than as part of a good plaque control program, elective dental care is best avoided during the first trimester because of potential vulnerability of the fetus (Table 20-1).

The second trimester is the safest period in which to provide routine dental care. Emphasis should be placed on controlling active disease and eliminating potential problems that could occur later in pregnancy or immediately after delivery, because attaining dental care during these periods is frequently difficult. Extensive reconstruction or significant surgical procedures are best postponed until after delivery; it should be borne in mind that pregnancy is a temporary condition.

The early part of the third trimester is still a good time to provide routine dental care; but after the middle of the third trimester, elective dental care is best postponed. This is only because of the increasing feeling of discomfort that the woman may have and is not necessarily applicable to all patients. Prolonged chair time should be avoided, to prevent the complication of supine hypotensive syndrome. If treatment becomes necessary during this period, problems can be minimized by scheduling short appointments, allowing the patient to assume a semireclining position, and encouraging frequent changes of position.

Dental radiographs

Dental radiography is one of the more controversial areas in the management of a pregnant patient. It is most desirable not to have any irradiation during pregnancy, especially during the first trimester, because the developing fetus is particularly susceptible to radiation damage. However, should dental treatment become necessary, radiographs will usually be required to provide an accurate diagnosis and to plan proper treatment. Therefore the dentist must be aware of how to proceed safely in this situation.

The safety of dental radiography has been well-established, provided features such as high-speed film, filtration, collimation, and lead aprons are used. Of all aids, the most important for the pregnant patient is the protective lead apron; studies[2,16] have shown that, when an apron is used during contemporary dental radiography, gonadal and fetal radiation is virtually unmeasurabe.

The dentist must keep in perspective the facts of radiation biology. Animal and human data[5-8,10,18] clearly support the conclusion that no increase in gross congenital anomalies or intrauterine growth retardation occurs as a result of exposures during pregnancy totaling less than 5 to 10 cGy.* For comparison purposes the following can be considered[10]: a medical chest radiograph results in an estimated fetal or embryonic dose of 0.008 cGy, a skull radiograph results in 0.004 cGy, and a full mouth series of

---

* One centigray (cGy) is the unit of absorbed radiation equivalent to a rad (roentgen, R).

TABLE 20-1
Treatment Timing During Pregnancy

First trimester	Second trimester	Third trimester
Plaque control	Plaque control	Plaque control
Oral hygiene instruction	Oral hygiene instruction	Oral hygiene instruction
Scaling, polishing, curettage	Scaling, polishing, curettage	Scaling, polishing, curettage
Avoid elective treatment; urgent care only	Routine dental care	Routine dental care

TABLE 20-2

Comparative Radiation Exposures to Fetal or Embryonic Tissues

Source of radiation	Absorbed exposure (cGy)
Upper gastrointestinal series	0.330
Chest radiograph	0.008
Skull radiograph	0.004
Daily (cosmic) background radiation	0.0004
Full mouth dental series (18 intraoral radiographs, D film, lead apron)	0.00001

Adapted from DiSaia PJ. In Scott JR, et al, editors: *Danforth's Obstetrics and gynecology,* ed 6, Philadelphia, 1990, JB Lippincott, p 1127.

dental radiographs with a lead apron results in 0.00001 cGy (Table 20-2).

When further assessing risks of dental radiography during pregnancy, it should be noted that the maximum risk attributable to 1 cGy (10% to 20% of the threshold dose) of in utero radiation exposure has been estimated[6] to be approximately 0.1%, a quantity thousands of times *less* than the normal anticipated risks of spontaneous abortion or malformation or genetic disease. From these figures it is evident that with use of the lead apron, one or two intraoral films are truly of no significance in terms of radiation effects to the developing fetus.

Even in light of the obvious safety of dental radiography, however, the dentist should not be cavalier in his approach to it during pregnancy (or at any other time, for that matter). Radiographs should be used selectively, and only when necessary and appropriate, to aid in diagnosis and treatment. When they are thus used, and when the lead apron is also applied, proper dental care can be given safely during pregnancy—in most instances using only bitewing, panoramic, or selected periapical films.

An additional consideration is the pregnant dental auxiliary or dentist. However, it is well-established that, as long as appropriate radiation safety measures are followed, there is no contraindication to these persons' operating the x-ray machine.

DRUG ADMINISTRATION
During pregnancy

Another controversial area in treating pregnant dental patients is drug administration. The principal concern is that a drug may cross the placenta and be toxic or teratogenic to the fetus. Also, any drug that is a respiratory depressant can cause maternal hypoxia, resulting in fetal hypoxia, injury, or death.

Ideally no drug should be administered during pregnancy, especially the first trimester; however, it is sometimes impossible to adhere to this rule. It is therefore fortunate that most of the commonly used drugs in dental practice can be given during pregnancy with relative safety, though there are a few exceptions. Table 20-3 is a suggested approach to drug usage for pregnant patients.

As an aid to the dentist who wishes to prescribe or administer a drug to a pregnant patient, the Food and Drug Administration[20] requires a categorization of prescription drugs for pregnant patients based on their risk of fetal injury.

Briefly, the format is as follows:

A. Controlled studies in humans have failed to demonstrate a risk to the fetus, and the possibility of fetal harm appears remote.

B. Animal studies have not indicated fetal risk, and there are no human studies; *or* animal studies have shown a risk, but controlled human studies have not.

C. Animal studies have shown a risk, but there are no controlled human studies; *or* no studies are available in humans or animals.

D. Positive evidence of human fetal risk exists, but in certain situations the drug may be used despite its risk.

X. Positive evidence of human fetal risk exists, and the risk outweighs any possible benefit of use.

Obviously, drugs in category A or B are preferable for prescribing. However, many drugs that fall into category C are administered during pregnancy and therefore these drugs will present the most difficulty for the dentist and physician in terms of therapeutic and medicolegal decisions.

It should be recognized that physicians may advise against the use of some of the approved drugs or, conversely, may suggest the use of a questionable drug. The listed guidelines are

TABLE 20-3
Drug Administration During Pregnancy and Breast-Feeding

Drug	FDA category (prescription drug)	During pregnancy	During breast-feeding
Local anesthetics			
Lidocaine	B	Yes	Yes
Mepivacaine	C	Use with caution; consult physician	Yes
Prilocaine	B	Yes	Yes
Bupivacaine	C	Use with caution; consult physician	Yes
Etidocaine	B	Yes	Yes
Procaine	C	Use with caution; consult physician	Yes
Analgesics			
Aspirin	C/D	Caution; avoid in third trimester	Avoid
Acetaminophen	B	Yes	Yes
Ibuprofen	B	Caution; avoid in third trimester	Yes
Codeine	C	Use with caution; consult physician	Yes
Hydrocodeine	C	Use with caution; consult physician	—
Oxycodone	C	Use with caution; consult physician	—
Propoxyphene	C	Use with caution; consult physician	Yes
Antibiotics			
Penicillins	B	Yes	Yes
Erythromycin	B	Yes; avoid estolate form	Yes
Clindamycin	Not assigned	Avoid	Yes
Cephalosporins	B	Yes	Yes
Tetracycline	D	Avoid	Avoid
Sedative-hypnotics			
Benzodiazepines	D	Avoid	Avoid
Barbiturates	D	Avoid	Avoid
Nitrous oxide	Not assigned	Avoid in first trimester; otherwise, use with caution; consult physician	Yes

general ones. An example of the occasional use of a questionable drug would be a narcotic for a frightened patient or a patient in severe pain.

Although it is unlikely that a single administration of nitrous oxide would be teratogenic, N_2O-O_2 inhalation analgesia is not recommended during the first trimester based on findings of animal studies relating chronic N_2O administration to birth defects. Although these results cannot be extrapolated to humans, it seems prudent to avoid its usage during organogenesis. If N_2O-O_2 is used in the second or third trimester, at least 50% O_2 should be delivered to ensure adequate oxygenation at all times and special precautions also should be taken to avoid diffusion hypoxia at the termination of administration. An additional consideration is for the female dentist or dental auxiliary who is pregnant. It is advisable that she not be exposed to persistent trace levels of N_2O in the operatory.

During breast-feeding

A potential problem arises when a nursing mother requires the administration of a drug in the course of dental treatment. The concern is that the administered drug will find its way into the breast milk and be transferred to the nursing infant, in whom exposure may result in adverse effects.

Unfortunately, the data on which to draw definitive conclusions about drug dosage and effects via breast milk are sparse; however, retrospective clinical studies and empiric observations, coupled with known pharmacologic pathways, allow recommendations to be made. A significant fact is that the amount of drug excreted in the breast milk is usually not more than 1% to 2% of the maternal dose; therefore it is highly unlikely that most drugs are of any pharmacologic significance to the infant.[23]

Agreement seems to exist that a few drugs, or categories of drugs, are definitely contraindicated for nursing mothers. These include lithium, anticancer drugs, radioactive pharmaceuticals, and phenindione.[1,19] Table 20-3 contains recommendations regarding the administration of commonly used dental drugs during breast-feeding. As with drug use during pregnancy, individual physicians may wish to modify these recommendations, which should be viewed only as general guidelines for treatment.

In addition to careful drug selection for the nursing mother, it is suggested that the mother take the drug just after breast-feeding and avoid nursing for 4 hours or more if possible. This will markedly decrease the drug concentration in her breast milk.[3]

TREATMENT PLANNING MODIFICATIONS

There are no technical modifications required for the pregnant patient. However, reconstructions, crown and bridge procedures, and signif-

icant surgery are best delayed until after pregnancy.

ORAL COMPLICATIONS

The most common oral complication of pregnancy (found in essentially 100% of patients) is a marked increase in gingival inflammation, which represents an exaggerated inflammatory response to local irritants as a result of hormonal influence. This is frequently labeled "pregnancy gingivitis" (Fig. 20-1).

On occasion a pyogenic granuloma may present as an exaggerated localized inflammatory hyperplastic tissue response; this is called a "pregnancy tumor" (Fig. 20-2). Gingival changes become apparent around the second month and continue until the eighth month, at which time the gingival tissues rapidly return to

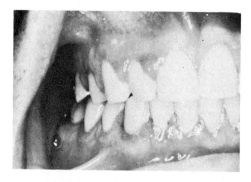

FIG. 20-1 Generalized gingivitis in a woman in the sixth month of pregnancy—"pregnancy gingivitis."

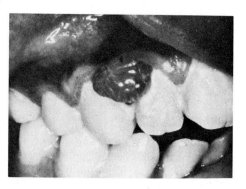

FIG. 20-2 Pyogenic granuloma occurring during pregnancy—"pregnancy tumor."

normal.[17] It should be stressed that pregnancy does not cause periodontal disease but only modifies and worsens what is already present.

The relationship between dental caries and pregnancy is not well-defined; however, it appears that pregnancy does not directly contribute to the carious process. More than likely, an increase in caries activity can be attributed to a poor diet and poor oral hygiene, which commonly result in sore and inflamed gingival tissues.

Many women are convinced that pregnancy causes tooth loss ("a tooth for every pregnancy") or that calcium is withdrawn from the maternal dentition to supply fetal requirements ("soft teeth"). Calcium is present in the teeth in a stable crystalline form and, as such, is not available to the systemic circulation to supply a calcium demand. However, calcium is readily mobilized from bone to supply these demands. Therefore, although calcium supplementation for the purpose of preventing tooth loss or "soft teeth" is unwarranted, the physician may prescribe calcium for general nutritional requirements of mother and infant.

A final dental finding is tooth mobility, which may be generalized. This sign is probably related to the degree of gingival disease and disturbance of the attachment apparatus as well as to some mineral changes in the lamina dura. The condition is reversible after delivery.

REFERENCES

1. American Academy of Pediatrics Committee on Drugs: Transfer of drugs and other chemicals into human milk, *Pediatrics* 84:924-936, 1989.
2. Bean LR Jr, Devore WD: The effects of protective aprons in dental roentgenography, *Oral Surg* 28:505-508, 1969.
3. Berlin CM: Pharmacologic considerations of drug use in the lactating mother, *Obstet Gynecol* 58(suppl):1755, 1981.
4. Bottoms SF, Scott JR: Transfusions and shock. In Scott JR, et al, editors: *Danforth's Obstetrics and gynecology,* ed 6, Philadelphia, 1990, JB Lippincott.
5. Brent RL: Environmental factors: radiation. In Brent RL, Harris MI, editors: *Prevention of embryonic, fetal and perinatal disease, Fogarty International Center series on preventive medicine,* vol 3, DHEW Publ. no. 76-853, pp 1799-197, 1976.
6. Brent RL: The effects of embryonic and fetal exposure to x-ray, micriwaves, and ultrasound, *Clin Obstet Gynecol* 26:484-510, 1983.
7. Brent RL: Ionizing radiation, *Contemp Obstet Gynecol* 30(2):20-29, 1987.
8. Brent RL, Gorson RO: Radiation exposure in pregnancy, *Curr Probl Radiol* 2:1-48, 1972.
9. Cunningham FG, MacDonald PC, Gant NF: *Williams Obstetrics,* ed 18, Norwalk Conn, 1989, Appleton & Lange.
10. DiSaia PJ: Radiation therapy in gynecology. In Scott JR, et al, editors: *Danforth's Obstetrics and gynecology,* ed 6, Philadelphia, 1990, JB Lippincott.
11. *Drug information for the health care professional,* vol IA and IB, ed 12, Rockville Md, 1992, United States Pharmacopeial Convention.
12. Glenn FB: Immunity conveyed by a fluoride supplement during pregnancy, *J Dent Child* 44:391-395, 1977.
13. Glenn FB, Glenn WD III, Duncan RC: Fluoride tablet supplementation during pregnancy for caries immunity: a study of the offspring produced, *Am J Obstet Gynecol* 143:560-564, 1982.
14. Hargreaves JA: The level and timing of systemic exposure to fluoride with respect to caries resistance, *J Dent Res* 71:1244-1248, 1992.
15. Hume RF, Killam AP: Maternal physiology. In Scott JR, et al, editors: *Danforth's Obstetrics and gynecology,* ed 6, Philadelphia, 1990, JB Lippincott.
16. Laws PW: *The x-ray information book. A consumer's guide to avoiding unnecessary medical and dental x-rays,* New York, 1983, Farrar, Straus & Giroux.
17. Löe H: Periodontal changes in pregnancy, *J Periodontol* 36:209-217, 1965.
18. Mole RH: Radiation effects on pre-natal development and their radiological significance, *Br J Radiol* 52:89-101, 1979.
19. Niebyl JR: Teratology and drugs in pregnancy and lactation. In Scott JR, et al, editors: *Danforth's Obstetrics and gynecology,* ed 6, Philadelphia, 1990, JB Lppincott.
20. Pregnancy categories for prescription drugs, *FDA Drug Bull* 12(3):24-25, 1982.
21. Scott JR: Spontaneous abortion. In Scott JR, et al, editors: *Danforth's Obstetrics and gynecology,* ed 6, Philadelphia, 1990, JB Lippincott.
22. Shrout MK, Comer RW, Powell BJ, McCoy BP: Treating the pregnant dental patient: four basic rules addressed, *J Am Dent Assoc* 123(5):75-80, 1992.
23. Wilson JT, Brown RD, Cherek DR, et al: Drug excretion in human breast milk: principles, pharmacokinetics and projected consequences, *Clin Pharmacokinet* 5:1-66, 1980.

21

Allergy

There are at least four reasons why it is important for the dentist to know about allergy: (1) to identify patients with a true allergic history so acute medical emergencies that might occur in the dental office because of an allergic reaction can be prevented, (2) to recognize oral soft tissue changes that might be caused by an allergic reaction, (3) to identify and plan appropriate dental care for patients who have severe alterations of their immune system because of radiation, drug therapy, or immune deficiency disorders, and (4) to recognize signs and symptoms of acute allergic reactions and manage these problems appropriately.

To accomplish these goals, it is first necessary to have a basic understanding of allergy.

GENERAL DESCRIPTION
INCIDENCE AND PREVALENCE

It is estimated[31] that 15% to 25% of all Americans are allergic to some substance—including about 4.5% who have asthma, 4% who are allergic to insect stings, and 5% who are allergic to one or more drugs. Allergic reactions account for about 6% to 10% of all adverse drug reactions[29,31,40]; of these, 46% consist of erythema and rash, 23% urticaria, 10% fixed drug reactions, 5% erythema multiform and 1% anaphylaxis.[29] There is about a 1% to 3% risk for an allergic reaction when using a drug. Fatal drug reactions occur in about 0.01% of surgical inpatients and 0.1% of medical inpatients.[31]

Drugs are the most common cause of urticarial reactions in adults, and food and infections are the most common cause of these lesions in children. Urticaria occurs in 15% to 20% of young adults. In about 70% of the patients with chronic urticaria no etiologic agent can be identified.[18]

Iodinated organic compounds used as radiographic contrast media result in about one death for every 1400 to 60,000 diagnostic procedures.[7] Animal insulin used to treat type I diabetic patients will cause an allergic reaction in about 10% to 56% of these individuals, and it has been reported[7] that some 25% of diabetic patients who are allergic to insulin will react to penicillin.

About 5% to 10% of the individuals given penicillin will develop an allergic reaction, and 0.04% to 0.20% of these an anaphylactic reaction, to the drug. Death will occur in about 10% of those individuals who had an anaphylactic reaction.[7,18,21]

In a report of 151 deaths worldwide from anaphylactic reactions to penicillin,[18] it was found that in 85% of the cases death occurred within 15 minutes following administration of the drug and in 50% the allergic reaction started immediately following the administration. Seventy percent of the individuals had a history of having been given penicillin[18] (Table 21-1). The most common causes of anaphylactic death are penicillin, bee stings, and wasp stings; individuals with an atopic history are more susceptible to anaphylactic death than are patients with no history of allergy.[7]

In rare cases antihistamines have been reported[7] to cause urticaria from an allergic response to the colored coating material of the capsule. In addition, azo and non-azo dyes used in toothpaste have been reported to cause anaphylactoid reactions. Also, analine dyes used to coat certain steroid tablets have caused serious allergic reactions.[7]

TABLE 21-1

Summary of 151 Cases of Penicillin-Related Anaphylactic Deaths

21 (14%)	Had history of allergies
106 (70%)	Had received penicillin before; 35 (1 of 3) had experienced sudden allergic reaction
128 (85%)	Died within 15 minutes of administration
75 (50%)	Experienced symptoms right after first administration of drug
3 (2%)	Were related to oral penicillin

From Idsoe O, et al: *Bull WHO* 38:159-188, 1968.

TABLE 21-2

Coombs and Gell Classifications of Immunologic Hypersensitivity Reactions

I and Type I — Anaphylactic or IgE-mediated
II and Type II — Cytotoxic
III and Type III — Immune complex-mediated
IV and Type IV — Cell-mediated or delayed

TABLE 21-3

The Immune System

1. Nonspecific
   a. Mechanical reflexes
      (1) Coughing, sneezing
      (2) Action of cila
      (3) Sphincter control of bladder
   b. Secretion of bactericidal substances
      (1) Stomach acid
      (2) Earwax (cerumen)
      (3) Enzymes in tears or saliva
   c. Phagocytic cells
      (1) Neutrophils
      (2) Monocytes
      (3) Macrophages
   d. Circulating chemicals
      (1) Complement
      (2) Interferon
2. Specific
   a. Humoral immunity
      (1) Protection against bacterial infection
      (2) Clones of B lymphocytes
      (3) Recognition of chemical configuration
      (4) Plasma cells produce antibodies
      (5) Eradication of antigen
   b. Cellular immunity
      (1) Protection against viral infection, tuberculosis, leprosy
      (2) Transplant rejection
      (3) T lymphocytes produce cytokines
      (4) Eradication of antigen

Based on Thomson NC, et al. In Thomson NC, et al, editors: *Handbook of clinical allergy*, Oxford, 1990, Blackwell Scientific, pp 1-36.

Parabens (used as preservatives in local anesthetics) have caused anaphylactoid reactions.[7] Seng and Gay[32] reported that the sulfites (sodium metabisulfite or acetone sodium bisulfite) used in local anesthetic solutions to prevent oxidation of the vasoconstrictors can cause serious allergic reactions. The group of patients most suscpetible to allergic reactions from sulfites are the 9 million to 11 million asthmatic persons in the United States.

ETIOLOGY

Allergic diseases are conditions that result from an immunologic reaction to a noninfectious foreign substance (antigen). They are actually a series of repeat reactions to a foreign substance. The reactions involve different types of immunologic hypersensitivity (Table 21-2) and involve elements of the nonspecific and specific branches of the immune system (Table 21-3). The functions of the humoral and cellular branches of the immune system are shown in Table 21-4.

The foreign substances that trigger hypersensitivity reactions are termed *allergens* or *antigens.* Table 21-5 shows some of the characteristics of antigens. Two types of lymphocytes play central roles in the two branches of the specific immune system. B lymphocytes are key in the humoral branch, and T lymphocytes key in the cellular branch. The three branches of the immune system do not operate independently. T lymphocytes play an important role in the regulation of B lymphocytes. The initial function of humoral and cellular branches of the immune system is the recognition of antigens; however, for the eradication of antigens, cells and chem-

TABLE 21-4
Functions of the Immune System

Function	Humoral	Cellular
Processing of antigen	T-helper cells and macrophages	Macrophages plus antigens of major histocompatibility complex (MHC)
Cellular recognition of antigen	Receptors on B lymphocytes sensitive to specific chemical configurations	T lymphocytes with receptors to specific subsets of MHC antigens
Cellular response to presentation of antigen	Specific clones of B lymphocytes multiply and produce plasma cells and memory cells	Specific clones of T lymphoctyes multiply and produce effector T cells and memory T cells
Cellular action against antigen	Plasma cells produce specific immunoglobulins (antibodies); memory cells become plasma cells, with later antigen contact	Effector T cells produce cytokines. Memory T cells become effector T cells, with later antigen contact
Eradication of antigen	Reaction with specific antibody facilitated by nonspecific branch of immune system; removed by cells of nonspecific branch	Destruction of antigen by cytokines and elements of nonspecific branch of immune system

Based on Thomson NC, et al. In Thomson NC, et al, editors: *Handbook of clinical allergy*, Oxford, 1990, Blackwell Scientific, pp 1-36.

TABLE 21-5
Antigens

Materials considered foreign by body
Large molecular size
Certain degree of molecular complexity
Polysaccharides rarely induce cell-mediated immune response (T-independent antigens)
Have multiple antigenic determinants or antibody binding sites (epitopes)
All humans will not show same reaction to antigen

Based on Thomson NC, et al. In Thomson NC, et al, editors: *Handbook of clinical allergy*, Oxford, 1990, Blackwell Scientific, pp 1-36.

icals from the nonspecific branch of the immune system are necessary.

Under some circumstances the repeated contact or exposure to an antigen may cause an inappropriate response (hypersensitivity) that can be harmful or destructive to the host's tissues; thus hypersensitivity reactions can involve either the cellular or humoral components of the immune system.

Reactions that involve the humoral system most often occur soon after contact with the antigen. Three types of hypersensitivity reaction involve elements of the humoral immune system (types I, II, and III).[37] Allergic reactions that involve the cellular immune system often are of delayed onset. Type IV hypersensitivity reactions involve the cellular immune system. Examples include contact dermatitis, graft rejection, graft-versus-host disease, some drug reactions, and some types of autoimmune disease.[37,38]

PATHOPHYSIOLOGY AND COMPLICATIONS
Humoral immune system

B lymphocytes recognize specific foreign chemical configurations via receptors on their cell membranes. For the antigen to be recognized by specific B lymphocytes, it must first be processed by T lymphocytes and marcrophages.

TABLE 21-6
Lymphocyte Response: B Cells

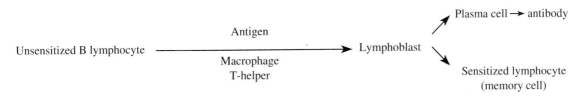

TABLE 21-7
Immunoglobulins (Antibodies)

Basic structure
   Two heavy chains (alpha, delta, epsilon, gamma, mu)
   Two light chains (kappa, lambda)
   Chains held together by disulfide bonds
Origin
   Plasma cells (from specific clones of B lymphocytes)
Classes
   IgG (gamma heavy chains)
   IgA (alpha heavy chains)
   IgM (mu heavy chains)
   IgD (delta heavy chains)
   IgE (epsilon heavy chains)
Functional structure
   Each chain has constant region
   Each chain has variable region
      Fab end—antibody (ab) end, highly variable, attaches to antigen
      Fc end—crystallizable (c) end, binds to complement and to effector cells

Based on Thomson NC, et al. In Thomson NC, et al, editors: *Handbook of clinical allergy*, Oxford, 1990, Blackwell Scientific, pp 1-36.

Each clone (family) of B lymphocytes recognizes its own specific chemical structure. Once recognition has taken place, the B lymphocytes differentiate and mulitply, forming plasma cells and memory B lymphocytes (Table 21-6). The memory B lymphocytes remain inactive until contact with the same type of antigen occurs. This contact will transform the memory cell into a plasma cell to produce immunoglobulins (antibodies) specific for the antigen involved.

TABLE 21-8
Functions of Immunoglobulins

1. IgG
   a. Most abundant immunoglobulin
   b. Small size allows diffusion into tissue spaces
   c. Can cross placenta
   d. Opsonizing antibody—facilitates phagocytosis of microorganisms by neutrophils
   e. Four subclasses—IgG1, IgG2, IgG3, IgG4
      (1) IgG4 can bind to mast cells
2. IgA
   a. Two types
      (1) Secretory (dimer, secretory component)—found in saliva, tears, nasal mucus; secretory component protects from proteolysis
      (2) Serum (monomer)
   b. Does not cross placenta
   c. Last immunoglobulin to appear in childhood
3. IgM
   a. Large molecule
   b. Confined to intravascular space
   c. First immunoglobulin produced
   d. Activates complement
   e. Good agglutinating antibody
4. IgE
   a. Very low concentration in serum (0.004%)
   b. Increased in parasitic and atopic diseases
   c. Binds to mast cells and basophils
   d. Key antibody in pathogenesis of type I hypersensitivity reactions
5. IgD
   a. Low concentration in serum
   b. Little importance

Based on Thomson NC, et al. In Thomson NC, et al, editors: *Handbook of clinical allergy*, Oxford, 1990, Blackwell Scientific, pp 1-36.

TABLE 21-9

Functions of the Humoral Immune System

1. First encounter with antigen (primary response)
   a. Latent period
      (1) Antigen is processed
      (2) B lymphocyte clone selected
      (3) Differentiation and proliferation
      (4) Plasma cells and memory cells
      (5) Plasma cells produce specific immuno-globulins
   b. Specific IgM level increases first in serum followed by IgG
   c. IgM levels will later fall to zero
   d. IgG levels will fall; however, some remain
2. Second encounter with antigen (secondary response)
   a. Latent period is shorter
      (1) Antigen is processed
      (2) Memory cells selected; become plasma cells
      (3) Plasma cells produce specific immuno-globulins
   b. IgM levels increase first
   c. IgG levels increase to 50 times level found in primary response
   d. IgM levels will later fall
   e. IgG levels will later fall but significant serum level is usually maintained

Based on Thomson NC, et al. In Thomson NC, et al, editors: *Handbook of clinical allergy*, Oxford, 1990, Blackwell Scientific, pp 1-36.

TABLE 21-10

Type I Hypersensitivity

1. IgE antibody–mediated
2. Immediate response
3. Usual allergens (antigens)
   a. Dust
   b. Mites
   c. Pollens
   d. Animal danders
   e. Food
   f. Drugs (haptens)
4. Symptoms
   a. Anaphylaxis
   b. Hay fever
   c. Asthma
   d. Urticaria, angioedema
   e. GI symptoms on occasion
5. Frequency—affects about 10% of population
6. Inherited tendency

Based on Thomson NC, et al. In Thomson NC, et al, editors: *Handbook of clinical allergy*, Oxford, 1990, Blackwell Scientific, pp 1-36.

Table 21-7 shows the structure, origin, classes, and functional components of the immunoglobulins produced by plasma cells. Table 21-8 lists the functions for the five classes of immunoglobulins. Note that IgE is the key antibody involved in the pathogenesis of type I hypersensitivity reactions. The normal functions of the humoral immune system are shown in Table 21-9.

Type I, type II, and type III hypersensitivities involve elements of the humoral immune system. Type I hypersensitivity is summarized in Table 21-10. These are IgE-mediated reactions leading to the release of chemical mediators from mast cells and basophils in various target tissues. Table 21-11 lists the sequence of events involved in type I hypersensitivity reactions. The role of IgE is clear in these reactions, but that of the other sensitizing antibody (IgG4) is not well-understood.

TYPE I HYPERSENSITIVITY REACTIONS

Type I hypersensitivity reactions are related to the humoral immune system. They usually occur soon after the second contact with an antigen; however, it is also common to find individuals who have had repeated contacts with a drug or material before finally becoming allergic to it (Fig. 21-1). *Anaphylaxis* is an acute reaction involving the smooth muscle of the bronchi in which the antigen-antibody complex formed causes histamine release from the mast cells. The smooth muscle contracts, and this may lead to acute respiratory distress or failure. *Atopy* is a hypersensitivity state influenced by hereditary factors. Hay fever, asthma, urticaria, and angioneurotic edema are examples of atopic reactions. The most common lesions associated with atopic reactions are urticaria (which is a superficial lesion of the skin) and angioneurotic edema (which is a lesion occurring in the deeper layer of the skin or in other tissues such as the larynx or tongue). In true allergic reactions these lesions result from the effect of antigens and their antibodies (IgE) on mast cells in various locations in the body. The antigen-antibody complex causes the release of mediators (histamine) from the mast cells; these mediators then produce an increase

TABLE 21-11

Sensitizing Antibodies in Hypersensitivity Reactions

1. Homocytotropic antibodies—attach to mast cells and basophils by Fc end of the molecule
   a. IgE
   b. IgG4
2. Type I hypersensitivity—setting the stage
   a. T cell–dependent antigens—stimulate IgE response
   b. Defect in suppressor controls
   c. Persistence of IgE
   d. Why B cell switches to IgE production rather than to one of other classes of immunoglobulins is not clear
   e. IgE binds to mast cell (thousands of IgE molecules can bind to surface of single mast cell)
3. Type I hypersensitivity—reaction
   a. New exposure of antigen
   b. Antigen cross-links with two or more IgE molecules
   c. Signal transmitted to inside of mast cell
   d. Activates cyclic nucleotides and influx of calcium ions (Ca^{++})
   e. Causes release of mediators and synthesis of new mediators
   f. Clinical symptoms of immediate hypersensitivity caused by action of mediators (histamine) on target tissues
4. Role of IgG4
   a. Will bind to mast cells and basophils
   b. Has low affinity for receptors of mast cells and basophils
   c. Symptoms in atopic individual more severe if both IgE and IgG4 are present
   d. Interpretation of high levels of IgG4 in given patient difficult in terms of clinical response

Based on Thomson NC, et al. In Thomson NC, et al, editors: *Handbook of clinical allergy*, Oxford, 1990, Blackwell Scientific, pp 1-36.

TABLE 21-12

Common Causes of Acute Urticaria (Type I Reactions), Usually IgE-Mediated*

Acute reaction to foods
  Shellfish
  Nuts
  Eggs
  Milk
Acute reaction to drugs
  Penicillin
  Sulfa
Acute reaction to insect stings
  Honeybees, bumblebees
  Yellow jackets, hornets, wasps

*Anaphylaxis may occur but is rare.

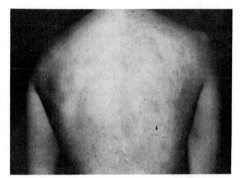

FIG. 21-1 This patient had taken penicillin a number of times without any problem. However, he developed a generalized urticarial reaction following the injection of penicillin for treatment of an acute oral infection.

in the permeability of adjacent vascular structures, resulting in a loss of intravascular fluid into the surrounding tissue spaces. This reaction accounts for the edematous lesions of urticaria, angioneurotic edema, and the secretions associated with hay fever. Table 21-12 shows some of the agents that can cause acute urticaria. The humoral antibodies involved in anaphylaxis and atopy are immunoglobulin E (IgE) antibodies that are fixed to and sensitize mast cells, so that when they encounter the antigen, they release histamine.[27,37]

TYPE II HYPERSENSITIVITY REACTIONS

The key elements involved in type II hypersensitivity are shown in Table 21-13. These reactions are IgG- or IgM-mediated. The classic example of type II (cytotoxic) hypersensitivity is transfusion reaction resulting from mismatched blood.

TYPE III HYPERSENSITIVITY REACTIONS

Type III hypersensitivity is summarized in Table 21-14. These reactions take place in blood

TABLE 21-13
Type II Hypersensitivity

1. Antibody-mediated
2. Cytotoxic hypersensitivity
   a. Antibodies combine with host cells recognized as foreign
   b. Foreign antigens bind to host cell membranes during induced hemolytic anemias or thrombocytopenia
3. Common examples
   a. Transfusion reactions from mismatched bloods
   b. Rhesus incompatibility
   c. Goodpasture's syndrome

Based on Thomson NC, et al. In Thomson NC, et al, editors: *Handbook of clinical allergy,* Oxford, 1990, Blackwell Scientific, pp 1-36.

TABLE 21-14
Type III Hypersensitivity

1. Antibody-mediated via immune complex formation
2. Also known as immune complex–mediated hypersensitivity
3. Local form is Arthus reaction
4. Immune complex formation
   a. Hypersensitivity state—complexes persist and lodge in blood vessel walls, initiating inflammatory reaction
   b. Large complexes
      (1) Removed by neutrophils and macrophages
   c. Soluble complexes (more antigen than antibody)
      (1) Most harmful
      (2) Penetrate vessel wall
      (3) Lodge on basement membrane
   d. Complement is activated
      (1) Vascular permeability increased
      (2) Neutrophils attracted
      (3) Neutrophils release enzymes
      (4) Vasculitis results
5. Sensitive sites
   a. Renal glomeruli
   b. Synovial membranes
6. Examples
   a. Systemic lupus erythematosus
   b. Poststreptococcal glomerulonephritis

Based on Thomson NC, et al. In Thomson NC, et al, editors: *Handbook of clinical allergy,* Oxford, 1990, Blackwell Scientific, pp 1-36.

vessels and involve soluble immune complexes. They constitute what is referred to as immune complex–mediated hypersensitivity. Their key feature is vasculitis. Clinical examples are systemic lupus erythematosus and streptococcal glomerulonephritis.

Cellular immune system

The cellular or delayed immune system has T lymphocytes playing the central role. The primary function of this system is to recognize and eradicate antigens that are fixed in tissues or within cells. This system is involved in protection against viruses, tuberculosis, and leprosy. Certain aspects of the cell-mediated immune system are shown in Table 21-15. Note that antibodies are not operative in this system. Effector T lymphocytes produce various cytokines that serve as the active agents of this system.

TYPE IV HYPERSENSITIVITY REACTIONS

Type IV hypersensitivity reactions involve the cellular immune system. They include contact dermatitis, transplant rejection, infections, and graft-versus-host disease (Table 21-16). The events in type IV hypersensitivity (contact dermatitis) are shown in Table 21-17. Dendritic cells and Langerhans cells are involved with processing and presenting the antigen to undifferentiated T lymphocytes. Table 21-18 lists some of the more common antigens causing contact

dermatitis. Type IV hypersensitivity reactions are usually delayed and will appear about 48 to 72 hours after contact with the antigen.

Infectious-type allergic reactions are exemplified by the tuberculin skin test, in which a person who has previously been exposed to *Myobacterium tuberculosis* will, with a second exposure in the form of an intradermal injection of altered bacteria, develop a delayed response, usually within 48 to 72 hours. The response is characterized by induration, erythema, swelling, and sometimes ulceration at the site of injection. *Contact allergy* occurs when a substance of low molecular weight that is not antigenic by itself comes in contact with a tissue component (primarily a protein) and forms an antigenic

TABLE 21-15
Cell-Mediated Immune Response

1. Cell types (T lymphocytes)
   a. T-suppressor cells (CD8 receptors)
      (1) Inhibit cell-mediated immune responses
      (2) Inhibit humoral immune responses
      (3) May be defective in atopic patients
      (4) Desensitization procedures, induce T-suppressor cells
      (5) Play role in preventing autoimmunity
   b. T-helper cells (CD4 receptors)
      (1) Stimulate other T lymphocytes and B lymphocytes into activity
      (2) Increase immune response
   c. T cytotoxic cells (CD8 receptors)
      (1) Destruction of viruses
      (2) Tumor immunity
   d. Tdth cells (delayed hypersensitivity cells)
      (1) Tuberculin skin test
      (2) Contact hypersensitivity
2. Cytokines produced by T lymphocytes
   a. Macrophage inhibition factor
   b. Macrophage activating factor
   c. B cell growth factor
   d. B cell differentiation factor
   e. Interleukin-2
   f. Interferons
   g. Others
3. Other cytotoxic cells
   a. Natural killer cells (part of nonspecific immune system)
      (1) Null lymphocytes (lack T or B markers)
      (2) Larger than other lymphocytes
      (3) Activated by interferon
      (4) Tumor surveillance
      (5) Destruction of virally infected cells
   b. K cells
      (1) Antibody-dependent cytotoxic cells (ADCC)
      (2) Uncertain lineage

Based on Thomson NC, et al. In Thomson NC, et al, editors: *Handbook of clinical allergy*, Oxford, 1990, Blackwell Scientific, pp 1-36.

TABLE 21-16
Type IV Hypersensitivity

1. Mediated by T lymphocytes
2. Antibodies not involved
3. Also called delayed-type hypersensitivity
   a. Response not seen until about 2 days following antigenic exposure
4. Examples
   a. Contact dermatitis
   b. Graft rejection
   c. Graft-versus-host reaction
   d. Some types of drug hypersensitivity
   e. Some types of autoimmune disease

Based on Thomson NC, et al. In Thomson NC, et al, editors: *Handbook of clinical allergy*, Oxford, 1990, Blackwell Scientific, pp 1-36.

TABLE 21-17
Type IV Hypersensitivity Reaction (Contact Dermatitis)

1. Allergen is usually a small chemical
   a. Remains in skin 18 to 24 hours
   b. Acts as hapten (most couple with protein)
2. Hapten-protein complex is processed by dendritic cells
3. Langerhans cells also involved as antigen presenting cells
   a. Migrate to local lymph nodes
   b. Processed antigen presented to undifferentiated T lymphocytes
   c. Differentiation and proliferation produce
      (1) T-effector cells
      (2) T-memory cells
4. T-effector and T-memory cells recirculate
   a. Patrol skin
   b. Reaction occurs if some antigen still present or when antigen is presented again; inflammatory mediators released
5. Clinical features of reaction
   a. Erythema
   b. Papulovesicular eruption
   c. Vesiculation and weeping
   d. Pruritis

Based on Thomson NC, et al. In Thomson NC, et al, editors: *Handbook of clinical allergy*, Oxford, 1990, Blackwell Scientific, pp 194-219.

complex. This small molecule is called a hapten (or one half of an antigen), and the resulting complex will cause sensitization of T lymphocytes. Poison ivy is an example of a contact allergy, wherein the reaction is delayed (with response occurring 48 to 72 hours after contact

TABLE 21-18
Common Allergens Causing Contact Dermatitis

Nickel
  Allergy more common in women
    10% to 30% sensitive to nickel
    Pierced ears, earrings
  Low-carat gold contains nickel
Perfumes and fragrances
  Shaving preparations
  Soaps, toiletries, washing powders, cosmetics
  Talcum powder
Rubber
  True allergy to rubber (latex) is rare; usually an
    immediate reaction (IgE-mediated)
  Allergy more common to other agents in rubber
    Accelerators
    Antioxidants
    Vulcanizing agents
  Rubber products reported to cause allergy
    Gloves
    Elastic band of underwear, bras, suspenders
    Shoes, slippers
    Condoms, diaphragms
    Sofas, beds, carpets
    Handles of tools, bikes
  Rubber exposure in hospital
    Tourniquets
    Blood pressure cuff
    Oxygen mask
    Gloves
    Drains, catheters
Formaldehyde
  Man-made fibers
  Shampoos, deodorants, nail polishes
  Cleaners, polishes, fabric conditioners
  Medical products
    Wart paints
    Disinfectants
    Tissue fixative
    Vaccines
Medicaments
  Neomycin, gentamicin
  Lanolin
  Benzocaine
  Merthiolate (eyedrops, contact lens solutions)

with the allergen). *Graft rejection* occurs when organs or tissues from one body are transplanted into another body. There is a cellular rejection of the transplanted tissue unless the donor and recipient are genetically identical or the host's immune response has been suppressed. *Graft-versus-host* reaction is an unusual phenomenon that occurs in bone marrow transplant patients whose cellular immune system has been rendered deficient by whole-body radiation. Lymphocytes transferred to the host attempt to destroy the host's tissues.

"Nonallergic" reactions

Other agents may cause mast cells to release their mediators without inciting a true allergic reaction—which is true in cases of chronic urticaria caused by certain drugs, temperature changes, and emotional states and in some reactions to drugs. In fact, most so-called "anaphylactic" reactions to local anesthetics do not involve an antigen-antibody reaction but are a result of damage to the mast cells through other mechanisms. These reactions are termed *anaphylactoid* or *anaphylaxis-like.*[7] Because the management of both anaphylactic and anaphylactoid reactions, from the clinical standpoint, is similar, we will deal with these types of drug reactions as if they were true allergic reactions. Certain cases of urticaria and angioneurotic edema can occur based on a similar pathogenesis and are not considered true "allergic" reactions.

The nonallergic cases of urticaria, angioneurotic edema, and anaphylactoid reactions are due to the nonspecific release of vasoactive amines from mast cells or the activation of some other form of nonspecific immunologic effector mechanisms.[7,31] The reader is referred to the text *Urticaria*[7] for an in-depth discussion of the origin of these reactions.

MEDICAL MANAGEMENT

Patients with atopy may receive injections to gradually desensitize them so they are no longer allergic to the antigen. Some individuals with severe asthma may be forced to move to an area of the country that does not contain the antigen (e.g., in the case of allergy to pollen).[1] Patients with asthma (Chapter 10), immune-complex injury, or cytotoxic immune reactions may be treated with systemic steroids whereas patients with hay fever or urticaria are treated with antihistamines.

Patients who have received an organ transplant often will be taking steroids and immunosuppressive drugs. A variety of treatments have been used for patients with contact dermatitis, including topical steroids. From a dental standpoint, the patient being treated for an allergic problem will have an increased chance of being allergic to another substance, and if this individual is taking steroids his or her reaction to stress may be impaired. (See Chapter 18.) Additionally, if the patient has received an organ transplant he may be susceptible to infection (Chapter 26).

DENTAL MANAGEMENT
MEDICAL CONSIDERATIONS

The dentist is frequently confronted with problems related to allergy. One of the most common concerns the patient who reports an allergy to a local anesthetic, antibiotic, or analgesic. The history must then be expanded, specifically trying to determine exactly what the offending substance was and exactly how the patient reacted to it. If the adverse reaction was of an allergic nature, one or more of the classic signs or symptoms of allergy should have been present (Table 21-19). If these signs or symptoms are not reported, the patient probably did not experience a true allergic reaction. Common examples of mislabeled "allergy" include syncope following injection of a local anesthetic and nausea or vomiting after the ingestion of codeine. Adverse drug reactions are listed in Table 21-20.

Local anesthetics

The most common reaction associated with local anesthetics is a toxic reaction, resulting usually from an inadvertent IV injection of the anesthetic solution (Table 21-21). Excessive amounts of an anesthetic can also cause a toxic reaction or a reaction to the vasoconstrictor. The signs and symptoms associated with toxic reactions to a local anesthetic are shown in Table 21-22. The signs and symptoms of a vasoconstrictor reaction include tachycardia, apprehension, sweating, and hyperactivity. Another common reaction to local anesthetics involves the anxious patient who, because of concern about receiving a "shot," will experi-

TABLE 21-19
Signs and Symptoms Suggestive of an Allergic Reaction

Urticaria
Swelling
Skin rash
Chest tightness
Dyspnea, shortness of breath
Rhinorrhea
Conjunctivitis

TABLE 21-20
Adverse Drug Reactions

Predictable
  Dose-related
  No immunologic basis
  Account for about 80% of all adverse reactions
    to drugs
  Direct toxicity
  Overdoses
  Drug interactions
  Side effects of drugs
Unpredictable
  Not dose-related
  Unrelated to expected pharmacologic effects
  Allergy
  Pseudoallergy (anaphylactoid reactions)
  Idiosyncrasy
  Intolerance
  Paradoxical reactions (cause histamine release
    but not IgE-mediated)
  Often underlying genetic defect present

Based on Weiler JM, Maves KK. In Lichtenstein LM, Fauci AS, editors: *Current therapy in allergy, immunology, and rheumatology*, ed 4, St Louis, 1992, Mosby–Year Book, pp 132-139.

TABLE 21-21
Adverse Reaction to Local Anesthetics

Toxic
  Central nervous system stimulation
  Central nervous system depression
Vasoconstrictor
Anxiety
Allergic

TABLE 21-22

Signs and Symptoms of a Toxic Reaction to Local Anesthetic

Talkativeness
Slurred speech
Dizziness
Nausea
Depression
Euphoria
Excitement
Convulsions

TABLE 21-23

Signs and Symptoms of a Psychomotor Response to the Injection of a Local Anesthetic

---

Hyperventilation
Vasovagal syncope
  Bradycardia
  Pallor
  Sweating
Sympathetic stimulation
  Anxiety
  Tremor
  Tachycardia
  Hypertension

TABLE 21-24

Local Anesthetics Used in Dentistry

Para-aminobenzoic acid (PABA) esters (cross-react)
  Procaine (Novocain)
  Tetracaine (Pontocaine)
Amides (usually do not cross-react)
  Lidocaine (Xylocaine)
  Mepivacaine (Carbocaine)
  Prilocaine (Citanest)

---

ence tachycardia, sweating, paleness, and syncope (Table 21-23). True allergic reactions to the local anesthetics (amides) most commonly used in dentistry are rare.[24]

If the patient's history supports a toxic or vasoconstrictor reaction, the dentist should explain the nature of the previous reaction (Table 21-19) and avoid injecting the local anesthetic solution IV by aspirating before the injection and by limiting the amount of solution to the recommended dose. If the patient's history supports an interpretation of fainting and not a toxic or allergic reaction, the dentist's primary task will be to work with the patient to reduce anxiety during dental visits. If the history supports a true allergic reaction to a local anesthetic, the dentist should try to identify the type of local anesthetic that was used. Once this has been done, a new anesthetic with a different basic chemical structure can be used. There are two main groups of local anesthetics in dentistry[2]: (1) paraaminobenzoic acid (PABA) esters (procaine [Novocain], tetracaine [Pontocaine]) and (2) amides (lidocaine [Xylocaine], mepivacaine [Carbocaine], prilocaine [Citanest]). It is not uncommon for the benzoic acid ester anesthetics to cross-react with each other, whereas the amide anesthetics usually do not cross-react. Cross-reaction does not occur between ester and amide local anesthetics[31] (Table 21-24).

Procaine is the local anesthetic with the highest incidence of allergic reactions. Its antigenic component appears to be PABA, one of the metabolic breakdown products of procaine. Cross-reactivity has been reported[12,22,30] between lidocaine and procaine; however, this could be traced to the presence of a germicide, methylparaben, which is used in small amounts as a preservative and is chemically similar to PABA. Thus a patient who is allergic to procaine may react to lidocaine solution if it contains methylparaben. Table 21-25 shows the various lidocaine preparations available for local anesthesia in dentistry. Lidocaine that does not contain methylparaben can now be readily obtained and should be used when dealing with a patient who has an allergic history to procaine.[12,22,30]

Patients with a history of being "allergic" to local anesthetics who cannot identify the specific agent used present more of a problem. The nature of the reaction must be established; and if it is consistent with an allergic reaction, the next step should be to attempt to identify the anesthetic that was used. When the patient is unable to provide this information, the dentist can attempt to contact the previous dentist involved. If this fails, there are two options: (1) an antihistamine (diphenhydramine [Benadryl]) can be used as the local anesthetic or (2)

TABLE 21-25

Lidocaine Preparations for Local Anesthesia in Dentistry[28]

1. With 1 mg methylparaben as preservative
2. Methylparaben-free (MPF)
3. With or without methylparaben
   a. Without epineprhine
   b. With epinephrine
      (1) Antioxidant (0.5 mg sodium metabisulfite)
      (2) Stabilizer (0.2 mg citric acid)

TABLE 21-26

Referral of Patient with a History of Anesthetic Allergy to an Allergist

1. If history shows reaction consistent with allergic response
   a. Allergic to anesthetic that is identified
   ?b. Allergic to anesthetic that cannot be identified
   ?c. Allergic to several anesthetics involving both amides and esters
?2. Skin testing not indicated because of variable results
3. Provocative dose testing (PDT)
4. Selection and recommendation of alternative local anesthetic based on results of PDT

the patient can be referred to an allergist for provocative dose testing (PDT). Frequently the use of diphenhydramine is the more practical option. A 1% solution of diphenhydramine that contains 1:100,000 epinephrine can be easily compounded by a pharmacist, but one must be certain that methylparaben is not used as a preservative. This solution induces anesthesia of about 30 minutes average duration and can be used for infiltration or block injection. When it is used for a mandibular block, 1 to 4 ml of solution is needed. Some patients have reported a burning sensation, swelling, and/or erythema following a mandibular block with 1% diphenhydramine, but these effects were not serious and cleared within 1 or 2 days. No more than 50 mg of diphenhydramine should be given during a single appointment. Diphenhydramine can also be used in the patient who gives a history of being allergic to both ester and amide local anesthetics.[23]

The dentist may also elect to refer the patient to an allergist for evaluation and testing, which will usually include both skin testing and PDT (provocative dose testing). Most investigators agree that skin testing alone for allergy to local anesthetics is of little benefit, because false-positive results are common; therefore the allergist will also perform PDT. It is a great help to have samples of your usual anesthetic agents without vasoconstrictors sent along for specific testing (Table 21-26).

Based on the patient's history, the allergist will select a local anesthetic for testing that is least likely to cause an allergic reaction, usually an anesthetic from the amide group because they do not usually cross-react with each other.[31]

At 15-minute intervals, 0.1 ml of test solution will be injected subcutaneously, with concentrations increasing from 1:10,000 to 1:1000 to 1:100 to 1:10, and then undiluted; next, 0.5 ml of undiluted test solution will be tried; and finally 1 ml of undiluted solution. During PDT the allergist will be prepared to deal with any adverse reaction that might occur and will report to the dentist on the drug selected, the final dose given, and the absence of any adverse reaction. Under these conditions, a local anesthetic with no reaction can be used in the tested patient and the risk of an allergic reaction will be no greater than in the general population.[19] Schatz and Greenberger[31] report that they have not dealt with a single patient for whom a safe local anesthetic could not be found using the PDT procedure.

When administering an alternative anesthetic to a patient with a history of a local anesthetic allergy, the dentist should follow these steps:

(1) Inject slowly, aspirating first to make sure that a vessel is not being injected. (2) Place one drop of the solution into the tissues. (3) Withdraw the needle and wait 5 minutes to see what reaction, if any, occurs. If there is no allergic reaction, as much anesthetic as needed for the procedure should be deposited. Be sure to aspirate before making the second injection (Table 21-27).

Penicillin

The use of penicillin has been increasing tremendously throughout the world, particu-

TABLE 21-27

Dental Management of a Local Anesthetic Allergy

1. Establish history of previous reaction following use of local anesthetic
2. Establish nature of previous reaction and type of anesthetic used
   a. Syncopal
   b. Allergic
      (1) Soft-tissue swelling
      (2) Skin rash
      (3) Rhinitis
      (4) Difficulty breathing
3. If reaction was consistent with allergic reaction
   a. Select anesthetic from different chemical group
      (1) Paraaminobenzoic acid (procaine)
      (2) Amide (lidocaine, mepivacaine)
   b. Aspirate, inject one drop of alternate anesthetic, and wait 5 minutes; if no reaction occurs, inject after aspirating rest of anesthetic needed (be prepared to deal with allergic reaction if one should occur)
   c. In cases of allergic reaction to several local anesthetic agents or if anesthetic used previously cannot be identified, diphenhydramine may be used
4. If history of multiple allergies is present or if type of local anesthetic used previously cannot be identified, refer patient to allergist for PDT

TABLE 21-28

Hypersensitivity Reactions to Penicillin in Order of Decreasing Frequency

1. Maculopapular rash (type IV)
2. Urticarial rash (type I)
3. Fever (type III)
4. Bronchospasm (type I)
5. Vasculitis (type III)
6. Serum sickness (type III)
7. Exfoliative dermatitis (type IV)
8. Anaphylaxis (type I)
9. Interstitial nephritis (type II)

Based on Kaplan MS. In Lichtenstein LM, Fauci AS, editors: *Current therapy in allergy, immunology, and rheumatology*, ed 4, St Louis, 1992, Mosby–Year Book, pp 126-132.

TABLE 21-29

Penicillin Reactions

Anaphylaxis
  In 0.04% to 0.2% of patients
  Fatal reaction in 1 per 100,000 treated individuals
  Atopic predisposition not risk factor for anaphylaxis, but is for fatal reaction
Risk of reaction dependent on
  History of prior reaction
  Time interval since prior reaction
  Persistence of specific IgE antibodies
  History of multiple drug sensitivities
Most useful parameter to assess risk in patients with history of penicillin reaction is skin testing with major and minor determinants
  Negative result
    Very little risk
  Positive result
    High risk for serious reaction to penicillin
    Risk for cross-reaction with cephalosporin

Based on Kaplan MS. In Lichtenstein LM, Fauci AS, editors: *Current therapy in allergy, immunology, and rheumatology*, ed 4, St Louis, 1992, Mosby–Year Book, pp 126-132.

larly in the United States, during the last 30 years. Approximately 2.5 million people in the United States are allergic to penicillin, and allergic reactions occur in 5% to 10% of patients who receive penicillin and related drugs. About 0.04% to 0.2% of the patients treated with penicillin develop an anaphylactic reaction, and about 10% of those individuals die, accounting for some 100 to 300 deaths per year. Table 21-28 lists the hypersensitivity reactions reported with penicillin. Table 21-29 shows the risk assessment of penicillin reactions.[7,17,18,21]

The possibility of sensitizing a patient to penicillin increases according to the route of administration as follows[2,41]: oral administration results in sensitization of only about 0.1% of patients; IM injection, 1% to 2%; and topical application, 5% to 12%. Based on these data, it is obvious that the use of penicillin in a topical ointment is contraindicated. Also, if the dentist has a choice, the oral route is preferable for administration whenever possible. Several authors[7,31] report that less serious reactions occur if oral administration of penicillin is used

TABLE 21-30
Penicillin Skin Testing

3% to 10% of adults will have positive results

Not cost-effective for all patients needing penicillin treatment

Preferable to use alternate antibiotic in patient with history of penicillin reaction and not to skin test

If penicillin must be used, skin test first with major and then with minor determinants

    If both test negative, penicillin can be used

    If either or both test positive, patient must be desensitized before using standard dose of penicillin

Based on Kaplan MS. In Lichtenstein LM, Fauci AS, editors: *Current therapy in allergy, immunology, and rheumatology*, ed 4, St Louis, 1992, Mosby–Year Book, pp 126-132.

TABLE 21-31
Skin Reactions to Penicillin

1. Reactivity declines with time
2. In patient with positive history of penicillin reaction
   a. Skin testing within 3 months of reaction will be 70% to 100% positive
   b. Skin testing within 5 years will be about 50% positive
   c. Skin testing within 10 years will be 20% to 30% positive
3. At any given time skin testing is 96% reliable
   a. 4% of patients with history of penicillin reaction and negative test will react to penicillin—25% of these are accelerated reactions, 75% mild cutaneous reactions
   b. Large study reported no anaphylaxis in patients with negative tests
   c. Negative testing to penicillin G excludes risk to semisynthetic penicillins

Based on Kaplan MS. In Lichtenstein LM, Fauci AS, editors: *Current therapy in allergy, immunology, and rheumatology*, ed 4, St Louis, 1992, Mosby–Year Book, pp 126-132.

instead of parenteral. However, Idsoe et al.[13] suggest that the early data on penicillin reactions involved primarily parenteral administration and thus are biased. They suggest the risk is equally great for a serious allergic reaction with both routes. Antibodies produced against penicillin will cross-react with the semisynthetic penicillins and can cause severe reactions in patients allergic to penicillin. Nevertheless, the synthetic penicillins do seem to cause fewer new sensitizations in patients who are not allergic to penicillin at the time of administration.[17] Patients with a history of penicillin allergy should be given erythromycin or clindamycin for the treatment of oral infections or prophylaxis against infective endocarditis.

Skin testing for allergy to penicillin is much more reliable than skin testing for allergy to a local anesthetic; however, there is some risk involved, and the allergist must be prepared for adverse reactions. Tables 21-30 and 21-31 show some of the points to be considered in the use of skin testing for pencillin sensitivity. To be cost-effective, the test should be conducted only on patients with a history of penicillin reaction who need penicillin for a serious infection. An important fact to remember is that penicillin reactivity declines with time; hence a patient may have reacted to the drug years ago but is now no longer sensitive (negative skin test). The length of time for retaining sensitivity is variable and is dependent on IgE levels.[21] Most anaphy-

lactic reactions to penicillin occur in patients who have been treated in the past with penicillin but reported no adverse reactions.[21]

When skin testing for penicillin sensitivity is performed, both metabolic breakdown products of penicillin—the major derivative, penicilloyl-polylysine (PP), and the minor derivative mixture (MDM)—must be tested. Ninety-five percent of penicillin is metabolized to the major determinant, and 5% to the minor determinants.[21] If skin tests are negative to both breakdown products, the patient is considered not allergic to penicillin; however, if positive tests are obtained for one or both of the breakdown products, the patient is considered to be allergic to penicillin and the drug should not be used.[17] When penicillin must be used, the patient with a positive skin test can be desensitized to it.[21] Patients with a positive skin test to MDM have a higher incidence of anaphylactic reactions than do patients with a positive test to PP.[17]

In dentistry, wherein alternative antibiotics can be selected, reactions to penicillin are preventable by merely not using penicillin in patients who have a history of penicillin allergy. Also drugs that may cross-react—including ampicillin, carbenicillin, and methicillin—should be avoided in these patients.[12]

Cephalosporins will cross-react in 5% to 10% of penicillin-sensitive patients. The risk is greatest with first- or second-generation drugs. Cephalosporins are metabolized to their major determinant, cephaloyl, which can cross-react with the major determinant of penicillin. Cephalosporins usually can be used in patients with a history of distant, nonserious reaction to penicillin.[17] However, skin testing is recommended by some authors for these patients. If the patient's skin test to penicillin is negative, then either penicillin or a cephalosporin may be used.

If the penicillin skin test is positive, a skin test for the specific cephalosporin selected should be performed. If this skin test is negative, the cephalosporin that was tested can be used. Table 21-32 summarizes the use of cephalosporins in patients with a history of penicillin hypersensitivity.[21]

Patients with a negative history of allergy to penicillin can be treated with the drug when indicated, and it should be given by the oral route. The patient is observed for 30 minutes after the first dose and is advised to seek immediate care if any of the signs or symptoms of an allergic reaction occur after he or she has left the dental office (Table 21-33).

Analgesics

Aspirin may cause gastrointestinal upset, but this can be avoided if it is taken with food or a glass of milk. The discomfort may include "heartburn," nausea, vomiting, or gastrointestinal bleeding. Aspirin should not be used in patients with an ulcer, gastritis, or a hiatal hernia and should be used with care in patients whose condition predisposes them to nausea,

---

TABLE 21-32

Use of Cephalosporins for Patients With a History of Penicillin Hypersensitivity

1. Cephalosporins metabolized to major determinant, cephaloyl
2. Cephaloyl can cross-react with major determinant of penicillin (penicilloyl polylycine)
3. Risk of adverse reaction to cephalosporin is controversial
   a. Greatest with first or second-generation drugs
      (1) Cephaloridin, 16.5%
      (2) Cephalothin, 5%
      (3) Cephalexin, 5.4%
   b. Anaphylaxis
      (1) Positive history of penicillin reaction, 0.1%
      (2) Negative history of penicillin reaction, 0.4%
   c. Urticaria
      (1) Positive history of penicillin reaction—1.3%
      (2) Negative history of penicillin reaction—0.4%
4. Patient with history of penicillin reaction—first skin test for penicillin sensitivity
   a. Negative
      (1) use either penicillin or cephalosporin
   b. If positive
      (1) Avoid penicillin
      (2) Skin test specific cephalosporin; use if result is negative

Based on Kaplan MS. In Lichtenstein LM, Fauci AS, editors: *Current therapy in allergy, immunology, and rheumatology*, ed 4, St Louis, 1992, Mosby–Year Book, pp 126-132.

TABLE 21-33

Procedures for Prevention of a Penicillin Reaction

1. Have emergency kit for treatment
2. Take medical history on all patients, including
   a. Previous contact with penicillin
   b. Reactions to penicillin
   c. Allergic reactions to other agents.
3. Do not use penicillin in patient with history of reactions to drug
4. Tell patient when you are going to give penicillin
5. Do not use penicillin in topical preparations
6. Do not use penicillinase-resistant penicillins unless infection is caused by penicillinase-producing staphylococci
7. Use oral penicillin whenever possible
8. Use disposable syringes for injection of penicillin
9. Have patient wait in office for 30 minutes following first dose of penicillin
10. Inform patient about signs and symptoms of allergic reaction to penicillin, and if these occur to seek immediate medical assistance

vomiting, dyspepsia, or gastric ulceration. Aspiration also is known to prolong the prothrombin time and to inhibit platelet function, which is usually of little clinical importance except in patients with a hemorrhagic disease or a peptic ulcer. In these patients it must be avoided. Many individuals, estimated at 2 per 1000, are allergic to salicylates.[17] Allergic reactions to aspirin can be serious, and deaths have been reported.[17]

Aspirin will provoke a severe reaction in some patients with asthma, who may react in the same way to other nonsteroidal antiinflammatory drugs (NSAIDs) that inhibit cyclooxygenase, which is the key enzyme in generating prostaglandin from arachidonic acid. The typical reaction consists of acute bronchospasm, rhinorrhea, and urticaria. Most asthmatic individuals who react to NSAIDs also have nasal polyps and lack IgE-mediated allergy to airborne allergens. The mechanism for this reaction does not appear to be allergic but is still undefined.[29]

The dentist should be aware of the many multiple-entity analgesic preparations that include aspirin or other salicylates (Table 21-34). These agents must be avoided in the patient who may be endangered by an adverse reaction associated with aspirin or other salicylates.

Many NSAIDs are now available (Table 21-35), and most can cause some degree of gastrointestinal irritation. NSAIDs also are inhibitors of prostaglandin formation, platelet aggregation, and prothrombin synthesis. Most have the potential for cross-sensitivity with patients who exhibit an asthma-like reaction to aspirin. NSAIDs should be avoided in certain asthma patients, in patients with an ulcer or hemorrhagic disease, and in patients who are pregnant or nursing.[17]

Codeine is a commonly used narcotic analgesic in dentistry. Emesis, nausea, and constipation may occur with analgesic doses of codeine. Miosis and adverse renal, hepatic, cardiovascular, and bronchial effects are not likely to occur with therapeutic doses, however. Most of the reported reactions to codeine consist of nonallergic gastrointestinal manifestations; nevertheless, these may be severe enough to preclude the use of codeine in certain patients. Alternate drug selections can be made by referring to a current pharmacology text, the *Physicians' Desk Reference,* or *Accepted Dental Therapeutics.*

Rubber products

A number of recent reports have demonstrated that certain health care workers and patients are at risk for hypersensitivity reactions to latex or agents used in the production of rubber gloves or related materials (rubber dam, blood pressure cuff, catheters). An obstetrics and gynecology physician[6] developed latex anaphylaxis from surgical gloves. Intraoperative cardiovascular collapse was reported in five patients because of latex gloves.[26] Sussman et al.[36] reported that latex caused hypersensitivity reactions in 14 subjects, including health care workers. All 14 cases had positive latex skin tests. Warpinski et al.[39] found allergic reactions to latex, including anaphylaxis, in four atopic patients. Gonzalez,[13] in a review of allergy to latex products, found that about 3% of hospital physicians and nurses were affected. Based on the above findings, it can be concluded that serious type I hypersensitivity reactions may occur in physicians, dentists, other health care workers, and patients from contact with latex products—such as gloves, rubber dam, balloons, or catheters.

TABLE 21-34
Analgesic Compounds That Contain Aspirin or Other Salicylates

Bufferin
Alka-Seltzer
Empirin
Excedrin
Fiorinal
Synalgos-DC

TABLE 21-35
NSAIDS Used in Dentistry

Etodolac (Lodine)
Fenoprofen (Nalfon)
Ibuprofen (Motrin)
Indomethacin (Indocin)
Nabumetone (Relafen)
Naproxen (Naprosyn)
Phenylbutazone (Butazolidin)
Piroxicam (Feldene)
Tolmetin (Tolectin)

Dentists should be aware that latex allergy can present as anaphylaxis during dental work when the patient or dentist has been sensitized to latex. Anaphylaxis may result in the sensitized individual following contact with rubber gloves, rubber dam material, blood pressure cuffs, or any other product containing latex. Studies[39] have shown that latex-allergic individuals have IgE antibodies for specific latex proteins. Latex skin tests are a satisfactory method to identify individuals who may be sensitized to latex.[36]

Dental Materials and Products

Type I, type III, and type IV hypersensitivity reactions have been reported to result from various dental materials and products. Topical anesthetic agents have been reported to cause type I reactions consisting of urticarial swelling. Mouth rinses and toothpastes containing phenolic compounds, antiseptics, astringents, or

TABLE 21-36

Type IV Hypersensitivity Reactions (Contact Dermatitis and Stomatitis) to Dental Materials and Dental Products

1. Dental amalgam
   a. Mercury content (rare)
   b. Relationship to nonspecific symptoms not established
2. Acrylic
   a. Free monomer will cause reaction
   b. Bench-cured acrylic temporary crowns and bridges
   c. Uncured acrylic
3. Composite resin
4. Nickel in chrome-cobalt prostheses, gold restorations, wire used in orthognatic surgery
5. Epimine-containing impression materials
6. Eugenol
7. Rubber dam material
8. Rubber gloves
9. Talcum powder
10. Toothpastes, mouth rinses

From Greenberg MS. In Rose LF, Kaye D, editors: *Internal medicine for dentistry*, ed 2, St Louis, 1990, Mosby–Year Book, pp 26-27; Guyuron B, Lasa CI Jr. *Plast Reconstr Surg* 89(3):540-542, 1992; Holmstrup P. *J Oral Pathol Med* 20(1): 1-17, 1991; Skoglund A, Egelrud T. *Scand J Dent Res* 99(4): 320-328, 1991; Stenman E, Bergman M. *Scand J Dent Res* 97(1):76-83, 1989; Sussman GL, Tarlo S, Dolvich J. *JAMA* 265(21):2844-2847, 1991.

flavoring agents have been known to cause type I, type III, and type IV hypersensitivity reactions involving the oral mucosa or lips. Hand soaps used by dental care workers have also been reported as a cause of type IV reactions. Table 21-36 lists some of the dental agents that can lead to type IV hypersensitivity (contact stomatitis).

Other conditions

Allergic patients being treated with steroids should be managed as described in Chapter 18. Patients who have had an organ transplant should be managed as described in Chapter 26.

The dental management of patients with asthma is primarily concerned with preventing severe asthma attacks from occurring in the dental office and dealing with an attack if one happens. In addition, certain important drug considerations must be taken for these patients[1] (Chapter 10).

TREATMENT PLANNING MODIFICATIONS

The dentist should obtain a history of any allergic reactions from each patient. If a patient has a history of allergy to drugs or materials that may be used in dentistry, a clear entry should be made in the dental record and any further contact or use of the antigen(s) avoided in that patient (Fig. 21-2).

Most allergic patients can receive any indicated dental treatment as long as the antigen is avoided and special preparations are made for those patients receiving steroids.

ORAL COMPLICATIONS
TYPE I HYPERSENSITIVITY

Oral lesions may be produced by type I hypersensitivity reactions. An *atopic reaction* to various foods, drugs, or anesthetic agents may occur within or around the oral cavity and is usually characterized by urticarial swelling or angioneurotic edema (Fig. 21-3). This reaction is generally rapid, the lesion developing within a short time after contact with the antigen. It is a painless, soft tissue swelling produced by transudate from the surrounding vessels that may lead to itching and burning. The lesion will usually be present for 1 to 3 days and then begin to resolve spontaneously. Oral antihistamines should be given; diphenhydramine, 50 mg every

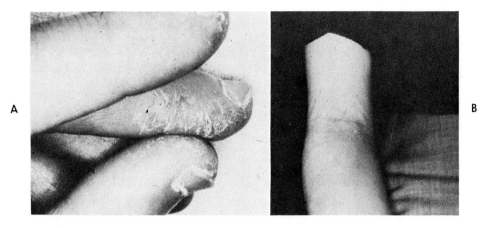

FIG. 21-2 Examples of contact dermatitis. **A,** Fingers of a dentist who developed an allergy to procaine. **B,** Arm of a patient who developed an allergy to soap.

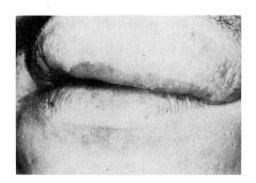

FIG. 21-3 Angioneurotic edema of the upper lip that occurred soon after the injection of a local anesthetic.

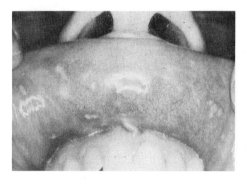

FIG. 21-4 Aphthous stomatitis that occurred in a man found to be allergic to the toothpaste he was using.

4 hours, orally, is the recommended regimen. Treatment is given for 1 to 3 days. Further contact with the antigen must be avoided.

TYPE III HYPERSENSITIVITY

Foods, drugs, or agents that are placed within the oral cavity can cause white, erythematous, or ulcerative lesions based on type III hypersensitivity or immune complex reactions. The lesions develop rather quickly, usually within a 24-hour period, after contact with the offending antigen. Some cases of aphthous stomatitis (Fig. 21-4) may be caused by type III hypersensitivity,

although most are related to lymphocyte dysfunction. Erythema multiforme represents an immune-complex reaction (Fig. 21-5).

About half the patients with erythema multiforme are found to have a predisposing factor — such as a drug allergy or herpes simplex infection — involved in the onset of their disease.[10,33] Sulfa antibiotics are the most common drug associated with the onset of erythema multiforme, and sulfonyl urea hypoglycemic agents (tolbutamide, tolazamide, glyburide, glipizide) used to treat some diabetics have been found to be associated with the onset of erythema multi-

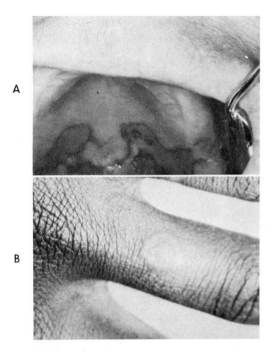

FIG. 21-5 Erythema multiforme that developed following oral adminstration of a drug used to treat an oral infection. **A,** Ulceration of the palatal mucosa. **B,** Target lesion of the finger.

TABLE 21-37
Type III Hypersensitivity Reactions

1. Usually occur within 24 hours following contact with antigen
2. Consist of
   a. Erythema
   b. Rash
   c. Ulceration
3. Treatment
   a. Topical steroids
   b. Systemic steroids (in severe cases)
   c. Identification of antigen
   d. Avoidance of any further contact with antigen

forme. Many patients with erythema multiforme can be managed by symptomatic therapy—including a bland mouth rinse, syrup of diphenhydramine, and/or triamcinolone acetonide (Kenalog) in Orabase. A few patients with more severe involvement may require systemic steroids. (See Appendix B for treatment regimens.) If a drug appears to be associated with the onset of the disease, any further contact with it should be avoided. Table 21-37 summarizes oral type III hypersensitivity reactions.

TYPE IV HYPERSENSITIVITY

Contact stomatitis is a delayed allergic reaction associated with the cellular immune response in most cases. Because of the delayed nature of the reaction following contact with the allergen in cases of contact stomatitis, the dentist must inquire about contacts with materials that may have occurred 2 to 3 days before the lesions appeared.[10] The antigen may be found in dental materials, toothpaste, mouth rinses, lipsticks, face powders, etc. In many cases no further treatment is necessary once the source of the antigen has been identified and removed from further contact with the patient; however, if the tissue reaction is severe or persistent, topical corticosteroids should be used. A good preparation to use topically is triamcinolone acetonide in Orabase. (See Appendix B for treatment regimens.)

Various dental materials have been reported as a cause of allergic reactions in patients. Impression materials containing an aromatic sulfonate catalyst (e.g., Scutan and Impregum) have been reported[8,9] to cause a delayed allergic reaction in postmenopausal women. The reaction consisted of tissue ulceration and necrosis that got progressively worse with each exposure.

A number of papers[4,5,16,20,34,35] have reported oral lesions found in close association with amalgam restorations. These (mucosal) lesions were described as whitish, reddish, ulcerative, or lichenoid and were thought to be due to toxic irritation or a hypersensitivity reaction to the silver amalgam restoration. When these restorations were removed, the lesions most often cleared. In some of the studies, skin testing for mercury sensitivity was performed. All the reports suggested that some of the oral lesions were a result of toxic injury to the mucosa and others were a result of type IV hypersensitivity reaction to mercury in the amalgams.

There are no well-done studies relating nonspecific symptoms—such as depression, fatigue, headaches—to the effects of mercury in amalgam restorations. The practice of avoiding use of amalgam restorations in patients with non-specific symptoms has at present no scientific basis.[14] However, it would seem rational to remove any amalgam restorations in contact with oral mucosa that shows lesions consistent with a toxic or hypersensitivity reaction to mercury.

On rare occasion, dental composite materials have been reported[25] to cause allergic reactions. The acrylic monomer used in denture construction has caused an allergic reaction[11]; however, the vast majority of tissue changes under dentures are from trauma and secondary infection with bacteria or fungi.[11] Gold, nickel, and mercury have all been reported[7,42] to cause allergic reactions resulting in tissue erythema and ulceration.

The dentist may want to test certain agents that are thought to be possible antigens causing oral lesions. Oral epimucous testing for contact stomatitis consists of placing the suspected antigen in contact with the oral mucosa and observing over a period of several days for any reaction (erythema, sloughing, ulceration) that might indicate an allergy to the test material. In most cases a reaction is not expected to develop for at least 48 to 72 hours. Various techniques have been used to conduct epimucous testing for suspected allergens. One of these is placing the suspected allergen in a rubber suction cup, placing the cup on the buccal mucosa, and observing at intervals for erythema or ulceration under the cup. Another technique is to place a sample of the suspected antigen in a depression on the palatal aspect of an overlay denture. The denture is inserted into the patient's mouth and holds the allergen in contact with the palatal mucosa. Another technique consists of incorporating the allergen into Orabase, applying the Orabase in the mucobuccal fold, and periodically observing for a reaction. Alternately, the antigen can be incorporated into an oral adhesive spray. Skin testing and oral epimucous testing for potential antigens are not foolproof, by any means; in certain patients they give unreliable tissue responses. The response in some cases may be due to trauma, and in others in which no tissue reaction occurs the patient may in fact still be allergic to the substance. The basic management of contact stomatitis is

to remove common sources of antigens known to cause hypersensitivity reactions to see if the lesions clear. Skin or mucosal testing for sensitivity can also be performed. Once the offending agent or antigen has been identified, the patient should be told to avoid any future contact with the antigen. Again, if the lesions persist, topical steroids can be applied. (See Appendix B.)

Lichenoid drug eruptions

Some patients with skin and/or oral lesions identical to those of lichen planus will be found to have taken certain drugs prior to the onset of their lesions. If these drugs are withdrawn, the lesions clear within several days (in most patients) or within a few weeks. The agents most commonly associated with the onset of the lichenoid lesions are levamisole (Levantine) and the quinidine drugs. Other agents found to be associated are the thiazide drugs, methyldopa, and photographic dyes (e.g., paraphenylenediamine).[10,43] Biopsy of a lichenoid lesion shows the same microscopic picture as seen in lichen planus, with the additional finding of eosinophils in the subepithelial infiltrate.[10] It would appear that these lesions are related to the cellular immune system and therefore could be placed under the heading of contact stomatitis; however, the true nature of the reactions is not clear at present.

MANAGEMENT OF SEVERE TYPE I HYPERSENSITIVITY REACTIONS

Even when the dentist has taken appropriate precautions, an allergic reaction may occur in the patient. Most of these will be mild and of a nonemergency nature; however, some may be severe and life-threatening (anaphylactic). The dentist must be ready to deal with either type. In handling the anaphylactic reaction it should be remembered that it has an allergic etiology. In other words, it should occur soon after (i.e., minutes) the injection, ingestion, or application of a topical anesthetic, medication, drug, local anesthetic, or dental product. The dentist must take the following actions immediately:

1. Place the patient in a head-down or supine position.
2. Make certain that the airway is patent.
3. Administer oxygen.
4. Be prepared to send for help and to support respiration and circulation. The

rate and depth of respiration should be noted, as should the patient's other vital signs.

Most reactions in dental patients will consist of simple fainting, which can be managed well by the preceding actions. In addition, the dentist may administer aromatic spirits of ammonia by inhalation, which will encourage breathing through reflex stimulation.

If the initial steps have not solved the emergency problem and it is indeed of an allergic cause, the dentist is faced with either an edematous-type reaction or an anaphylactic reaction.

Angioneurotic Edema

If the immediate type I hypersensitivity reaction has resulted in edema of the tongue, pharyngeal tissues, or larynx, the dentist will have to take additional emergency steps to prevent death from respiratory failure. At this point, if the patient has not responded to the initial procedures and is in acute respiratory distress, the dentist should do the following:

1. Inject 0.5 ml of 1:1000 epinephrine IM (into the tongue) or SC.
2. Support respiration, if indicated, by mouth-to-mouth breathing or bag and mask; be sure the chest moves when either of these methods is used.
3. Check the carotid or femoral pulse; if a pulse cannot be detected, closed chest cardiac massage should be initiated.
4. By this time someone in the office should have called a nearby physician or hospital (Table 21-38).

Anaphylaxis

An anaphylactic reaction usually takes place within minutes. The signs and symptoms associated with anaphylactic reactions are listed in Table 21-39. In contrast to the severe edematous reaction, in which respiratory distress occurs first, both respiratory and circulatory depression occurs early in the anaphylactic reaction. Anaphylaxis is often fatal unless vigorous, immediate action is taken. Because it occurs within minutes after contact with the antigen, the dentist should take the following steps[2] (Table 21-40):

1. Have someone in the office call for medical aid — a nearby physician or hospital.

TABLE 21-38

Oral or Paraoral Type I Hypersensitivity Reactions

---

1. Urticarial swelling (or anginoeurotic edema)
   a. Reaction occurs soon after contact with antigen
   b. Reaction consists of painless swelling
   c. Itching and burning may occur
   d. Lesion may remain for 1 to 3 days
2. Treatment
   a. Reaction not involving tongue, pharynx, or larynx and no respiratory distress present
      (1) 50 mg of diphenhydramine four times a day until swelling diminishes
   b. Reaction involving tongue, pharynx, or larynx with respiratory distress present
      (1) 0.5 ml of 1:1000 epinephrine, IM or SC
      (2) Oxygen
      (3) Once immediate danger over, 50 mg of diphenhydramine four times a day until swelling diminishes

---

TABLE 21-39

Signs and Symptoms of Anaphylaxis

Itching of soft palate
Nausea, vomiting
Substernal pressure
Shortness of breath
Hypotension
Pruritus
Urticaria
Laryngeal edema
Bronchospasm
Cardiac arrhythmias

---

2. Place the patient in a supine position.
3. Make certain the airway is patent.
4. Administer oxygen.
5. Check the carotid or femoral pulse and respiration; if no pulse is present and the respiration is depressed
   a. Inject 0.5 ml of 1:1000 epinephrine IM (into the tongue) or SC.
   b. Support circulation by closed chest cardiac massage.
   c. Support respiration by mouth-to-mouth breathing.

TABLE 21-40
Anaphylaxis

Basis

1. First contact with antigen results in formation of antibodies by plasma cells
2. Antibodies circulate in bloodstream (IgE antibodies)
3. Antibodies attach to target tissues (mast cells near smooth muscle of bronchi)
4. Next contact with antigen may result in combining of antigen and antibody
5. Antigen-antibody complex causes degranulation of mast cell(s) with release of histamine
6. Smooth muscle contracts and vessels lose fluid, etc
7. Acute respiratory distress and cardiovascular collapse may occur within minutes

Management

1. Call for medical help
2. Place patient in supine position
3. Check for open airway
4. Administer oxygen
5. Check pulse, blood pressure, respiration
   a. If depressed or absent, inject 0.5 ml epinephrine IM in tongue
   b. Provide cardiopulmonary resuscitation if needed
   c. Repeat injection of 0.5 ml epinephrine if no response

d. Repeat the injection of epinephrine if no response occurs.

REFERENCES

1. Aaronson DW, Rosenberg M: Asthma, general concepts. In Patterson R, editor: *Allergic diseases,* ed 3, Philadelphia, 1985, JB Lippincott.
2. American Dental Association: *Accepted dental therapeutics,* Chicago, 1986, The Association.
3. Austen, KF: Diseases of immediate type hypersensitivity. In Wilson JD, et al, editors: *Harrison's Principles of internal medicine,* ed 12, New York, 1991, McGraw-Hill, pp 1422-1428.
4. Bergman M: Side-effects of amalgam and its alternatives: local, systemic, and environmental, *Int Dent J* 40(1):4-10, 1990.
5. Bolewska J, Jansen, HJ, Holmstrup P, et al: Oral mucosal lesions related to silver amalgam restorations, *Oral Surg* 70:55-58, 1990.
6. Chen MD, Greenspoon JS, Long TL: Latex anaphylaxis in an obstetrics and gynecology physician, *Am J Obstet Gynecol* 166:968-969, 1992.
7. Czarnetzki BM: *Urticaria,* New York, 1986, Springer-Verlag.
8. Dahl BL: Tissue hypersensitivity to dental materials, *J Oral Rehabil* 5:117-120, 1978.
9. Duxbury AJ: Hypersensitivity to epimine containing dental materials, *Br Dent J* 147:331-333, 1979.
10. Eversole LR: Allergic stomatitis, *J Oral Med* 34:93-102, 1979.
11. Fernstrom AL: Location of the allergenic monomer in warm-polymerized acrylic dentures. I, *Swed Dent J* 4:253-260, 1980.
12. Giovannitti JA, Bennett CR: Assessment of allergy to local anesthetics, *J Am Dent Assoc* 98(5):701-706, 1979.
13. Gonzalez E: Latex hypersensitivity: a new and unexpected problem, *Hosp Pract* 27(2):145-148, 1992.
14. Greenberg MS: Dental correlations: immunological and allergic diseases. In Rose LF, Kaye D, editors: *Internal medicine for dentistry,* ed 2, St Louis, 1990, Mosby–Year Book, pp 26-27.
15. Guyuron B, Lasa CI Jr: Reaction to stainless steel wire following orthognathic surgery, *Plast Reconstr Surg* 89(3):540-542, 1992.
16. Holmstrup P: Reactions of the oral mucosa related to silver amalgam: a review, *J Oral Pathol Med* 20(1):1-17, 1991.
17. Holroyd SV, Wynn RL: *Clinical pharmacology in dental practice,* ed 4, St Louis, 1987, CV Mosby.
18. Idsoe O, Guthe T, Willcox RR, et al: Nature and extent of penicillin side-reactions, with particular reference to fatalities from anaphylactic shock, *Bull WHO* 38:159-188, 1968.
19. Incaudo G, Schatz M, Patterson R, et al: Administration of local anesthetics to patients with a history of prior adverse reaction, *J Allergy Clin Immunol* 61:339-345, 1978.
20. James J, Fergusen MM, Forsyth A, et al: Oral lichenoid reactions related to mercury sensitivity, *Br J Oral Maxillofac Surg* 25(6):474-480, 1987.
21. Kaplan MS: Penicillin allergy. In Lichtenstein LM, Fauci AS, editors: *Current therapy in allergy, immunology, and rheumatology,* ed 4, St Louis, 1992, Mosby–Year Book, pp 126-132.
22. Larson CE: Methylparaben, an overlooked cause of local anesthetic hypersensitivity, *Anesth Prog* 24:72-74, 1977.
23. Malamed SF: Diphenhydramine hydrochloride, its uses as a local anesthetic in dentistry, *Anesth Prog* 20:76-82, 1973.
24. Milan SB, Giovannitti JA, Bright D: Hypersensitivity to amide local anesthetics? *Oral Surg* 56:593-596, 1983.
25. Nathanson D: Delayed extra-oral hypersensitivity to dental composite materials, *Oral Surg* 47:329-333, 1979.
26. Nguyen DH, Burns MW, Shapiro GG, et al: Intraoperative cardiovascular collapse secondary to latex allergy, *J Urol* 146(2):571-574, 1991.

27. Norman PS, Lichtenstein LM: Immune responses in man. In Harvey A, et al, editors: *The principles and practice of medicine,* ed 19, New York, 1976, Appleton-Century-Crofts.

28. *Physicians' desk reference,* ed 46, Monvale NJ, 1992, Medical Economics, pp 637-645.

29. Reed CE: Drug allergy. In Wyngaardin JB, Smith LH, editors: *Cecil textbook of medicine,* ed 17, Philadelphia, 1985, JB Lippincott.

30. Reuben BM: A current practical review of local anesthesia, *Dent Surv* 56:38-43, 1980.

31. Schatz M, Greenberger PA: Drug allergy. In Patterson R, editor: *Allergic diseases,* ed 3, Philadelphia, 1985, JB Lippincott.

32. Seng GF, Gay BJ: Dangers of sulfites in dental local anesthetic solutions: warming and recommendations, *J Am Dent Assoc* 113:769-770, 1986.

33. Shafer WG, Hine MK, Levy BM: *A textbook of oral pathology,* ed 4, Philadelphia, 1983, WB Saunders.

34. Skoglund A, Egelrud T: Hypersensitivity reactions to dental materials in patients with lichenoid oral mucosal lesions and in patients with burning mouth syndrome, *Scand J Dent Res* 99(4):320-328, 1991.

35. Stenman E, Bergman M: Hypersensitivity reactions to dental materials in a referred group of patients, *Scand J Dent Res* 97(1):76-83, 1989.

36. Sussman GL, Tarlo S, Dolvich J: The spectrum of IgE-mediated responses to latex, *JAMA* 265(21):2844-2847, 1991.

37. Thomson NC, Kirkwood EM, Lever RS: Basic immunological mechanisms. In Thomson NC, et al, editors: *Handbook of clinical allergy,* Oxford, 1990, Blackwell Scientific, pp 1-36.

38. Thomson NC, Kirkwood EM, Lever RS: Contact dermatitis. In Thomson NC, et al, editors: *Handbook of clinical allergy,* Oxford, 1990, Blackwell Scientific, pp 194-219.

39. Warpinski JR, Folgert J, Cohen J, Bush RK: Allergic reaction to latex: a risk factor for unsuspected anaphylaxis, *Allergy Proc* 12(2):95-102, 1991.

40. Weiler JM, Maves KK: Drug reactions. In Lichtenstein LM, Fauci AS, editors: *Current therapy in allergy, immunology, and rheumatology,* ed 4, St Louis, 1992, Mosby–Year Book, pp 132-139.

41. Weinstein L: Chemotherapy of microbial diseases. In Goodman LS, Gilman A, editors: *The pharmacological basis of therapeutics,* ed 5, New York, 1975, Macmillan Publishing.

42. Wiesenfeld D, Ferguson MM, Forsyth A, MacDonald DG: Allergy to dental gold, *Oral Surg* 57:158-160, 1984.

43. Williams BG: Oral drug reaction to methyldopal, *Oral Surg* 56:375-377, 1983.

22

Bleeding Disorders

A number of procedures that are performed in dentistry may cause bleeding. Under normal circumstances these procedures can be performed with little risk to the patient; however, the patient whose ability to control bleeding has been altered by drugs or disease may be in grave danger unless the dentist identifies the problem before performing any dental procedure. In most cases, once the patient with a bleeding problem has been identified, steps can be taken to greatly reduce the risks associated with dental procedures.

This chapter is designed to provide the dentist with an understanding of the mechanisms involved in the normal control of bleeding, to describe the common causes of bleeding problems, to present an approach for identifying patients with possible bleeding abnormalities, and to describe in general terms the management of these patients once they have been identified.

GENERAL DESCRIPTION
INCIDENCE AND PREVALENCE

Most bleeding disorders are iatrogenic. Every patient who receives coumarin to prevent recurrent thrombosis has a potential bleeding problem. Most of these patients are receiving anticoagulant medication because they have had a recent myocardial infarction, a cerebrovascular accident, or thrombophlebitis. Patients who have had open heart surgery to correct a congenital defect, to replace diseased arteries, or to repair or replace damaged heart valves also may be receiving long-term anticoaulgation therapy. In addition, some individuals treated with aspirin for chronic illnesses — such as rheumatoid arthritis — have potential bleeding problems.

von Willebrand's disease is the most common inherited bleeding disorder. It affects one out of every 800 to 1000 individuals in the United States. The disease is usually inherited as an autosomal dominant trait.[10] True hemophilia, Factor VIII deficiency, is the most common of the inherited coagulation disorders. The overall prevalence of hemophilia in the United States is about 1 case for every 20,000 people; however, because of its genetic mode of transfer, certain areas of the United States are found to contain many more persons with hemophilia than other areas. About 80% of all genetic coagulation disorders are true hemophilia, 13% are Christmas disease (Factor IX deficiency), and 6% are Factor XI deficiency.[13,15]

Patients with acute or chronic leukemia may have clinical bleeding tendencies because of thrombocytopenia, which may result from overgrowth of malignant cells in the bone marrow that leaves no room for red blood cells or platelet precursors. In addition, leukemic patients may develop thrombocytopenia from the toxic effects of the various chemotherapeutic agents used to treat the disease.

The incidence of acute leukemia in the United States for all ages is about 3 to 4 cases per 100,000 persons. Chronic lymphocytic leukemia is rare in children but increases in incidence to about 10 cases per 100,000 persons over the age of 75 years, whereas chronic myeloid leukemia is rare in those under the age of 30 years and over the age of 70.[19,32,33]

The incidence of acute leukemia does not vary much among races. By contrast, chronic

TABLE 22-1
Classification of Bleeding Disorders

1. Nonthrombocytopenic purpuras
   a. Vascular wall alteration
      (1) Scurvy
      (2) Infections
      (3) Chemicals
      (4) Allergy
   b. Disorders of platelet function
      (1) Genetic defects (Bernard-Soulier disease)
      (2) Drugs
         (a) Aspirin
         (b) NSAIDs
         (c) Alcohol
         (d) Beta-lactam antibiotics
         (e) Penicillin
         (f) Cephalothins
      (3) Allergy
      (4) Autoimmune disease
      (5) von Willebrand's disease
      (6) Uremia
2. Thrombocytopenic purpuras
   a. Primary
   b. Secondary
      (1) Chemicals
      (2) Physical agents (radiation)
      (3) Systemic disease (leukemia)
3. Disorders of coagulation
   a. Inherited
      (1) Hemophilia (deficiency of Factor VIII)
      (2) Christmas disease (deficiency of Factor IX)
      (3) Others
   b. Acquired
      (1) Liver disease
      (2) Vitamin deficiency
         (a) Biliary tract obstruction
         (b) Malabsorption
         (c) Excessive use of broad-spectrum antibiotics
      (3) Anticoagulation drugs
         (a) Heparin
         (b) Coumarin
      (4) Disseminated intravascular coagulation (DIC)
      (5) Primary fibrinogenolysis

leukemia is rare in eastern countries, less common in black Africa, and more common in northern countries.[32,33]

It is difficult to obtain accurate information about the incidence of other systemic conditions that may render the patient susceptible to prolonged bleeding following injury or surgery. However, when considering the prevalence of the drug-influenced or disease-produced defects in the normal control of blood loss, it is clear that a busy dental practice will contain a large number of patients who may be "bleeders."

ETIOLOGY

A pathologic alteration of blood vessel walls, a significant reduction in the number of platelets, defective platelets or platelet function, a deficiency of one or more coagulation factors, the administration of anticoagulant drugs, a disorder of platelet release, or the inability to destroy free plasmin can result in significant abnormal clinical bleeding. This can occur even following minor injuries and may lead to death in some patients if immediate action is not taken.

The classification given in Table 22-1 is based on bleeding problems in patients with normal numbers of platelets (nonthrombocytopenic purpuras), decreased numbers of platelets (thrombocytopenic purpuras), and disorders of coagulation.

Infections, chemicals, collagen disorders, or certain types of allergy can alter the structure and function of the vascular wall to the point at which the patient may have a clinical bleeding problem. A patient may have normal numbers of platelets, but they may be defective or unable to perform their proper function in the control of blood loss from damaged tissues. If the total number of circulating platelets is reduced below 50,000 to 100,000/mm^3 of blood, the patient may be a bleeder.[10,19,32] In some cases the total platelet count is reduced by unknown mechanisms — this is called primary or idiopathic thrombocytopenia. Chemicals, radiation, and various systemic diseases (e.g., leukemia) may have a direct effect on the bone marrow and result in secondary thrombocytopenia.

Patients may be born with a deficiency of one of the factors needed for blood coagulation — for example, Factor VIII deficiency (hemophilia) or Factor IX deficiency (Christmas disease).

Acquired coagulation disorders are the most common cause of prolonged bleeding. Liver disease and disseminated intravascular coagulation (DIC) can lead to severe bleeding problems. Many of the other acquired coagulation disorders may become apparent in patients only after trauma or surgical procedures.

The liver produces all the protein coagulation factors except Factor VIII and possibly Factor XIII; thus any patient with significant liver disease may have a bleeding problem. In addition to a possible disorder in coagulation, the patient with liver disease who develops portal hypertension with hypersplenism may be thrombocytopenic as a result of splenic overactivity, which may destroy circulating platelets.

Any condition that so disrupts the intestinal flora that vitamin K is not produced in sufficient amounts will result in a decreased plasma level of prothrombin, because vitamin K is needed by the liver to produce prothrombin (Factor II) and Factors VII, IX, and X. Biliary tract obstruction, malabsorption syndrome, and excessive use of broad-spectrum antibiotics can lead to low levels of prothrombin on this basis.

Other drugs, such as heparin and coumarin derivatives, can cause a bleeding disorder because of disruption of the coagulation process. Aspirin, penicillin, cephalosporins, and alcohol also can interfere with platelet function.

PATHOPHYSIOLOGY

Under normal conditions any spontaneous bleeding (with the exception of menstruation) is abnormal — even large injuries can result in relatively little blood loss; however, when the body's ability to control bleeding is altered, a slight injury may result in massive blood loss. For hemostasis to be maintained, the blood vessels must be normal, an adequate number of functional platelets must be present, and the coagulation mechanisms must be intact; in addition, the clot, once it has served its function, must be removed by the fibrinolytic system. Thus the control of bleeding can be described as involving four phases[32] (Table 22-2): vascular, platelet, coagulation, and fibrinolysis (metabolism).

Table 22-3 shows the functions of the vascular system in hemostasis.

The *vascular* phase begins immediately fol-

TABLE 22-2
Normal Control of Bleeding

1. Vascular phase
   a. Vasoconstriction in area of injury
   b. Begins immediately after injury
2. Platelet phase
   a. Platelets and vessel wall wall become "sticky"
   b. Mechanical plug of platelets seals off openings of cut vessels
   c. Begins seconds after injury
3. Coagulation phase
   a. Blood lost into surrounding area coagulates through extrinsic and common pathways
   b. Blood in vessels in area of injury coagulates through intrinsic and common pathways
   c. Takes place more slowly than other phases
4. Metabolic (fibrinolytic) phase
   a. Release of antithrombotic agents
   b. Spleen and liver destroy these

TABLE 22-3
Functions of the Vascular System in Hemostasis

1. Prevention of excessive bleeding
   a. Vasoconstriction
   b. Diversion of flow abound injury
   c. Contact activation of platelets
      (1) Adhesion
      (2) Aggregation
   d. Contact activation of coagulation system
2. Maintenance of fluidity of blood
   a. Nonwettable surface (glycocalyx)
   b. Physiologic anticoagulant (antithrombin-III [AT-III])
   c. Thrombomodulin (endothelial cell membrane) neutralizes thrombin, activates protein C (fibrinolytic agent)
   d. Tissue plasminogen activator (TPA) initiates fibrinolysis
   e. Prostacyclin (PGI_2) (vasodilator) inhibits fibrinolysis
3. Endothelial cells synthesize
   a. Type IV collagen
   b. Fibronectin
   c. von Willebrand's factor (vWF)
4. Endothelial cells metabolize
   a. Angiotensin
   b. Serotonin
   c. Bradykinin

lowing injury and involves vasoconstriction of arteries and veins in the area of injury, retraction of arteries that have been cut, and buildup of extravascular pressure by blood loss from cut vessels. This pressure aids in collapsing the adjacent capillaries and veins in the area of injury. Vascular wall integrity is important to maintain the fluidity of blood. The smooth endothelial lining consists of a nonwettable surface that under normal conditions will not activate platelet adhesion or coagulation.

Disruption of the endothelial lining exposes subendothelial tissues (collagen and basement membrane) that activate *platelets* and *coagulation* by surface activation. In addition, injured endothelial cells release ADP and tissue thromboplastin. ADP induces platelet adhesion, and tissue thromboplastin activates coagulation through the extrinsic pathway.

Endothelial cells also have *metabolic* functions—the release of antithrombotic agents. Glycocalyx, a mucopolysaccharide, coats the luminal surface and can stimulate the release of antithrombin III (AT-III), a physiologic anticoagulant. Prostacyclin, a vasodilator and inhibitor of platelet response, is secreted by endothelial cells. An enzyme (ADPase) is produced that degrades ADP. Tissue plasminogen activator (TPA) is secreted to activate firbinolysis.[11] Endothelial cells also contribute to normal hemostasis and vascular integrity by synthesis of type IV collagen, fibronectin, and von Willebrand's factor.[11] Platelets are cellular fragments from the cytoplasm of megakocytes that last 9 to 12 days in the circulation. About 30% of the platelets are sequestered in the microvasculature or spleen and serve as a functional reserve. Aged or nonviable platelets are removed and destroyed by the spleen and liver.

Platelet structure consists of three areas (Table 22-4): (1) a peripheral zone, (2) a sol-gel zone (cytoskeleton), and (3) an organelle zone.

The peripheral zone serves as a stimulus receptor and stimulus transmitter region. The plasma membrane contains receptors for von Willebrand's factor (glycoprotein Ib), fibrinogen and fibronectin (glycoproteins IIb and IIIa), ADP, thrombin, epinephrine, and serotonin. The phospholipid portion of the plasma membrane contains Factor V, Factor VIII, platelet Factor 3 (PF3), and platelet Factor 4 (PF4).

TABLE 22-4
Platelet Structure and Function

---

1. Peripheral zone (stimulus receptor-transmitter region)
   a. Exterior coat (glycocalyx, blood groups, HLA)
   b. Plasma membrane (receptors)
      (1) Glycoprotein Ib (von Willebrand's factor) (vWF/GP-Ib)—adhesion to subendothelium
      (2) Glycoproteins IIb and IIIa (fibrinogen, fibronectin)
      (3) ADP, thrombin, epinephrine, serotonin
   c. Phospholipid portion of plasma membrane
      (1) Factor V
      (2) Factor VIII
      (3) Platelet Factors 3 and 4
   d. Open canalicular system (OCS)—allows pathway for granules to exterior
2. Sol-gel zone (cytoskeleton)
   a. Submembranous filaments
   b. Microtubules—contraction facilitates secretion
      (1) Actin
      (2) Myosin
3. Organelle zone (metabolic and secretory)
   a. Dense granules (ADP)
   b. Alpha granules (PF4, growth factor)
   c. Lysosomes (acid hydrolases)
   d. Dense tubular system
      (1) *Prostaglandin* synthesis
      (2) Calcium secretion
   e. Mitochondria (ATP generation for energy)

Based on Harmening DM: *Clinical hematology and fundamentals of hemostasis*, ed 2, Philadelphia, 1992, FA Davis, pp. 415-439.

The sol-gel zone contains filaments and microtubules that, when stimulated, contract to facilitate the secretion of granules of the organelle zone through the open canalicular system to the exterior.

The organelle zone contains dense granules (ADP), alpha granules (PF4, growth factor), lysosomes (acid hydroplases), a mechanism for prostaglandin synthesis and calcium secretion (dense tubular system), and mitochondria for ATP generation.

The functions of platelets include maintenance of vascular integrity, formation of a platelet plug to aid the initial control of bleeding, and stabilization of the platelet plug by involvement in the coagulation process. About 10% of the platelets are used to nurture endothelial cells, allowing for endothelial and smooth muscle regeneration.

Subendothelial tissues at the site of injury are exposed and, through contact activation, cause the platelets to become sticky and adhere to the subendothelial tissues (vWF/GP-Ib). ADP released by damaged endothelial cells initiates aggregation of platelets (primary wave); and when the platelets release their secretions, a second wave of aggregation results. The platelet plug is stabilized by binding with fibrinogen that is converted to fibrin. The result of the above processes is a clot of platelets and fibrin attached to the subendothelial tissue.[11] Tables 22-4 and 22-5 summarize the structure and functions of platelets.

A product of platelets, thromboxane, is needed to induce platelet aggregation. The enzyme cyclooxygenase is key in the process for generation of thromboxane. Endothelial cells, through a similar process (also dependent on cyclooxygenase), generate prostacyclin, which inhibits platelet aggregation. Aspirin acts as an inhibitor of cyclooxygenase, and this causes irreversible damage in the platelets.

However, endothelial cells can synthesize cyclooxygenase; thus aspirin has only a short effect on the availability of prostacyclin from these cells. The net result of aspirin therapy is to inhibit platelet aggregation. This effect will last about 9 days (time needed for old platelets to be cleared from the blood).[11]

In summary: The platelet phase begins only seconds following injury and consists, first, of the platelets' becoming "sticky." This allows them to adhere to endothelial tissues of the damaged vessels and to collagen in the surrounding injured tissue. Soon the platelets begin to stick to each other, and this produces platelet "plugs" that seal off the openings of cut vessels. The whole process is helped by the slowing of blood flow, which occurs soon after injury. The adhesion and aggregation of platelets are influenced by the plasma factor ADP, which is released from the injured tissues, the red blood cells, and the platelets themselves. Platelet prostaglandin activity (thromboxane)[5] will stimulate the aggregation of platelets. Thus the role of platelets in hemostasis is both mechanical and biochemical: the platelet plug seals the damaged vessels mechanically, and various substances associated with platelets play important physical as well as biochemical roles in the coagulation phase.

The process of the fibrin-forming (coagulation) system is shown in Figure 22-1. The overall time involved from injury to a fibrin-stabilized clot is about 9 to 18 minutes. Platelets, blood proteins, lipids, and ions are involved in the process.[11] Thrombin is generated on the surface of the platelets, and bound fibrinogen is converted to fibrin.[11]

Coagulation of blood involves the factors shown in Tables 22-6 and 22-7. Coagulation proceeds through two pathways, the intrinsic and the extrinsic. Both utilize a common pathway to form the end product, fibrin. Figure 22-2 shows these coagulation pathways. The intrinsic pathway is initiated through surface contact activation of Factor XII by exposed subendothelial tissues at the site of injury. The (faster) extrinsic pathway is initiated through tissue thromboplastin released by injured tissues, which activates

TABLE 22-5
Platelet Functions and Activation

1. Maintain vascular integrity
   a. Nurturing endothelial cells
   b. Endothelial and smooth muscle regeneration
2. Initial control of bleeding (platelet plug)
   a. Contact activation (subendothelial)
   b. Stickiness
   c. Adhesion (vWF/GP-Ib)
   d. Aggregation (ADP-initiated)
      (1) Platelet changes shape (spherical)
      (2) Calcium and fibrinogen (GP-IIb and GP-IIIa) form bridges between platelets
   e. Secretion release (second-wave aggregation)
      (1) ADP, serotonin, calcium (dense granules)
      (2) Irreversible changes in platelets
3. Stabilization of platelet plug—contributes to coagulation process
   a. Binding of fibrinogen
   b. Exposure of Platelet Factor 3 on surface
   c. Factor V and Factor VIII complexes on surface
   d. Thrombin generated on surface
   e. Conversion of fibrinogen to fibrin

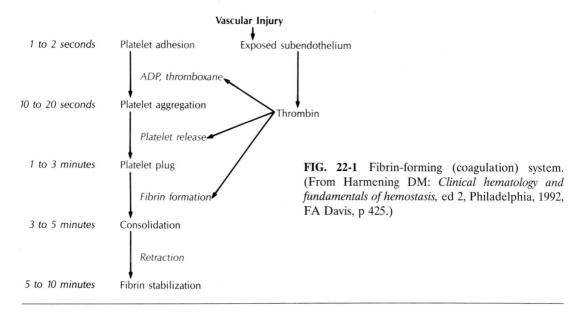

Vascular Injury

1 to 2 seconds	Platelet adhesion
10 to 20 seconds	Platelet aggregation
1 to 3 minutes	Platelet plug
3 to 5 minutes	Consolidation
5 to 10 minutes	Fibrin stabilization

ADP, thromboxane

Platelet release

Fibrin formation

Retraction

Exposed subendothelium

Thrombin

FIG. 22-1 Fibrin-forming (coagulation) system. (From Harmening DM: *Clinical hematology and fundamentals of hemostasis,* ed 2, Philadelphia, 1992, FA Davis, p 425.)

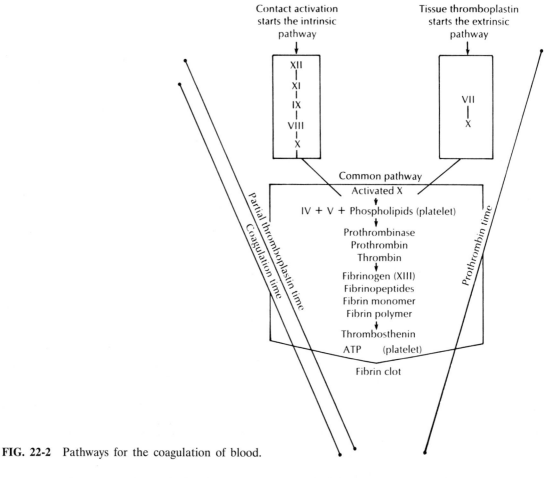

FIG. 22-2   Pathways for the coagulation of blood.

TABLE 22-6
Blood Coagulation Factors

Factor	Name
I	Fibrinogen
II	Prothrombin
III	Thromboplastin
IV	Calcium
V	Labile factor, proaccelerin, accelerator (Ac) globulin
(VI)	Not assigned
VII	Proconvertin, serum prothrombin conversion accelerator (SPCA), cothromboplastin, autoprothrombin I
VIII	Antihemophilic factor (AHF), antihemophilic globulin (AHG), von Willebrand's factor (vWF)
IX	Plasma thromboplastin component (PTC) (Christmas factor)
X	Stuart-Prower factor
XI	Plasma thromboplastin antecedent (PTA)
XII	Hageman factor
XIII	Fibrin-stabilizing factor
Fitzgerald factor	High–molecular weight kininogen (HMWK)
Fletcher factor	Prekallikrein

Based on Harmening DM: *Clinical hematology and fundamentals of hemostasis*, ed 2, Philadelphia, 1992, FA Davis, pp 415-439.

TABLE 22-7
Classification of the Coagulation Factors

1. Substrates
   Factor I — Fibrinogen
2. Cofactors—accelerate enzymatic reactions
   Factor III — Tissue factor (thromboplastin)
   Factor V — Labile factor
   Factor VIII — Antihemophilic factor
   Fitzgerald factor — HMWK (high–molecular weight kininogen)
3. Enzymes
   a. Serine proteases
      Factor II — Prothrombin
      Factor VII — Proconvertin
      Factor IX — Plasma thromboplastin component
      Factor X — Stuart-Prower factor
      Factor XI — Plasma thromboplastin antecedent
      Factor XII — Hageman factor
   b. Transamidase
      Factor XIII — Fibrin-stabilization factor
4. Contact proteins
   Factor XI — Plasma thromboplastin antecedent
   Factor XII — Hageman factor
   Fletcher factor — Prekallikrein
   Fitzgerald factor — HMWK
5. Prothrombin proteins (vitamin K–dependent)
   Factors II, VII, IX, X
6. Fibrinogen group (high–molecular weight)
   Factors I, V, VIII, XIII

Based on Harmening DM: *Clinical hematology and fundamentals of hemostasis*, ed 2, Philadelphia, 1992, FA Davis, pp 415-439.

Factor VII. Many of the coagulation factors are proenzymes that become activated in a "waterfall" or cascade manner[2,11,25,27,32]—that is, one factor becomes activated and it, in turn, activates another, and so on in an ordered sequence.

Thrombin generated by the faster extrinsic common pathway is used to accelerate the slower intrinsic common pathway. The activation of Factor XII acts as a common link between the component parts of the hemostatic mechanism: coagulation, fibrinolytic, kinin, and complement systems. The interactions of these systems are shown in Figure 22-3. Other functions of generated thrombin are shown in Table 22-8.

The fibrin-lysing (fibrinolytic) system is needed to prevent coagulation of intravascular blood away from the site of injury and to dissolve the clot once it has served its function in hemostasis (Fig. 22-4). This system involves plasminogen (a proenzyme for the enzyme plasmin) and various plasminogen activators and inhibitors of plasmin (Table 22-9). The fibrin-forming and fibrin-lysing systems are intimately related; activation of the fibrin-forming (coagulation) system also activates the fibrinolytic system. Tissue plasminogen activator (TPA), released by injured endothelial cells,

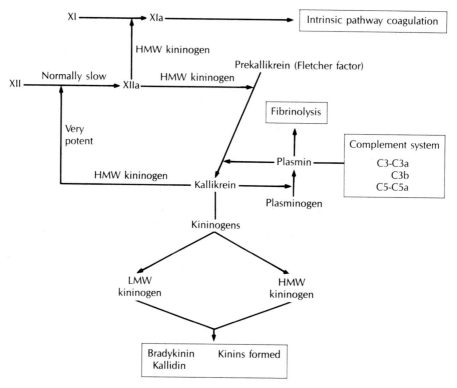

FIG. 22-3 Interactions of the coagulation, fibrinolytic, kinin, and complement systems. (From Harmening DM: *Clinical hematology and fundamentals of hemostasis,* ed 2, Philadelphia, 1992, FA Davis, p 429.)

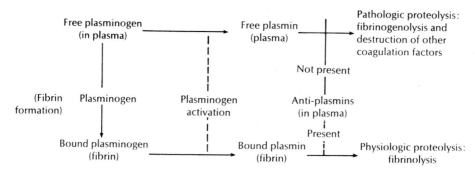

FIG. 22-4 Plasminogen system.

TABLE 22-8
Functions of Thrombin

1. Converts fibrinogen to fibrin
   a. Alpha and beta chains cleaved
   b. Fibrin monomer formed
   c. Monomer polymerizes to fibrin with weak hydrogen bonding
   d. Factor XIIIa combines with calcium; induces cross-linking covalent bonding
   e. Fibrin clot
2. Activates Factor XIII
3. Enhances Factor V and Factor VIII activity
4. Stimulates aggregation of more platelets

Based on Harmening DM: *Clinical hematology and fundamentals of hemostasis*, ed 2, Philadelphia, 1992, FA Davis, pp 415-439.

TABLE 22-9
Actions of Plasmin

1. Destroys fibrin and fibrinogen
2. Produces fibrin degradation products
3. Destroys Factors V and VIII
4. Indirectly enhances conversion of Factor XII to XIIa
5. Enhances or amplifies conversion of prekallikrein to kallikrein, liberating kinins from kininogen (Fig. 22-3)
6. Cleaves complement-3 (C3) into fragments

Based on Harmening DM: *Clinical hematology and fundamentals of hemostasis*, ed 2, Philadelphia, 1992, FA Davis, pp 415-439.

binds to fibrin as it activates the conversion of fibrin-bound plasminogen to plasmin. Circulating plasminogen (i.e., not fibrin-bound) is not activated by TPA. Thus TPA is efficient in dissolving a clot without causing systemic fibrinolysis.[11]

The action of plasmin on fibrin in the clot is to split off large pieces of alpha and beta chains and smaller pieces of gamma chains. The remaining fragments are termed *X* and *Y monomers*. These are split further to *D* and *E fragments*. The final split products from each molecule of fibrin are 2D and 1E fragments. The split products are known as fibrin-split or fibrin-degradation products (FDPs). These can be important clinically if they are allowed to accumulate. FDPs increase vascular permeability and interfere with thrombin-induced fibrin formation.[11] The actions of plasmin are shown in Table 22-10. Table 22-9 summarizes the fibrin-lysing system.

The kinin system is important in inflammation—to increase vascular permeability and for chemotaxis. It is activated by both the coagulation system and the fibrinolytic system (Fig. 22-3). Contact activation of the intrinsic pathway (Factor XII) does not occur without kallikrein or Fitzgerald factor (HMWK). The activation of Factor XI is also dependent on the presence of Fitzgerald factor.

Twenty-two serum proteins form the complement system. These proteins work together with antibodies and clotting factors. The comple-

TABLE 22-10
Fibrin-Lysing (Fibrinolytic) System

1. Activation of coagulation also activates fibrinolysis
2. Active enzyme: plasmin
3. Plasminogen activated to plasmin
   a. Tissue plasminogen activator (TPA)
   b. Kallikrein (Fig. 22-3)
   c. Urokinase, streptokinase, staphylokinase
4. Tissue plasminogen activator (TPA)
   a. Produced by endothelial cells
   b. Released by injury
   c. Activates plasminogen bound to fibrin
   d. Circulating plasminogen not activated
   e. TPA will dissolve clot, not cause systemic fibrinolysis
5. Action of plasmin
   a. Splits large pieces of alpha and beta polypeptides from fibrin
   b. Splits small pieces of gamma chains
   c. First product is X monomer
   d. Each X monomer splits into one E fragment and two D fragments
   e. Split products are called fibrin split products (FSP) and fibrin degradation products (FDP)
6. Action of fibrin degradation products
   a. Increase vascular permeability
   b. Interfere with thrombin-induced fibrin formation

Based on Harmening DM: *Clinical hematology and fundamentals of hemostasis*, ed 2, Philadelphia, 1992, FA Davis, pp 415-439.

ment proteins play an important role as mediators of immune and allergic reactions. Plasmin is an important activator of complement. C3 is activated by plasmin to C3a, C3b, and C3c. C3a is an anaphylatoxin that causes the degranulation of mast cells, resulting in increased vascular permeability. Plasmin also activates C5 to C5a, which functions as both an anaphylatoxin and a platelet aggregator (Table 22-11).

A significant disorder in either the vascular or the platelet phase will lead to an immediate clinical bleeding problem following injury or surgery. These phases are concerned with controlling blood loss immediately after an injury; and if they are defective, this will lead to an early problem. However, if the vascular and platelet phases are normal and the coagulation phase is abnormal, the bleeding problem will not be detected until several hours after the injury or surgical procedure. In the case of small cuts, for example, little bleeding would occur until several hours after the injury, and then a slow trickle of bleeding would start. If the coagulation defect were severe, this slow loss of blood could continue for days. Even with this "trivial" rate a significant loss of blood might occur—0.5 ml per minute or about 3 units per day.[2]

Various antiplasmin factors also are present in circulating blood, and these rapidly destroy free plasmin but are relatively ineffective against plasmin that is bound to fibrin (Table 22-12). Thus under normal conditions, once an injury has occurred, coagulation will proceed to the formation of fibrin. At the same time both bound plasminogen and free plasminogen become activated to plasmin. The free plasmin is rapidly destroyed; thus it does not interfere with the formation of a clot. The bound plasmin is not inactivated, and it is free to dispose of the fibrin clot after its function in hemostasis has been fulfilled. In a sense, the clot is "programmed" to self-destruct at the time of its formation.

TABLE 22-11
Complement System

1. Over 22 serum proteins involved
2. Function of complement system
   a. Immune system
   b. Coagulation system
   c. Allergic reactions
3. Plasmin is important activator of complement
   a. Complement-3 activated by plasmin to
      (1) C3a (anaphylatoxin)—degranulation of mast cells
      (2) C3b (opsonin)—increases immune adherence
   b. Complement-5 activated by plasmin to C5a (anaphylatoxin)—platelet aggregator
   c. Role of C-1 esterase inhibitor

Based on Harmening DM: *Clinical hematology and fundamentals of hemostasis*, ed 2, Philadelphia, 1992, FA Davis, pp 415-439.

TABLE 22-12
Protease Inhibitors

1. Plasmin and kallikrein in circulation eliminated by
   a. Liver
   b. Lymphoid system
   c. Serine protease inhibitors in blood
2. Plasma protease inhibitors
   a. Antithrombin III (AT-III)
   b. Alpha 2 macroglobulin
   c. Alpha 2 antiplasmin
   d. Alpha 2 antitrypsin
   e. C1 esterase inhibitor
   f. Protein C and S inhibitors*
3. Antithrombin III (AT-III)
   a. Also called heparin cofactor or Factor Xa inhibitor
   b. Major physiologic inhibitor of thrombin and Factor Xa
   c. In natural state a slow inhibitor
   d. Activity increased 100 times with heparin
   e. Deficiency causes thrombosis
4. Protein C (serine protease)
   a. Cleaves Factor V and VIII
   b. Increases release of TPA
   c. Acts as cofactor with protein S*
   d. Deficiency causes thrombosis

*Protein S (a vitamin K–dependent fibrinolytic agent manufactured in the liver) is needed, along with protein C (another fibrinolytic agent from the liver), for the destruction of Factors V and VIII.
Based on Harmening DM: *Clinical hematology and fundamentals of hemostasis*, ed 2, Philadelphia, 1992, FA Davis, pp 415-439.

PHYSICAL EXAMINATION (SIGNS)

It is important that the exposed skin and oral mucosa be examined for objective signs that might indicate the presence of a bleeding disorder. Jaundice, spider angiomas, and ecchymoses may be seen in the person with liver disease. A fine tremor of the hands when held out also may be observed in these patients. In about 50% of persons with liver disease there is a reduction of platelets secondary to hypersplenism that results from the effects of portal hypertension, and these individuals may show petechiae on the skin and mucosa.[2,32,33]

The most common objective findings in patients with genetic coagulation disorders are ecchymoses, hemarthrosis, and dissecting hematomas (Fig. 22-5). The signs seen most commonly in patients with abnormal platelets or thrombocytopenia are petechiae and ecchymoses (Fig. 22-6).

Patients with acute or chronic leukemia may reveal one or more of the following signs: ulceration of the oral mucosa, hyperplasia of the gingivae, petechiae of the skin or mucous membranes, ecchymoses of skin or mucous membranes, and lymphadenopathy (Figs. 22-7 and 22-8).

A number of patients with bleeding disorders may show no objective signs that suggest their underlying problem.

LABORATORY TESTS

Several tests are available to evaluate patients for bleeding disorders and to pinpoint the specific deficiency.

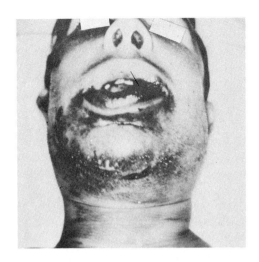

FIG. 22-5 Patient with hemophilia who has massive areas of ecchymosis secondary to trauma.

The PTT (partial thromboplastin time) test is used to check the intrinsic system and the common pathways. For the PTT test, activation is accomplished by the glass wall of the test tube or by adding a contact activator such as kaolin. When a contact activator is added, the test is referred to as the "activated PTT." A control must be run with the test sample, and the results can be interpreted only if the control value falls within the normal range of results for the laboratory performing the test. The activated PTT varies from laboratory to laboratory; hence, the dentist must be aware of the normal

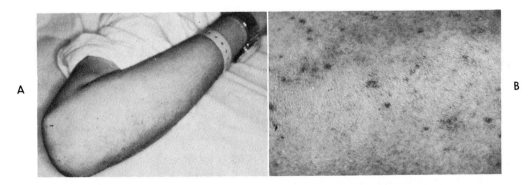

FIG. 22-6 A, Arm of a patient with thrombocytopenia snowing numerous petechiae. **B,** Close-up view of the petechiae.

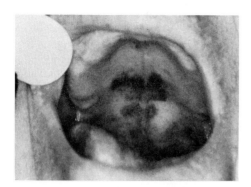

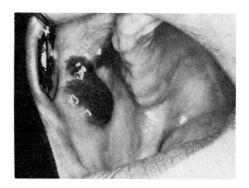

FIG. 22-7 Areas of ecchymosis on the mucosa of the hard and soft palate in a patient with chronic lymphocytic leukemia.

FIG. 22-8 Cheek lesion that might appear to be an area of ecchymosis. However, the lesion blanched with pressure and was determined to be a capillary hemangioma.

range for the laboratory being used. In general, the activated PTT ranges from 25 to 35 seconds, and results in excess of 35 seconds are considered abnormal or prolonged.

The PT (prothrombin time) test is used to check the extrinsic system (Factor VII) and the common pathways. For this test, tissue thromboplastin is added to the test sample to serve as the activating agent. Again, a control must be run and results vary from one laboratory to another. In general, the normal range is 11 to 15 seconds and results in excess of 15 seconds are considered abnormal or prolonged.

In the TT (thrombin time) test, thrombin is added as the activating agent. It converts fibrinogen in the blood to insoluble fibrin, which constitutes the essential portion of a blood clot. Again, a control must be run, and results vary from laboratory to laboratory. Generally, the normal range for the TT test is 9 to 13 seconds and results in excess of 16 to 18 seconds are considered abnormal or prolonged.

The Ivy bleeding time (BT [Ivy]) is used to evaluate the platelet and vascular phases from a functional standpoint. It is a crude but valuable screen and is performed by measuring how long it takes for bleeding to stop from a fresh cut of defined size. A blood pressure cuff is placed on the arm and the pressure is raised to 30 mm Hg. A wound is made on the inner surface of the forearm with a sterile lancet, and every 15 seconds it is blotted with a piece of sterile filter paper. The test is finished when no blood can be absorbed by the filter paper. The normal range

for the bleeding time is 1 to 6 minutes with a time greater than 6 minutes considered abnormal or prolonged.

A platelet count is often used to screen for possible bleeding problems. The normal platelet count is 140,000 to 400,000/mm³ of blood; however, clinical bleeding problems are usually associated with platelet counts of less than 50,000/mm³. A peripheral blood smear is also used to examine for the presence of platelets.

Accelerated fibrinolysis can be diagnosed by demonstrating fibrin split products in the serum or by finding increased plasminogen activation in the circulation. Fibrin split products can be tested for by using direct measurements or paracoagulation.[1]

In the staphylococcus clumping assay (a direct test) *Staphylococcus aureus* is agglutinated by fibrin split products. If no fibrin split products are present, no agglutination takes place; the more concentrated the amount of fibrin split products, the greater will be the amount of staphylococcal agglutination.

The ethanol paracoagulation test also can be used to measure for the presence of fibrin split products. This test is based on the fact that fibrin split products can form soluble complexes with fibrin monomers, preventing the bound monomers from polymerizing into a fibrin clot. When ethanol is added to serum containing such complexes, the complexes degenerate, releasing their fibrin monomers. The liberated monomers polymerize in normal fashion, forming a visible clot.

The euglobulin lysis time test is used to demonstrate increased plasminogen activation in the circulation. In this test the patient's plasma is treated with diluted acid. Fibrinogen is precipitated out, carrying with it other clotting factors, plasmin, plasminogen, and any circulating plasminogen activators; however, circulating inhibitors of the fibrinolytic system are left in the solution. The precipitate is called euglobulin fraction, and it can be isolated and redissolved in neutral buffer containing a calcium-binding anticoagulant. Calcium is then added to the solution of euglobulin fraction and a fibrin clot is formed that will dissolve over the next few hours if plasminogen activators are present. The rate at which the clot dissolves is related to the quantity of circulating plasminogen activators in the original plasma. The time required for the euglobulin precipitate to dissolve (euglobulin lysis time) is thus a measure of plamsa fibrinolytic activity; therefore the shorter the euglobulin lysis time, the greater must be the fibrinolytic activity.

Platelet adhesion can be evaluated by measuring platelet aggregation in response to ristocetin.[1] Although ristocetin causes a completely artificial type of aggregation, it happens to be a good index of platelet adhesion in vivo. Ristocetin aggregation is defective in von Willebrand's disease and Bernard-Soulier disease but is generally normal in other platelet diseases.

The last laboratory test to be considered is the measurement of Platelet Factor 3 (PF3) to evaluate platelet release reaction.[1] For this test, blood that has been anticoagulated with a calcium binder (citrate or oxalate) is divided into two separate test tubes. One test tube is centrifuged and the serum separated from the platelets and other cellular elements. The other test tube is left unspun and contains platelets left in suspension. Next, kaolin is added to both test tubes (the one "without" and the one with platelets); this causes the platelets to become fully potent as promotors of coagulation (i.e., to make available their PF3). Finally, calcium is added to each test tube, and the time required for the samples to clot is measured. The platelet-rich plasma should clot more rapidly than the platelet-poor plasma because PF3 is present. The difference in clotting times between the two samples is used as the index of PF3 activity. The most common cause of a defective release reaction is aspirin ingestion. The greater the effect, the less will be the differences in clotting time between the platelet-rich and platelet-poor samples.

The dentist will be apprised of the screening test results—PT, PTT, BT, TT, and platelet count. If an abnormal result is reported, the patient should be referred for more specific testing to pinpoint the exact deficiency or problem.

MEDICAL MANAGEMENT

In this section conditions that may cause clinical bleeding are considered. The emphasis is placed on the detection of patients with a potential bleeding problem and the management of these patients if surgical procedures are needed.

Hemophilia, von Willebrand's disease, Bernard-Soulier disease, DIC, disorders of platelet release, and primary fibrinogenolysis will be described in some detail to demonstrate the nature of certain genetic and acquired bleeding disorders. These diseases show the role of various factors involved in the control of excessive bleeding following injury and what happens when these factors are defective.

von Willebrand's disease

von Willebrand's disease is an inherited defect involving platelet adhesion. The affected gene has been localized to chromosome 12. The disease has several variants depending on the severity of genetic expression. Most of the variants are transmitted as autosomal dominant traits (types IA, IIA, and IIIB). These variants of the disease tend to result in mild to moderate clinical bleeding problems. Two of the variants, type IIC and type III, are transmitted as autosomal recessive traits. They usually cause moderate to severe clinical bleeding problems.[10,30]

The cause of the platelet dysfunction is a deficiency of von Willebrand's factor (vWF), which is made from a group of glycoproteins. These glycoproteins are produced by megakaryoctes and endothelial cells. They form into a single monomer that polymerizes into huge complexes, which are needed to carry Factor VIII and to allow platelets to adhere to surfaces. Nonbound Factor VIII does not survive long in blood. Thus a deficiency of vWF results in a similar decrease in plasma Factor VIII levels. The complex of vWF and Factor VIII attaches to the surface of circulating platelets, and it is from this location that the factors contribute to hemostasis.[10,20]

Patients with von Willebrand's disease usually give a family history of more or less severe bleeding and may also report having had problems with bleeding following injury or surgery. Laboratory investigation is needed to make the diagnosis. Laboratory findings consist of a prolonged BT, impaired adhesion of platelets with failure to aggregate with ristocetin, and decreased Factor VIII activity.

Bernard-Soulier disease

Bernard-Soulier disease also represents a disorder of platelet adhesion; however, in this disease the platelets are defective and unable to interact with vWF. The basic defect is the absence of a glycoprotein (GP-Ib) from the membrane of the platelet. GP-Ib appears to function as a receptor for vWF. Laboratory tests show a low platelet count, large platelets, faulty platelet adhesion, and poor aggregation with ristocetin.

Disseminated intravascular coagulation

DIC is a condition that results when the clotting system is activated in all or a major part of the vascular system. Despite widespread fibrin production, the major clinical problem is bleeding, not thrombosis. DIC is caused when large quantities of thromboplastic substances are introduced into the vascular system and "trip" the clotting cascade. Acute DIC can be caused by obstetric complications (abruptio placentae, missed abortion, amniotic fluid embolism), infection, injuries and burns, antigen-antibody complexes, shock, and acidosis. Symptoms include severe bleeding from small wounds, purpura, and spontaneous bleeding from the nose, gums, gastrointestinal tract, or urinary tract. Traumatic hemolytic anemia can occur because the red blood cells are "sliced" by fibrin strands. On rare occasion, bilateral necrosis of the renal cortex has developed. Chronic DIC may occur in association with certain types of cancer. Malignant cells can release thromboplastic material as they die within the tumor mass. Antigen-antibody complexes associated with systemic lupus erythema-

tosus may cause chronic DIC. In the chronic form of the disease, thrombosis is more common than bleeding.

Thromboplastic substances can be aided by tissue acidosis and circulatory stasis and when released in large quantities may swamp the body's defenses — antithrombin III, protein C, and phagocytes. The thromboplastic substances act on Factor XII, Factor VII, and platelets and the result is triggering every component of the coagulation system. Plasmin is generated by Factor XIIa, thrombin, and plasminogen activators released by monocytes and endothelial cells.

The excessive generated plasmin splits both fibrinogen and newly generated fibrin, releasing fibrin split products (which have strong anticoagulation properties of their own). Platelets are activated by thrombin, exposed collagen, and tissue thromboplastic substances. This activation releases PF3, which feeds back to accelerate the clotting cascade; in addition, the activated platelets are consumed as they aggregate and adhere to damaged tissue.

The net effect of the above processes involved in acute DIC is to reduce the levels of fibrinogen, reduce Factors V, VIII, and XIII, decrease the platelet count, and cause numerous fibrin split products to appear in the blood. The end result is a complex bleeding disorder due to clotting factors and platelet deficiencies and complicated by the anticoagulant effects of fibrin split products. The classic laboratory findings with DIC are shown in Table 22-13.

Disorders of platelet release

Platelets participate directly in the clotting cascade by serving as constituents of Factor X and prothrombin-converting complexes through the release of PF3. The potency of this release effect is increased the more often platelets participate in the clotting process. In certain cases the platelets can fail to complete the release reaction of PF3. Sometimes this is due to a defective production of thromboxane, other times to a deficiency in the production of dense granule adenosine disphosphate (ADP).

Defective thromboxane production almost always results from the administration of anti-inflammatory drugs. The best example is aspirin, which inactivates cyclooxygenase, the first enzyme of the prostaglandin-thromboxane syn-

TABLE 22-13
Laboratory Findings in DIC

Test	Findings
Prothrombin time (PT)	Prolonged
Partial thromboplastin time (PTT)	Prolonged
Thrombin time (TT)	Prolonged
Platelet count	Decreased
Fibrinogen level	Decreased
Presence of fibrin split products	Marked increase
Bleeding time (BT[Ivy])	Prolonged

thetic pathway. Other drugs that interfere with thromboxane formation include indomethacin, phenylbutazone, ibuprofen, and sulfinpyrazone. All platelet-release defects produce about the same clinical picture. Usually little in the way of bleeding occurs unless the defect is superimposed upon some other "clotting" disorder—such as hemophilia or thrombocytopenia. Bleeding time may be normal or prolonged, and platelet function studies often show an absence of secondary-wave aggregation. Patients can be screened with the standard screening tests; if these are normal, surgical procedures can be performed, and if no other defects are present surgery can be performed even though the bleeding time is moderately prolonged (6 to 20 minutes).

Uremia may interfere with platelet function. This effect can be severe with prolonged bleeding times and grossly abnormal platelet function tests. These patients are in danger of bleeding to death if injury occurs or surgery is performed. They respond to dialysis, cryoprecipitate, or kidney transplant but not to platelet replacement. Although beta lactam antibiotics (penicillin and cephalothins) can cause platelet dysfunction, usually no treatment is required. Alcohol can, in some undetermined way, impair platelet function, which may be severe enough to contraindicate surgery unless corrective measures are taken.

Primary fibrinogenolysis

Primary fibrinogenolysis may develop if active plasmin is generated in the circulation at a time when the clotting cascade is not in operation. It can occur in patients with liver disease, cancer of the lung, cancer of the prostate, or heat stroke. Severe bleeding results from the depletion of fibrinogen (split by plasmin) and the formation of fibrin split products (with their anticoagulant properties) from the fibrinogen.

Laboratory test results are similar to those in DIC, with the following important exceptions: (1) platelet count is normal; (2) euglobulin lysis time is shortened in primary fibrinogenolysis and is normal in DIC (the euglobulin lysis test is a crude measurement of circulating plasmin); and (3) the fibrin split products of primary fibrinogenolysis clump with the staphylococcal clumping assay (same for DIC), but no fibrin monomers can be released by paracoagulation with ethanol (in DIC a loose complex of fibrin monomers is released from fibrin split products and then polymerizes to form a gel).

Fibrinogenolysis can be treated with epsilon-aminocaproic acid (EACA) or tranexamic acid, which inhibits both plasmin and plasmin activators[3,17]; however, these drugs can be dangerous if used in DIC because diffuse thromboses may result.

Hemophilia

In this discussion hemophilia will be used to demonstrate some of the problems involved in dealing with the medical management of patients who have a coagulation disorder. Hemophilia is caused by a serum deficiency of Factor VIII, and severe forms of the disease occur when the level is less than 1% of normal. The level tends to remain constant in a given hemophiliac patient. Patients with a Factor VIII level greater than 10% of normal usually have less severe problems with bleeding complications. A complication that poses great difficulties in the management of patients with hemophilia is the appearance of so-called inducible inhibitors. About 10% of individuals with hemophila have Factor VIII neutralizing antibodies. Half of these patients will have stable levels of inhibitors (remaining constant over time) and half will have inducible inhibitors (whose level increases in response to Factor VIII replacement therapy).[2]

Treatment regimens for bleeding problems in patients with hemophilia are shown in Table 22-14. All types of general surgical procedures

TABLE 22-14
Medical Treatment for the Patient with
Hemophilia

1. Without inhibitors of Factor VIII (antihemophilic factor, AHF)
   a. Factor VIII stimulant—1-desamino-8-D-arginine vasopressin (DDAVP)
   b. Antifibrinolytic agents
      (1) Epsilon-aminocaproic acid (EACA)
      (2) Tranexamic acid
   c. Replacement factors
      (1) Cryoprecipitate
      (2) Frozen fresh plasma
      (3) Purified heat-treated AHF
      (4) New ultrapure preparations of AHF
         (a) Monoclonal antibody technique
         (b) Recombinant DNA–produced AHF
2. With mild or moderately stable levels of AHF inhibitors
   a. High doses of purified AHF
   b. Porcine Factor VIII concentrate
   c. Steroids
3. With inducible or high levels of AHF inhibitors
   a. Porcine Factor VIII concentrate
   b. Prothrombin complex concentrate
   c. Activated Factor IX
   d. Plasmapheresis
   e. Steroids

TABLE 22-15
Medical Treatment of the Patient with
von Willebrand's Disease

1. Increase Factor VIII and vWF (type I cases)—1-desamino-8-D-arginine vasopressin (DDAVP)
2. Replace missing vFW and Factor VIII*
   a. Fresh frozen plasma
   b. Cryoprecipitate
3. Oral contraceptive agents to suppress menses

*Factor VIII concentrates are not effective because vWF is destroyed or removed during processing.

replacement. Plasmapheresis has been used to remove the inhibitors.[13,15,20,22]

von Willebrand's disease

Medical treatment to prevent excessive bleeding in patients with von Willebrand's disease does not include Factor VIII concentrates (Table 22-15). The Factor VIII concentrates are not effective because vWF is destroyed or removed during processing. Many patients with the more mild type I and some with type II forms of the disease can be controlled when DDAVP is used.[26] In patients with severe deficiency of vWF activity either fresh frozen plasma or cryopreciptate is required. Women often are given oral contraceptive agents to suppress menses and avoid excessive physiologic loss of blood.[10,20]

Risk of infection with replacement products

The use of cryoprecipitates, Factor VIII concentrates, and fresh frozen plasma carries several important risks. For example, transmission of hepatitis B virus (HBV), hepatitis C virus (HCV), and the human immune deficiency virus (HIV) can occur.

In one study of 190 patients with hemophilia in western Pennsylvania[23] 62.5% were found to have antibodies to HIV. The first two seroconversions occurred in 1978, but the vast majority have taken place from 1982 to 1984. In 27 patients who had been seropositive for at least 3 years, 4 (15%) developed AIDS, 7 (26%) developed AIDS-related complex (ARC), and 16 were symptom-free. In 16 patients who had been seropositive for less than 3 years, 3 developed ARC and 13 were symptom free. A

can now be performed in these individuals without inducible inhibitors of antihemophilic factor (AHF).[13,15,20] The expected rate of postoperative bleeding problems is 6% to 23%, with orthopedic surgery on the knee resulting in up to 40% of these.[13,15] Patients with mild deficiency of AHF often can undergo surgical procedures when DDAVP is used alone or in combination with EACA. Patients with more severe AHF deficiency will require Factor VIII replacement. EACA also is given to patients receiving factor replacement.

Patients with high titers of inducible inhibitors still present too great a risk for most elective surgical procedures. If surgery must be performed, high doses of porcine Factor VIII concentrate can be given or activated Factor IX. Prothrombin complex concentrate may be effective in some patients. Steroids are often given to reduce the inhibitor response to Factor VIII

significantly greater amount of Factor VIII concentrate had been used in seropositive hemophiliacs than in seronegative hemophiliacs,[23] although there was no difference in the use of cryoprecipitate between the seropositive and seronegative groups.

The ability of the AIDS virus to be spread by heterosexual sexual activities was demonstrated in a report by Kreiss et al.[16] in which 42 patients with hemophila and their wives were studied. Twenty-one of the individuals with hemophilia had seroconverted and were found to have antibodies to HIV. One of these patients had AIDS, nine had persistent generalized lymphadenopathy (PGL), and eleven were asymptomatic. Two of the wives were found to have antibodies to HIV, and both of their husbands were asymptomatic but HIV antibody—positive.

The identification of an etiologic agent for AIDS, the development of a screening test to determine exposure to the AIDS virus, and the heating of blood concentrates all have enabled the blood pool in the United States to be "safe." However, because of the risk to individuals needing repeated replacement of blood products, alternate sources and substitutes for therapeutic blood components are used.[10,12,20] Porcine Factor VIII concentrate is used for patients with lower levels of inhibitor to Factor VIII. Ultrapure preparations of AHF are now available, produced by recombinant DNA or monoclonal antibody techniques.[20]

DENTAL MANAGEMENT
PATIENT IDENTIFICATION

There are four methods by which the dentist can detect the patient who may have a bleeding problem. The skill developed with these methods will determine how well dentists can protect certain patients from the danger of excessive bleeding following dental surgical treatment. The four methods are (1) a good history, (2) physical examination, (3) screening clinical laboratory tests, and (4) observation of excessive bleeding following a surgical procedure (Table 22-16).

History (symptoms)

A good history is the best single screening procedure to identify the patient with a possible bleeding disorder. The history should include

TABLE 22-16
Detection of the Patient Who Is a "Bleeder"

1. History
   a. Bleeding problems in relatives
   b. Bleeding problems following operations and tooth extractions
   c. Bleeding problems following trauma (cuts, etc)
   d. Medications that may cause bleeding problems
      (1) Aspirin
      (2) Anticoagulants
      (3) Long-term antibiotic therapy
   e. Presence of illnesses that may have associated bleeding problems
      (1) Leukemia
      (2) Liver disease
      (3) Hemophilia
      (4) Congenital heart disease
   f. Spontaneous bleeding from nose, mouth, ears, etc
2. Examination findings
   a. Jaundice, pallor
   b. Spider angiomas
   c. Ecchymosess
   d. Petechiae
   e. Oral ulcers
   f. Hyperplastic gingival tissues
   g. Hemarthrosis
3. Screening laboratory tests
   a. PT
   b. PTT
   c. TT
   d. BT
   e. Platelet count
4. Surgical procedure—excessive bleeding following surgery may be first clue to underlying bleeding problem

PT, Prothrombin time; *PTT*, partial thrombplastin time; *TT*, thrombin time; *BT*, bleeding time (Ivy).

questions concerning the following six topics:
1. Presence of bleeding problems in relatives
2. Excessive bleeding following operations
3. Excessive bleeding following trauma
4. Use of drugs for prevention of coagulation or chronic pain
5. Past and present illness
6. Occurrence of spontaneous bleeding

BLEEDING PROBLEMS IN RELATIVES

Hemophilia and Christmas disease, the two most common inherited coagulation disorders, will be discussed here to show how a history of bleeding in a patient's relatives can give a clue to the presence of a congenital bleeding problem. These coagulation disorders are transmitted by a sex-linked recessive mode of inheritance. The X chromosome contains the altered gene; in most cases the female serves as the carrier and the disease manifest itself only in the male.[2,32] To demonstrate the various possibilities of inheritance of these diseases, the following symbols will be used:

---

xx Normal female
xy Normal male
x* Abnormal recessive gene for disease
x*y Affected male
xx* Female carrier
x*x* Affected female

An affected male cannot transmit the disease to his sons; however, his daughters will be carriers.

Half the sons of a female carrier who is married to a normal male will be affected by the disorder, and half the daughters will be carriers.

One combination that could produce a daughter with such a coagulation disorder[2,32] would be when a female carrier marries an affected male. Half their daughters would have the disorder, and half would be carriers. Half the sons would be affected, and half would be normal. However, the probabilities for this type of union are small, which explains why so few females are affected.

About 25% of patients with a proven hereditary coagulation disorder have a negative family history.[13] The reason is the relatively high rate of mutation producing new cases; therefore a negative family history does not, in itself, always preclude a genetic coagulation disorder.

BLEEDING PROBLEMS FOLLOWING OPERATIONS AND TOOTH EXTRACTIONS

Each new patient should be questioned concerning excessive bleeding following major or minor operations. The number of individuals who have had an appendectomy, tonsillectomy, or tooth extraction is large. Persons who have had such procedures without a bleeding problem do not have a significant inherited coagulation disorder. However, although they did not have a significant acquired bleeding problem at the time the operative procedure was performed, this does not mean that they are free of such a problem that could have been acquired since the last surgery.

BLEEDING PROBLEMS FOLLOWING TRAUMA

All new patients should be asked if they have experienced any recent trauma and if so whether it was followed by excessive bleeding. The more severe the trauma, the more likely it is to reveal the presence of an underlying bleeding disorder. Small cuts in patients with coagulation disorders may not cause excessive bleeding initially because the vascular and platelet phases may be sufficient to control blood loss even if there is a defect in coagulation. However, small cuts in patients with platelet or vascular deficiencies usually will result in excessive bleeding and in patients with severe coagulation disorders may lead to bleeding several hours after the injury.

When excessive bleeding does occur following trauma in patients with coagulation disorders, it is usually delayed because the immediate control of blood loss by vasoconstriction, extravascular pressure, and platelet plugging proceeds normally. However, when these effects begin to lessen, they are not replaced by the formation of a good clot of fibrin as happens in normal coagulation. This is when the bleeding occurs in the patient who has a coagulation defect.

MEDICATIONS THAT MAY CAUSE BLEEDING PROBLEMS

All new patients should be asked if they are taking an anticoagulant drug—such as heparin or a coumarin derivative. If the patient is receiving one of these drugs, the dentist should contact the patient's physician to determine the degree of anticoagulation being maintained and the purpose for which the drug is being used. All patients should be asked if they have been taking aspirin or drugs that contain aspirin and in what dosage and over what length of time. Patients also should be asked if they have had recent treatment with a broad-spectrum antibiotic and asked about excessive use of alcohol.

PRESENCE OF ILLNESSES WITH ASSOCIATED BLEEDING PROBLEMS

The past and current medical status of patients needs to be reviewed. They should be questioned concerning a history of liver disease, biliary tract obstruction, malabsorption problems, infectious diseases, genetic coagulation disorders, chronic inflammatory diseases, chronic renal disease, or leukemia or other types of cancer and whether they have received radiation therapy or been exposed to large amounts of radiation. It must be determined if patients with cancer are being treated with chemotherapy, for this can cause significant suppression of platelet production.

SPONTANEOUS BLEEDING

Each patient should be asked about a history of spontaneous bleeding—including gingival, nasal, urinary, rectal, gastrointestinal, oral, pulmonary, and vaginal sources of bleeding. If spontaneous bleeding has occurred, the frequency, amount of blood lost, appearance of the blood, and steps that were necessary to stop it should be determined.

Screening laboratory tests

Five clinical laboratory tests can be used by the dentist to screen patients for bleeding disorders. These tests are the platelet count, the BT (Ivy), PTT, PT, and TT[14,18] (Table 22-17).

From a functional viewpoint the platelet count does not have to be obtained to screen a patient, because the bleeding time will reflect problems with both the number and the quality of platelets. However, by ordering a platelet count the dentist can gain better insight into the nature of the problem in patients with a prolonged bleeding time. For example, if the BT was prolonged and the platelet count within normal limits, a problem in platelet function would be indicated. The BT (Ivy) is the best test to measure for the presence of adequate platelet function (Fig. 22-9).

In the past we recommended that the tourniquet test be used to screen for abnormalities in the vascular phase. However, this test has been found too insensitive to be of any real value in the screening procedure, although it may show abnormal results in patients with vascular or platelet phase disorders. The BT is now used to screen these phases.

TABLE 22-17

Screening Laboratory Tests for the Detection of a Potential "Bleeder"

---

1. PT—activated by tissue thromboplastin
   a. Tests extrinsic and common pathways
   b. Control should be run
   c. Normal (11 to 15 seconds, depending on laboratory)
   d. Control must be in normal range
2. Activated PTT—activated by addition of contact activator (kaolin)
   a. Tests intrinsic and common pathways
   b. Control should be run
   c. Normal (25 to 35 seconds, depending on laboratory)
   d. Control must be in normal range
3. TT—activated by thrombin
   a. Tests ability to form initial clot from fibrinogen
   b. Controls should be run
   c. Normal (9 to 13 seconds)
4. BT
   a. Tests platelet and vascular phases
   b. Normal if adequate number of platelets of good quality present with intact vascular walls
   c. Normal (1 to 6 minutes)
5. Platelet count
   a. Tests platelet phase
   b. Normal (140,000 to 400,000/mm³)
   c. Clinical bleeding problem can occur if less than 80,000/mm³

PT, Prothrombin time; *PTT,* partial thromboplastin time; *TT,* thrombin time; *BT,* bleeding time (Ivy).

The PTT test is used to measure the status of the intrinsic and common pathways of coagulation. This test reflects the ability of blood still within vessels in the area of injury to coagulate. It will be prolonged in coagulation disorders affecting the intrinsic and common pathways (hemophilia, liver disease) and also in cases of excessive fibrinolysis.

The PT test is used to measure the status of the extrinsic and common pathways of coagulation. This test reflects the ability of blood lost from vessels in the area of injury to coagulate. It will be prolonged in cases of Factor VII deficiency and disorders affecting the common pathway and fibrinolysis. This test usually is

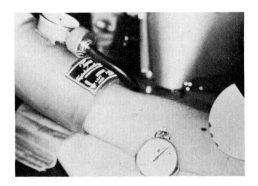

FIG. 22-9 Ivy bleeding time. Midway through the test, blood can still be blotted onto filter paper.

normal in patients with intrinsic pathway defects (hemophilia).[14,18]

The TT test uses thrombin as the test activating agent; hence it measures only the ability of fibrinogen to form an initial clot. Since fibrin degradation products tend to prolong the TT, this test becomes reasonably sensitive for fibrinolysis disorders. When done with the PT and PTT tests, it allows for the identification of coagulation disorders involving the last "stage" of the sequence. For example, if the PT, PTT, and TT are all prolonged, the problem in the coagulation system would be at the point of conversion of fibrinogen to the initial clot.

The results of these screening tests direct the hematologist to the possible source of a bleeding disorder and allow for the selection of more specific tests to identify the nature of the defect.[5,32,33]

DENTAL MANAGEMENT
MEDICAL CONSIDERATIONS

No surgical procedures should be performed on a patient suspected of having a bleeding problem based on history and examination findings. Such a patient should be screened with the appropriate clinical laboratory tests and, if indicated, referred to a hematologist for diagnosis and treatment. Patients under medical management who may have a bleeding problem should receive no dental treatment until consultation with the patient's physician has taken place and appropriate preparations have been

TABLE 22-18

Selection of Screening Laboratory Tests for Detecting the Patient with a Potential Bleeding Problem Based on History and Examination Findings

---

No clinical or historical clues to bleeding problem—problem develops following surgical procedure

History or clinical findings or both suggest possible bleeding problem but no clues to cause
  PT
  PTT
  TT
  BT
  Platelet count

Aspirin therapy
  BT
  PTT

Coumarin therapy
  PT

Possible liver disease
  BT
  PT

Chronic leukemia
  BT

Malabsorption syndrome or long-term antibiotic therapy
  PT

Renal dialysis (heparin)
  PTT

Vascular wall alteration
  BT

Primary fibrinogenolysis (active plasmin in circulation), cancers (lung, prostate)
  TT

BT, Bleeding time (Ivy); *PTT*, partial thromboplastin time; *PT*, prothrombin time; *TT*, thrombin time.

made to avoid excessive bleeding following dental procedures.

Nine clinical situations often present the dentist with the problem of whether or not a given patient has a bleeding problem. Each of these situations will be discussed in detail (Tables 22-18 and 22-19).

No clinical or historical clues to bleeding problem

A person with a potential bleeding problem may have no subjective or objective findings that

TABLE 22-19
Results of Screening Tests

Condition	Platelet count	BT	PTT	PT	TT
			Screening tests		
Thrombocytopenia	+ +	+ +	−	−	−
Dicumarol therapy	−	−	+ +	+ +	−
Liver disease	+	+	+ +	+ +	+ +
Vascular wall defect	−	+	−	−	−
Hemophilia	−	−	+ +	−	−
Aspirin therapy	+	+	+	+	−
Leukemia	+	+	−	−	−
Malabsorption syndrome or long-term antibiotic therapy	−	−	+ +	+ +	+ +
Factor VII deficiency	−	−	−	+ +	−
Renal dialysis (heparin)	+	+	+ +	−	−
Fibrinogenolysis	−	−	+	+	+ +

BT, Bleeding time (Ivy); *PTT*, partial thromboplastin time; *PT*, prothrombin time; *TT*, thrombin time.
−, Normal; +, may be abnormal; + +, abnormal.

suggest the condition. The first indication may be prolonged bleeding following a dental surgical procedure, and for this local measures should be taken to control the bleeding; if these fail, a hematologist may have to be consulted. Once the problem is under control, the patient should be screened with the appropriate laboratory tests—PT, PTT, BT, platelet count, and TT—because there are no clues as to the cause of the problem. The screening can be done by the dentist through a commercial clinical laboratory or by referring the patient to a hematologist.

History or clinical findings, or both, suggest a possible bleeding problem but no clues to its cause

When there are no clues regarding the cause of a potential bleeding problem in a patient, all five screening laboratory tests should be performed. The patient's physician can order these tests, or the dentist can order them from a clinical laboratory facility (Table 22-17).

Aspirin therapy

Patients receiving aspirin therapy may have a bleeding problem based on the drug's effect on platelets. Usually these patients have been receiving high doses (20 gr or more) of aspirin each day for a prolonged period (more than a week). Not all patients taking aspirin as described will have a bleeding problem, but all of them should be screened to make certain of this. Although aspirin affects the coagulation process through its effect on platelet release, it does not usually lead to a significant bleeding problem unless there is some other defect present. Tests should be ordered to screen this type of patient: a BT to screen for platelet function and a PTT to screen for platelet-associated coagulation disorders. If these tests are abnormal, the patient's physician should be consulted before any dental surgical procedure is performed.

Coumarin therapy

If the history establishes that a patient is receiving one of the coumarin drugs, the dentist should consult the patient's physician concerning the reason for taking the drug, the level of anticoagulation (reported in terms of the PT—most patients are held at about 1½ to 2½. Most physicians are aware of the recommendations of the American Medical Association and the American Dental Association suggesting that the patient be at a level of anticoagulation of about 1½ to 2½ times the normal PT before a surgical procedure is attempted. If bleeding occurs, local measures can be used to control it.[19] If the physician agrees to this approach, he or she will reduce the dosage of anticoagulant; and some physicians may have the patient discontinue anticoagulant therapy entirely before surgery. In either case it will take at least 2 to 3 days for the effect of the reduced dosage to be reflected in a decrease in the PT.[32] On the day of surgery the physician or dentist should order a PT before the procedure to be certain that the desired degree of anticoagulation reduction has occurred. If the PT is still greater than twice normal, the dosage of anticoagulant should be reduced again by the physician and the surgery should be postponed for 2 or 3 more days, at which time the PT should be repeated. A recent study[3] suggests that dental surgery can be performed without major bleeding complications in patients on anticoagulation therapy at higher than 1½ to 2½ times the normal PT.

If infection is present, no surgery should be done until the patient has been treated with antibiotics. When the patient is free of acute infection and the PT is in the acceptable range (1½ to 2½ times normal), surgery can be performed. The procedure should be done with as little trauma as possible, and the patient can be administered antibiotics to prevent postoperative infection (although, in most cases, this may not be necessary). Patients free of chronic dental or periodontal infection do not need prophylaxis. Prophylaxis can be considered for patients with active periodontal disease and/or conditions that might render the patient more susceptible to postoperative infection. If excessive postoperative bleeding occurs, Gelfoam with thrombin can be used to control it. In some patients it may be helpful to construct a splint before surgery to cover the surgical area, which will protect the clot, and Gelfoam with thrombin can be packed beneath the splint. In addition, primary closure over the sockets is desirable.

Oxcel, Surgicel, or microfibrillar collagen may be used in place of Gelfoam. However, thrombin should not be used with these agents because it is inactivated as a result of pH factors, thus representing an additional cost with no real benefits (Table 22-20).

TABLE 22-20
Dental Management of the Patient Taking Dicumarol

1. Detection by history
2. Consultation with physician
   a. Status of underlying problems
   b. Level of anticoagulation expressed in PT
      (1) If greater than 2½ times normal, request that dicumarol dosage be reduced
      (2) Effects of reduction in dicumarol dosage will take 2 to 3 days
      (3) On day of procedure, check to see if PT is 2½ times normal or less
3. If scaling or surgical procedures are planned, patient should be free of active infection
4. Prophylactic antibiotics are suggested following surgery to prevent postoperative infection, which may complicate control of bleeding problem
5. If excessive bleeding should occur following surgery, it can be controlled by local measures
   a. Splints
   b. Gelfoam with thrombin
   c. Oxcel, Surgicel, microfibrillar collagen
   d. Pressure packs
6. Have patient return in 4 to 5 days; if healing is normal, call physician and have patient returned to usual dosage of anticoagulant
7. Avoid aspirin and aspirin-containing compounds

Possible liver disease

A patient with a history of jaundice or heavy alcohol use may have significant liver disease. Most of the coagulation factors are produced in the liver; therefore, if enough liver damage has occurred, the patient could have a serious bleeding problem because of a defect in the coagulation phase. In addition, about 50% of patients with significant liver disease will have a defect in the platelet phase as a result of platelet destruction by the spleen. Alcohol also can have a direct effect on hemostasis by interfering with platelet function. The PT test can be used to screen for a defect in the coagulation phase in patients with a history that indicates liver disease. A bleeding time also should be obtained to see if the platelet phase has been affected. It is possible that the amount of liver damage would not be great enough to affect the coagulation phase, but the effect on the platelet phase could be severe enough to lead to a serious bleeding problem. If both the PT and the bleeding time are normal, surgery can be performed on these patients with little risk of a postoperative bleeding problem.

Chronic leukemia

Patients with chronic leukemia should have their platelet status checked before they undergo dental surgery. A bleeding time should be performed on the day of surgery, and if abnormal results are obtained, surgery should be postponed if possible. If the surgery must be done, platelet replacement will have to be considered before the procedure. The patient's physician must be involved with this evaluation and preparation.

Malabsorption syndrome or long-term antibiotic therapy

In patients with malabsorption syndrome or patients receiving long-term antibiotic therapy, the bacteria in the intestine that produce vitamin K may be adversely affected. Vitamin K is needed by the liver for the production of prothrombin. The PT test can be ordered to screen for a possible bleeding problem; and if it is normal, surgery can be performed on these patients without risk of a bleeding problem. The patient's physician should be consulted regarding the patient's health status before surgery, because there may be complicating factors in addition to the possible bleeding problem that would contraindicate surgery.

Renal dialysis (heparin)

During hemodialysis the patient is usually given heparin, a short-acting anticoagulant. Heparin has a half-life of 4 hours; therefore its effects may be variable for up to 24 hours after administration. If such a patient reports for dental care on the day of hemodialysis treatment, the appointment should be postponed until the following day to be certain that the effect of heparin has worn off.

Vascular wall alteration

Some patients with autoimmune disease may have alterations of the vessel wall that result in excessive bleeding following surgical procedures. The BT (Ivy) test can be used to identify the presence of significant vascular wall changes in these patients.

MANAGEMENT OF THE PATIENT WITH A SERIOUS BLEEDING PROBLEM

Before any dental treatment is performed for a patient with a bleeding disorder, the dentist must consult with the patient's physician to determine the severity of the disorder and the need for special preparations for dental treatment. Patients with significant bleeding disorders are at increased risk for spontaneous gingival bleeding or excessive bleeding following minor trauma to the oral tissues. They can be at even greater risk if surgical procedures are performed without special preparations. Good oral hygiene is a must for these patients. Care should be taken in the placement of intraoral radiographic films to avoid trauma to the oral tissues. In general, block anesthesia and intramuscular injections must be avoided unless appropriate replacement factors have been used.[7,18,31]

Infiltration anesthesia can usually be given without replacement therapy. Simple restorative procedures can often be performed without replacement therapy as well as endodontic treatment of nonvital teeth. However, overinstrumentation and overfilling must be avoided. Complex restorative procedures when performed usually will require replacement therapy. Orthodontic treatment can be considered, but care must be taken with the placement of bands and arch wires.[7,18]

Conservative periodontal procedures—including polishing with a prophy cup and supragingival calculus removal—can often be done without replacement therapy. In children, primary teeth should be removed soon after they become loose. Local bleeding control can usually be obtained by use of pressure, thrombin, or microfibrillar collagen. If bleeding continues, topical AHF (Factor VIII) can be applied to the "wounds."[7,18,31]

THROMBOCYTOPENIA

Patients found to have severe thrombocytopenia or a severe coagulation disorder will most often require hospitalization and special preparation for surgery. A hematologist should be involved with the diagnosis, presurgical evaluation, preparation, and postsurgical management of these patients.

Surgical treatment (including extractions) requires special preparation. For patients with thrombocytopenia the platelet count should be at least 50,000/mm³ before surgery is attempted. Continuous transfusion of platelets may be required, or a single preoperative platelet transfusion can be given 30 minutes prior to the dental surgery. All bleeding sites should be packed with microfibrillar collagen and EACA (100 mg/kg orally) given just before surgery and then continued for 8 days (50 mg/kg every 6 hours, orally).[7,28,29]

In children with idiopathic thrombocytopenia, prednisone (4 mg/kg per day for 1 week, orally) or IV gamma globulin (1 g/kg per day in two doses) will increase the platelet count to over 50,000/mm³ within 48 hours in about 90% of the cases.[18] In patients whose platelet count increases, the needed surgical procedures can be performed (Table 22-21).

HEMOPHILIA

The patient with hemophilia (Factor VIII deficiency) can be used to illustrate some of the management problems involved in dealing with a serious coagulation disorder. Consultation with a hematologist is necessary. The hematologist first establishes the diagnosis and determines the degree of Factor VIII deficiency and whether any Factor VIII inhibitors are present. The type of replacement material is selected (Table 22-14) and the dosage of the replacement material determined.[7,17,21]

Extractions have been performed for patients

TABLE 22-21
Medical Treatment for the Patient With Idiopathic Thrombocytopenic Purpura

---

1. None indicated unless platelet count less than 20,000/mm³ or there is extensive bleeding
2. High doses of steroids
3. IV gamma globulin
4. Elective splenectomy for steroid nonresponders
5. Azathioprine, cyclophosphamide, vincristine, or vinblastine
6. Danazol (Androgen)

---

with a mild deficiency of Factor VIII using only DDAVP and EACA, and postoperative bleeding problems have been few[8]; also, tranexamic acid has been used.[24] In patients with mild hemophilia without inhibitors, DDAVP can be given by IV infusion at a dose of 4 to 5 mg/kg in 50 ml of isotonic saline over 15 minutes just prior to surgery. EACA (epsilon-aminocaproic acid) should also be given to prevent fibrinolysis.[7,9,18] Patients with moderate Factor VIII deficiency and no inhibitors can be given a single dose of Factor VIII concentrate 10 to 30 minutes before the procedure. Factor VIII has a half-life of 8 to 12 hours. EACA also is given orally (100 mg/kg) every 6 hours for 3 to 5 days. If bleeding occurs after the first 8 to 12 hours, additional infusions of Factor VIII will be needed. If the risk for postoperative infection is increased due to local or systemic factors, prophylactic antibiotics should be given.[18,29]

Patients with more severe deficiencies of Factor VIII without Factor VIII inhibitors can receive most oral surgical procedures if proper Factor VIII replacement is effectively achieved. Even patients with stable levels of Factor VIII inhibitors can have oral surgery performed if large doses of Factor VIII replacement are used. However, patients with inducible Factor VIII inhibitors still present great problems and are at high risk for serious bleeding if surgery is attempted. Elective surgery is not recommended for these patients. Periodontal surgery is not suggested, and extractions are performed only when no alternate treatment is available. Both nonactivated and activated prothrombin-complex concentrates with EACA have been tried in patients with high titers of Factor VIII inhibitors, but success has been limited.[25] Porcine Factor VIII concentrate has been used, with some success.[10,20] Cortisone has also been tried in patients with inducible inhibitors to interfere with their action. Plasmapheresis may clear the blood of inhibitors for a short time.[19,32,22]

Splints can be made by the dentist before surgery so mechanical displacement of the clot in wounds healing by secondary intention is prevented. All extraction sites should be packed with microfibrillar collagen and the wound closed with absorbable sutures for primary healing whenever possible. Electrosurgery should not be used in these patients. Endodontic procedures should be done rather than extractions whenever possible since the risk for serious bleeding is less.[19,30-32]

The administration of local anesthetics is a major concern in dental treatment for the patient with hemophilia. Hematomas, airway obstruction, and death have occurred as complications of block anesthesia in these individuals. Block injections or intramuscular injections should not be given unless the patient has a plasma Factor VIII level of 50% or greater, and patients with severe hemophilia (2% or less of Factor VIII) must be given replacement therapy before any local anesthetic is administered[7] (Table 22-22).

In many cases the patient must be hospitalized for surgical procedures. This decision should be made in consultation with the patient's hematologist. Patients with a mild to moderate form of hemophilia without inhibitors can be managed on an outpatient basis using replacement therapy or DDAVP (l-desamino-8-D arginine vasopressin) and EACA or tranexamic acid. When replacement therapy is used, the dentist and hematologist must observe the patient for any signs of allergic reaction and be prepared to take appropriate action.

VON WILLEBRAND'S DISEASE

Surgical procedures can be performed in patients with mild von Willebrand's disease (type I and some type II variants) by using DDAVP and EACA. Patients with more severe types of von Willebrand's disease will require fresh frozen plasma or cryoprecipitate replacement for vWF and Factor VIII. As stated earlier, the Factor VIII concentrates do not contain active vWF and are ineffective in correcting the basic deficiency (Table 22-15).

TREATMENT PLANNING MODIFICATIONS

With proper preparation, most indicated dental treatment can be provided for patients with various bleeding problems. Patients with congenital coagulation defects must be encouraged to improve and maintain good oral health, because most dental treatment for these patients at present is complicated by the need for replacement of the missing factor. Dental treatment often requires hospitalization. Patients with bleeding problems secondary to diseases that may be in the terminal phase should, in general, be offered only conservative dental treatment. Aspirin should not be used for pain relief in patients who have known bleeding disorders or who are receiving anticoagulant medication. This includes the various compounds that contain aspirin—such as Anacin, Synalgos-DC, Fiorinal, Bufferin, Alka-Seltzer, Empirin with Codeine, and Excedrin.

ORAL COMPLICATIONS

Patients with bleeding disorders may complain of spontaneous gingival bleeding. Oral tissues may show petechiae, ecchymoses, jaundice, pallor, and ulcers. Spontaneous gingival bleeding and petechiae are usually found in patients with thrombocytopenia. Hemarthrosis of the TMJ is a rare finding in patients with coagulation disorders and is not found in

TABLE 22-22
Dental Management of the Patient With Hemophilia

1. Detection and referral
2. Consultation with hematologist regarding
   a. Diagnosis
   b. Level of Factor VIII deficiency
   c. Presence of Factor VIII inhibitors
   d. Selection of replacement factor
   e. Dosage of replacement factor
   f. Need for epsilon-aminocaproic acid (EACA) (or tranexamic acid) for clot maintenance
   g. Need for steroids to interfere with action of inhibitors
   h. Hospitalization for surgical procedures
3. Construction of splints if multiple extractions or flap procedures are planned
4. Patient should be free of active infection
5. Use of good surgical techniques and sutures for closure whenever possible (at extraction site); packing of extraction sockets with microfibrillar collagen
6. Use of local measures to assist in control of excessive bleeding
   a. Splints
   b. Microfibrillar collagen
   c. Gelfoam with thrombin
7. Prophylactic antibiotics to prevent postoperative infection
8. Avoid aspirin and aspirin-containing compounds

patients with thrombocytopenia. Individuals with leukemia may reveal a generalized hyperplasia of the gingiva. Patients with neoplastic disease may show osseous lesions on radiographs, oral ulcers, or tumors. These patients may also have drifting and loosening of teeth and may complain of paresthesias (e.g., burning of the tongue, numbness of the lip).[19,26,30]

REFERENCES

1. Babior BM, Stossel TP, editors: *Hematology: a pathophysiological approach,* New York, 1984, Churchill Livingstone.
2. Barber A, Green D, Galluzzo T, Ts'ao CH: The bleeding time as a preoperative screening test, *Am J Med* 78:761-765, 1985.
3. Benoliel R: Dental treatment for the patient on anticoagulant therapy: prothrombin time—what difference does it make? *Oral Surg* 62:149-151, 1986.
4. Capitanio AM, Sacco R, Mannucci PM: Pseudopathologies of hemostasis and dental surgery, *Oral Surg* 71:184-186, 1991.
5. Catalano PM: Hemostatic disorders. In Rose LF, Kaye D, editors: *Internal medicine for dentistry,* ed 2, St Louis, 1990, CV Mosby, pp 346-360.
6. Cohen SG, Glick M: Dental correlations, platelet and vascular disorders. In Rose LF, Kaye D, editors: *Internal medicine for dentistry,* ed 2, St Louis, 1990, CV Mosby, pp 369-371.
7. Cohen SG, Glick M: Dental correlations, factor defiencies. In Rose LF, Kaye D, editors: *Internal medicine for dentistry,* ed 2, St Louis, 1990, CV Mosby, pp 371-374.
8. Eastman JR, Nawakowski AR, Triplett MD: DDAVP: a review of indications for its use in treatment of factor VIII deficiency and a report of a case, *Oral Surg* 56:246-250, 1983.
9. Ghirardini A, Chistolini A, Tirindelli MC, et al: Clinical evaluation of subcutaneously administered DDAVP, *Thromb Res* 49(3):363-372, 1988.
10. Handin RI: Clotting disorders. In Wilson JD, et al, editors: *Harrison's Principles of internal medicine,* ed 12, New York, 1991, McGraw-Hill, pp 1500-1511.
11. Harmening DM: Introduction to hemostasis—an overview of hemostatic mechanism, platelet structure and function, and extrinsic and intrinsic systems. In Harmening DM, editor: *Clinical hematology and fundamentals of hemostasis,* ed 2, Philadelphia, 1992, FA Davis, pp 415-439.
12. Kahn RA, Allen RW, Baldassare J: Alternate sources and substitutes for therapeutic blood components, *Blood* 66:1-12, 1985.
13. Kasper CK, Boylen AL, Ewing NP, et al: Hematologic management of hemophilia A for surgery, *JAMA* 253:1279-1283, 1985.
14. Kelly MA: Common laboratory tests: Their use in the detection and management of patients with bleeding disorders, *Gen Dent* 38(4):282-285, 1990.
15. Kitchens CS: Surgery in hemophilia and related disorders, *J Med* 65:34-45, 1986.
16. Kreiss JK, Kitchen LW, Prince HE, et al: Antibody to human T-lymphotrophic virus type III in wives of hemophiliacs, *Ann Intern Med* 102:623-626, 1985.
17. Lucas DN, Albert TW: Epsilon amino caproic acid in hemophiliacs: a concise review, *Oral Surg* 51:115-120, 1981.
18. Luke KH: Comprehensive care for children with bleeding disorders: physicians perspective, *J Can Dent Assoc* 58(2):115-118, 1992.
19. Lynch MA: Hematologic diseases and related problems. In Lynch MA, editor: *Burket's Oral medicine diagnosis and treatment,* ed 7, Philadelphia, 1977, JB Lippincott.
20. McGlasson DL: Defects of plasma clotting factors. In Harmening DM, editor: *Clinical hematology and fundamentals of hemostasis,* ed 2, Philadelphia, 1992, FA Davis, pp 462-486.
21. Nossel HL: Bleeding. In Petersdorf RG, et al, editors: *Harrison's Principles of internal medicine,* ed 10, New York, 1983, McGraw-Hill.
22. Perkin NA: Transfusion-associated AIDS, *Am J Hematol* 19:307-313, 1985.
23. Ragni MV, Tegtmeier GE, Levy JA, et al: AIDS retrovirus antibodies in hemophiliacs treated with Factor VIII or Factor IX concentrates, cryoprecipitate, or fresh frozen plasma, *Blood* 67:592-595, 1986.
24. Recent drug approvals. Tranexamic acid. *FDA Drug Bull* 17(1):9, 1987.
25. Redding SW, Stiegler KE: Dental management of the classic hemophiliac with inhibitors, *Oral Surg* 56:145-148, 1983.
26. Rodeghiero F, Castaman G, Di Bona E, et al: Hyperresponsiveness to DDAVP for patients with type I von Willebrand's disease and normal intra-platelet von Willebrand factor, *Eur J Haematol* 40(2):163-167, 1988.
27. Shafer WG, Hine MK, Levy BM: *A textbook of oral pathology,* ed 4, Philadelphia, 1983, WB Saunders.
28. Sindet-Pedersen S: Haemostasis in oral surgery, *Dan Med Bull* 38(6):427-443, 1991.
29. Speirs RL: Haemostasis, *Dent Update* 18(4):166-171, 1991.
30. Stajcic Z, Baklaja R, Elezovic I, Bolovic Z: Primary wound closure in hemophiliacs undergoing dental extractions, *Int J Oral Maxillofac Surg* 18(1):14-16, 1989.
31. Ublansky JH: Comprehensive dental care for children with bleeding disorders, *J Can Dent Assoc* 58(2):111-114, 1992.
32. Wintrobe MM, Lee GR, Boggs DR, et al: *Clinical hematology,* ed 8, Philadelphia, 1981, Lea & Febiger.
33. Zieve PD: Bleeding disorders. In Harvey A, et al, editors: *The principles and practice of medicine,* ed 19, New York, 1976, Appleton-Century-Crofts.

23

Blood Dyscrasias

The purpose of this chapter is to present the most common disorders of the white and red blood cells that may influence dental treatment (Table 23-1). The dentist should be able to detect patients with these diseases by history, clinical examination, and screening laboratory tests. Patients with disorders of the white or red blood cells may be susceptible to abnormal bleeding, delayed healing, infection, or mucosal ulceration. In addition, some of these diseases can be fatal; thus they must be detected and affected patients referred to a physician for diagnosis and treatment before any dental procedure is performed. Patients with known disorders who are under medical care should

TABLE 23-1
Classification of Blood Dyscrasias

1. Red blood cell disorders
   a. Anemia
   b. Polycythemia
2. White blood cell disorders
   a. Leukocytosis
   b. Leukopenia
   c. Myeloproliferative disorders
      (1) Acute myeloid leukemia (AML)
      (2) Chronic myeloid leukemia (CML)
   d. Lymphoproliferative disorders
      (1) Acute lymphoblastic leukemia (ALL)
      (2) Chronic lymphocytic leukemia (CLL)
      (3) Lymphomas
         (a) Hodgkin's disease
         (b) Non-Hodgkin's disease
         (c) Burkitt's lymphoma
      (4) Multiple myeloma

have no dental care until consultation with the physician is obtained.

Anemia

GENERAL DESCRIPTION

Anemia is defined as a reduction in the oxygen-carrying capacity of the blood and is usually related to a decrease in the number of circulating red blood cells or to an abnormality in the hemoglobin contained within the red blood cells. Anemia is not a disease but rather a symptom complex that may result from iron deficiency, decreased production of red blood cells, or increased rate of destruction of circulating red blood cells.

About 1% of the circulating erythrocyte mass is generated by the bone marrow each day. The normal reticulocyte count (immature red blood cell) is 1% of the total red cell count. The normal red cell is about 33% hemoglobin. The need for oxygen serves as the stimulus for erythropoiesis. This occurs through the kidney, which releases erythropoietin; erythropoietin then stimulates the bone marrow to release red blood cells. About 95% of erythropoietin is produced by cortical cells in the kidney. The other 5% is produced by the liver. The liver secretion of erythropoietin increases with hypoxia.[3]

Excessive blood loss from menses or bleeding from the gastrointestinal tract can lead to iron deficiency anemia. Individuals with gastrectomy or malabsorption syndrome may have reduced absorption of iron from the gastrointestinal tract, which can result in anemia. Children and pregnant women may have an inadequate dietary intake of iron, which also can lead to anemia.

Factors that reduce the capacity of the bone marrow to produce red blood cells will cause anemia. Patients with gastric changes that result in the failure to produce enough intrinsic factor for absorption of vitamin B_{12} (cobalamin) will be unable to produce adequate numbers of red blood cells and will become anemic. Leukemia and metastatic tumors to bone can lead to replacement of the red blood cell precursors in the bone marrow and result in decreased production of red blood cells. The bone marrow cells may be destroyed by radiation or by the effects of drugs or chemicals, resulting in decreased production of red blood cells as well as white blood cells and platelets. The bone marrow may be functioning normally, but the red blood cells may be destroyed at an increased rate once in circulation because of the effects of toxins, transfusion reactions, hyperactivity of the spleen, or defectively constructed red blood cells. The increased rate of destruction of red blood cells can lead to anemia. This form of anemia is termed *hemolytic anemia.* The hemolytic anemias can be due to extracorpuscular or intracorpuscular defects. Two diseases caused by intracorpuscular defects — glucose-6-phosphate deficiency and sickle cell anemia — will be described in this chapter to demonstrate the problems presented by the hemolytic anemias.[5]

All the various causes of anemia are not covered in detail in this chapter. Examples have been selected to demonstrate the clinical problems involved in the management of patients with anemia.

MENSES AND PREGNANCY

It is common for women who are menstruating or pregnant to develop a mild iron deficiency anemia. The repeated loss of blood associated with menses can lead to depletion of iron and result in a mild state of anemia. On occasion when taking a history from a female patient, it may be appropriate for the dentist to ask if she is having periods, when the periods first started, if they have been regular, the number of days involved, and the number of pads used. Patients with a history of regular periods but with heavy flow may be anemic and should receive medical advice and treatment. A patient with a change in the pattern, onset, length, or rate of flow of her periods should be encouraged to seek medical evaluation. Patients who have stopped having periods long before expected should be referred for medical evaluation, as should those who have had bleeding in between regular periods.

During pregnancy there is an increased demand on the expectant mother for additional iron and vitamins to support the growth of her fetus; and unless sufficient amounts of these nutrients have been provided in some form, she may become anemic. In fact, approximately 20% of pregnant women have iron deficiency anemia. In obtaining the health history, the dentist should establish if the patient has other children and when they were born, because the closer together the pregnancies were the greater will be the chances for the patient to have developed iron deficiency anemia. Once the baby is born, the mother may lose additional iron if she breast-feeds her baby.

By contrast, mild anemia in men usually indicates the presence of a serious underlying medical problem. Under normal conditions men lose little iron, and iron deficiency anemia on a physiologic basis is rare; therefore any man found to be anemic must be referred for medical evaluation.

PERNICIOUS ANEMIA

Vitamin B_{12} (cobalamin) and folic acid are needed for the maturation of red blood cells in the bone marrow. A deficiency in the daily intake or absorption of these vitamins can result in anemia. Pernicious anemia is due to a deficiency of intrinsic factor, the substance secreted by the parietal cells of the stomach that is necessary for the absorption of vitamin B_{12}, which is needed for the maturation of red blood cells.

Pernicious anemia is usually a disease of late adult life. It most often occurs in 40-to-70-year-old northern Europeans of fair complexion, with one notable exception. An early onset in black American women, 21% of whom were under the age of 40, has been observed.[3] Most patients with pernicious anemia have chronic atrophic gastritis with decreased intrinsic factor and HCl secretion. Fifty to seventy percent of the patients also have binding or blocking intrinsic factor antibodies in their serum. This finding would suggest that the disease may be related to an autoimmune process.

Patients with pernicious anemia are at increased risk for gastric carcinoma, myxedema, or rheumatoid arthritis.[3] Early symptoms include weakness, fatigue, palpitations, syncope, tingling of the fingers and toes (paresthesias), numbness, uncoordination, and muscular weakness. The Schilling test with radioactive cyanocobalamin is used to establish the diagnosis of pernicious anemia.[3] Early detection is important so treatment, which involves vitamin B_{12} injections, can be started before neurologic symptoms have progressed so far that they cannot be corrected. Folic acid will correct the anemia but will not stop the progression of neurologic symptoms. The vitamin B_{12} deficiency will still exist but be undetected, which is why federal regulations have stated that vitamins sold over the counter cannot contain a significant amount of folic acid.

A form of megaloblastic anemia similar to pernicious anemia has been reported[12] as a consequence of gastric bypass surgery.

GLUCOSE-6-PHOSPHATE DEHYDROGENASE DEFICIENCY

The search during World War II for a substitute quinine led to the discovery of glucose-6-phosphate deficiency. Since that time, the glucose metabolism of red blood cell has been established. Glucose enters the red blood cell by a carrier mechanism independent of insulin. About 90% of the glucose is metabolized by the glycolytic pathway. The remaining glucose is metabolized by the hexose monophosphate shunt pathway. The byproduct of the glycolytic pathway is ATP, which is used for the energy needs of the cell. The byproduct of the hexose monophosphate shunt pathway is NADPH, which is used to reduce various cellular oxidants.[5]

Glucose-6-phosphate dehydrogenase (G-6-PD) is an enzyme needed for the hexose monophosphate shunt pathway. There are over 350 G-6-PD variants. The G-6-PD gene is located on the X chromosome; thus the disease inheritance is sex-linked. G-6-PD A is the most common variant associated with hemolysis and is found in 11% of American blacks. G-6-PD

MED is the second most common variant associated with hemolysis, and it is found in ethnic groups of Mediterranean origin.[5]

Blockage of the hexose monophosphate shunt pathway in individuals with glucose-6-phosphate deficiency allows the accumulation of oxidants in the red blood cells. These substances, which produce methemoglobin and denatured hemoglobin, precipitate to form Heinz bodies; the Heinz bodies attach to cell membranes. Alteration of the cell membranes leads to hemolysis of the cell.[5]

The clinical features of glucose-6-phosphate deficiency involve acute intravascular hemolysis, which can be severe. Jaundice, palpitations, dyspnea, and dizziness may result. Infection is the most common event that triggers hemolysis in G-6-PD A deficiency. Drugs are the most common trigger for hemolysis in G-6-PD MED deficiency. Drugs that can lead to hemolysis include acetylsalicyclic acid, acetophenetidin (phenacetin), dapsone, ascorbic acid, and vitamin K.[5]

Screening tests for NADPH can be used to detect individuals with G-6-PD. More sensitive tests use direct spectrophotometric measurement of NADPH. Other tests used are the cyanide-ascorbate assay and the cytochemical estimation.[5]

SICKLE CELL ANEMIA

More than 400 human hemoglobin variants have been reported. Over 90% of these are single amino acid substitutions in the hemoglobin chain. Sickle cell hemoglobin (S) was the first hemoglobin variant to be recognized. Sickle cell hemoglobin results in the substitution of a single amino acid, valine, for glutamic acid at the sixth residue of the beta chain. Hemoglobin variants, including sickle cell anemia, are inherited as codominant traits.[7,19]

Sickle cell trait is the heterozygous state in which the affected individual carries one gene for hemoglobin S. It is estimated that 8% to 10% of American blacks carry the trait. In central Africa up to 25% of the population may carry it. Sickling crises are rare in individuals with sickle cell trait.[7] Sickle cell anemia is the homozygous state. A gene from each parent contributes to formation of the hemoglobin S molecule responsible for the disease. The red blood cell with hemoglobin S becomes sickle-shaped when blood has a lowered oxygen tension or increased pH or becomes dehydrated.[17,19,26]

Distortion of the red blood cell into a sickled shape is the result of low oxygen tension or increased blood pH, causing partial crystallization of Hb S and realignment of the defective hemoglobin molecule. Cellular rigidity and membrane damage occur, with irreversible sickling the final result. The net effect of these changes is erythrostasis, increased blood viscosity, reduced blood flow, hypoxia, increased adhesion of red blood cells, vascular occlusion, and further sickling.[7,26]

In patients with sickle cell anemia over 80% of the hemoglobin is Hb S. About 0.003% to 0.15% of the black population in America has sickle cell anemia.[7,18,26,28] Fifty percent of those individuals with sickle cell anemia die before the age of 20, and most of the others before the age of 40. Clinical signs and symptoms of sickle cell anemia include jaundice, pallor, cardiac failure, leg ulcers, stroke, and attacks of abdominal and bone pain (Table 23-2). Aplastic crises — in which the patient becomes acutely ill, the production of red cells stops, and severe anemia occurs — may develop from infection, hypersensitivity reactions, hypoxia, systemic disease, acidosis, dehydration, or trauma. Folic acid deficiency may play a role in the cause of the crises,

TABLE 23-2
Signs and Symptoms in the Patient with Anemia

Symptoms

Weakness
Fatigue
Palpitations
Tingling of fingers and toes
Numbness of fingers and toes
Burning of tongue, oral tissues
Bone pain
Shortness of breath

Signs

Pallor
Spooning of nails
Brittle nails
Loss of filiform papillae (smooth red tongue)
Cracking and splitting of nails

---

and for this reason folic acid dietary supplements are given to most patients with sickle cell anemia. New therapeutic strategies are now being tested. One approach is to induce the production of hemoglobin F. Hydroxyurea and erythropoietin are being tested in combination to induce F reticulocytes.[7] Once a crisis develops, high doses of folic acid, analgesia for pain, and hydration are used to treat the patient.[7]

Dental findings in patients with a history of sickle cell anemia include pallor of the oral mucous membranes, delayed eruption of teeth, and hypoplasia of enamel. Dental radiographs may show a loss of the bony trabecular pattern, with decreased radiodensity of the jaws reflecting the increased size of marrow spaces and the loss of fine bone structure from erythroblastic hyperplasia. Some patients may complain of pain in the mandible followed by paresthesias of the mental nerve during acute crises.[12]

Most blacks with sickle cell anemia are aware of their problem. The dentist must ask all blacks in the health history if they have sickle cell anemia.

Sickle cell trait is the heterozygous form of sickle cell disorder, wherein only one parent contributes a gene to Hb S. These individuals have no symptoms unless they are placed in situations in which abnormally low concentrations of oxygen are present (e.g., in an unpressurized airplane or through the injudicious administration of general anesthesia). Patients with sickle cell trait are much more resistant to sickling stimuli because only 20% to 45% of their hemoglobin is Hb S. Patients with sickle cell trait are not at risk during dental treatment unless severe hypoxia or dehydration occurs.[7,18,26,28]

RENAL DISEASE

The kidney produces the hormone erythropoietin, which stimulates red blood cell production by the bone marrow. If there is significant renal damage, the lack of production of this hormone will result in anemia. (See Chapter 11.)

CLINICAL PRESENTATION
SIGNS AND SYMPTOMS

Symptoms of anemia include fatigue, palpitations, shortness of breath, abdominal pain, bone pain, tingling of fingers and toes, and muscular weakness. Signs of anemia may include jaundice, pallor, cracking and splitting of the fingernails, increased size of the liver and spleen, lymphadenopathy, and blood in the stool. Patients with anemia may complain of a sore or painful tongue, smooth tongue, or redness of the tongue. Some patients may complain of a loss of taste sensation (Table 23-2).

SCREENING LABORATORY TESTS

If the dentist identifies a patient with signs or symptoms that suggest anemia, this patient should be sent to a commercial laboratory for screening tests or referred to a physician for evaluation. The hemoglobin level and hematorocrit are the tests used to screen the patient; in addition, a total white blood cell count and platelet count should be obtained (Chapter 1).

Black patients can be screened for the sickle cell trait by use of the *Sickledex Test* (distributed by Johnson & Johnson).[25] This is a simple test that uses a small amount of blood, and it can be performed in the dental office.

All blacks should be questioned about the presence of sickle cell disease in their family. If there is no history of an individual having been screened for sickle cell disease, the dentist should arrange for the patient to be tested. This can be done in the dental office using the Sickledex Test, in a commercial clinical laboratory, or by a physician.

White blood cell disorders

GENERAL DESCRIPTION

Three groups of white blood cells are found in the peripheral circulation: granulocytes, lymphocytes, and monocytes. There are three types of granulocytes—neutrophils, eosinophils, and basophils. Circulating lymphocytes are also of three types—thymus mediated (T lymphocytes), those originating from lymphoid tissue in association with the gastrointestinal tract (B lymphocytes), and null lymphocytes.

The primary function of neutrophils is to defend the body against certain infectious agents by phagocytosis and enzymatic destruction. The eosinophils and basophils are involved with inflammatory allergic reactions. The thymus-mediated lymphocytes (T cells) are involved with the delayed, or cellular, immune reaction whereas the B lymphocytes (B cells) play an important role in the immediate, or humoral, immune system. The monocytes serve as phagocytes and appear to be involved in some way with the immune response. (See Chapter 21.)

The majority of white blood cells are produced primarily in the bone marrow (granulocytes and monocytes [Chapter 1]), and there are several "pools" of these cells in the marrow: (1) the mitotic pool, which consists of immature precursor cells; (2) a maturing pool, which consists of cells that are undergoing maturation; and (3) a storage pool of functional cells, which can be released as needed.

The white blood cells released by the bone marrow that are found circulating in the peripheral blood form two pools of cells, a marginal one and a circulating one. Cells in the marginal pool adhere to vessel walls and are readily available. When infection threatens the body, the storage and marginal pools can be called on to help fight the invading organisms.

Growth-promoting substances called colony-stimulating factors (CSFs) are responsible for the growth of committed granulocyte-monocyte stem cells. The major function of CSFs seems to be to amplify leukopoiesis rather than recruit new stem cells into the granulocyte-monocyte differentiation pathway. Thus, by the local release of CSFs, the bone marrow can increase the production of granulocytes and monocytes. This process occurs as a response to infection.[23]

LEUKOCYTOSIS AND LEUKOPENIA

The number of circulating white blood cells is expressed as the number of cells found in a cubic millimeter of blood, which normally ranges from 4500 to $11,000/mm^3$ in adults.[28] The differential white cell count is an estimation of the percentage of each cell type per cubic millimeter of blood. A normal differential count would be as follows: neutrophils, 50% to 60%; eosinophils, 3%; basophils, less than 1%; lymphocytes, 20% to 30%; and monocytes, 3% to 7%. The term *leukocytosis* is defined[28] as an increase in the number of circulating white blood cells to more than $11,000/mm^3$, and *leukopenia* as a reduction in the number of circulating white cells (usually to less than $4500/mm^3$).

There are many causes of leukocytosis. Exercise, pregnancy, and emotional stress can lead to increased numbers of white blood cells in the peripheral circulation. Leukocytosis resulting from these causes is called physiologic leukocytosis. Pathologic leukocytosis can be caused by infections, neoplasia, and necrosis. Pyogenic infections induce a type of leukocytosis characterized by an increased number of neutrophils. If excessive numbers of immature neutrophils (stab cells) are released into the circulation in response to a bacterial infection, a shift to the left is said to have occurred. Viral infections often produce a type of leukocytosis characterized by increased numbers of lymphocytes. Tuberculosis and syphilis also primarily cause a lymphocytosis. Protozoan infections often produce a type of leukocytosis that appears as an increase in the numbers of monocytes. Allergies and infections caused by certain helminths usually result in a leukocytosis caused primarily by an increase in the number of circulating eosinophils. Cellular necrosis will result in a type of leukocytosis brought about by increased numbers of circulating neutrophils. Leukemia (cancer of the white blood cells) usually is characterized by a great increase in the numbers of circulating leukocytes. Carcinomas of glandular tissues may cause an increase in the number of circulating neutrophils. Acute bleeding also can result in a leukocytosis (Table 23-3).

There are also many causes of deficient numbers of leukocytes (less than 4500/mm³) in the blood. A leukopenia may occur in the early phase of leukemia and lymphoma and can be found in both agranulocytosis (reduction and granulocytes) and pancytopenia (decrease in white and red blood cells).[25] An important form of leukopenia involves the cyclic depression of circulating neutrophils—a disorder called cyclic neutropenia, in which patients have a periodic decrease in the number of neutrophils (about every 28 days). During the period in which few circulating neutrophils are present, the patient is susceptible to infection.[18,24] These patients often show progressive forms of periodontal disease and may develop recurrent oral ulcers. A patient with severe leukopenia is susceptible to infection (Table 23-3). Many patients with leukocytosis or leukopenia can manifest thrombocytopenia from direct or indirect effects on platelet precursor cells in the bone marrow. Toxic effects are from drugs, chemicals, or

TABLE 23-3
Causes of Leukocytosis and Leukopenia

1. Leukocytosis
   a. Physiologic
      (1) Exercise
      (2) Pregnancy
      (3) Emotional stress
   b. Pathologic
      (1) Infection
      (2) Allergies
      (3) Necrosis
      (4) Leukemia
      (5) Acute blood loss
2. Leukopenia
   a. Early phase of leukemia and lymphoma
   b. Agranulocytes (reaction to drugs, chemicals)
   c. Cyclic neutropenia
   d. Radiation
   e. Metastatic tumor to bone

replacement by excessive proliferation of white blood cells and red blood cells.

INFECTIOUS MONONUCLEOSIS

Infectious mononucleosis is a viral infection that results in a marked lymphocytic response. It is caused by the Epstein-Barr virus, which is a lymphotropic herpesvirus. Large reactive lymphocytes are found in normal blood smears, representing about 1% to 2% of the cells. In infectious mononucleosis they constitute at least 10% of the cells. The reactive lymphocytes are not the Epstein-Barr (EBV)–infected B lymphocytes but are T lymphocytes reacting to the infection.[6] The classic disease description includes clinical symptoms of fever, sore throat, and cervical lymph node enlargement, with an absolute lymphocytosis (greater than 10% reactive lymphocytes) and a positive heterophil antibody test.[6] Patients with a negative heterophil antibody test should be retested in 7 to 10 days. If the second test is negative, then tests for EBV-IgM antibody should be performed. If these tests are positive, the patient has heterophil-negative infectious mononucleosis.[6] A few patients with the classic disease description may be heterophil antibody–negative and EBV-IgM–negative. For these patients tests for CMV (cytomegalovirus)-IgM should be performed, and if these tests are positive the patient has CMV mononucleosis. If these tests are negative, then toxoplasma titer and viral cultures should be performed.[6] Infectious mononucleosis is usually asymptomatic when found in children; however, when young adults are affected, about 50% will be symptomatic. The virus is transmitted via the oropharyngeal route during close personal contact and has an incubation time of 30 to 50 days. A prodromal period of 3 to 5 days precedes the clinical phase, which lasts 7 to 20 days. About 10% to 20% of asymptomatic, seropositive adults (antibodies to the Epstein-Barr virus) carry the virus in their oropharyngeal region.[21]

During the prodromal period the patient may complain of headache, malaise, myalgia, and fatigue; by contrast, the clinical phase consists of fever, sore throat, and cervical lymphadenopathy.

About a third of the patients will develop palatal petechiae during the first week of the illness, and about 10% will have a generalized skin rash. Laboratory studies reveal a reactive lymphocytosis, heterophil antibodies, and antibodies to the Epstein-Barr virus. Many of these clinical findings can be confused with the symptoms of leukemia; hence the importance of the laboratory tests.[21]

Treatment of infectious mononucleosis is symptomatic and consists of bed rest, salicylates for pain control, and gargling and irrigation with saline solution to provide symptomatic relief of pharyngitis and stomatitis. In some patients with severe toxic exudative pharyngotonsillitis and pharyngeal edema, a short course of prednisone may be given. About 20% of the patients with symptomatic infectious mononucleosis will have concurrent beta-hemolytic streptococcal pharyngotonsillitis and should be treated with 500 mg of penicillin V four times a day for 10 days if they are not allergic to penicillin. Ampicillin should be avoided because of the high incidence of skin rash in patients with infectious mononucleosis treated with this drug.[21]

Patients with infectious mononucleosis may come to the dentist because of oral signs and symptoms. Patients with clinical findings of fever, sore throat, petechiae, and cervical lymphadenopathy must be evaluated to establish a diagnosis of their condition. Screening clinical laboratory tests can be ordered by the dentist (complete blood count [CBC], heterophil [monospot or monosticon] antibody test, and EBV-IgM antibody test), or the patient can be referred to a physician for evaluation and treatment.[6,21]

LEUKEMIA AND LYMPHOMA

Leukemia is cancer of the white blood cells. It can involve myeloid or lymphoid cell proliferation and occurs in both an acute and a chronic form. Six types of leukemia will be described in this section: acute lymphocytic, acute myeloid, chronic lymphocytic, chronic myeloid, hairy cell, and acute T-cell leukemia. Lymphoma is cancer of the lymphoid organs, although it can be found in extranodal locations. Three types of lymphoma will be described in this section: Hodgkin's disease, non-Hodgkin's lymphoma, and Burkitt's lymphoma. These diseases are of importance to the dentist because often the initial signs occur in the mouth and in the head and neck region, and precautions must be taken before any dental treatment is provided.

Leukemia and lymphoma account for about 8% of all new malignancies each year in the United States, which amounts to approximately 65,000 cases per year.[24] These patients are usually immunosuppressed because of the disese itself or secondary to the treatment used to control it; hence they are prone to develop serious infections and often are bleeders.

Leukemia

Leukemia can occur in all races and at any age. There are some 27,000 new cases per year in the United States.[23,25] About 50% of all leukemia is the acute form. Acute lymphocytic leukemia is the type most commonly found in children. Chronic lymphocytic leukemia is the most common type in adults.[23,25] Table 23-4 lists some of the terms used to describe acute or chronic leukemia. The cause is unknown; however, an increased risk is found to be associated with large doses of ionizing radiation, certain chemicals, and a few viruses.[25] Table 23-5 lists the various factors that have been implicated in the etiology of human leukemias. There are acute and chronic forms of leukemia based on the degree of maturation of cells and survival time of the patient. Hemorrhage and infection are the chief causes of death.

TABLE 23-4
Leukemia Terminology

Term	Abbreviation	Definition
Acute leukemia	AL	Rapid onset
Chronic leukemia	CL	Slow onset
Acute lymphocytic leukemia	ALL	Immature neoplastic lymphocytes
Acute myelogenous leukemia	AML	Immature neoplastic myeloid cells
Chronic lymphocytic leukemia	CLL	Mature neoplastic lymphocytes
Chronic myelogenous leukemia	CML	Mature neoplastic myeloid cells
Terminal deoxynucleotidyl transferase	Tdt	Nuclear enzyme found in leukemic lymphoblasts
Common acute lymphocytic leukemia antigen	CALLA	Found on surface of leukemic lymphoblasts
Multidrug-resistant phenotype	MDR	Expression of P-glycoprotein often associated with drug resistance

ACUTE LEUKEMIA

Acute leukemia has a sudden onset and will lead to death in 1 to 3 months if untreated. It consists of increased numbers of immature white blood cells in the peripheral circulation. There are two types of acute leukemia, acute lymphocytic (ALL) and acute myelogenous (AML).

The incidence of leukemia has remained somewhat stable in the United States since about 1956; and the mortality rate also has remained stable, at about 6.8 deaths per 100,000 population per year, with 50% to 60% of the deaths caused by acute leukemia. All types of leukemia are somewhat more common in males than females. The male/female ratio for acute leukemia is about 3:2, and for chronic leukemia about 2:1.

Symptoms of acute leukemia include fever, bleeding, pallor, weakness, recurrent infection, enlargement of tonsils, lymph nodes, spleen, and gingiva, oral ulcerations, and small hemorrhages of the skin and mucous membranes (Table 23-6). Patients with acute leukemia are susceptible to excessive bleeding, poor healing, and infection following dental surgical procedures.[11]

Acute lymphocytic leukemia (ALL) accounts for about 50% of all neoplasms in children. It is found most often in 2-to-4-year-old children. Seventy-five percent of the cases are in this age group, and 25% are in teenagers and adults.

ALL is classified based on the type and size of the lymphocytes found. The classification system consists of three groups: L-1 (small cells), L-2 (large cells), and L-3 (Burkitt type, large homogeneous B marker cells). Over 90% of the leukemic lymphoblasts in ALL contain a nuclear enzyme, terminal deoxynucleotidyl transferase (Tdt), which serves as a marker for this disease. Tdt can be found in leukemic lymphoblasts of AML but this is rare.[10] The leukemic cells in 60% of the patients with ALL, in addition to being Tdt-positive, have a common ALL antigen (CALLA) and no T cell antigens and they come from B cell lineage.[10] The leukemic cells in 20% of the patients with ALL are T cell types, Tdt-positive, and CALLA-negative. In 15% of the patients, leukemic lymphocytes are the null cell type and are negative for Tdt, CALLA, and T cell or B cell antigens. In less than 5% of the patients with ALL the cells are B cell–type lymphocytes.[10,23]

The prognosis for children with ALL is very good, with cures now being obtained in 50% to 70% of the cases. The prognosis is not good for adults with ALL, however (Table 23-6). Although a 50% to 70% remission rate can be achieved with current therapy, the duration of remission is short. The overall long-term survival (cure) rates for adults are less than 20%.[10,23]

Acute myelogenous leukemia (AML) accounts for over 85% of the cases in adults, with only about 15% occurring in children. Seven subtypes have been identified. They are M-1

TABLE 23-5
Etiology of the Leukemias

1. Host factors
   a. Heredity
      (1) Generally not inherited disease
      (2) High concordance among identical twins if one twin develops disease early
      (3) A few leukemic families have been reported
   b. Chromosome abnormalities — increased risk in
      (1) Down's syndrome
      (2) Turner's syndrome
      (3) Klinefelter's syndrome
      (4) Fanconi's anemia
   c. Immunodeficiency syndromes (hereditary types)
   d. Chronic bone marrow dysfunction
2. Environmental factors
   a. Ionizing radiation
      (1) Radiation therapy
      (2) Occupation exposure
      (3) Atomic bomb survivors
   b. Chemical and drugs
      (1) Benzene
      (2) Chloramphenicol
      (3) Phenylbutazone
      (4) Alkylating chemotherapeutic agents
   c. Viruses
      (1) HTLV-I (adult T-cell leukemia)
      (2) HTLV-II (atypical hairy-cell leukemia)

Based on Champlin R, Golde DW. In Wilson JD, et al, editors: *Harrison's Principles of internal medicine*, ed 12, New York, 1991, McGraw-Hill pp 1552-1561; List AF, et al. In Hiddeman W, et al, editors: *Haematology and blood transfusion: acute leukemias*, ed 34, New York, 1992, Springer-Verlag, pp 3-10; O'Mura GA. In Rose LF, Kaye D, editors: *Internal medicine for dentistry*, ed 2, St Louis, 1990, CV Mosby, pp 317-324; Perkins ML. In Harmening DM, editor: *Clinical hematology and fundamentals of hemostasis*, ed 2, Philadelphia, 1992, FA Davis, pp 266-292.

TABLE 23-6
Signs and Symptoms of Leukemia

Signs

Pallor
Lymphadenopathy
Petechiae
Ecchymoses
Gingival enlargement
Oral ulcerations
Loose teeth
Pulpal abscess
Enlarged tonsils
Gingival bleeding

Symptoms

Dyspnea
Palpitations
Fever
Weakness
Recurrent infections
Spontaneous gingival bleeding
Weight loss
Sore throat
Body pains

tramedullary involvement of the gingiva, skin, and CNS.[10,22,23]

A preleukemia syndrome is found in about 25% of adult patients with AML. The syndrome consists of anemia and cytopenia. Patients who have this syndrome and develop AML have a poorer prognosis than do those who develop AML without a preceding preleukemia syndrome.[10] Chemotherapy is not started during the preleukemia stage. Retinoic acid treatment may be used in an attempt to mature the cells.[10]

The prognosis for adults with AML is poor. Treatment can produce remission in 60% to 80% of the patients, but the duration is short (Table 23-5). Children with AML also have a poor prognosis, with less than 20% to 40% long-term survival (cure) occurring with the best of treatment.

TREATMENT OF AN ACUTE LEUKEMIA

The treatment strategy for acute leukemia involves the arithmetic leukemia concept:

The normal bone marrow consists of 0.3% to 5% blast cells. Under normal conditions, this would represent

(myeloblastic without differentiation), M-2 (myeloblastic with differentiation), M-3 (promyelocytic), M-4 (myelomonocytic), M-5 (monocytic well-differentiated [A] or poorly differentiated [B]), M-6 (erythrocytic), and M-7 (megakaryoblastic). There appears to be little difference in the clinical findings among the seven subtypes except that disseminated intravascular coagulation is found associated most often with M-3 and M-4 whereas M-5 is more likely to have ex-

about 5 to 10 billion cells. In patients with acute leukemia there are about a trillion blast cells. Once effective chemotherapy has been given and no signs or symptoms of leukemia can be found, the patient is said to be in remission. The number of blast cells will be reduced from trillions to billions and leukemic cells can no longer be detected. With a 5-day generation time for the remaining undetectable leukemic cell mass, ten doublings in 50 days could restore the leukemic cell mass to a trillion cells and the patient would again shows signs and symptoms of leukemia. This would constitute a short remission with a relapse.[22]

Based on the above, there are three phases in the chemotherapy of acute leukemias. The first phase is to hit hard and induce a state of remission. The second phase is to consolidate the kill of remaining leukemic cells. The third phase is to provide maintenance treatment to prevent any remaining leukemic cell mass from

TABLE 23-7

Clinical Factors in Acute and Chronic Leukemias

Factor	Type of Leukemia			
	ALL	**AML**	**CLL**	**CML**
Age	Children (75%)	Adults (85%)	Over 40 years	30 to 50 years
Prognosis	Very good	Poor	Good	Poor
Survival (mean)		2 years	Stage 1 (19 months) Stage IV (12 years)	3 to 4 years
Remissions	90%	60% to 80%	—	—
Duration	Usually long-term	9 to 24 months		
Cures	50% to 70%	10% to 30%	—	—
Main Rx				
Induction	Vincristine + Prednisone	Daunorubicin + Cytarabine	Chlorambucil + Prednisone	Busulfan
Maintenance	Methotrexate + Mercaptopurine BMT for failures	Mitoxantrone + Cytarabine BMT	— —	— BMT
	ALL	**AML**	**CLL**	**CML**
Age	Adults (25%)	Children (15%)	Children (rare)	Children (rare)
Prognosis	Poor	Poor	—	—
Survival (mean)	26 months	—	—	—
Remissions	50% to 70%	56% to 66%	—	—
Duration	10 to 19 months	8 to 12 months		
Cures	20%	20% to 40%	—	—

ALL, Acute lymphocytic leukemia; *AML*, acute myelogenous leukemia; *CLL*, chronic lymphocytic leukemia; *CML* chronic myelogenous leukemia.
Based on Canellos GP. In Petersdorf RG et al, editors: *Principles of internal medicine*, ed 10, New York, 1983, McGraw-Hill; Champlin R, Golde DW. In Wilson JD, et al, editors: *Harrison's Principles of internal medicine*, ed 12, New York, 1991, McGraw-Hill pp 1552-1561; Clarkson, B. In Petersdorf R, et al, editors: *Harrison's Principles of internal medicine*, ed 10, New York, 1983, McGraw-Hill; O'Mura GA. In Rose LF, Kaye D, editors: *Internal medicine for dentistry*, ed 2, St Louis, 1990, CV Mosby pp 317-324; Perkins ML. In Harmening DM, editor: *Clinical hematology and fundamentals of hemostasis*, ed 2, Philadelphia, 1992, FA Davis, pp 266-292.

expanding. Patients are cured of leukemia when no leukemic cells remain. Long-term survival occurs when the leukemic cell mass is greatly reduced and kept from increasing over a long period. A relapse occurs when the leukemic cell mass again becomes about a trillion cells. In general, once a patient relapses, a second remission is more difficult to induce and, if it occurs, will be of a shorter duration.[10]

Another concept involved in the treatment of patients with an acute leukemia is that leukemic cells can migrate to areas in the body where chemotherapeutic agents cannot reach them. These areas are called sanctuaries and they require special treatment. The most important sanctuary in patients with ALL is the central nervous system. Thus patients with ALL will be treated by cranial irradiation plus intrathecal methotrexate in addition to the usual antileukemic agents. Another important sanctuary (in males) is the testes.[10]

Agents used to treat the acute leukemias are shown in Tables 23-7 and 23-8. When bone marrow transplantation is selected for treating an acute leukemia, the patient should be in remission. Because of the high long-term survival (cure) rates following initial treatment of ALL in children, bone marrow transplantation is usually considered only for children who relapse. In these patients a second remission is

induced and then the bone marrow transplantation can be performed.[10]

CHRONIC LEUKEMIAS

There are two types of chronic leukemia, chronic myelogenous (CML) and chronic lymphocytic (CLL). The more common form in the United States is CLL. The chronic leukemias have a slower onset of symptoms, a better prognosis, and more mature white blood cells than do acute leukemias.

In general, patients with a chronic leukemia have anemia and bleeding problems associated with thrombocytopenia. These can be caused by the leukemia itself and the effects of chemotherapy. Infection is less of a problem in patients with a chronic leukemia than in those with an acute leukemia because the cells are more mature and functional in chronic leukemias. However, in the later stages of both CML and CLL, infection does become a serious complication.[9] Table 23-9 lists parameters in comparison of acute and chronic leukemias.

The majority of patients with *chronic myelogenous leukemia* (CML) are 30 to 50 years of age at the onset. Their white blood cell count is usually around 200,000/mm³ at the time of diagnosis, and the symptoms include an enlarged and painful spleen, pallor, weight loss, fever, bleeding problems, and increased serum vitamin B_{12} levels. Lymphadenopathy is rare in the early phase of CML. About 20% of the patients with CML are asymptomatic at the time

TABLE 23-8
Classes of Drugs Used To Treat Childhood Leukemias

Class	Agent
Steroids	Prednisone
Plant alkaloids	Vincristine
Folic acid analogs	Methotrexate
Purine analogs	6-Mercaptopurine
	Thioguanine
Alkylating agents	Cyclophosphamide
Enzymes	Asparaginase
Pyrimidine nucleoside analogs	Arabinosyl cytosine
Anthracycline antibiotics	Daunorubicin
	Doxorubicin

Based on O'Mura GA. In Rose LF, Kaye D, editors: *Internal medicine for dentistry*, ed 2, St Louis, 1990, CV Mosby, pp 317-324.

TABLE 23-9
Comparison of Acute and Chronic Leukemias

Parameter	Acute	Chronic
Clinical onset	Sudden	Insidious
Course (untreated)	Less than 6 months	2 to 6 years
Leukemic cells	Immature	Mature
Anemia	Mild to severe	Mild
Thromocytopenia	Mild to severe	Mild
WBC	Variable	Increased
Organomegaly	Mild	Prominent
Age	Adults and children	Adults

Based on Perkins ML: *Clinical hematology and fundamentals of hemostasis*, Philadelphia, 1992, FA Davis, pp 266-292.

of diagnosis. They are identified by the marked elevation of their white cell count during routine examinations. After the first 6 to 12 months following diagnosis, 25% of the patients per year undergo a transformation to the blastic stage of the disease. The blastic stage consists of acute lymphoid or myeloid leukemia. Over 85% of the patients with CML die in the blastic stage. The overall prognosis for CML is poor, with survival from time of diagnosis being about 3.5 years.[1,10,22]

Ninety-five percent of the leukemic cells in CML have the Philadelphia chromosome marker, which can be found in the metaphyses. Those patients without the Philadelphia chromosome appear to have a poorer prognosis. The leukemic cell in CML is functional; thus infection is not a major problem during the chronic stage of the disease. However, once transformation to the blastic stage has occurred, the leukemic cells are immature and nonfunctional; infection then becomes a major problem. CML is treated using busulfan or other alkylating agents. If bone marrow transplantation is considered, it must be done within 1 year of the diagnosis. Once transformation to the blastic stage has occurred, bone marrow transplantation is no longer an option.[1,10]

Patients with *chronic lymphocytic leukemia* (CLL) are older than those with CML (mean age 60 years). Both CML and CLL are rare in children. The white cell count is usually lower in patients with CLL than in patients with CML. CLL patients have an enlarged spleen and lymphadenopathy, and some CLL patients develop associated anemia and thrombocytopenia. Again, about 25% of the patients are identified during routine examinations.[10,22]

CLL is classified using an international staging system. Three stages are identified: stage A (two or fewer lymph node groups, no anemia or thrombocytopenia), stage B (three or more lymph node groups, no anemia or thrombocytopenia), and stage C (anemia and thrombocytopenia, any number of lymph node groups). The lymph node groups include cervical, axillary, inguinal, liver, and spleen. The mean survival time for patients with stage A disease is more than 10 years, with stage B about 5 years, and with stage C only about 2 years. Treatment of CLL has had little effect on survival times. Patients in the asymptomatic phase are usually

not treated. Only moderate effectiveness has been reported for some treatments in the reduction of lymphocyte counts and palliation of symptoms. Prednisone, chlorambucil, and ionizing radiation have been used in the treatment of CLL, with some benefit.[10,22]

Ninety-five percent of the patients with CLL have neoplastic B lymphoctyes. A trisomy 12 chromosomal abnormality is usually present as a marker in these leukemic cells. Also, in most cases, monoclonal immunoglobulin can be demonstrated on the cell surface. Less than 5% of the patients with CLL have leukemic cells of T cell origin.

A form of chronic lymphocytic leukemia called hairy-cell leukemia has been described. These patients have leukemic B cell lymphocytes with hairlike cytoplasmic projections. This form of chronic leukemia is usually found in men over the age of 40. The patient may have an enlarged spleen, a hemocytopenia, and an associated vasculitis-like disorder (e.g., erythema nodosum or polyarteritis nodosa). More than 50% of affected patients will survive longer than 8 years from the time of diagnosis. Patients with atypical hairy-cell leukemia appear to have a viral etiology for their disease (HTLV-II). Other human leukemias caused by virus infection are African Burkitt's (EBV) and acute T cell (HTLV-I).[1,10,22]

Lymphomas

Three types of lymphoma will be considered in this section: Hodgkin's disease, non-Hodgkin's lymphoma, and Burkitt's lymphoma. In addition, multiple myeloma will be described because it represents a lymphoproliferative disorder of clinical importance to the dentist.

HODGKIN'S DISEASE

Hodgkin's disease is a lymphoproliferative disorder of unknown cause. There are two peaks of incidence, one in early adulthood and one around the fifth decade of life.[20,25] Hodgkin's disease affects about 7500 Americans per year.[20,25] Signs and symptoms include fever, weight loss, sweating, pruritus, fatigue, and firm nontender swelling of the lymph nodes (Table 23-10). Fifty to sixty percent of the patients present with mediastinal nodes.[20] Survival time varies from short- to long-term, and radiation and chemotherapy are used for treatment;

TABLE 23-10
Signs and Symptoms of Lymphoma

Signs
 Lymphadenopathy
 Extranodal soft tissue tumors
Symptoms
 Fever
 Weight loss
 Sweating
 Pruritis
 Fatigue

TABLE 23-11
Comparison of Non-Hodgkin's and Hodgkin's Lymphomas

Parameter	Non-Hodgkin's	Hodgkin's
Cellular derivation	90% B cell 10% T cell	Unresolved
Site		
Localized	Uncommon	Common
Nodal	Discontiguous	Contiguous
Extranodal	Common	Uncommon
Abdominal	Common	Uncommon
Mediastinal	Uncommon	Common
Bone marrow	Common	Uncommon
Symptoms (fever, night sweats, weight loss)	Uncommon	Common
Curability	Less than 25%	Greater than 75%

From Nadler LM. In Wilson JD, et al, editors: *Harrison's Principles of internal medicine,* ed 12, New York, 1991, McGraw-Hill, pp 1599-1612.

however, there is an increased risk for developing acute leukemia with combined-modality treatment. Patients with Hodgkin's disease are prone to infection and inflammations. During chemotherapy they are susceptible to infection, oral ulcerations, and excessive bleeding following minor trauma or surgical procedures.

NON-HODGKIN'S LYMPHOMA

Non-Hodgkin's lymphoma is a lymphoproliferative disorder of unknown cause that can occur in all races and age groups. Unlike Hodgkin's disease which often begins with a single focus of tumor, non-Hodgkin's lymphoma is usually multifocal when first detected.[20,25] Each year about 30,000 new cases are reported. The condition has been reported[20,25] in association with AIDS, being found in about 10% of AIDS patients. Classification of non-Hodgkin's lymphoma is based on pattern of distribution (diffuse or nodular), cell type (lymphocytic, histocytic, mixed), and degree of differentiation of the cells (well, moderate, poor). Ninety percent of all cases on non-Hodgkin's lymphoma are of B cell derivation.[20] Signs and symptoms include fever, weight loss, malaise, sweating, painful lymphadenopathy, and on occasion extranodal tumors.[14,15,25] However, two thirds of the patients present with painless lymphadenopathy.[20] Lymphoma in the oral cavity is uncommon, but head and neck manifestations occur fairly often.[14,15] These lymphomas are radiosensitive. Radiation and chemotherapy are used in their treatment; survival is variable, though usually poor. Extranodal lymphomas in the oral-pharyngeal region have a poor prognosis. Table 23-11 compares the findings of Hodgkin's disease and non-Hodgkin's lymphoma.

BURKITT'S LYMPHOMA

Burkitt's lymphoma is a B cell lymphoid proliferation associated in some way with the Epstein-Barr virus; it also has been reported[25] as a complication in some AIDS cases. Burkitt's lymphoma is found most often in Central Africa, where it usually is seen as a tumor of the jaws; in America the disease initially involves lymph nodes and bone marrow. The American form has a worse prognosis than the African form. Radiation and chemotherapy are used for treatment of Burkitt's lymphoma.

Multiple myeloma

Multiple myeloma is a lymphoproliferative disorder consisting of plasma cell dyscrasias. Incidence is equal among men and women, and mean survival is only 2 years. Each year about 10,000 new cases occur.[25] The disease consists of plasma and myeloma cell proliferation with bone marrow replacement. The bone marrow replacement leads to anemia, leukopenia, thrombocytopenia, hypercalcemia, and a decrease in plasma immunoglobulins. Signs and symptoms include weakness, weight loss, recurrent infections, bone pain, anemia, pathologic fractures, and excessive bleeding following minor trauma.

Dental radiographs may show "punched-out" lesions or mottled areas representing areas of tumor. Extramedullary plasma cell tumors can occur in the oral pharynx. An amyloid-like protein is sometimes found in oral soft tissues as a result of multiple myeloma, and these areas may be swollen and painful. Biopsy and special amyloid stains can be used for diagnosis.[25] Treatment of multiple myeloma consists of chemotherapeutic agents. Patients being treated are susceptible to infection and excessive bleeding.

DENTAL MANAGEMENT
MEDICAL CONSIDERATIONS

The dentist should search for signs and symptoms of anemia or white blood cell disorders in patients who are seen for dental treatment. A patient with the classic signs or symptoms of anemia, leukemia, or lymphoma, for example, should be referred directly to a physician. Patients with signs and symptoms less suggestive of these disorders should be screened by appropriate laboratory tests and/or biopsy of soft tissue and osseous lesions. Screening laboratory tests can be obtained by sending the patient to a commercial clinical laboratory or to a physician. Screening tests should include a total white blood cell count, a differential white cell count, a smear for cell morphologic study, a hemoglobin or hematocrit count, a Sickledex Test (blacks), and a platelet count. If the screening tests are ordered by the dentist and one or more are abnormal, the patient should be referred for medical evaluation and treatment.

Patients with anemia may have a serious underlying disease, such as peptic ulcer or carcinoma, in which early detection may be lifesaving. Patients with sickle cell anemia may be in grave danger if the disease is not detected before dental treatment is started. Undetected leukemic patients may develop serious bleeding problems following any surgical procedure, may have problems with healing of surgical wounds, and are prone to postsurgical infections. Thus it is important for the dentist to attempt to identify these patients before starting any treatment.

White blood cell disorders

New dental patients under medical treatment for leukemia, lymphoma, and multiple myeloma must be identified by their health history and

TABLE 23-12
Dental Management of the Leukemic Patient

1. Detection
   a. History
   b. Examination
   c. Screening laboratory tests
      (1) White cell count
      (2) Differential white cell count
      (3) Smear for cell morphologic study
      (4) Hemoglobin or hematocrit level
      (5) Platelet count
2. Referral
   a. Medical diagnosis
   b. Treatment
3. Consultation before any dental care is rendered
   a. Current status
   b. Review of dental treatment needs
   c. Dental management plan
4. Routine dental care
   a. None for patient with acute symptoms
   b. Once disease is under control, patient may receive indicated dental care
   c. Scaling and surgical procedures
      (1) Bleeding time on day of procedure; if normal, proceed; if prolonged, delay or obtain platelet replacement
      (2) Prophylactic antibiotic therapy to prevent postoperative infection (if severe neutropenia is present)
5. Emergency dental care
   a. Treatment of oral ulcers (see Appendix B)
      (1) Antibiotics
      (2) Bland mouth rinse
      (3) Antihistimin solutions
      (4) Orabase
   b. Oral moniliasis—treat with antifungal medication (see Appendix B)
   c. Conservative management of pain and infection
      (1) Antibiotic sensitivity testing
      (2) Antibiotics, heat for infection
      (3) Strong analgesics for pain

their current status established by consultation with the physician. With special considerations, the patient who is in a state of remission can receive most indicated dental treatment (Table 23-12). Patients with acute signs or symptoms of the disease in general should receive only conservative emergency dental care.

If scaling or surgical procedures are planned for a patient who has leukemia that is under good medical control, a bleeding time should be obtained on the day of the procedure. This is done to establish that an adequate number of functional platelets are present. The number of platelets can be depressed in these patients, by the leukemic process or by the agents used to treat the process. If the bleeding time is abnormal, the procedure should be canceled and the patient's physician consulted. In patients whose disease is under good control but who are still thrombocytopenic, platelet re-

TABLE 23-13

Prophylactic Antibiotic Regimens for Postoperative Infection in the Patient with Leukemia, Lymphoma, Sickle Cell Anemia, or Multiple Myeloma

1. Penicillin—for most situations
   a. 2 g of penicillin V, orally, at least 30 minutes before surgical procedure
   b. 500 mg of penicillin V, orally, every 6 hours for remaining part of appointment day
   c. 500 mg of penicillin V, orally, every 6 hours for following 2 to 5 days; length of coverage based on absence of postoperative infection and rate of healing
2. Erythromycin—for penicillin allergy
   a. 1 g orally 1 to 1½ hours before surgical procedure
   b. 500 mg orally every 6 hours for remaining part of appointment day
   c. 500 mg orally every 6 hours for following 2 to 5 days; length of coverage based on absence of postoperative infection and rate of healing
3. Under special conditions (poor control of disease, recurrent infection, antibiotic sensitivity)
   a. Consult with physician concerning selection of drugs, dosage, and duration of treatment
   b. Consider following drugs: amoxicillin, cephalosporins, gentamincin, ampicillin, vancomycin, etc.

placement by the physician can be instituted if a dental procedure must be done. Prophylactic antibiotic therapy should be considered for leukemic patients if the functional neutrophil count is depressed and surgical treatment is planned (Table 23-13). Dental management of the patient receiving radiation or chemotherapy is covered in Chapter 24.

Anemias

Patients with glucose-6-phosphate dehydrogenase deficiency have an increased incidence of drug sensitivity—with sulfonamides, aspirin, and chloramphenicol being the prime offenders.[2,18] Dental infection and drugs that contain phenacetin may accelerate the rate of hemolysis in patients with this type of anemia[2,18]; thus dental infections should be avoided and, if they occur, must be dealt with effectively. Drugs containing phenacetin should not be used in these patients.

Blacks with sickle cell anemia can receive routine dental care during noncrisis periods; however, long and complicated procedures should be avoided. Good dental repair and preventive dental care are important, since an oral infection could precipitate a crisis. If infection occurs, it must be treated as soon as possible using local and systemic measures—incision and drainage, heat, high doses of appropriate antibiotics, pulpectomy, extraction, etc. If cellulitis develops, the patient's physician must be consulted and hospitalization considered.[18,26] The important points in dental management of the patient with sickle cell anemia are shown in Table 23-14.

For routine dental care the appointments should be short for patients with sickle cell anemia. The use of a local anesthetic is indicated (avoid general anesthesia); however, inclusion of small amounts of epinephrine in the local anesthetic is controversial, in that some authors believe it may impair circulation and cause vascular occlusion. Smith et al.[26] suggest that for the short appointment to render routine dental care, a local anesthetic without a vasoconstrictor be used. When a surgical procedure must be performed, they recommend using a local with epinephrine 1:100,000 to obtain hemostasis and profound anesthesia. The use of nitrous oxide–oxygen also is controversial; however, if $N_2O\text{-}O_2$ is given with 50% oxygen

TABLE 23–14
Dental Management of the Patient with Sickle Cell Anemia

1. Arrange short appointments
2. Avoid long and/or complicated procedures
3. Maintain good dental repair
4. Institute aggressive preventive dental care
   a. Oral hygiene instruction
   b. Diet control
   c. Toothbrushing and flossing
   d. Fluoride gel application
5. Avoid oral infection; treat aggressively when present
6. Use local anesthetic without epinephrine for routine dental care; for surgical procedures use 1:100,000 epinephrine in local anesthetic
7. Avoid barbiturates and strong narcotics; sedation with diazepam (Valium) can be used
8. Use prophylactic antibiotics for surgical procedures
9. Avoid liberal use of salicylates; pain control with acetaminophen and codeine
10. Use nitrous oxide–oxygen with great care; 50% oxygen, high flow rate, good ventilation

concentration, using a high flow rate and proper ventilation, it appears to have a good margin of safety.[26]

IV sedation must be used with extreme caution in patients who have a history of sickle cell anemia. Barbiturates and narcotics must be avoided because suppression of the respiratory center by these agents leads to acidosis, which could precipitate an acute crisis. Light sedation with diazepam (Valium) or nalbuphine hydrochloride can be used.[26]

The liberal use of salicylates should be avoided since the "acid" effect could (again) cause a crisis. Pain control can be attempted with codeine and acetaminophen.[26]

Prophylactic antibiotics are recommended for surgical procedures to prevent wound infection or osteomyelitis (Table 23-5). Dehydration must be avoided during surgery and the postoperative period. Consultation with the patient's physician is a must prior to any surgical procedure. The dentist needs to establish the patient's current status and, if blood transfusion is indicated, to correct severe anemia or its complications prior to surgery[26] (Table 23-7).

TREATMENT PLANNING MODIFICATIONS

Patients with acute leukemia should receive only conservative treatment for emergency dental problems. Routine dental treatment is not indicated for these patients. Special attention should be given to oral hygiene procedures for patients with leukemia to avoid dental caries and gingival inflammation and infection. Leukemic patients whose disease is in a state of remission or control can receive any indicated dental treatment, as long as the preceding special considerations are followed. Leukemic patients with acute infections should not receive routine dental care until the infection has been treated and the patient has returned to a "normal" state.

Elective surgical procedures are best avoided in patients with sickle cell anemia. Routine dental care can be rendered for patients with sickle cell trait and disease. Special emphasis should be placed on oral hygiene procedures to avoid dental caries and gingival inflammation and infection.

Patients with lymphoma that is in a state of remission can receive routine dental care as indicated. Patients with advanced disease should receive emergency care only; complex restorative procedures, etc., are usually not indicated. A platelet count or bleeding time should be obtained before any surgical procedure; if abnormal, platelet replacement may be indicated.

Because of the limited prognosis in many cases of acute leukemia and multiple myeloma, complex and extensive dental restorations are usually not indicated for patients with these conditions.

Prophylactic antibiotics are often recommended to prevent infection following a surgical procedure that must be performed in a patient with leukemia, lymphoma, sickle cell anemia, or multiple myeloma. The need for prophylaxis depends on the type of medical treatment the patient is receiving and the status of the disease. Patients in remission usually do not require prophylaxis. If adequate numbers of functional neutrophils are present, there usually is no need for prophylaxis. A modification of the current

American Heart Association recommended standard regimen for endocarditis prevention is presented in Table 23-13.

ORAL COMPLICATIONS
White blood cell disorders

Patients with leukemia may develop multiple oral ulcers that can be painful and are prone to secondary infection (Fig. 23-1). Signs of infection are often masked in patients with untreated leukemia, those who were nonresponsive to treatment, or those who have relapsed following treatment. The swelling and erythema usually associated with oral infection are often less marked. In these patients severe infection can be present with minimal clinical signs. Such infections often develop from invasion by bacteria that do not cause oral infections in most patients seen by the dentist. Unusual infections may be due to *Pseudomonas, Klebsiella, Proteus, Escherichia coli,* or *Enterobacter.* Often these infections will present as oral ulcerations. The most common cause in patients receiving chemotherapy is recurrent herpes simplex infection, whose lesions tend to be larger and take longer to heal than herpetic lesions found in nonleukemic patients. Oral candidiasis is also common in symptomatic patients and those undergoing chemotherapy. Oral ulcerations should be cultured to establish the diagnosis. Large ulcers should be cultured and, in addition, biopsied. Thus any unusual bacterial or fungal infection can be identified and the best treatment selected.[16]

Patients with leukemia are usually prone to infection because of the immaturity of the malignant leukocytes. When oral infection develops in such patients, a specimen of exudate should be sent for diagnosis and antibiotic sensitivity testing, and penicillin therapy should be begun (if the patient is not allergic to penicillin). If the clinical course shows little or no improvement in several days, the antibiotic sensitivity testing data may be used to select an antibiotic that may be more effective.

Leukemic patients are prone to oral moniliasis. When this complication occurs, the patient can be treated with one of the topical antifungal medications listed in Appendix B. Patients with an oral ulceration should receive symptomatic treatment for the ulcer. (See Appendix B for suggested regimens.) A bland mouth rinse can be used to clean the surface of the ulcer (commercial mouth rinses are not recommended because they tend to irritate ulcerated tissues). Following the bland mouth rinse, a topical anesthetic can be used to make the mouth more comfortable. Various solutions of antihistamines are effective for this. Many of the antihistamines have local anesthetic properties that will provide relief from the pain. A lesion in the mucobuccal fold or under the tongue can then be coated with a thin layer of Orabase, which will protect its surface from irritation. This sequence can be repeated four to six times a day.

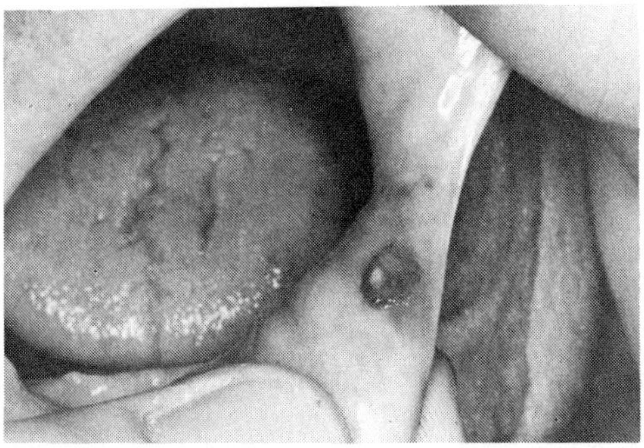

FIG. 23-1 Multiple intraoral ulcers involving the mucosa of the lower lip in a patient with chronic lymphocytic leukemia.

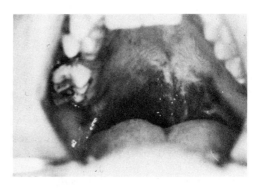

FIG. 23-2 Palatal ecchymoses in a leukemic patient.

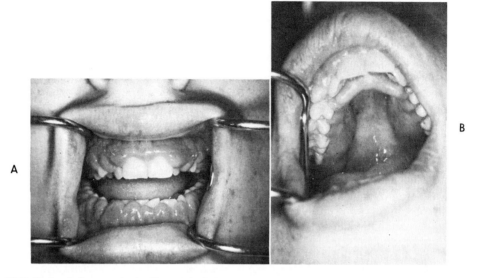

FIG. 23-3 A, Severe gingival hyperplasia in a patient with acute nonlymphoblastic leukemia. Gingival biopsy revealed numerous immature white blood cells in the tissues. **B,** Palatal view of the hyperplasia.

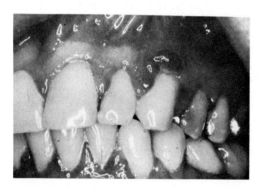

FIG. 23-4 Localized area of gingival inflammation in a patient with only moderately good oral hygiene. The lesion would not clear up following removal of the local irritants. Biopsy revealed immature white blood cells compatible with leukemic infiltrate. The patient was referred, and a diagnosis of acute nonlymphoblastic leukemia established.

Small or large areas of submucosal hemorrhage may be found in the leukemic patient (Fig. 23-2). These lesions result from minor trauma and are related to the thrombocytopenia. Leukemic patients also may complain of spontaneous gingival hemorrhage and some will complain of paresthesias resulting from leukemic infiltration of the peripheral nerves.

Leukemic patients with active disease often have severe gingival bleeding if significant thrombocytopenia is present. The dentist should use local measures to control the bleeding. A gelatin sponge with thrombin or microfibrillar collagen can be placed over the area. An oral rinse of an antifibrinolytic agent can also be used. If local measures fail, medical help will be needed and may involve platelet transfusion.[16]

Leukemic patients with poor oral hygiene are prone to develop localized or generalized gingival inflammation (Figs. 23-3 and 23-4), which is most common in patients who have CML. Chlorhexidine rinses are recommended to promote the healing of oral ulcerations and prevent oral infections.[12,16,18,24]

Patients with Hodgkin's disease or non-Hodgkin's lymphoma may be seen with cervical lymphadenopathy or extranodal tumors (Figs. 23-5 to 23-7). The dentist should refer patients with chronic enlargement of head and neck lymph nodes for needle biopsy or excisional biopsy; extranodal tumors can be biopsied by the dentist or referred to an oral surgeon for biopsy. Patients with lymphomas treated by

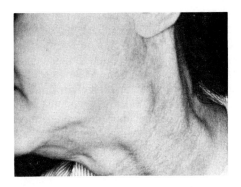

FIG. 23-5 Lymphadenopathy involving the cervical lymph nodes in a patient with Hodgkin's disease.

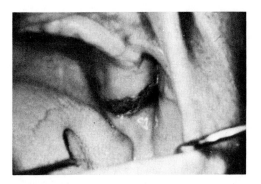

FIG. 23-6 Non-Hodgkin's lymphoma in a patient who came to the dentist complaining of loose maxillary denture.

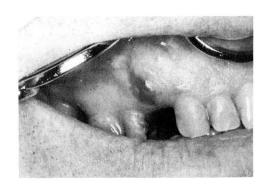

FIG. 23-7 Lesion on the alveolar ridge that was found on radiographs to involve the underlying alveolar bone. The patient had non-Hodgkin's lymphoma.

radiation usually are not at increased risk for osteoradionecrosis, because the radiation dosage seldom exceeds 6000 rads, but they can develop xerostomia.[25]

Patients with lymphoma sometimes complain of burning mouth symptoms similar to those noted in patients with leukemia—which may be related to drug toxicity, xerostomia, candidiasis, or anemia.[11] (See Appendix B for management regimens.)

Patients with multiple myeloma may have jaw lesions, soft tissue lesions, and soft tissue deposits of amyloid. The bone and soft tissue lesions are often painful.[25]

As mentioned earlier, patients with leukemia, lymphoma, or multiple myeloma are usually treated by radiation, chemotherapy, or a combination of radiation and chemotherapy. The complications associated with these treatments and their management are covered in Chapter 24.

Anemia

The oral findings in patients with anemia usually relate to the underlying cause of the anemia. The oral mucosa will often appear pale. Patients with nutritional causes of anemia (e.g., vitamin B_{12} or iron deficiency) may show loss of papillae from the tongue and atrophic changes of the oral mucosa (Fig. 23-8). An angular cheilitis may be found. These patients also may complain of burning or sore tongue. Some patients with iron deficiency anemia may have

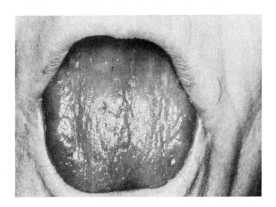

FIG. 23-8 Smooth red tongue in a patient found to have pernicious anemia (vitamin B_{12} deficiency caused by lack of intrinsic factor).

Plummer-Vinson syndrome — a sore mouth, dysphagia (resulting from muscular degeneration in the esophagus with esophageal stenosis), and an increased frequency of carcinoma of the oral cavity and pharynx. Patients with this syndrome should be followed up closely for any oral or pharyngeal tissue changes that might be early indicators of carcinoma.[18,24]

Patients with hemolytic anemia may show, in addition to pallor, oral evidence of jaundice caused by hyperbilirubinemia secondary to excessive erythrocyte destruction. The trabecular pattern of the bone on dental radiographs may be affected because of hyperplasia of marrow elements in response to the increased destruction of red blood cells. The bone will appear more radiolucent with prominent lamellar striations.[18,24]

Patients with sickle cell anemia also may slow, in addition to pallor, evidence of jaundice in the oral tissues. Erythropoietic activity is increased, and dental radiographic findings associated with the bone marrow hyperplasia may be present. The trabeculae between teeth may appear as horizontal rows (Fig. 23-9), and the lamina dura may seem more dense and distinct. Areas of sclerosis have been reported. Patients with sickle cell anemia often have delayed eruption of teeth, with hypoplasia of teeth.[18,24,26]

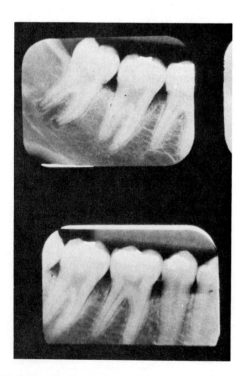

FIG. 23-9   Radiographs of the mandible in a patient with sickle cell anemia. Note the prominent horizontal trabeculations and dense lamina dura.

REFERENCES

1. Adamson JW: The myeloproliferative diseases. In Wilson JD, et al, editors: *Harrison's Principles of internal medicine,* ed 12, New York, 1991, McGraw-Hill, pp 1561-1567.
2. American Dental Association: *Accepted dental therapeutics,* ed 39, Chicago, 1982, The Association.
3. Beck WS: Megaloblastic anemias. I. Cobalamin deficiency. In Beck WS, editor: *Hematology,* ed 5, Cambridge Mass, 1991, MIT Press, pp 83-111.
4. Beck WT, Funabiki T, Danks MK: The role of DNA topoisomerase II in multidrug resistance in human leukemia. In Hiddemann W, et al, editors: *Haematology and blood transfusion: acute leukemias,* ed 34, New York, 1992, Springer-Verlag, pp 11-15.
5. Beck WS, Tepper RI: Hemolytic anemias. IV. Metabolic disorders. In Beck WS, editor: *Hematology,* ed 5, Cambridge Mass, 1991, MIT Press, pp 283-299.
6. Best ML: Infectious mononucleosis and reactive lymphocytes. In Harmening DM, editor: *Clinical hematology and fundamentals of hemostasis,* ed 2, Philadelphia, 1992, FA Davis, pp 258-265.
7. Bunn HF: Hemoglobin. II. Sickle cell anemia and other hemoglobinopathies. In Beck WS, editor: *Hematology,* ed 5, Cambridge Mass, 1991, MIT Press, pp 187-205.
8. Cadman EC, Durivage HJ: Cancer chemotherapy. In Wilson JD, et al, editors: *Harrison's Principles of internal medicine,* ed 12, New York, 1991, McGraw-Hill, pp 1587-1599.
9. Canellos GP: The chronic leukemias. In Petersdorf RG, et al, editors: *Harrison's Principles of internal medicine,* ed 10, New York, 1983, McGraw-Hill Book Co.
10. Champlin R, Golde DW: The leukemias. In Wilson JD, et al, editors: *Harrison's Principles of internal medicine,* ed 12, New York, 1991, McGraw-Hill, pp 1552-1561.
11. Clarkson B: The acute leukemias. In Petersdorf RG, et al, editors: *Harrison's Principles of internal medicine,* ed 10, New York, 1983, McGraw-Hill.
12. Dreizen S, McCredie KB, Keating MJ, Luna MA: Malignant gingival and skin "infiltrates" in adult leukemia, *Oral Surg* 55:572-579, 1983.
13. Drummond JF, White DK, Damm DD: Megaloblastic anemia with oral lesions: a consequence of gastric bypass surgery, *Oral Surg* 59:149-152, 1985.
14. Eisenbud L, Sciubba J, Mir R, Sachs SA: Oral presentations in non-Hodgkin's lymphoma: a review of thirty-one cases. I, *Oral Surg* 56:151-156, 1983.

15. Eisenbud L, Sciubba J, Mir R, Sachs SA: Oral presentations in non-Hodgkin's lymphoma: a review of thirty-one cases. II, *Oral Surg* 57:272-280, 1984.

16. Greenberg MS: Leukemia, dental correlations. In Rose LF, Kaye D, editors: *Internal medicine for dentistry,* ed 2, St Louis, 1990, CV Mosby, pp 365-366.

17. List AF, Spier CM, Dalton WS: Multidrug resistance and its circumvention in acute leukemia. In Hiddemann W, et al, editors: *Haematology and blood transfusion: acute leukemias,* ed 34, New York, 1992, Springer-Verlag, pp 3-10.

18. Lynch MA: Hematologic diseases and related problems. In Lynch MA, editor: *Burket's Oral medicine; diagnosis and treatment,* ed 7, Philadelphia, 1977, JB Lippincott.

19. May DA: Dental management of sickle cell anemia patients, *Gen Dent,* May-June, pp 182-184, 1991.

20. Nadler LM: The malignant lymphomas. In Wilson JD, et al, editors: *Harrison's Principles of internal medicine,* ed 12, New York, 1991, McGraw-Hill, pp 1599-1612.

21. Niederssam JC: Epstein-Barr infection, including infectious mononucleosis. In Petersdorf RG, et al, editors: *Harrison's Principles of internal medicine,* ed 10, New York, 1983, McGraw-Hill.

22. O'Mura GA: The leukemias. In Rose LF, Kaye D, editors: *Internal medicine for dentistry,* ed 2, St Louis, 1990, CV Mosby, pp 317-324.

23. Perkins ML: Introduction to leukemia and the acute leukemias. In Harmening DM, editor: *Clinical hematology and fundamentals of hemostasis,* ed 2, Philadelphia, 1992, FA Davis, pp 266-292.

24. Shafer WG, Hine MK, Levy BM: *A textbook of oral pathology,* ed 4, Philadelphia, 1983, WB Saunders.

25. Silverman S, editor: *Oral cancer,* ed 2, New York, 1985, American Cancer Society.

26. Smith HB, McDonald DK, Miller RI: Dental management of patients with sickle cell disorders, *J Am Dent Assoc* 114:85-87, 1987.

27. Trippett T, Lin JT, Elisseyeff Y, et al: Development of sensitive assays to detect antifolate resistance. In Hiddemann W, et al, editors: *Haematology and blood transfusion: acute leukemias,* ed 34, New York, 1992, Springer-Verlag, pp 16-22.

28. Wintrobe MM, Lee GR, Boggs DR, et al: *Clinical hematology,* ed 8, Philadelphia, 1981, Lea & Febiger.

24

Oral Cancer

The emphasis in this chapter is on the role of the dentist in management of a patient with oral cancer. However, the dental management recommendations dealing with chemotherapy and/or radiotherapy apply also to patients with other forms of cancer, such as leukemia and lymphoma.

The effective management of the patient with oral cancer requires a team approach that involves dental, medical, surgical, radiotherapeutic, chemotherapeutic, reconstructive, and psychiatric considerations. The management of such patients presents many of the same types of problems to the dentist that the management of patients with a systemic medical condition (e.g., diabetes mellitus) does; however, the emphasis on the various roles of the dentist is different with the patient who has cancer. For example, the dentist plays a more primary role in the detection of a cancerous lesion and carries a more active part in the pretreatment and posttreatment phases for the patient who needs reconstruction following surgery or preparation for radiotherapy or chemotherapy. In addition, dentists play an important role in the maintenance phase of dental care for the postsurgical, postirradiation, and postchemotherapy patient.

All patients who have lesions involving the oral cavity require a diagnosis. Often a final or definitive diagnosis can be made by the dentist based on history and clinical findings. This is usually true of conditions such as geographic tongue, lichen planus, and aphthous stomatitis. When the dentist is unable to make a final diagnosis based on clinical findings, however, additional steps must be taken—which may include biopsy or referral to a specialist (e.g., an oral surgeon or oral pathologist).

If the initial clinical impression of a lesion is that it is cancerous, the best course under most circumstances is to refer the patient directly to a cancer treatment center for diagnosis and therapy (Fig. 24-1). There are two reasons for this recommendation: (1) it minimizes the time from the finding to the initiation of therapy and (2) it allows the individuals who will make decisions concerning the selection of treatment an opportunity to see the lesion before it has been altered by the biopsy procedure. In some cases this is important in determining the stage of the tumor, on which the selection of therapy may be based. In general, if any patient has a lesion for which the suspicion of cancer is low, the lesion should be biopsied by the dentist or the patient referred to an oral surgeon for biopsy to establish a definitive diagnosis (Fig. 24-2). When a diagnosis of cancer is established by the biopsy, the patient can then be referred for appropriate therapy.

GENERAL DESCRIPTION
INCIDENCE AND PREVALENCE

During 1978 about 660,000 cases of cancer were identified, excluding superficial skin cancers.[28] Sixty-seven thousand of these involved the head and neck region. Excluding cancers of the central nervous system, eyes, and thyroid as well as sarcomas, lymphomas, and cutaneous melanomas (all of which accounted for roughly 30,000 cases), there were about 37,000 new cases of squamous cell carcinoma involving the head and neck (5.5% of all cancers); 17,400 of these were oral carcinomas, which accounted for about 2.6% of all new cancers for the year (Table 24-1). In 1984, 870,000 new cancer cases were recorded in the United States, including

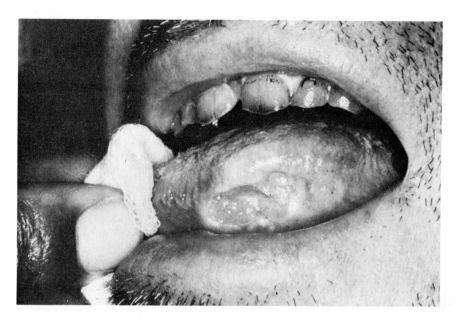

FIG. 24-1 Tongue lesion with a high chance of being cancerous, based on its clinical appearance (size, margins, induration). Direct referral to a cancer treatment center for diagnosis and therapy would be indicated. This lesion was diagnosed as squamous cell carcinoma.

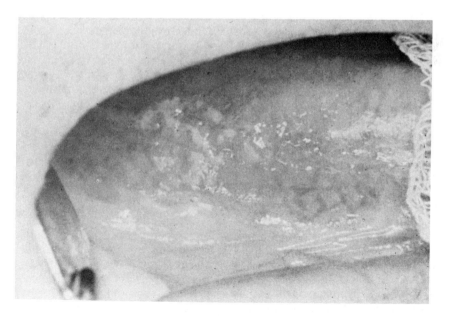

FIG. 24-2 No clinical cause for this tongue lesion could be identified. Its appearance was not highly suggestive of cancer. Nevertheless, it was diagnosed as early squamous cell carcinoma by histopathology. In such cases it would be appropriate for the dentist to biopsy the lesion.

TABLE 24–1

Location and Incidence of Head and Neck Cancer*

Location	Incidence	Percent	Percent all cancers
Oral cavity (including salivary glands)	17,400	48	2.6
Nasopharynx	1300	4	0.2
Oropharynx	3500	10	0.5
Hypopharynx	1800	5	0.5
Larynx	9200	25	1.4
Maxillary sinus	1100	3	0.2
Nose and paranasal sinuses	400	1.3	0.1
Esophagus (cervical)	800	2	0.1
Trachea (cervical)	100	1	0.1
Ear	300	1	0.1
Unknown primary	800	2	0.1
TOTAL	36,700	100%	5.5%

*Does not include thyroid, CNS, eye, or soft tissue melanomas or lymphomas; accounts for another 30,600 cases (or 4.6%) of all cancers.
From US Department of Health, Education, and Welfare: *Management guidelines for head and neck cancer*, Public Health Service Publ. no. 80-2037, 1979.

TABLE 24–2

1992 Estimated Cancer Incidence by Site and Sex

Site	Males (%)	Females (%)
Skin (melanoma)	3	3
Oral cavity	4	2
Lung	18	12
Breast	—	32
Pancreas	2	3
Stomach	3	—
Colon and rectum	14	14
Leukemia and lymphomas	9	7
Urinary tract	10	4
Prostate	23	—
Ovary	—	4
Uterus	—	8
All others	14	11

From Boring CC: *CA* 42(1):19–38, 1992.

27,500 new cases of oral cancer.[2] In 1985 there were about 900,000 new cancer cases with 29,000 cases of oral cancer.[25] If cancers of the nasopharynx, hypopharynx, sinuses, and major salivary gland were included with oral cancers, the total would represent 5% of all new cancers recorded for 1985.[25] The death rate from all types of cancer has risen, from 101 per 100,000 in 1930 to 191 per 100,000 in 1984.[25]

The American Cancer Society has estimated that 1,130,000 cases of cancer would occur in 1992.[5] Over thirty thousand of these would be cancers of the oral cavity and pharynx, representing 2.7% of all cancers projected for 1992. The 1992 estimated cancer incidence by site and sex is shown in Table 24-2. The 1992 estimated cancer death total (520,000 with 7950 due to oral cavity and pharyngeal cancer[5]) is shown in Table 24-3.

The most common location for oral cancer reported in 1979 by the Public Health Service was the tongue (4600 cases),[30] followed by the lip (4200 cases). The least common location was the palate (Table 24-4). The 1985 data showed that the tongue was the most common location for oral cancer.[25] The male/female incidence ratio was over 3 to 1 for head and neck cancer in the 1979 data. The male/female ratio for lip cancer was 11 to 1, and for the other oral locations it was 2.2 to 1.[30] In 1985 the male/female ratio for oral cancer was 2 to 1.[25] About 6000 cases of tongue cancer and 3600 cases of lip cancer were projected for 1992.[5] The vast majority of head and neck cancers, including those in the oral cavity, are in patients over the age of 50, and the incidence increases with each decade over age 40 for men and women.[30] Cancer in American blacks is increasing faster than in whites,[5,25] with blacks having a higher rate of oropharyngeal cancer than other racial groups. Nasopharyngeal cancer is about 20 to 30 times more prevalent in Chinese than whites.[25]

Table 24-5 shows the 5-year survival rates for selected sites by race based on 1981 to 1987 data.[5] The survival rates for all stages of oral cavity and pharyngeal cancer were lower for blacks than for whites. The 5-year survival rate for localized oral cavity and pharyngeal cancer in blacks was only 57%. Table 24-6 demonstrates the trends in survival for all cancers and for oral cavity and pharyngeal cancer. All the sites listed in Tables 24-1 and 24-2, except the oral cavity and pharynx and the liver, had

TABLE 24–3
1992 Estimated Cancer Deaths by Site and Sex

Site	Males (%)	Females (%)
Skin (melanoma)	1	1
Oral cavity	2	1
Lung	34	22
Breast	—	19
Pancreas	4	5
Stomach	3	—
Colon and rectum	11	12
Leukemia and lymphomas	9	9
Urinary tract	5	3
Prostate	12	—
Ovary	—	5
Uterus	—	4
All others	19	19

From Boring CC: *CA* 42(1):19–38, 1992.

TABLE 24–4
Location and Frequency of Oral Cancer

Location	Incidence	Percent
Lip	4200	24
Tongue	4600	26
Floor of mouth	2200	13
Buccal cavity	1500	9
Gingivae	1500	9
Palate	900	5
Salivary gland	2400	14
TOTAL	17,300	100

From US Department of Health, Education, and Welfare: *Management guidelines for head and neck cancer,* Public Health Service Publ. no. 80–2037, 1979.

TABLE 24–5
Five-year Survival Rates for Selected Sites by Race, 1981–1987

Site	Whites (%)	Blacks (%)
Oral cavity and pharynx		
All stages	54	31
Localized	77	57
Regional	42	28
Distant	19	13
Esophagus		
All stages	9	6
Localized	21	16
Regional	6	4
Distant	0	1
Liver		
All stages	5	4
Localized	13	14
Regional	5	1
Distant	2	0
Colon and rectum		
All stages	57	47
Localized	88	83
Regional	58	50
Distant	6	4

From Boring CC: *CA* 42(1):19–38, 1992.

TABLE 24–6
Trends in Survival for All Cancers and for Oral Cavity and Pharyngeal Cancers — Expressed as Percent of 5-year Survival

Periods	All Sites		Oral Cavity and Pharynx	
	Whites	Blacks	Whites	Blacks
1960-1963	39	27	45	—
1970-1973	43	31	43	—
1974-1976	50	39	55	35
1977-1980	51	39	54	34
1981-1987	53*	38	54	31

*The difference in rates between 1974-1976 and 1981-1987 is statistically significant (*p* less than 0.05).
From Boring CC: *CA* 42(1):19-38, 1992.

statistically significant improvement in 5-year survival rates from 1974-1976 to 1981-1987.[5]

ETIOLOGY

The cause of oral cancer is not known at the present time. Little evidence has been found for a genetic role[5,25]; however, several factors have been found to be associated with the development of oral cancer (Table 24-7). In the case of lip cancer, exposure to the sun and smoking have been found to have a strong association in the development of cancer. Smokeless tobacco use,[33] smoking, and/or excessive alcohol intake have been found to be associated with most cases of intraoral squamous cell carcinoma. An increased incidence of cancer has been reported in patients with congenital or acquired defects in the immune system. Organ transplant patients have an increased incidence of lower lip cancer and oral lymphoma.[21] Patients with AIDS have a high incidence of Kaposi's sarcoma, including lesions in the oral cavity, and also a higher incidence of non-Hodgkin's lymphoma.[25] There is increasing evidence[6,13,14,28,32] that human papilloma virus and herpes simplex virus play a role in the etiology of oral cancer.

Other viruses have been implicated in the cause of Burkitt's lymphoma and Kaposi's sarcoma. Other factors suggested to play a minor role in the cause of oral cancer include arsenic compounds used in the treatment of syphilis, nutritional deficiencies, and heavy exposure to materials such as wood and metal dusts.[24,30] An association of *Candida* and oral cancer has been suggested. In one review[17] the more rarely occurring biotypes of *C. albicans* were reported to play a role through the production of nitrosamine. Certain oral lesions — including leukoplakias and erythroplakias — appear to be precancerous. The malignant transformation rate for leukoplakias could be as high as 1% to 2% per year, and leukoplakias with areas of erythema have a 3 to 5 times greater risk for developing into oral cancer than do homogeneous leukoplakias.[25] Other oral lesions may appear clinically as cancer but are benign on histologic examination. Proliferative verrucous leukoplakia (PVL), is an example of such a lesion. PVL is a rare but progressive lesion that requires aggressive early surgical treatment.[25]

PATHOPHYSIOLOGY AND COMPLICATIONS

The vast majority of oral cancers are of epithelial origin, with most developing from the lining tissues of the oral cavity (Table 24-8); hence about 90% of the oral cancers seen by dentists will be squamous cell carcinomas. The remaining primary lesions are carcinomas arising from salvary gland tissues and lesions of other tissue types such as sarcomas and lymphomas.[30] About 1% of the cancers found in the oral cavity are metastatic from elsewhere in the body.[34] In a review of 422 metastatic cancers to

TABLE 24-7

Predisposing Factors in Oral Cancer Development

Age
Tobacco use (cigarettes, pipes, cigars, smokeless tobacco)
Excessive alcohol intake
Actinic radiation
Nutritional deficiencies (iron, vitamin A, zinc, copper)
Syphilis
   Tertiary syphilis
   Arsenic compounds used to treat syphilis
Poor oral hygiene
Chronic physical and thermal trauma
Defective immune system (congenital, acquired)
Viruses
   Papillomavirus
   Herpes simplex virus
   Epstein-Barr virus
   Cytomegalovirus
   Human immunodeficiency virus (HIV)

TABLE 24-8

Classification of Oral Carcinomas

Squamous cell carcinoma
   Carcinoma in situ
   Well-differentiated
   Moderately well-differentiated
   Poorly differentiated
   Undifferentiated
Verrucous carcinoma
Glandular epithelial tumors
Unclassified carcinoma

the oral cavity[34] 22% of them were the first indication of a primary lesion. The balance of this chapter will deal primarily with squamous cell carcinoma, although many of the management recommendations may apply to a patient with other types of oral cancer.

Squamous cell carcinoma can develop in normal-appearing tissue or, as is more often the case, in preexisting benign white or red lesions involving the oral mucosa (Fig. 24-3). Various studies have shown that white lesions that cannot be scraped off and that are nonspecific clinically (leukoplakia) may be benign, premalignant, or malignant at the time of initial biopsy. About 19% of these white epithelial lesions show evidence of dyskeratosis at the time of initial biopsy, and some 4% are squamous cell carcinoma. Patients with white epithelial lesions that were not cancerous when first biopsied will have about a 6% chance of the lesion developing into cancer when followed up over time[24]; thus the incidence of squamous cell carcinoma in nonspecific white epithelial lesions found in the oral cavity is close to 10%. A few investigators[25] have reported malignant transformation rates as high as 17.5% for homogeneous and mixed leukoplakias. Leukoplakias with areas of erythema have a 3-to-5-times greater chance of being cancerous at initial biopsy or developing into cancer with time than do homogeneous leukoplakias.[25] Nonspecific red lesions involving the oral mucosa (erythroplakia) are much less common than the white lesions. However, at initial biopsy far more nonspecific red lesions (51%) than leukoplakias with erythema (14%) or homogeneous leukoplakias (6%) are found to be malignant.[24]

Squamous cell carcimona of the oral cavity may spread by local infiltration into surrounding tissues or may metastasize to regional lymph nodes through the lymphatic system. Distant metastasis of oral cancer is rare but does occur. Most commonly sites for distant metastases are the lung, liver, and bone. Lesions of the floor of the mouth and tongue tend to metastasize much earlier than do carcinomas located in other parts of the oral cavity.

Usually squamous cell carcimona is asymptomatic in the early stages, which often delays its identification and early treatment. Oral cancer can often lead to death by (1) local obstruction of the pathway for food, (2) infiltration into major vessels of the head and neck (resulting in significant blood loss), (3) secondary infections,

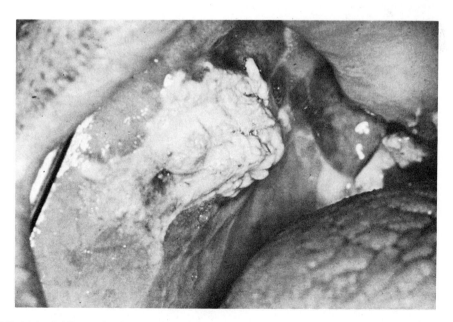

FIG. 24-3 Diffuse white lesion involving the buccal mucosa. Histopathology revealed one area of squamous cell carcinoma.

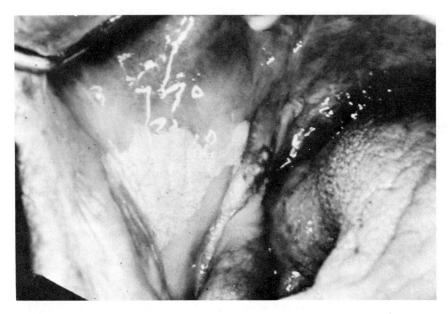

FIG. 24-4   Squamous cell carcinoma appearing as a red patch in a diffuse white lesion (hyperkeratosis).

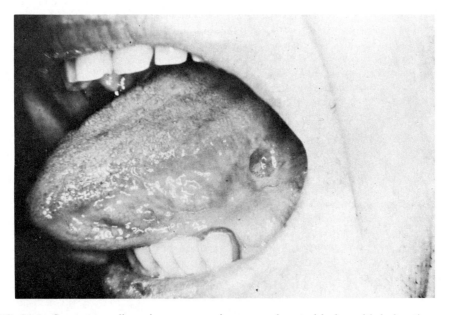

FIG. 24-5   Squamous cell carcinoma appearing as an ulcerated lesion with induration and raised margins.

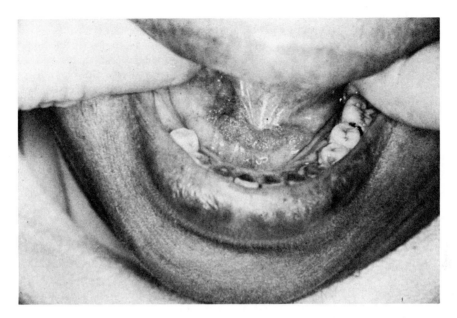

FIG. 24-6 Squamous cell carcinoma appearing as a raised, granular lesion.

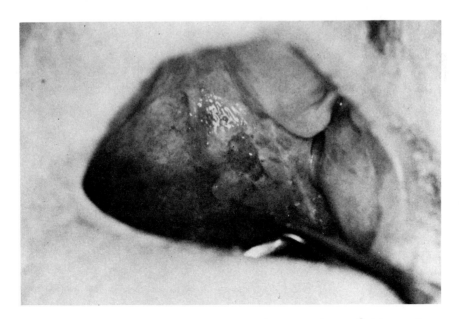

FIG. 24-7 Squamous cell carcinoma appearing as an ulcerated white patch.

(4) impaired function of other organs through distant metastases, (5) general wasting, or (6) complications of therapy.

CLINICAL PRESENTATION
SIGNS

Squamous cell carcinoma may appear as a white and/or red patch, an exophytic mass, an ulceration, a granular raised lesion, or combinations of these (Figs. 24-2 to 24-7). Ulcerated lesions often will have raised margins that are indurated on palpation. White lesions with areas of erythema tend to have a higher incidence of being cancerous than do homogenous white lesions[24-26] (Fig. 24-8).

Over 90% of patients with lip cancer have no clinical evidence of regional or distant metastases; by contrast, about 50% of patients with carcinoma of the tongue have clinical evidence of regional or distant spread of the lesions at the time of diagnosis. About 35% to 40% of patients with squamous cell carcinoma of the tongue and floor of the mouth have no clinical evidence of metastases at the time of treatment but will develop metastatic disease later.[30] In advanced cases of carcinoma of the tongue, the hypoglossal nerve may be involved and the tongue may become atrophic and develop a tremor on the side of involvement. When the patient is asked to stick his or her tongue out, the tongue will "point" to the side of involvement—that is, if the right hypoglossal nerve is involved, the tongue will deviate to the right. Carcinomas of the palate can involve the glossopharyngeal and/or vagus nerves, resulting in unilateral paralysis of the soft palate and loss of the gag reflex on the involved side. This can also be found in association with "hidden" head and neck tumors in the nasopharynx and pharynx. Areas of leukoplakia, leukoplakia with erythema, and erythroplakia must be examined histologically for evidence of premalignant change or cancer.[24,25]

SYMPTOMS

As previously mentioned, symptoms of squamous cell carcinoma tend to develop late in the course of the disease. In patients with more advanced lesions, pain may become a significant problem. Large lesions in the posterior portions of the oral cavity may interfere with the passage of food and air; hence the patient may complain of weight loss and difficulty in breathing. Other symptoms that may be found in association with

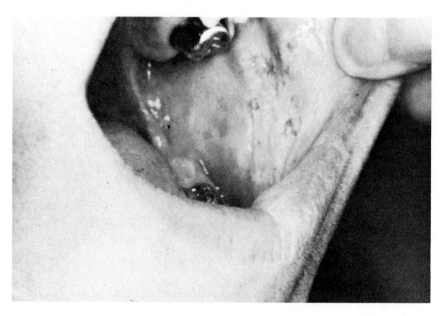

FIG. 24-8 Diffuse white lesion of the buccal mucosa with several areas of erythema. The diagnosis was squamous cell carcinoma.

oral cancer include pain, hoarseness, dysphagia, intractable ulcers, bleeding, numbness, loosening of teeth, and a change in the fit of a denture.

LOCATION

Tables 24-1 and 24-2 summarize the incidence and location of head and neck cancers and oral cancer. Carcinoma of the upper lip is rare compared with carcinoma of the lower lip. Carcinoma of the dorsum of the tongue is rare and when found tends to be related to previous treatments (e.g., the use of arsenic compounds). The vast majority of cases of oral cancer are found in the floor of the mouth, on the lateral (posterior) and ventral (anterior) surfaces of the tongue, and on the soft palate and surrounding tissues. Carcinomas that develop next to bone tend to be generally more difficult to manage because of their tendency to infiltrate into the bone. Lesions in the maxillary region have more of a tendency to metastasize than do those in the mandibular region. In general, the more posterior the location of a primary lesion in the oral cavity, the poorer is the patient's prognosis.

LABORATORY FINDINGS

The diagnosis of oral cancer is dependent on a microscopic examination by an oral or general pathologist of tissue taken from the lesion. The more undifferentiated the lesion, the more difficult it is to identify the tissue's origin.

Attempts have been made to use the nuclear DNA pattern of benign white lesions to predict which lesions might become malignant. In one study[21] image cytometry was used and three variables of chromatin pattern had an 86% predictive value for lesions that became malignant or remained benign.

MEDICAL AND SURGICAL MANAGEMENT

If an attempt for a cure or long-term survival is indicated, the lesion is best treated by surgery or irradiation, and, at times, a combination of these two techniques may be implemented. In a patient with an advanced lesion, for whom there is no chance for a cure or long-term survival, palliation may be gained through radiation therapy or chemotherapy. Some cancer treatment centers use a combination of radiation and chemotherapy for palliation, but it is not clear if significant benefits are provided by a combination of modalities.[30]

Other techniques are being evaluated for their effectiveness in treating oral cancer. Topical 5-fluorouracil and laser surgery have been used to treat carcinoma in situ.[18] Photodynamic therapy (PDT), using a photosensitizing drug, photofrin II, and 630 nm light from an argon dye laser has been in phase III of trials for several years.[4] PDT is being evaluated for treatment of early laryngeal carcinomas, carcinomas in situ, T1 tumors, and Kaposi's sarcoma of the oral cavity.

The selection of treatment method is based on the following: (1) size of the lesion, (2) location of the lesion, (3) presence of regional or distant spread, (4) general health status of the patient, and (5) degree of differentiation of the lesion based on histopathologic evaluation. In addition, the functional and cosmetic problems involved in rehabilitation may influence the selection of treatment, as may the acceptance of recommended procedures by the patient.

The international tumor-node-metastases (TNM) system of classification and staging of head and neck lesions is used to evaluate and classify a tumor's status.[3,16,30] This classification helps in the selection of treatment and allows for the comparison of treatment results from one center to another. Tables 24-9 and 24-10 summarize the international TNM system for classification and staging of oral carcinomas.

The goal in management of a patient with oral cancer is to provide maximum length of survival and improved quality of survival. This goal is achieved by the following means: (1) early detection of the primary lesion, (2) sound management of precancerous lesions, (3) use of effective therapeutic measures that will produce the least disabling and disfiguring changes, (4) early application of measures to facilitate full rehabilitation, and (5) selection of effective palliation procedures for the patient who cannot be cured.

The fact that little improvement in 5-year survival rates for oral cavity and pharyngeal cancers has occurred since 1970 is discouraging.[5] This may be due, in large part, to the greater number of patients still coming to treatment centers with advanced lesions. The early detection and referral of the patient with

TABLE 24-9

International TNM System of Classification and Staging of Oral Carcinomas

T—Size of primary tumor
  T1S, Carcinoma in situ
  T_1, Lesion less than 2 cm in diameter
  T_2, Lesion 2 to 4 cm in diameter
  T_3, Lesion greater than 4 cm in diameter
  T_4, Massive lesion with deep invasion
N—Regional lymph node involvement
  N_0, No palpable nodes
  N_1, Single node, homolateral, 3 to 6 cm, *or*
    Multiple nodes, homolateral, none over 6 cm
  N_3, Single or multiple homolateral nodes, one
    greater than 6 cm in diameter, *or* Bilateral
    nodes (stage each side of neck), *or*
    Contralateral node(s)
M—Metastases
  M_0, No known distant metastasis
  M_1, Distant metastasis—PUL (pulmonary), OSS
  (osseous), HEP (hepatic), BRA (brain)

TABLE 24-10

International TNM System for Staging of Oral Carcinomas

Stage	Classification
I	T_1, N_0, M_0
II	T_2, N_0, M_0
III	T_3, N_0, M_0
	T_1, T_2, or T_3, N_1, M_0
IV	T_4, N_0, N_1, M_0
	Any T, N_2, N_3, M_0
	Any T, any N, M_1

T, tumor; *N*, node; *M*, metastasis.

oral cancer must be a high priority for all physicians and dentists.

The pretreatment management of the patient with oral carcinoma involves procedures to rule out the presence of distant metastases to the liver, lung, bone, brain, etc. The patient's general health status is determined, as is his or her nutritional status. If surgery is indicated, a preoperative evaluation regarding the construction of a prosthodontic appliance may be needed, which would include impressions, etc. The method of treatment selected depends on a number of factors, as previously described. Each of the treatment methods will be discussed in general terms.

SURGERY

Surgical treatment for oral cancer is indicated for tumors that are not radiosensitive, for recurrences in already irradiated areas where the side effects of radiation would be more severe than surgical defects, and when the tumor involves bone, lymph nodes, or salivary glands.[25,29] The primary advantage in the surgical removal of a cancerous lesion is that the margins can be examined to ensure that the lesion has been removed completely. Other advantages are that the treatment is given at a

single time and usually results in few problems to the patient once healing has occurred. The major disadvantage of surgery for the treatment of oral cancer occurs when the extent of surgery needed to remove the lesion results in major functional and cosmetic problems to the patient. In addition, surgery carries certain risks in terms of morbidity and mortality.

In general, a patient with a small- to moderate-sized lesion that shows no evidence of metastasis is treated by surgery. Primary closure is performed with small lesions located in movable tissue; secondary healing will occur with lesions over bone, such as on the hard palate, as long as there was no evidence of bone involvement by the tumor. Larger lesions may require grafting to manage the surgical defect.[3,29]

A patient with a small- to moderate-sized lesion that has invaded bone is usually treated by surgical means. A patient with a small- to moderate-sized lesion with regional metastases will be treated by surgical removal of the primary tumor in continuity with a radical neck dissection. However, those individuals with a large primary lesion for whom no chance of long-term survival is possible are not candidates for surgery; in addition, those with bilateral node involvement or distant metastases are not treated by surgical means. In a few selected patients with large lesions, surgery may be used as a palliative measure.

A patient with squamous cell carcinoma of the tongue or floor of the mouth who has no clinical evidence of metastases is often treated by surgical removal of the primary tumor and a "prophylactic" neck dissection. The neck dissection also may be done when the primary tumor is treated by radiation techniques.

The reason for the prophylactic neck dissection is that studies indicate about 30% to 35% of the patients who initially are seen with no clinical evidence of metastasis develop metastases following treatment of the primary tumor. A patient who under these circumstances has had a prophylactic neck dissection has about a 40% chance of one or more lymph nodes being microscopically positive for squamous cell carcinoma. If the primary lesion is treated by radiation, the neck dissection is usually performed about 2 weeks following completion of the radiotherapy.[3,30]

In general, patients with oral cancer presenting with a clinically negative neck who are initially treated with elective neck dissections show better survival rates than do similar patients undergoing a later (salvage) neck dissection.[19]

RADIATION

The primary advantage of radiotherapy for treatment of oral cancer is the preservation of normal tissues and function. However, disadvantages include the following[30]: (1) treatment is prolonged over several weeks; (2) radiation injury may occur to surrounding normal tissues; and (3) there is a long-term potential for induction of a new lesion. The larger and deeper the lesion, the more radiation needed to treat the patient.

Squamous cell carcinomas of the lip, buccal mucosa, soft palate, tongue, and/or floor of the mouth are often treated by radiation; primary lesions of the alveolar ridge and hard palate are less often treated by radiation. A patient with a recurrent tumor following surgery is usually treated by radiation. Combination therapy using radiation and surgery is used, but at present it is not clear if increased survival is obtained. A patient with advanced oral cancer often undergoes radiotherapy for palliation.[20,30]

Three methods of radiation therapy are used[6]: (1) interstitial, (2) implantation, and (3) external beam. Implantation techniques are used for small, superficial lesions. Interstitial methods can be used with carcinoma of the tongue or with large primary lesions prior to treatment with external beam cobalt-60. A protective prosthesis can be used during certain forms of radiation therapy (interstitial and implantation) to reduce radiation exposure to noncancerous tissues.[22] External beam techniques (Table 24-11) are the most common method of radiotherapy used for oral cancer. The superficial lesions are treated through a single field, whereas larger and/or deeper lesions are usually treated with multiple fields to reduce the amount of radiation to normal tissues and to concentrate a maximum amount of radiation on the tumor site. Cobalt-60 is the most common source used for external beam irradiation of large and/or deep oral cancers.

The usual dosage ranges from 5000 to 7000 rads, given in separate doses of 150 to 200 rads over a 6-to-7-week period with 4 or 5 treatment days followed by 2 or 3 nontreatment days.[16,20] Radiotherapy can be followed by some significant complications depending on the normal tissues that are in the path of the radiation beam. Table 24-12 lists the effects of radiother-

TABLE 24-11
Types of External Beams Used for the Treatment of Oral Cancer

Energy level	Terminology	Source	Clinical use
80 to 150 kV	Low voltage	X-ray	Superficial lesions
150 to 400 kV	Orthovoltage	X-ray	Skin tumors
500 kV to 8 meV	Supervoltage	Cobalt-60	Deeper lesions
8 to 200 meV	Megavoltage	Linear accelerator, betatron	Larger lesions
10 to 15 meV	Electron beam	Electrical	Superficial lesions

From Rothwell BR. In Hooley JR, Daun LC, editors: *Hospital dental practice*, St Louis, 1980, CV Mosby, p 265.

TABLE 24-12

Radiation Effect on Normal Tissues in the Path of the External Beam

Mucosa
    Epithelial changes (atrophy)
    Vascular changes
    Intimal thickening
    Luminal stenosis
    Obliteration
    Decreased blood flow
Muscle
    Fibrosis
    Vascular changes
Bone
    Decreased numbers of osteocytes
    Decreased numbers of osteoblasts
    Vascular changes (decreased blood flow)
Salivary glands
    Atrophy of acini
    Vascular changes
    Fibrosis
Pulp (necrosis [orthovoltage])

TABLE 24-13

Complications of Radiotherapy

Nausea and vomiting (early onset)
Mucositis—starts about second week
Taste alteration—starts about second week
Xerostomia—starts about third week
Secondary infections (fungal, bacterial, viral)
Radiation caries (delayed onset)
Hypersensitive teeth (early and delayed onset)
Muscular dysfunction (delayed onset)
Osteoradionecrosis (delayed onset)
    More common in mandible
    Less common in maxilla
Pulpal pain and necrosis (delayed onset)
    (orthovoltage, not found with cobalt-60)

apy on different tissues, and Table 24-13 describes the complications that can result. These will be discussed in detail in the section on dental management of the cancer patient.

Several new techniques are being used in radiotherapy for head and neck lesions.[25] Treatment with a beam of heavy charged particles (neutrons) termed *linear energy transfer* is now being tested. Radiosensitizers are being used to sensitize hypoxic tumor cells to the effects of irradiation, and analogs of thymidine are being used in an attempt to increase the sensitivity of tumor cells to radiation. Radioprotective compounds are being tested in an attempt to decrease radiation injury to normal tissues; in addition, hyperthermia is being tested in an attempt to reduce the radiation dosage needed to kill tumor cells.[25]

CHEMOTHERAPY

Chemotherapy is used for palliative care in a patient with advanced squamous cell carcinoma. The agents are given systemically or infused on a local or regional basis. Most chemotherapeutic agents will cause breakdown of the mucous membranes (mucositis) and depression of the bone marrow (infection, bleeding, anemia), produce gastrointestinal changes (diarrhea, malabsorption), and induce cardiac and pulmonary dysfunctions (Table 24-14). The drugs most often used for treatment of advanced squamous cell carcinoma are methotrexate, 5-fluorouracil, cisplatin, and bleomycin. Agents that have been used in combination with radiation include hydroxyurea, bleomycin, or 5-fluorouracil. Several agents have been tried in combination— such as 5-fluorouracil and cisplatin, methotrexate and 5-fluorouracil, and cisplatin and bleomycin.[20,23,25]

PRETREATMENT PREPARATION

The larger cancer treatment centers have a team that deals with head and neck cancer patients. The head and neck tumor board usually consists of a radiation oncologist, a head and neck surgeon, a dentist, and a medical oncologist, who evaluate the patient and recommend the most appropriate treatment. Alternatives, if available, also are discussed with the patient, and the risks and complications of treatment are explained. Once the patient has accepted the recommendations, he or she is prepared for receiving treatment. In cases with small superficial lesions that require only local excision, this step is simple; however, for the patient needing major surgical resection and reconstruction, thorough counseling becomes much more complex and important.

The patient needing extensive surgery will be sent for consultation to a maxillofacial prosth-

TABLE 24-14
Effects of Chemotherapy

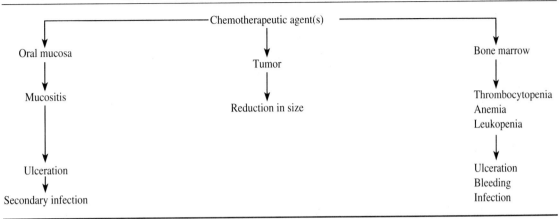

odontist, dentist, speech pathologist, and psychologist. Presurgical casts will be made and recommendations explained to the patient as to the types of prostheses that can be constructed and the types of surgical preparation that might be needed. The patient is told about the problems that will occur with speech, etc. and what steps will be taken after surgery to help overcome these problems. A psychologic evaluation of the patient will be made to serve as a basis for counseling concerning any emotional problems to be faced during rehabilitation.

Following surgery, the psychologist will help the patient deal with psychologic problems that are common to major cancer surgery — including (1) concern about recurrence of the tumor, (2) disappointment over the changes in body function and body image, (3) mourning for the lost body part, (4) alarm at the disfigurement, (5) a tendency to withdraw from friends and family, and (6) a loss of self-esteem. The psychologist will also help the patient cope with the anxiety and/or depression these problems cause.[30]

All members of the treatment team can help patients during the surgical and postsurgical periods by letting them know that it is acceptable to resent the way they feel and that these feelings are normal and appropriate. The anxiety or depression needs to be acknowledged and legitimized. The patient must feel supported and accepted as a person of worth and value. Every attempt should be made to restore function or replace the lost part. Finally, voca-

tional counseling and contact with a social worker may be needed to help the patient return to society as a contributing, worthwhile person.[30]

A patient who needs radiotherapy must be seen by a dentist before the start of treatment. The status of the dentition and oral hygiene level must be evaluated, necessary extractions performed, and large carious lesions restored. The role of the dentist will be discussed in the following section of this chapter.

Once treatment has been completed, the oral cancer patient must be placed on a recall program. Usually, the patient is seen once every month during the first year, once every 2 months during the second year, once every 4 months during the third year, and once every 6 months during the fourth and fifth years. After 5 years the patient should be examined at least once per year. This recall program is important for the following reasons[20,24,25,30]: (1) a patient with one oral cancer tends to develop additional lesions because of the "field" effect, (2) latent metastases may develop, (3) the initial lesions may recur, and (4) complications related to therapy can be detected and managed.

DENTAL MANAGEMENT OF THE ORAL CANCER PATIENT
GENERAL CONSIDERATIONS

One of the most important roles the dentist plays in the management of a cancer patient relates to early detection of the lesion. A head and neck examination and an intraoral soft tissue examination should be performed on each dental patient as he or she enters the practice. This exam, which takes only a few minutes and may save the life of the patient with an "early" cancerous lesion, should be repeated on a regular basis as often as possible but at least during dental recall visits.

A patient who comes in with a lesion that appears clinically to be cancerous or a patient who has a less obviously cancerous lesion but has hard, fixed, and/or matted lymph nodes should be referred directly to a cancer treatment center or to a head and neck surgeon in the community (Fig. 24-1). The patient should be told of the concern that he or she may have a serious problem and immediate evaluation by specialists is necessary. If the patient seems willing to talk, the concern about cancer should be discussed, with the benefits of prompt diagnosis and treatment strongly emphasized. The patient should be dealt with in an honest and direct manner, with as many questions answered as possible. The patient should be asked if he or she has a preference concerning a cancer treatment center; if not, the dentist should be prepared to recommend one and, if possible, phone the center to make an appointment for the patient. This should be followed by a letter to the physician in charge to introduce the patient and describe the findings and clinical impression. If the spouse is present, it is usually advisable to share your findings; however in rare cases it may be best to withhold the clinical diagnosis from the patient and share it with a member of the family.

TREATMENT PLANNING MODIFICATIONS

Dental treatment planning for the patient with oral cancer begins when the lesion has been found and a diagnosis established. Planning involves the pretreatment evaluation and preparation of the patient, the posttreatment management of the patient, and the long-term management from a dental standpoint.

Pretreatment evaluation

The dentist needs to become aware of the type of treatment being selected for the patient and whether the lesion stands a good chance of being controlled (Table 24-15). A patient who is going to receive palliative therapy may not want replacement therapy for missing teeth; however, it is important that this patient be free of active dental disease. By contrast, a patient who has an early lesion with no evidence of regional spread that will be treated by local excision can be managed for future dental care as a normal patient. An exception is that the dentist will recall this patient for more frequent examinations for evidence of metastases, recurrence of

TABLE 24-15
Distribution and Relative 5-Year Survival by Subsite and Extent of Disease*

	Cases†	Localized		Regional		Distant		Total survival (%)
		Distribution (%)	Survival (%)	Distribution (%)	Survival (%)	Distribution (%)	Survival (%)	
Lip	2645	90	89	7	57	1	‡	86
Tongue	3414	44	52	40	22	12	7	33
Floor of mouth	2146	44	65	44	31	8	18	45
Other oral cancers	2362	49	61	36	29	11	18	44

*Ratio of survival rate to rate expected of individuals in the general population with the same age, sex, race, and calendar year of observation.
†White patients only.
‡Number of cases too small to yield reliable data.
From US Department of Health, Education, and Welfare: *Management guidelines for head and neck cancer*, Public Health Service Publ. no. 80-2037. 1979.

the lesion, or presence of a new cancer. Studies[25] have shown that a patient with cancer of the oral cavity is at increased risk for a second primary cancer in the respiratory system, upper digestive tract, or oral cavity. The risk for a second oral cancer in smokers whose habits remained unchanged is about 30% as compared with 13% for those who quit.

PRETREATMENT CONSIDERATIONS FOR RADIATION PATIENTS

There are several important dental considerations for the patient with oral cancer who is going to receive radiation therapy. If the beam will pass through the jaws and/or major salivary glands, the patient will be liable to development of osteoradionecrosis and radiation caries. Potential sources of infection to the radiated bone must be treated or removed prior to initiation of radiation therapy.

Before radiotherapy the following recommendations apply:

The patient with broken-down teeth that are nonrestorable or a patient who has no interest in saving teeth should have them extracted.

The patient with advanced periodontal disease should have the teeth removed. Nonvital teeth should be endodontically treated or extracted, and all active carious lesions should be restored.

Chronic inflammatory lesions in the jaws should be examined and treated. To allow for adequate wound healing, extractions and other surgical procedures should be performed at least 2 weeks before the start of radiotherapy.

There still appears to be some risk for osteoradionecrosis if teeth are extracted 14 days before the start of radiotherapy.[8] This risk may be reduced to zero if extractions are performed 21 or more days before the therapy is started. The bone at the wound margins should be trimmed to eliminate sharp edges and allow for primary closure of the wound.[8]

Patients who will be retaining their teeth must be informed concerning the problems associated with decreased salivary function, which includes xerostomia and radiation caries[16,30] (Table 24-16). Radiation caries (Fig. 24-9) can progress quickly; and if pulpal tissues become

TABLE 24-16
Causes of Radiation Caries

Decreased salivary flow
Change in quality of saliva (decreased buffering capacity)
Poor oral hygiene
Changes in oral flora

infected and the infection extends to the surrounding irradiated bone, extensive infection and necrosis can result. The importance of effective hygiene procedures and the maintenance of good oral hygiene must be emphasized.

Impressions should be made so custom trays can be constructed of soft flexible mouth guard material. These trays are used to hold 5 to 10 drops of a 1% to 2% acidulated fluoride gel, which should be inserted into the mouth for 5 minutes each day, with the fluoride application following cleaning by a toothbrush and dental floss. When the tray is taken out of the mouth, any excess gel left in the mouth can be spit out. If the 1% to 2% acidulated gel is found to be irritating to the tissues, an equal amount of 0.5% neutral sodium fluoride gel should be substituted.[10,16,20] A major weakness of the above approach is poor patient compliance. Attempts must be made to educate patients concerning the complications associated with radiotherapy and to motivate them in use of the aforementioned preventive techniques.[8]

PRETREATMENT CONSIDERATION FOR SURGICAL PATIENTS

Dental preparation of the oral cancer patient who is going to be treated by surgery is not as critical as for the radiation patient. However, active oral infection should be treated, teeth that are broken down should be removed, and teeth that may be utilized for the retention of a prosthetic appliance can be restored as needed. The better the dental health of the patient, the lower will be the risk of dental infection complicating the healing process. When possible, the dentist should be in direct consultation with the maxillofacial prosthodontist so proper coordination of the patient's dental and tool-replacement needs can occur during the presurgical and postsurgical phases.

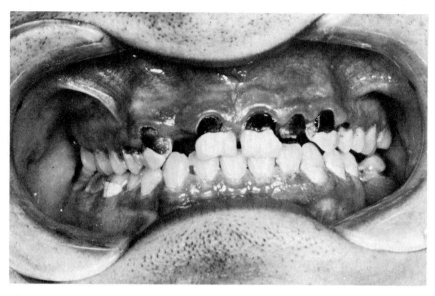

FIG. 24-9 Note the extensive cervical caries in a patient who received radiotherapy. (Courtesy R. Gorlin, D.D.S., Minneapolis Minn.)

ORAL COMPLICATIONS AND THEIR MANAGEMENT

In this section the oral complications associated with the treatment of oral cancer will be considered from the standpoint of what the dentist can offer to minimize discomfort of the patient and how future dental complications related to the altered oral environment can be prevented and/or dealt with if they occur. The section on radiation complications applies to all head and neck tumors treated by radiation in which the oral mucosa, jaw bones, or major salivary glands have been irradiated. The section on chemotherapy complications has been expanded to include the complications associated with agents used in the treatment of leukemia, lymphoma, and squamous cell carcinoma.

Surgical complications

The functional and cosmetic problems caused by major surgical procedures can be best managed by presurgical preparation and planning. Prosthetic appliances can be constructed once healing has occurred, and transitional appliances can be fabricated if additional surgical procedures are needed to prepare the site for

construction of the "final" prosthetic replacement device.

Radiation complications and their management

MUCOSITIS

Table 24-12 lists the effects of radiotherapy on different oral tissues, and Table 24-13 presents the complications that may result. A radiation dose of 180 rads per week will usually not cause a mucositis; by contrast, a dose of 220 rads per week will almost always cause mucositis.[26] During radiotherapy the patient often will develop a mucositis (Fig. 24-10). Breakdown of the oral mucosa begins about the second week and usually subsides a few weeks following the completion of treatment. The mucositis results in ulceration, pain, dysphagia, loss of taste, and difficulty in eating. If the major salivary glands have been irradiated, xerostomia will follow the initial onset of mucositis. This complication of mucositis and xerostomia makes the patient uncomfortable and increases the difficulty of maintaining proper nutritional intake. During this acute phase the patient can be managed by use of the following[8,10,20,23,26]: (1) a bland mouth rinse to keep ulcerated areas as clean as possi-

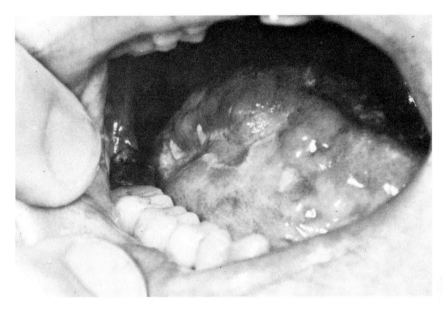

FIG. 24-10 Extensive mucositis that developed from the effects of radiation on the oral mucosa. (Courtesy R. Gorlin, D.D.S., Minneapolis Minn.)

ble, (2) an antihistamine solution to serve as a topical anesthetic agent (for pain control) combined with milk of magnesia or Kaopectate to serve as a coating agent (for protection of the ulcerated areas), (3) topical steroids to reduce the inflammatory reaction, (4) adequate hydration, (5) no alcohol or tobacco, (6) a diet with soft foods, protein supplements, and vitamin supplementation at therapeutic levels, (7) oral lubricants (Xero-Lube), (8) no irritating food (e.g, citrus fruits and juices, hot spicy dishes), (9) humidified air (humidifiers or vaporizers), (10) small portable filtering appliances to remove smoke from rooms, and (11) no lip balms that are petrolatum based; instead, a water-based, beeswax-based, or vegetable oil–based lubricant (e.g., Surgi-Lube) should be used. A patient who wears dentures will be much more comfortable if the dentures are not worn during this acute phase (Table 24-17).

Once the mucositis has healed, long-term management of the patient involves dealing with the chronic xerostomia, loss of taste, altered bone, and related problems.

XEROSTOMIA

Salivary function will return to normal in many irradiated patients in several months following completion of radiotherapy; however, in some patients it may take 6 to 12 months, and in others salivary function does not return.

Chronic xerostomia can be managed first by using techniques to attempt to stimulate the endogenous secretion of saliva (e.g., sugarless lemon drops or a sorbitol-based chewing gum). If the radiation damage to the salivary glands is too extensive, salivary substitutes such as a buffered solution of glycerin and water, Xero-Lube, Saliv-Aid, or Moistior can be used.[8,10,25,30,31] However, most investigators[25] find that the synthetic saliva solutions are not satisfactory for relief of the complaints associated with chronic xerostomia.

Silverman[25] has stated that patients with severe chronic xerostomia have improved using 5 mg of pilocarpine four times per day. Recent studies[8] have shown pilocarpine to be effective in relieving symptoms and improving salivary flow. In these studies the dosage ranged from 15 to 30 mg per day. Epstein[12] reported significant increase in parotid salivary flow rate and improved subjective symptoms in patients with severe chronic xerostomia treated with antholetrithrone (ANTT) 25 mg three times per day followed 1 week later by adding 2 drops of a 1% solution of pilocarpine four times a day on

TABLE 24-17

Management of the Patient with Oral
Complications of Radiotherapy*

Mucositis
  Sodium bicarbonate mouthwash
  Elixir of diphenhydramine (Benadryl)
  Topical steroids
  Milk of magnesia
  Orabase
  Avoid tobacco and alcohol
  Soft diet
  Maintain hydration
  Avoid irritating foods
  Use humidifier, vaporizer
Xerostomia
  Sugarless lemon drops
  Sorbitol-based chewing gum
  Buffered solution of glycerine and water
  Salivary substitutes
  Pilocarpine
Radiation caries
  Oral hygiene procedures
  Topical fluoride gel
  Frequent dental recall
  Restore early carious lesions
Secondary infection
  Culture
  Cytologic study
  Antibiotics
  Antifungal agents
  Acyclovir
Sensitivity of teeth
  Topical fluorides
Loss of taste
  Zinc supplementation
Osteoradionecrosis
  Avoid trauma to mucosa
  Avoid extractions
  Irrigate with saline, antibiotics
  Hyperbaric oxygen, tetracycline antibiotics
  Resection
Muscular dysfunction
  Tongue blades to help retain maximum
    opening of jaws and access to oral cavity

*See Appendix B for medications, dosage, and duration
of use.

the tongue. ANTT and pilocarpine were suggested[12] to act synergistically to improve salivary flow; however, more thorough clinical studies are needed to establish the real benefit of any of these combination agents.

Patients should avoid wearing their dentures during the first 6 months following completion of the radiotherapy because mild trauma to the altered mucosa can result in ulcerations and possible necrosis of underlying bone. Once they start to wear the dentures, they must be told to come to the dentist if any sore spots develop so the dentures can be adjusted. Ill-fitting dentures should be replaced by new ones. In severe cases of chronic xerostomia a small amount of petrolatum can be applied to the mucosal surface of the denture.

SECONDARY INFECTIONS

During radiation therapy patients may develop secondary oral infections. Candidiasis is a common complication. Ctyologic study and/or culture should be used to confirm secondary infection with *Candida albicans.* Nystatin oral suspension, nystatin vaginal tablets, clotrimazole (Mycelex), ketoconazole tablets, or fluconazole tablets may be prescribed to treat candidiasis. (See Appendix A for dosages and duration of therapy.) Bacteria and viruses also may be the cause of secondary infections in patients undergoing radiotherapy. Culture techniques should be used to identify the causative organism(s) and then appropriate treatment should be rendered, including antibiotics or acyclovir for extensive secondary viral infection. Antibiotic sensitivity testing may be considered in patients with extensive infection or for those in poor general health.

SENSITIVITY OF TEETH

During and following radiotherapy the teeth may become hypersensitive, which could be related to the decreased secretion of saliva and the lowered pH of secreted saliva. The topical application of a fluoride gel may be of benefit in reducing these symptoms.[10]

TASTE

In most patients the ability to taste will return in 3 to 4 months following completion of radiotherapy. In cases of chronic loss of taste, zinc supplementation has been reported to improve taste perceptions. Silverman[25] recommends 220 mg of zinc two times per day for patients with severe chronic loss of taste.

OSTEONECROSIS

The risk for osteonecrosis following radiotherapy increases with largers doses of radiation to bone and especially with doses in excess of 7000 rads. Edentulous patients have a lower risk for osteonecrosis than do dentulous patients. The greatest risk is for patients whose mandible has received large doses of radiation and who require tooth extraction some time following the completion of radiotherapy.

A patient who has retained his or her teeth following radiotherapy must continue the maintenance of good oral hygiene, which includes a daily brushing, flossing, and in some cases the continued use of daily fluoride gel applications using the custom trays made prior to irradiation. All carious lesions should be treated when first detected. Frequent recall of the patient is a must for reinforcement of hygiene procedures and detection of oral disease that could involve bone and lead to necrosis. The risk of bone infection and necrosis is much greater with extraction of teeth than with endodontic therapy. Thus, if the pulp has become infected, endodontic therapy is the preferred treatment, assuming that the tooth is restorable.

The use of prophylactic antibiotics to prevent infection following surgical procedures in postradiation patients is suggested; however, the effectiveness of such coverage can be greatly reduced because of altered blood flow to the affected bone. The reduction in blood flow following radiotherapy is much greater in the mandible than the maxilla because of the limited source and lack of collateral circulation, which accounts for the greater frequency and severity of osteoradionecrosis in the mandible. The use of hyperbaric oxygen treatment at the time of extraction is gaining more support, but its benefit remains to be proven.[8]

Once necrosis occurs, conservative management is usually indicated. The exposed bone can be irrigated with a saline or antibiotic solution and the patient directed to use oral irrigating devices to clean the involved area; however, extreme pressures should be avoided when these devices are prescribed. Severe cases may benefit from hyperbaric oxygen treatment (in a hyperbaric "chamber"). Tetracycline antibiotics also can be prescribed. Cases that do not respond to conservative measures may require surgical resection of the involved bone.[3,8,16,20,25]

In one study[25] 16 of 22 cases of osteonecrosis were managed with nonsurgical techniques. Four cases (18%) healed within 3 to 24 months, ten cases (63%) persisted but did not progress, and two cases (9%) required surgical resection because of progression of the necrosis. Six (27%) of the twenty-two cases required surgical resection as the initial treatment, and three of these patients had recurrence of osteonecrosis.[25]

MUSCLE TRISMUS

To minimize the effects of radiation on the muscles around the face and the muscles of mastication, a mouth block should be placed when the patient is receiving external beam irradiation; the patient should also be given a number of tongue blades to place in the mouth several times each day. These procedures will minimize muscle contracture and allow for more normal function and access to the oral cavity.[30]

CHEMOTHERAPY COMPLICATIONS AND MANAGEMENT

Bone marrow suppression and mucositis associated with chemotherapy are predictible, dose-dependent, and usually manageable. The patient receiving chemotherapy for treatment of leukemia, lymphoma, or palliation of oral cancer may manifest erythema and ulceration of the oral mucosa, infection of the surrounding tissues, excessive bleeding with minor trauma, xerostomia, anemia, and neurotoxicity.[8,10,20,23,25]

Before starting chemotherapy, all areas of infection or sources of oral infection—such as teeth with pulpal and periapical pathologic findings, periodontal abscesses, pericoronitis, advanced carious lesions, or advanced periodontal disease—need to be treated. Measures such as plaque control, calculus removal, and a complete prophylaxis with oral hygiene instructions must be initiated before chemotherapy is started. In children being treated for leukemia, mobile primary teeth and those expected to be lost during chemotherapy should be extracted, and gingival opercula should be surgically removed to prevent entrapment of food debris.

Orthodontic bands should be removed prior to starting chemotherapy.

Once chemotherapy begins, the dentist must consult with the oncologist before any invasive dental procedures are performed. The white blood cell count and platelet status must be determined. In general, routine dental procedures can be performed if the granulocyte count is greater than 2000/mm³ and the platelet count greater than 40,000/mm³.[11]

When the granulocyte count is less than 2000/mm³, antibiotic prophylaxis is recommended[11] if invasive dental procedures must be performed. These levels usually occur when the patient is in the hospital and will not be encountered in the general practice setting. If the white cell count is declining (patient has just started chemotherapy) and the granulocyte count is already below 2000/mm³, invasive dental procedures are contraindicated. The use of prophylactic antibiotics for these patients is rational but without scientific evidence of effectiveness. The potential adverse effects of antibiotics should be kept in mind when making the decision to use them. There is no standard antibiotic regimen recommended for prophylaxis. The drug(s), duration, and dosage to be used for prophylaxis should be established in consultation with the patient's oncologist. Penicillin V, 500 mg, every 6 hours starting at least 1 hour before any procedure that involves bone, pulp, or periodontium and continuing for 2 to 3 days has been recommended.[9,10] The American Heart Association endocarditis prophylaxis regimen has been suggested for patients with indwelling catheters.[16] By contrast, other authors[11] have suggested 30 minutes before the dental procedure giving the patient ticarcillin disodium, 75 mg/kg, by intravenous infusion and gentamicin sulfate, 1.5 mg/kg, by intravenous infusion. This regimen is then repeated 6 hours after the first dose.

Care must be taken to prevent excessive blood loss following invasive dental procedures in patients with platelet counts below 40,000/mm³.[11] Again, consultation with the patient's oncologist is a must. Platelet replacement may be indicated if the dental procedure must be performed, and topical therapy using pressure, thrombin, microfibrillar collagen, and splints may be required.

In general, routine dental care when needed is best provided on the day before the patient is to receive a drug treatment.[10] Mucosal mouth guards may be constructed to help control spontaneous gingival bleeding and to facilitate patient comfort. Custom-made carriers for fluoride gel application in caries control should be utilized and patients encouraged to maintain excellent oral hygiene, brushing teeth with a soft nylon brush and flossing on a regular basis. When the gingivae bleed easily and/or the white cell count is low, the patient should stop

TABLE 24-18

Dental Management of the Patient Receiving Chemotherapy for Leukemia, Lymphoma, or Oral Squamous Cell Carcinoma*

Prior to starting chemotherapy

Eliminate infection (periapical, gingival, periodontal)
Treat advanced carious lesions
Institute periodontal disease control
Provide oral hygiene instructions
Remove mobile primary teeth in children
Remove gingival opercula in children and young adults

During chemotherapy

Consult with oncologist before any invasive dental procedure
Administer antibiotic prophylaxis if granulocyte count less than 2000/mm³
Consider possible platelet replacement if platelet count less than 40,000/mm³
Culture areas of suspected infection
Control spontaneous bleeding (gauze, periodontal packing, mouth guard)
Prescribe topical fluoride for caries control
Provide home care instructions (modify based on oral status)
Provide symptomatic relief of mucositis and xerostomia
Avoid general anesthesia, etc if severe anemia present

Following chemotherapy

Watch patient until all side effects to therapy have cleared
Place patient on dental recall schedule

*See Appendix B for medications, dosage, and duration of use.

brushing the teeth and clean them using gauze wrapped around the finger and dampened in warm water. During this stage patients should be instructed not to use toothpicks, water-irrigating appliances, or dental floss[10] (Table 24-18).

Dentures must not be worn at night or while sleeping, and should be brushed daily with a dental brush and denture cleaner. When not being used, they should be cleaned, rinsed, and stored in a denture-soaking solution. If denture sores develop or the mucosa is ulcerated, the dentures should not be worn until adjusted by a dentist or until the mucositis has healed.[10]

There is little evidence for taste or olfactory losses produced by chemotherapy. However, many patients receiving these agents complain of bitter tastes, unpleasant odors, and conditioned aversions to foods.[8] The bitter taste and odors may be due to the chemotherapeutic agents themselves. To avoid conditioned aversion to foods, the following are suggested: (1) eat a novel food not important to the diet about 10 to 15 minutes before chemotherapy; (2) nutritionally important foods should not be consumed until the nausea completely ends; (3) before treatment, fast for about 4 hours; (4) educate the patient about food aversions.

For the management of complications associated with mucositis and xerostomia, refer to the section dealing with these problems in the radiation section above (pp. 476 to 479).

REFERENCES

1. Abdel-Salam M, Mayell BH, Chew K, et al: Which oral white lesions will become malignant? An image cytometric study, *Oral Surg* 69:345-350, 1990.
2. American Cancer Society: *Cancer—facts and figures,* New York, 1984, The Society.
3. Archer WH: *Oral and maxillofacial surgery,* ed 5, Philadelphia, 1975, WB Saunders.
4. Biel MA: Photodynamic therapy, phase III trial for treatment of various cancers. Personal communication, 1992.
5. Boring CC, Squires TS, Tong T: Cancer statistics, 1992, *CA* 42(1):19-38, 1992.
6. Chang F, Syrjanen S, Kellokoski J, Syrjanen K: Human papillomavirus (HPV) infections and their association with oral disease, *J Oral Pathol Med* 20(7):305-317, 1991.
7. Christen AG, McDonald JL, Christen JA: *The impact of tobacco use and cessation on non-malignant and precancerous oral and dental diseases and conditions,* Indianapolis, June 1991, Indiana University School of Dentistry, pp 25-41.
8. Consensus Development Conference: *Oral complications of cancer therapies: diagnosis, prevention, and treatment.* National Cancer Institute monograph no. 9, Washington DC, 1990, United States Department of Health and Human Services.
9. Council on Scientific Affairs: Health effects of smokeless tobacco, *JAMA* 256:1038-1043, 1986.
10. Curators of the University of Missouri: *Oral management of the cancer patient: a guide for the health care professional,* Kansas City, 1981, The University.
11. DePaola LG, Peterson DE, Overholser CD Jr, et al: Dental care for patients receiving chemotherapy, *J Am Dent Assoc* 112:198-203, 1986.
12. Epstein JB: Synergistic effect of sialogogues in management of xerostomia following radiation therapy, *Oral Surg* 64:179-182, 1987.
13. Eversole R: The human papillomaviruses and oral mucosal disease. (Editorial.) *Oral Surg* 71:700, 1991.
14. Gerson SJ: Oral cancer, *Crit Rev Oral Biol Med* 1(3):153-166, 1990.
15. Harrison LB, Fass DE: Radiation therapy for oral cavity cancer, *Dent Clin North A* 34:205-222, 1990.
16. Hooley JR, Daun G: *Hospital dental practice,* St Louis, 1980, CV Mosby.
17. Krogh P: The role of yeasts in oral cancer by means of endogenous nitrosation, *Acta Odontol Scand* 48:85-88, 1990.
18. Maxson BB, Scott RF, Headington JT: Management of oral squamous cell carcinoma in situ with topical 5-fluorouracil and laser surgery, *Oral Surg* 68:44-48, 1989.
19. Mayers EN, Cunningham MJ: Treatments of choice for early carcinoma of the oral cavity, *Oncology* 2(2):18-31, 1988.
20. Million RR, Cassisi MJ, editors: *Management of head and neck cancer,* Philadelphia, 1984, JB Lippincott.
21. Penn I: Occurrence of cancers in immunosuppressed organ transplant recipients. In Terasaki P, ed: *Clinical transplants,* Los Angeles, 1990, UCLA Tissue Typing Laboratory, pp 53-62.
22. Poole TS, Flaxman NA: Use of protective prostheses during radiation therapy, *J Am Dent Assoc* 112:485-488, 1986.
23. Rosenberg SW: Oral care of chemotherapy patients, *Dent Clin North Am* 34:239-250, 1990.
24. Shafer WG, Hine MK, Levy BM: *A textbook of oral pathology,* ed 4, Philadelphia, 1983, WB Saunders.
25. Silverman S Jr, editor: *Oral cancer,* ed 2, New York, 1985, American Cancer Society.
26. Silverman S Jr, Gorsky M, Lozada F: Oral leukoplakia and malignant transformation; a follow-up study of 257 patients, *Cancer* 53:563-568, 1984.
27. Silverman S Jr, Migliorati C, Barbosa J: Toluidine blue staining in the detection of oral precancerous and malignant lesions, *Oral Surg* 57:379-383, 1984.
28. Steele C, Shillitoe EJ: Viruses and oral cancer, *Crit Rev Oral Biol Med* 2(2):153-175, 1991.

29. Strong E: Surgical management of oral cancer, *Dent Clin North Am* 34:185-203, 1990.
30. US Department of Health, Education, and Welfare: *Management guidelines for head and neck cancer.* Public Health Service Publ. no. 80-2037, 1979.
31. Vergo TJ, Kadish SP: Dentures as artificial saliva reservoirs in the irradiated edentulous cancer patient with xerostomia, *Oral Surg* 51:229-233, 1981.
32. Watts SL, Brewer EE, Fry TL: Human papillomavirus DNA types in squamous cell carcinomas of the head and neck, *Oral Surg* 71:701-707, 1991.
33. Winn DM: Smokeless tobacco and cancer: the epidemiologic evidence, *CA* 38(4):236-243, 1988.
34. Zacharides N: Neoplasms metastatic to the mouth, jaws and surrounding tissues, *J Craniomaxillofac Surg* 17(6):283-290, 1989.

25

Behavioral and Psychiatric Disorders

Problems may be encountered in dental practice that stem from a patient's behavioral patterns rather than from physical conditions. A good dentist-patient relationship can reduce the number of behavioral problems encountered in practice as well as modify the intensity of emotional reactions to many problems. A positive dentist-patient relationship is based on mutual respect, trust, understanding, cooperation, and empathy. Role conflicts between the dentist and the patient should be avoided or identified and dealt with effectively. The anxious patient should be offered support that will minimize the damaging effects of anxiety, and the angry or uncooperative patient should be accepted and encouraged to share reasons for feelings and behavior and thus become a more peaceful and cooperative individual. Patients with emotional factors that contribute to oral or systemic diseases or symptoms and patients with more serious mental disorders can be managed in an understanding, safe, and empathetic manner.

The dentist may see patients with a variety of behavioral and mental disorders. The *Diagnostic and Statistical Manual of Mental Disorders*[11] presents a classification system with which the dentist should be familiar to be better able to understand psychiatric diagnoses and associated symptoms. This system consists of five axes (axis I through axis V) or categories used to describe mental disorders. Table 25-1 lists the five specific areas used to evaluate a patient's psychosocial health.[11] Table 25-2 lists the most frequent diagnoses encountered in axis I disorders[11]; and Table 25-3 shows the most frequent diagnoses encountered in axis II disorders.[11]

In this chapter certain aspects of the dentist-patient relationship will be explored as well as patients' reactions to illness and to the dentist. The identification and management of patients with anxiety, depression, and mental illness outlined in Table 25-4 also will be considered.

GENERAL DESCRIPTION
INCIDENCE AND PREVALENCE

Mental disorders are common in today's society. It is estimated that one third of the population in the United States will have at least one psychiatric disorder during their lifetime, and 20% of adults in the United States will suffer from one or more psychiatric disorders during a 6-month period. Six percent of the population suffer from serious affective or mood disorders. About 7% of the adult population have a serious drug abuse or dependency problem. Based on this data it is clear that the dentist will see patients not only with behavioral problems but also with more serious mental disorders. The dentist needs to be able to identify these individuals and deal with their specific dental needs, which in many cases may be significant.[15]

ANXIETY DISORDERS

Anxiety disorders constitute the most frequently found psychiatric problem in the general population. Simple phobia is the most common of the anxiety disorders; however, panic disorder is the most common anxiety disorder in people seeking medical treatment. About 1% to 2% of the population experience one or more panic attacks. Panic disorder, phobic disorders, and obsessive-compulsive disorders occur more frequently among first-

TABLE 25-1

System for Classification of Psychosocial Health

	Description
Axis I	Clinical syndromes
Axis II	Personality disorders
Axis III	Physical disorders and conditions
Axis IV	Severity of psychosocial stressors
Axis V	Highest level of adaptive functioning during last year

From *Diagnostic and statistical manual of mental disorders*, ed 3, revised, Washington DC, 1987, American Psychiatric Association.

degree relatives of people with these disorders than among the general population.[11] Also 4 million Americans served in the military in Asia from 1964 to 1975; of these individuals 1 million saw active combat. Over 500,000 veterans now have emotional problems, the most common being posttraumatic stress disorder (PTSD).[18]

MOOD DISORDERS

At any time about 5% of the adults in the United States have a significant mood disorder. Mood disorders are more common among women. Major depression may begin at any age and is evenly distributed throughout adult life. Twenty percent of the adult female population and 10% of the adult male population at some time will experience a major depressive episode. About one third of these individuals will require hospitalization, and 30% will develop a chronic course with residual symptoms and social impairment.[12] The 1-month prevalence of major depression is 2.9% in women and 1.6% in men. The prevalence of dysthymia, a chronic, milder form of depression, in women is 3.3%.[22] It is also estimated that 0.4% to 1.2% of the adult population in the United States have bipolar disorder.[9] In contrast to major depression, which is twice as common in females as in males, bipolar disorder occurs with equal frequency among both sexes.[11]

SOMATOFORM DISORDERS

Body dysmorphic disorder is more common than was previously thought. Conversion disorder was common 10 to 20 years ago but is now rarely seen.[11]

TABLE 25-2

Frequently Encountered Axis I Diagnoses

Diagnosis	Specifics
Organic mental disorders	Dementia
	Delirium
Substance use disorders	Cocaine
	Narcotics
	Alcohol
Schizophrenia	Affective disorders
	Major depression
	Bipolar disorder
Anxiety disorders	Phobias
	Panic disorders
	Posttraumatic stress disorder (PTSD)
Somatoform disorders	Conversion disorder
	Somatoform pain disorder

From *Diagnostic and statistical manual of mental disorders*, ed 3, revised, Washington DC, 1987, American Psychiatric Association.

TABLE 25-3

Frequently Encountered Axis II Personality Traits

	Specifics
Histrionic	Excess emotionality, attention seeking
Narcissistic	Grandiosity, hypersensitivity to evaluation by others, lack of empathy
Antisocial	Irresponsibility, antisocial behavior
Dependent	Dependency, submissiveness
Compulsive	Perfectionism, inflexibility
Passive-aggressive	Resistance to demands for adequate social and occupational performance

From *Diagnostic and statistical manual of mental disorders*, ed 3, revised, Washington DC, 1987, American Psychiatric Association.

PSYCHOLOGIC FACTORS AFFECTING PHYSICAL CONDITIONS

It is difficult to estimate the prevalence of physical conditions affected by psychologic factors. The list of examples of psychophysiologic conditions is long. Included in it would be disorders that are relatively common, like mi-

TABLE 25-4
Classification of Behavioral and Psychiatric Disorders

	Specifics
Anxiety disorders	Panic disorders
	Agoraphobia
	Social phobia*
	Obsessive-compulsive disorder*
	Posttraumatic stress disorder
	Generalized anxiety disorder
	Anxiety with organic disease
	Anxiety with other psychiatric disorders
	Drug-associated anxiety*
Mood disorders	Depressive disorder
	Bipolar disorder
	Dysthymia
Somatoform disorders	Body dysmorphic disorder*
	Conversion disorder
	Hypochondriasis
	Somatoform pain disorder
Psychologic factors affecting physical condition	Psychophysiologic duodenal ulcer, tension headache, ulcerative colitis
Psychoactive substance use disorders	Alcohol dependence
	Alcohol abuse
	Amphetamine dependence and abuse
	Cannabis dependence and abuse
	Cocaine dependence and abuse
Organic mental syndromes	Delirium
	Dementia
	Primary (Alzheimer's type)
	Vascular
	CNS infection
	Brain trauma
	Toxic-metabolic disturbances
Schizophrenia	Catatonic type
	Disorganized type
	Paranoid type
	Undifferentiated type
Delusional (paranoid) disorder	Erotomania, grandiosity, jealousy, persecution complex, somatic delusions

*Conditions not covered in this chapter.
From *Diagnostic and statistical manual of mental disorders*, ed 3, revised, Washington DC, 1987, American Psychiatric Association, and Judd LL, Braff DL, Britton KT, et al. In Wilson JD, et al, editors: *Harrison's Principles of internal medicine*, ed 12, New York, 1991, McGraw-Hill, pp 2123-2151.

graine and tension headaches or gastric and duodenal ulcers, as well as disorders that are relatively uncommon, like neurodermatitis.

PSYCHOACTIVE SUBSTANCE USE DISORDERS

Alcohol dependence tends to cluster in families. Approximately 13% of the adult population have abused or been dependent on alcohol at some time in their lives. One in five male dental patients and one in ten female dental patients are alcoholics.

Cannabis is the most widely used illicit psychoactive substance in the United States. A study conducted from 1981 to 1983 showed that approximately 4% of the adult population had abused cannabis at some time in their lives. The same study also indicated that approximately 0.2% of the adult population had abused cocaine. However, based on broadened criteria for dependence and a definite increase in cocaine use in recent years, the prevalence of cocaine dependence is now thought to be much higher.[11] It is now estimated[16] that over 22 million Americans have tried cocaine, and about 2 million use it on a regular basis. About 500,000 Americans have serious problems directly related to the chronic use of cocaine. Cocaine can be injected into a vein, snorted through the nose, smoked in a free base form, or smoked as "crack" (cocaine base pre-made into solid pellet form).[16]

SCHIZOPHRENIA

The lifetime prevalence rate for schizophrenic disorders is about 1% (this includes all cultures and both sexes). The age at onset is usually during adolescence or early adulthood. Studies have suggested an earlier onset in males than in females.

DELUSIONAL (PARANOID) DISORDER

Delusional (paranoid) disorder is uncommon. Its prevalence in the United States is about 0.03%. Age at onset is usually in middle or late adult life with the mean age of 50 years. Delusional disorder is slightly more common in females.[11,22]

ORGANIC MENTAL SYNDROMES

Dementia is found in about 2% to 3% of individuals 65 to 79 years of age, and in approximately 20% who are 80 years or older. There are an estimated 2 to 3 million Americans with dementia, and more than half of these are confined to nursing homes.[17]

ETIOLOGY

The etiology of behavioral and psychiatric disorders is complex and not well understood. In some conditions there appears to be an interaction between genetic makeup and the individual's environment. In others, the stresses of life appear to play the dominant role. The etiologic factors identified for the major psychiatric disorders will be discussed.

ANXIETY DISORDERS

Anxiety represents a threatened emergence into consciousness of painful, unacceptable thoughts, impulses, or desires (anxiety results from psychologic conflicts of the past and present). These psychologic conflicts or feelings stimulate physiologic changes that lead to clinical manifestations of anxiety.[21,22] Anxiety disorders may occur in persons under emotional stress, in those with certain systemic illnesses, or as a component of various psychiatric disorders.

Panic disorders, in particular, tend to be familial. If one first-degree relative has a panic disorder other relatives have about an 18% chance of developing a panic disorder.

Patients with generalized anxiety disorder have persistent diffuse anxiety. Gamma-aminobutyric acid (GABA) is an inhibitory amino acid neurotransmittor. It appears to play a central role in the development of anxiety. The action of an antianxiety medication, such as benzodiazepine, is to selectively, but indirectly, enhance GABA neurotransmission. This may occur by increasing neuronal receptor sensitivity to GABA.[14,18] However, exactly what role GABA plays in the etiology of generalized anxiety disorder and other forms of anxiety still remains to be established.

Anxiety states may also be associated with organic diseases, other psychiatric disorders, and certain drugs. Patients with hyperthyroidism and mitral valve prolapse often have associated anxiety. Anxiety is also associated with mood disorders, schizophrenia, or personality disorders.[21-23]

MOOD DISORDERS

These disorders appear to be caused by an interaction between genetic and environmental factors. The mode of genetic transmission has not been established. Concordance rates in identical twins range from 33% to 75% with a mean of 65%. Concordance rates in nonidentical twins range from 9% to 23% with a mean of 15%. Family studies involving first-degree relatives of patients with mood disorders[22] also show increased risk for mood disorders. If a patient has bipolar disorder, 17.7% of relatives are at risk for bipolar disorder and 2.8% for unipolar disorder. However, if a patient has unipolar disease, 22.4% of the relatives are at risk for unipolar disease. Adoption studies show a trend for mood disorders in adoptees to be related to their biologic parents rather than their adopted parents. Again, noting strong association from a genetic standpoint as opposed to environmental, the etiology of mood disorders suggests an inherited predisposition that is triggered by stresses in life.[22]

SOMATOFORM DISORDERS (CONVERSION)

In this group of disorders a psychologic conflict or need is expressed as an alteration or loss of physical function, suggesting a physical disorder. The symptoms of the disturbance are not intentionally produced. Following appropriate investigation, the symptoms cannot be explained by a physical disorder or known pathophysiologic mechanism. A person who views a traumatic event, for example, but has a conflict about acknowledging that event, may develop a conversion disorder of blindness. In this case the symptom of blindness has symbolic value and is a representation and partial solution to the underlying psychologic conflict.[11,22]

PSYCHOLOGIC FACTORS AFFECTING PHYSICAL CONDITIONS

In the past, this group of disorders has been referred to as psychophysiologic disorders. Psychologic factors may contribute to the initiation or exacerbation of a physical condition. Common examples of physical conditions in which psychologic factors play an important role are migraine and tension headaches, duodenal ulcer, ulcerative colitis, neurodermatitis, asthma, and sacroiliac pain. The physical condition involves either demonstrable organic pathology (duodenal ulcer) or a known pathophysiologic process (migraine headache).[11]

SCHIZOPHRENIA

The etiology of schizophrenia also appears to involve the interaction of genetic and environmental factors. The risk for schizophrenia in the general population is about 1% to 2%. However, if both parents are schizophrenic, 46% of the children will develop the disease. The risk for developing schizophrenia for first-degree relatives is 5% to 10% and for second-degree relatives 2% to 4%. Concordance in identical twins for schizophrenia is 65% for identical twins and 12% for non-identical twins. However, 89% of the individuals with schizophrenia do not have a parent with the disease and 81% do not have either a parent or a sibling with the disease. Recent studies have suggested that the defect in schizophrenia involves chromosome 5.[22]

Schizophrenia appears to be triggered by environmental events operating in a genetically predisposed individual. Drugs, medical illnesses, stressful psychosocial events, viral infections, and family situations characterized by conflicting and self-contradictory forms of communication have been reported to precipitate schizophrenia in susceptible individuals.[10,21]

ORGANIC MENTAL SYNDROME

The etiology of Alzheimer's disease or dementia is unknown; however, several possibilities are under investigation including genetics, nutrition, environment, and infectious agents. Current evidence suggests chromosomal factors are involved in some cases of the disease although certain environmental elements (e.g., aluminum) are also suspected. There has been no support to date for an infectious etiology.

Major mental disorders: pathophysiology, complications, signs and symptoms, and medical management

ANXIETY DISORDERS

Anxiety can be defined as emotional pain or a feeling that all is not well—a feeling of impending disaster. The source of the problem usually is not apparent to the person with anxiety. The feeling is the same as that of the patient with fear but that person is aware of what the problem is and why he or she is "fearful."

The physiologic reaction to anxiety and fear is the same and is mediated through the autonomic nervous system. Both sympathetic and parasympathetic components may be involved. Symptoms of anxiety caused by overactivation of the sympathetic nervous system include increased heart rate, sweating, dilated pupils, and muscle tension. Symptoms of anxiety resulting from stimulation of the parasympathetic system include urination and diarrhea.

PANIC DISORDER

A panic disorder consists of the sudden, unexpected, overwhelming feeling of terror with symptoms of dyspnea, palpitations, dizziness, faintness, trembling, sweating, choking, flushes or chills, numbness or tingling sensations, or chest pains. The panic attack peaks in about 10 minutes and usually lasts for about 20 to 30 minutes. About 15% of patients seen by cardiologists come to the doctor because of symptoms associated with a panic attack. The major complication of repeated panic attacks is a restricted lifestyle adopted to avoid situations that might trigger an attack. Some patients develop *agoraphobia,* an irrational fear of being alone in public places, which can lead to being house-bound for years. Sudden loss of social supports or disruption of important interpersonal relationships appear to predispose an individual to the development of panic disorder. Tricyclic antidepressants, monomine oxidase inhibitors, alprazolam, propranolol, and clonidine have all been used in the treatment of panic disorder. Follow-up psychotherapy may be needed in more severe cases.[11,22]

GENERALIZED ANXIETY DISORDER

Some patients develop a persistent diffuse form of anxiety with symptoms of motor tension, autonomic hyperactivity, and apprehension. There appears to be no familial or genetic basis for the disorder. It has a better outcome than panic disorder; however, it can lead to depression and substance abuse. Anxiolytic drugs are not used to treat patients with generalized anxiety disorder unless symptoms are significant. Nondrug management includes modification of maladaptive lifestyles, cognition and avoidance behaviors, relaxation training, biofeedback, and desensitization. Drug treatment includes the use of benzodiazepines or buspirone.[11,22] The commonly used benzodiazepines are shown in Table 25-5.

POSTTRAUMATIC STRESS DISORDER

Posttraumatic stress disorder (PTSD) may appear following traumatic events that are anticipated or not anticipated, acute or chronic, constant or repetitive, natural or malevolent. If the onset of symptoms occurs within 6 months of the trauma or if the duration of symptoms is less than 6 months, the patient has acute PTSD. Chronic PTSD occurs when the onset of symptoms occurs at least 6 months after the trauma or the disorder has a duration longer than 6

TABLE 25-5
Commonly Used Benzodiazepines

	Range for daily oral dose (mg)	Half-life (hr)
Anxiolytics*		
Chlordiazepoxide (Librium)	20 to 100	7 to 23
Diazepam (Valium)	5 to 40	20 to 90
Lorazepam (Ativam)	1 to 10	10 to 12
Oxazepam (Serax)	30 to 120	3 to 20
Prazepam (Centrax)	20 to 60	40 to 70
Alprazolam (Xanax)	0.75 to 10.0	12 to 15
Sedative-hypnotics†		
Flurazepam (Dalmane)	15 to 30	24 to 100
Temazepam (Restoril)	30	8 to 10
Triazolam (Halcion)	0.125 to 0.5	2 to 3

*Prescribed in a three or four times daily regimen—lorazepam, oxazepam, alprazolam.
†Prescribed in a daily or bedtime regimen—flurazepam, temazepam, triazolam.
From Judd LL. In Wilson JD, et al, editors: *Harrison's Principles of internal medicine,* New York, 1991, McGraw-Hill, pp 2139-2154.

months. Factors that influence the development of PTSD are extent of life-space affected, duration of the impact, extent of perception that human malevolence was behind the traumatic event (fire due to arson), and the degree of social isolation present at the time of stress. The traumatic event is outside the range of usual human experience. It may be a serious threat to one's life or physical integrity; serious threat to one's children, spouse, or other loved ones; sudden destruction of one's home or community; or seeing an accident or physical violence that seriously injures or kills another person(s).[11]

The disorder consists of re-experiencing the event in one of the following ways: (1) recurrent and intrusive distressing recollections of the event; (2) recurrent distressing dreams of the event; (3) sudden acting or feelings as if the event was recurring; or (4) intense psychologic distress at events that symbolize or resemble an aspect of the traumatic event. Patients with PTSD may avoid thoughts or feelings associated with the trauma, avoid activities or situations that arouse recollections of the trauma, be unable to recall an important aspect of the trauma, have feelings of detachment or estrangement from others, have a restricted range of affect, or have a sense of a foreshortened future. These individuals will often have persistent symptoms of increased arousal shown by difficulty sleeping, irritability or outbursts of anger, difficulty concentrating, exaggerated startle response, or hypervigilance. The complications associated with this disorder include anxiety, depression, substance abuse, and impaired social and interpersonal relations.[11,22]

Medical treatment includes behavioral techniques, psychotherapy, and medications including heterocyclic antidepressants, monoamine oxidase (MAO) inhibitors, lithium, propranolol, and clonidine. (See Tables 25-7, 25-15, and 25-19.)

MOOD DISORDERS

Mood disorders represent a heterogeneous group of mental disorders characterized by extreme exaggeration and disturbance of mood and affect. These disorders have associated physiologic, cognitive, and psychomotor dysfunctions. Mood disorders tend to be cyclic — they clear and then tend to recur.[11,22]

MAJOR DEPRESSION

Major depression (unipolar) is one of the main mood disorders. Patients with major depression are depressed most of the day, show a marked decrease in interest or pleasure in most activities, have a marked gain or loss in weight, and manifest insomnia or hypersomnia. These symptoms must be present for at least 2 weeks for a diagnosis of major depression. About 50% to 80% of individuals who have had a major depressive episode will have at least one more depressive episode. Twenty percent of the individuals will have a subsequent manic episode and should be reclassified as bipolar. A major depression usually will last about 8 to 9 months if the individual is not treated. *Dysthymia* represents a chronic, more mild form of depression with symptoms lasting at least 2 years.[11,22]

BIPOLAR DISORDER

Bipolar disorder consists of manic and depressive episodes occurring at different times in the patient or a mixture of symptoms occurring at the same time. The essential feature of a manic episode is a distinct period during which the person's mood is either elevated and expansive or irritable. Associated symptoms of the manic syndrome include inflated self-esteem, grandiosity, decreased need for sleep, excessive speech, flight of ideas, distractibility, psychomotor agitation, and excessive involvement in pleasurable activities. During a manic episode the mood is often described as euphoric, cheerful, or "high" (Table 25-6). The expansive quality of the mood is characterized by unceasing and unselective enthusiasm for interacting with people. However, the predominant mood disturbance may be irritability. The speech is often loud, rapid, and difficult to interpret.[11,22]

Men tend to have more manic episodes and women more depressive episodes. Untreated individuals with bipolar disorder will have a mean of nine affective episodes during their lifetime. Each cycle's length tends to decrease although the number of cycles increases with age. Each affective episode lasts about 8 to 9 months. Bipolar patients have more episodes, hospitalizations, divorce, and suicides than unipolar patients.

The etiology of mood disorders appears to be related to a malfunction of the neurotransmittor

TABLE 25-6

Clinical Findings Suggestive of a Manic Component in a Bipolar Disorder

Unusual involvement in activities
Involvement in multiple activities
Colorful and strange style of dress
Intrusive and demanding behavior
Extreme anger
Loud, rapid, and dramatic manner of speaking
Inability to sleep
Drug and alcohol abuse
Lack of judgment resulting in financial and legal problems

TABLE 25-7

Commonly Used First-Generation Antidepressants

Drug	Daily oral dose (mg)
Tricyclic derivatives	
Amitriptyline (Elavil)	150 to 300
Nortriptyline (Aventyl)	50 to 150
Imipramine (Tofranil)	150 to 300
Desipramine (Norpramin)	150 to 250
Doxepin (Sinequan)	150 to 300
Monoamine oxidase inhibitors	
Phenelzine (Mardil)	15 to 60
Tranylcyproimine (Parnate)	20 to 30
Isocarboxazid (Marplan)	10 to 30

From Judd LL. In Wilson JD, et al, editors: *Harrison's Principles of internal medicine*, New York, 1991, McGraw-Hill, pp 2139-2154.

TABLE 25-8

Selected Second-Generation Antidepressants

Drug	Daily oral dose (mg)
Tricyclic derivatives	
Trimipramine (Surmonil)	100 to 250
Amoxapine (Asendin)	150 to 300
Tetracyclic derivatives	
Maprotiline (Ludiomil)	100 to 225
Derivatives of other chemical classes	
Fluoxetine (Prozac)	10 to 40
Bupropion (Wellbutrin)	200 to 300
Trazodone (Desyrel)	100 to 600

From Judd LL. In Wilson JD, et al, editors: *Harrison's Principles of internal medicine*, New York, 1991, McGraw-Hill, pp 2139-2154.

system in the brain, resulting in increased secretion of norepinephrine and decreased release of serotonin and dopamine. Current research has focused on the role of the post-synaptic receptor systems, involving underactivity and downregulation. A dysregulation of biologic rhythms may also occur during the winter months in northern states and has been reported to be associated with depression. White light has been effective in treating some individuals with this type of depression.[11,22]

Patients with major depression may show increased cortisol secretion and abnormal circadian secretion of cortisol. The origin of the secretion problem appears to be in the CNS. About 50% of patients with major depression have a positive (nonsuppression) dexamethasone suppression test. Borderline hypothyroidism is suggested in about 25% to 30% of the patients with major depression. These patients have a blunted TSH response to TRH.[22]

Sleep disruption occurs in almost all patients with major depression. Over 60% of the patients show short REM (rapid eye movement) latency with increased number of eye movements. Monoamine oxidase (MAO) levels in platelets from patients with a bipolar disorder is lowered. Platelet MAO levels are high in patients with anxiety associated with their mood disorder.[22]

A high degree of specificity and success can be obtained by the use of potent psychotropic drugs for the treatment of mood disorders. The drugs used are antidepressants and lithium. Table 25-7 shows the commonly used first-generation antidepressants. Table 25-8 shows selected second-generation antidepressants. Mood disorders have a tendency to recur. Affective episodes may occur spontaneously or be triggered by adverse events. Individuals with mood disorders and their families need to become aware of the early signs and symptoms of affective episodes so that treatment can be initiated by their physician. These individuals also must be aware of the need for medication compliance and be aware of the medication's side effects and possible complications.[22]

During the acute phase of an affective episode, the physician sees the patient for short visits, one to three times per week. The focus during these visits is on monitoring medications and side effects. The physician should be reassuring and supportive so that the episode can be abated with the right drug and dosage. Most of the antidepressant drugs have a delay (10 to 21 days) before full therapeutic benefits are achieved.[22]

An estimated 30,000 suicides occur each year in the United States. About 70% of these involve individuals with major depression. The physician must consider suicidal lethality in the management of patients with depression. In general, the risk for suicide is increased with the following: alcoholism, drug abuse, social isolation, being an elderly male, terminal illness, and undiagnosed/untreated mental disorders. Once the patient with a mood disorder undergoes medical control, insight-oriented psychotherapy is often initiated as an adjunct to the patient's management.[11,22]

Lithium has some antidepressant effects but its real benefit is in the treatment of manic episodes in bipolar disorders. The mode of action of lithium is not clear. It takes about 7 to 10 days to reach full therapeutic effectiveness. Carbamazepine (an anticonvulsant drug) also has been used in the treatment of manic episodes in bipolar patients.[21]

PSYCHOACTIVE SUBSTANCE USE DISORDERS

This group of disorders deals with symptoms and maladaptive behavioral changes associated with the regular use of psychoactive substances that affect the CNS. These disorders involve substance dependence, abuse, tolerance, and withdrawal symptoms.[11]

Substance dependence occurs when an individual takes a substance in larger amounts or over a longer period than was originally intended. A great deal of time may be spent in activities needed to get the substance, taking the substance, or recovering from its effects. The person gives up important social, occupational, and recreational activities because of substance use. A marked tolerance may develop to the substance (more than 50% increase); hence larger amounts are needed to achieve intoxication or the desired effect. The person continues to take the substance despite having persistent or recurrent social, psychologic, and/or physical problem(s) resulting from its use.

Substance abuse is a category denoting substance use that does not meet the criteria for dependence. This diagnosis is most likely to be applicable to people who have just started taking psychoactive substances. Examples of substance abuse may include the following: a middle-aged man who repeatedly drives his car while intoxicated (the man has no other symptoms) or a woman who keeps drinking although her physician has warned her it is responsible for exacerbating the symptoms of a duodenal ulcer (she has no other symptoms).[11]

Withdrawal symptoms occur when the person with substance dependence stops or reduces intake of the substance. Withdrawal symptoms vary based on the substance involved. Physiologic signs of withdrawal are common with alcohol, opioids, sedatives, hypnotics, and anxiolytics. Such signs are less obvious in withdrawal from cocaine, nicotine, amphetamines, and cannabis.[11]

COCAINE USE

Cocaine intoxication is defined as a substance-induced organic mental disorder caused by the drug's effect on the CNS. The mental and physiologic changes involved with cocaine intoxication are listed in Table 25-9. Frequent or high-dose use of cocaine can produce psychiat-

TABLE 25-9

Signs and Symptoms Associated with Cocaine Intoxication

Sense of well-being
Heightened awareness of sensory input
Anorexia
Decreased desire to sleep
Restlessness
Elation, grandiosity, agitation
Tachycardia, cardiac arrhythmias
Pupillary dilation
Elevated blood pressure
Chills, nausea, vomiting
Headache
Psychotic states

ric states similar to acute schizophrenic episodes.[16] Cocaine abuse can produce physical dependence, increased tolerance, and withdrawal symptoms. Chronic cocaine use decreases brain catecholamines and increases catecholamine receptor sensitivity.[16]

IV cocaine abusers are at increased risk for hepatitis B and exposure to the human immunodeficiency (AIDS) virus. Some IV cocaine abusers develop a pruritic rash on the chest (allergic reaction to a benzoic acid ester), and ester-type local anesthetics must be avoided in these patients.[16]

AMPHETAMINE USE

Amphetamines and related drugs are CNS stimulants. Their psychoactive effects last longer than those of cocaine. Their peripheral sympathomimetic effects may also be more potent than those of cocaine. Many people develop dependence when first using amphetamines for their appetite suppressant effect in an attempt at weight control. Intravenous administration of amphetamine can lead to rapid development of dependence. Progressive tolerance is common in amphetamine dependence.[11]

CANNABIS USE

Delta-9-tetrahydrocannabinol (THC) is the major psychoactive ingredient in substances causing cannabis dependence. These substances are marijuana and hashish. They are usually smoked but can be taken orally or are sometimes mixed with food. Current marijuana supplies are much more potent than those available in the 1960s. Social and occupational impairment occurs but is less than that seen with alcohol and cocaine use. Cannabis is the most widely used illicit psychoactive substance in the United States.[11]

ALCOHOL DEPENDENCE

Most alcohol is consumed by a small percentage of people. Ten percent of alcohol drinkers consume 50% of the total amount consumed. Most adults in the United States are light drinkers. Fifty-five percent drink fewer than three alcoholic drinks a week. About 35% of adults abstain from alcohol. Drinking patterns vary by age and sex. For both sexes, the prevalence of drinking is highest in the 21- to 34-year range. At all ages two to five times more males than females are heavy drinkers.[11]

Three patterns of alcohol use in cases of abuse or dependence are seen: regular daily intake of large amounts, regular heavy drinking limited to weekends, or long periods of sobriety interspersed with binges of daily heavy drinking. Alcoholism can be divided into two "species." One species is termed *gamma* alcoholism. Gamma alcoholism involves problems with control. Once a person with gamma alcoholism begins to drink, he or she is unable to stop until poor health or depleted financial resources prevent further drinking. In the other group, the person with alcoholism is not aware of the amount consumed or lacks control and thus drinks a given quantity of alcohol every day but there seems to be no compulsion to exceed that amount. Although these two pure types of alcoholism exist, either group can conform to the three drinking patterns just mentioned and seen in most people in the United States with alcohol abuse or dependence.[11]

Patients suffering from alcoholic withdrawal delirium (delirium tremens [DTs]) will have clouding of consciousness, disorientation, impaired attention and memory, incoherent speech, perceptual disturbances, illusions, and grand hallucinations.[19] An episode of DTs is a serious medical event with a 5% mortality rate, and it requires immediate treatment in a medical intensive care unit.[19] Alcohol withdrawal symptoms are listed in Table 25-10.

Chronic heavy alcohol intake can result in cognitive impairment even when the person is sober. Some individuals will develop an alcohol amnestic disorder and are unable to learn new

TABLE 25-10
Symptoms Associated with Alcohol Withdrawal

Hand tremors
Malaise
Weakness
Anxiety, irritability
Depression
Tachycardia
Sweating
Increased blood pressure
Hallucinations
Delirium

material or to recall known material. An alcoholic blackout occurs in some individuals, which is an amnesic period for events occurring while intoxicated. A few individuals can develop an alcohol-induced dementia, which involves the loss of intellectual abilities, and the loss of abstract thinking, language, and judgment. Severe personality changes may also occur.[19] See Chapter 12 for a discussion concerning dental findings and dental management of chronic heavy alcohol abusers.

ORGANIC MENTAL SYNDROME

Dementia is a clinical condition characterized by a general decline in memory, intellect, and personality from a previously normal intellectual level occurring in the presence of an otherwise normal consciousness (Table 25-11). There are many causes of dementia. A relatively small percentage of cases are due to reversible causes and include such conditions as intoxication, infection, metabolic diseases, nutritional disorders, and intracranial lesions. The majority of cases, however, are the result of irreversible processes, Alzheimer's disease, especially in the elderly, being a prime example.

ALZHEIMER'S DISEASE

This disease was first described in 1907 by Alois Alzheimer. It predominantly affects the elderly; however, the process is seen in younger individuals as well. It is estimated that approximately 4 million people in the United States suffer from dementia and more than half of these are the Alzheimer's type.[9,23]

TABLE 25-11
Clinical Findings Suggestive of Dementia

Apathy
Lack of spontaneity
Withdrawal from social interactions
Inability to recall important dates
Inability to learn or recall new information
Aphasic defects
Poor judgment
Inability to identify friends or family members
Disorientation as to time and place
Inability to feed or clothe self
Weight loss

Alzheimer's disease is the fourth leading cause of death in the United States — after heart disease, cancer, and stroke. Over 40 billion dollars is spent annually in care for its victims. It affects men and women equally and occurs predominantly in persons over the age of 65. In individuals over 65, approximately 11% have Alzheimer's and this figure is increasing yearly. Over 100,000 deaths/year are attributed to this disease. Approximately 60% of residents of nursing homes have Alzheimer's disease or related dementias.[2]

The definitive diagnosis of Alzheimer's can be made only at autopsy. Gross examination of the brain reveals cortical atrophy and ventricular enlargement. Characteristic microscopic features include neurofibrillary tangles, senile plaques, amyloid angiopathy, granulovacuolar degeneration, and Hirano bodies. It is interesting to note that these changes are also present but to a lesser degree in patients who do not have dementia. On a biochemical level there is a deficiency of acetylcholine and its associated enzymes.[29] This is significant since cholinergic neurons are intimately involved in cognition.

The onset of this disease is usually subtle and insidious, with the first sign being recent memory loss or a personality or behavioral change. Depression, anxiety, or apathy is common in the early stages. Progression is typically slow and changes may go unrecognized for long periods unless the person is challenged by a new or unusual situation, at which point he or she typically becomes confused.

The diagnosis of the disease is based solely on patient history and clinical findings. Criteria for making a definitive diagnosis include the confirmation of dementia, at least two cognitive deficits, progressive worsening of memory, normal consciousness, onset between ages of 40 and 90, and the absence of any other condition that could account for the deficits.[25]

As the disease progresses, there is continued deterioration in cognitive processes, including memory, judgment, learning, and language skills, as well as further disorientation, personality changes, and the inability to perform routine tasks. This disease eventually renders its victims incapable of caring for themselves.

There are no clinical laboratory tests that are diagnostic of Alzheimer's disease; however, conducting a battery of tests is useful in an attempt to identify correctable causes of dementia. These tests include a complete blood count, electrolyte panel, screening metabolic panel, thyroid function, vitamin B_{12} and folate levels, tests for syphilis and HIV antibodies, urinalysis, ECG, and chest x-ray. A CT scan or MRI of the brain, positron emission tomography, EEC, and lumbar puncture are also included when warranted.[23] Of significant aid in diagnosis are neuropsychiatric tests, which are part of the necessary criteria for diagnosis.

Once it is determined that the dementia is Alzheimer's and not the result of a treatable condition, management is directed toward symptomatic relief. Unfortunately, nothing has been found to retard or reverse the process of dementia; however, noncognitive symptoms do respond to therapy. Although efforts are made to use nonpharmacologic approaches to manage symptoms such as anxiety, depression, irritability, and sleep disturbances, medications inevitably are required. Antidepressants, sedative-hypnotics, and antipsychiatrics are all used, with varying degrees of success. A small percentage of patients experience seizures and are treated with standard anticonvulsants.

Early in the disease, patients are capable of providing much of their own care but this ability ultimately deteriorates and patients require an increasingly greater degree of care and supervision. The burden on caregivers is given much attention in overall management, and their continued support and periodic relief are necessary. Patients ultimately become completely helpless and cannot help with their toilet and feeding. Transfer to a nursing facility or hospice is often necessary, but economics may prohibit or limit this option.

SCHIZOPHRENIA

Patients with schizophrenia show psychotic symptoms consisting of delusions, hallucinations, incoherence, catatonic behavior, or flat or grossly inappropriate affect (Table 25-12). The delusions are usually bizarre such as thought broadcasting or being controlled by a dead person. The hallucinations are prominent and occur throughout the day for several days or several times a week for several weeks. Signs of the disturbance must be continuous over a 6-month period. The four types of schizophrenic

TABLE 25-12
Clinical Findings Associated with Schizophrenia

Confusion
Depression
Withdrawal
Anxiety
Marginal social and economic adjustment
Persecutory delusions
Reference delusions
Psychomotor hyperactivity
Grimacing
Pacing
Psychomotor hypoactivity—catatonic rigidity
Feelings of having thoughts broadcast
Feelings of being controlled by others
Hallucinations
Absense of emotions
Monotonous speech

disorders are catatonic, disorganized, paranoid, and undifferentiated. Patients with schizophrenic disorders show deterioration in their level of functioning regarding work, social relations, and self-care. The vulnerability to a schizophrenic disorder is inherited and life stresses trigger the disorder.[11,22]

Overactivity of dopamine remains the central hypothesis in explaining schizophrenic behavior. Dopamine plays a role in attentional mechanisms and stimulus filtering. Alterations in dopamine can lead to cognitive fragmentation, thought disorder, and clinical impairment. The potency of all antipsychotic medications is roughly predicted by their dopaminergic-blocking capacity.[11,22]

Neuropathologic changes have been demonstrated in patients with schizophrenic disorders.[22] CT scan and MRI have shown an increase in ventricular size, indicating brain atrophy in such patients. Positron emission tomography has demonstrated decreased frontal lobe activity.

Treatment of schizophrenic disorders consists of using antipsychotic medications that act selectively against specific target symptoms. These drugs are effective for symptoms such as hallucinations and psychotic agitation but are noneffective for other symptoms such as social withdrawal or anhedonia.

DELUSIONAL (PARANOID) DISORDERS

The essential feature of a delusional disorder is the presence of a persistent, nonbizzarre delusion that is not due to any other mental disorder. The following delusional themes are commonly found[11]: erotomanic, jealous, persecutory, and somatic. Individuals with delusional disorder may manifest more than one delusional theme. The main theme of an erotic delusion is that one is loved by another. The delusion usually concerns idealized romantic love and spiritual union rather than sexual attraction. The persecutory type of delusion is the most common. It usually involves the belief that one is being conspired against, cheated, spied on, followed, poisoned, or harassed. Individuals with percusatory delusions are often resentful and angry and may become violent to those they believe are hurting them. Somatic types of delusions include the conviction that a foul odor is being emitted from the skin, mouth, rectum, or vagina, or that an infestation of insects is occurring in the skin.[11]

Impairment in daily functioning is rare in patients with delusional disorder. Intellectual and occupational functioning is usually satisfactory. However, social and marital functioning is often impaired.

DRUGS USED TO TREAT PSYCHIATRIC DISORDERS

ANTIDEPRESSANT MEDICATIONS

The major group of drugs used to treat depression are tricyclics. The first tricyclic used to treat depression was imipramine. Tricyclics inhibit neural re-uptake of norepinephrine and 5-hydroxytryptamine (5-HT) resulting in down-regulation of their respective receptors. The tricyclics are all equally effective in the management of depression, but they differ in their associated side effects. Amitriptyline and doxepin are the most sedating, and this side effect is taken advantage of by using these drugs just before bedtime. Two combinations of drugs are available for treating depression and other psychotic symptoms. Triavil (amitriptyline and perphenazine) is used to treat patients with depression and agitation or psychotic behavior. Limbitrol (amitriptyline and chlordiazepoxide) is used to treat patients with depression and anxiety.[21,22,31]

The adverse side effects associated with tricyclics include dry mouth, constipation, blurred vision, tachycardia, allergic reactions, and important drug interactions (Tables 25-13 and 25-14). Tricyclic drugs should not be used in patients with cardiac conditions because there is a risk of atrial fibrillation, A-V block, or

---

TABLE 25-13

Common Side Effects of Tricyclic Antidepressants

---

1. Anticholinergic (atropine-like) responses
    a. Dry mouth
    b. Nausea and vomiting
    c. Constipation
    d. Urinary retention
    e. Blurred vision
2. Cardiovascular effects
    a. Postural hypotension
    b. Tachycardia
    c. Cardiotoxic side effects — arrhythmias
3. Obstructive jaundice
4. Drowsiness and sleepiness
5. Fine rapid tremor
6. Dizziness, ataxia
7. Leukopenia

From Judd LL. In Wilson JD, et al, editors: *Harrison's Principles of internal medicine*, New York, 1991, McGraw-Hill, pp 2139-2154.

TABLE 25-14

Adverse Effects Caused by Antipsychotic Drug Blockage of Various Neuronal Receptors

Type of receptor blockage	Adverse effects
Muscarinic	Urinary retention
	Memory dysfunction
	Dry mouth
	Blurred vision
	Constipation
	Speech blockage
Histamine H_1	Sedation
	Possible hypotension
	Possible weight gain
Histamine H_2	Possible depression
L_1 adrenergic	Postural hypotension
	Light-headedness
	Reflex tachycardia
L_2 adrenergic	?

ventricular tachycardia. Tricyclics can lower the seizure threshold and must be used with care in patients with a history of seizures. They can increase intraocular pressure in patients with glaucoma. Urinary retention can be increased if they are used in patients with prostate hypertrophy. If used in certain patients with bipolar disorder, tricyclics can reduce the time between episodes, induce manic episodes, and cause rapid cycling of episodes. Drug interactions reported with the use of tricyclics include the following: (1) tricyclics potentiate the effects of other CNS depressants such as ethanol and benzodiazepines; (2) they also potentiate the actions of anticholinergic drugs such as antihistamines; and (3) they produce other drug interactions, including potentiation of the pressor effects of sympathomimetic agents, blockage of the antihypertensive effect of guanethidine, and induction of a hypertensive crisis if taken with or soon after a monoamine oxidase inhibitor. Overdosage with a tricyclic can cause death from cardiac arrhythmias or respiratory failure.[21,31]

MONOAMINE OXIDASE INHIBITORS

The monoamine oxidase (MAO) inhibitors were the first effective drugs used in the treatment of depression. There are now only three drugs on the market that are MAO inhibitors: phenelzine (Nardil), tranylcypromine (Parnate), and isocarboxazid (Marplan). These drugs act by inhibiting the two forms of MAO, type A and type B. Inhibition of type A MAO results in the antidepressant effect seen with MAO inhibitors. Over 80% of type A MAO must be bound before the drug effects can be seen clinically. Resynthesis of new enzyme takes 10 to 14 days. If a patient is changing from a MAO inhibitor drug to a tricyclic drug, 2 weeks or more must elapse after stopping the MAO inhibitor before starting the tricyclic. Significant drug interactions occur between MAO inhibitors and opioids and sympathomimetic amines. MAO inhibitors potentiate the depressant activity of the opioids. They can produce a hypertensive crisis if combined with sympathomimetic amines (Table 25-15). Phenylethanolamine and phenylephrine must not be given to patients taking MAO inhibitors. These agents are metabolized by MAO, and their use with an MAO inhibitor could lead to significant potentiation of

their pressor effects (Chapter 6). Many over-the-counter cold remedies contain phenylephrine and should be avoided in patients taking MAO inhibitors. Several foods contain high concentrations of tyramine and also must be avoided in these patients. Food with high tyramine levels include bananas, cheeses, chocolate, and red wines.[21,31]

SECOND-GENERATION ANTIDEPRESSANT DRUGS

These drugs are not tricyclics or MAO inhibitors. Second-generation drugs include maprotiline (Ludiomil), amoxapine (Asendin), trazodone (Desyrel), bupropion (Wellbutrin), and fluoxetine (Prozac) (Table 25-16). Bupropion lacks cardiac toxicity but its use is limited because of other side effects and drug interactions. Fluoxetine inhibits neuronal re-uptake of 5-HT. Among its adverse reactions has been an increase in frequency of suicide attempts.[21,31]

TABLE 25-15

MAO Inhibitors—Side Effects and Drug Interactions

1. Examples of agents used
   a. Phenelzine (Nardil)
   b. Isocarboxazid (Marplan)
   c. Tranylcypromine (Parnate)
2. Significant side effects
   a. Hypotension
   b. Xerostomia
   c. Manic reactions
   d. Nausea, constipation, anorexia
3. Significant drug interactions
   a. Prolongation and intensification of effects of following drugs that can lead to severe respiratory depression
      (1) General anesthetics
      (2) Sedatives
      (3) Antihistamines
      (4) Narcotics
      (5) Nonnarcotic analgesics
      (6) Atropine
   b. Hypertensive crisis—myocardial infarction, etc
      (1) Epinephrine (very slight risk)
      (2) Levonordefrin (Carbocaine with Neo-Cobefrin) (very slight risk)
      (3) Phenylephrine (significant risk)

TABLE 25-16
Heterocyclic Antidepressants — Side Effects and Drug Interactions

1. Examples of agents used
   a. Tricyclics
      1. Amitriptyline (Elavil)
      2. Imipramine (Tofranil)
   b. Modified tricyclics
      Amoxapine (Asendin)
   c. Tetracyclics
      Maprotiline (Ludiomil)
2. Significant side effects
   a. Xerostomia
   b. Orthostatic hypotension
   c. Tachycardia, cardiac arrhythmias
3. Significant drug interactions
   a. Severe respiratory depression
      1. General anesthetics
      2. Sedatives, hypnotics
      3. Narcotics
   b. Increased ocular pressure
      Atropine
   c. Hypertensive crisis — myocardial infarction, etc
      Epinephrine

LITHIUM

Lithium has some antidepressant effects, but its main role is in the treatment of bipolar disorders. Its mode of action is unclear. Lithium is used to treat acute manic episodes and to prevent manic episodes in a patient with bipolar disorder. Lithium should not be used if renal disease is present. Lower doses must also be used in older patients. The dose ranges from 600 to 3000 mg/day. It takes 7 to 10 days to reach full therapeutic effect. The patient on maintenance therapy should be evaluated every 3 to 6 months for serum levels of lithium, sodium, potassium, creatinine, T_4, TSH, and free T_4 index. Medical complications associated with chronic lithium use include nontoxic goiters and hypothyroidism, arrhythmias, T-wave depression, and a vasopressin-resistant nephrogenic diabetes insipidus. All these complications are related to the effect of lithium on adenylate cyclase activity. The common side effects of lithium are shown in Table 25-17.

TABLE 25-17
Common Lithium Side Effects

Type	Specifics
Side effects commonly seen	
Very mild	Thirst
	Nausea
	Fine tremor of hand
Mild to moderate	Anorexia
	Vomiting
	Diarrhea
	Polydipsia-polyuria
	Muscular weakness and fatigue
Side effects indicating toxicity	
Mild to moderate	Muscle hyperirritability with twitching
	Sedation
	Giddiness
	Coarse tremor, ataxia
Moderate to severe	Hypertonic muscles
	Hyperextension of arms and legs
	Chorea
	Impairment of consciousness
	Seizures
Very severe	Coma
	Death

From Judd LL. In Wilson JD, et al, editors: *Harrison's Principles of internal medicine*, New York, 1991, McGraw-Hill.

CARBAMAZEPINE

This anticonvulsant drug has been successful in the treatment of manic episodes in bipolar patients who do not respond to lithium or who can not take lithium because of its complications. The dose is 600 to 1600 mg/day. Side effects include nausea, blurred vision, ataxia, leukopenia, and/or aplastic anemia.

ANTIANXIETY (ANXIOLYTIC) DRUGS

The benzodiazepines are used to treat the various anxiety states. These drugs selectively but indirectly enhance gamma-aminobutyric acid (GABA) neurotransmission. This may occur by the drugs' increasing neuronal receptor sensitivity to GABA. The benzodiazepines are very effective for short-lived reactive states of tension and anxiety. They are the drugs of choice for generalized anxiety disorders. Tricyclics and MAO inhibitors are the drugs of choice for panic disorders. Benzodiazepines are used for the treatment of anticipatory anxiety associated with panic disorders. They are also utilized in the treatment of other forms of anxiety associated with panic disorders and for anxiety symptoms found in patients with phobic disorders.[21,33]

Diazepam is the standard for antianxiety therapy. No other anxiolytic drug has shown better anti-anxiety efficacy. Treatment with anxiolytic drugs should continue only for a period of 4 weeks or less. In order to avoid the development of drug tolerance, these drugs are often given for 7 to 10 days, followed by a 2- to 3-day period without the drug. An early sign of drug tolerance occurs when increased dosage is required.[21,33] Symptoms of drug withdrawal include muscle aches, agitation, restlessness, insomnia, confusion, delirium, and, on rare occasions, grand mal seizures. Some patients may experience rebound anxiety after the drug has been stopped. Drug side effects include daytime sedation, mild cognitive impairment, and aggressive and impulsive behavior responses. The benzodiazepines can potentiate the CNS effects of opioids, barbiturates, and alcohol. Benzodiazepines are hazardous or contraindicated in the following cases: driving or operating machinery; patients with depressive mood disorders or psychosis; and in moderate-to-heavy drinkers, pregnant women, and the elderly. Tolerance and habitual and physical dependence can occur with therapeutic doses. Actions of the benzodiazepines are additive and usually synergistic with psychotropic agents. Drug interactions have been reported with cimetidine and erythromycin.[21,33]

Propranolol can dampen the peripheral physiologic symptoms of anxiety, but it does not effect the psychologic components such as fear. Buspirone is a new drug that appears to be effective and produces less sedation and motor impairment than the benzodiazepines.[21]

ANTIPSYCHOTIC (NEUROLEPTIC) DRUGS

The introduction of chlorpromazine in the 1950s revolutionized the practice of psychiatry. Other agents have been introduced since chlor-

TABLE 25-18

Antipsychotic Agents of Choice for Various Conditions

Conditions	Recommended drug
Psychiatric	
Agitation and psychosis	Chlorpromazine
	Mesoridazine
	Thioridazine
Withdrawal and psychosis	Fluphenazine
	Haloperidol
	Molindone
	Trifluoperazine
Suicidal tendency	Avoid mesoridazine and thioridazine
Tendency for parkinsonism or acute dystonia	Chlorpromazine
	Mesoridazine
	Thioridazine
Tendency for akathisia	Chlorpromazine
	Loxapine
	Mesoridazine
Elderly, medical history unknown, dehydration	Fluphenazine
	Haloperidol
	Molindone
Neurologic	
Parkinson's disease	Chlorpromazine
	Mesoridazine
	Thioridazine
Delirium	Fluphenazine
	Haloperidol
	Molindone
	Perphenazine
Dementia with behavior disorganization	Fluphenazine
	Haloperidol
	Perpherazine
	Thiothixene

promazine but none represent any real improvement beyond this prototypic agent. Two thirds of all prescriptions for antidepressant and antipsychotic drugs are written by physicians other than psychiatrists. The antipsychotic drugs appear to work by antagonizing the effects of dopamine in the basal ganglia and limbic portions of the forebrain. The antipsychotic drugs should be used only when they are clearly the drug of choice (Table 25-18). This is because of significant adverse reactions associated with use of these drugs.[21,39]

TABLE 25-19
Commonly Used Antipyschotic Medications

	Range of oral dosage (mg)	Potency ratio compared to 100 mg of chlorpromazine
1. Phenothiazines	400 to 800	1 : 1
a. Aliphatics		
Chlorpromazine (Thorazine)		
Piperazines	4 to 20	1 : 50
(1) Fluphenazine (Prolixin)	8 to 32	1 : 10
(2) Perphenazine (Trilafon)	6 to 20	1 : 20
(3) Trifluoperazine (Stelazine)		
c. Piperidines	200 to 600	1 : 1
Thioridazine (Mellaril)		
2. Butyrophenones		1 : 50
Haloperidol (Haldol)	8 to 32	
3. Thioxanthenes		1 : 1
(1) Chlorprothixene (Taractan)	400 to 800	1 : 25
(2) Thiothixene (Navane)	15 to 30	
4. Oxoidoles		1 : 10
Molindone (Moran, Lidone)	40 to 200	
5. Dibenzoxazepines		1 : 10
Loxapine (Loxitane, Dazolin)	60 to 100	

From Judd LL. In Wilson JD, et al, editors: *Harrison's Principles of internal medicine*, New York, McGraw-Hill, pp 2139-2154.

The antipsychotic drugs sedate, tranquilize, blunt emotional expression, attenuate aggressive and impulsive behavior, and cause disinterest in the environment. They leave higher intellectual functions intact but ameliorate the bizarre behavior and thinking of psychotic patients. They all have significant anticholinergic side effects and produce dystonias and extrapyramidal symptoms.[21,39] The commonly used antipsychotic drugs are shown in Table 25-19.

Side effects of the antipsychotic drugs are numerous and often significant (Table 25-20). Patients become sedated, lethargic, and drowsy when first placed on these drugs; however, after several days they develop a tolerance to these effects. The anticholinergic actions produced by these drugs include dry mouth, postural hypotension, constipation, and urinary retention. Other side effects observed include obstructive jaundice, retinal pigmentations, lenticular opacities, skin pigmentation, hypersensitivity to light, and male impotence.[21,39]

The extrapyramidal side effects include acute

TABLE 25-20
Side Effects and Drug Interactions of Antipsychotic Drugs

1. Significant side effects
   a. Agranulocytosis
   b. Visual impairment
   c. Cholestatic jaundice
   d. Excessive or abnormal involuntary movements
   e. Parkinson-like symptoms
   f. Xerostomia
   g. Hypotension
   h. Tachycardia
2. Significant drug interactions
   a. Prolong and intensify effects of following drugs, which can lead to severe respiratory depression
      (1) Sedatives
      (2) Hypnotics
      (3) Opioids
      (4) Antihistamines
   b. Produce hypertensive crisis — myocardial infarction, etc.
      Epinephrine

and chronic conditions. During the first 5 days of treatment with an antipsychotic agent, acute muscular dystonic reactions or a parkinson-like syndrome may occur. Akathisia, or extreme motor restlessness, may also develop early in treatment. Symptoms consist of involuntary repetitive movements of the lips (lip smacking), the tongue (tongue thrusting), the extremities, and the trunk. The risk increases for patients over 60 and those with preexisting CNS pathology (70% risk). The overall risk for tardive dyskinesa is 20% to 40% with the chronic use of antipsychotic drugs.[21,39]

The effects of neuroleptic drugs on the fetus are unknown.[4] There is thought to be a slightly increased risk for developmental defects if the fetus is exposed to these drugs during the first trimester; however, untreated psychotic women also have an increased risk for damage to the fetus. Thus all factors must be considered in deciding whether or not to use drug therapy during pregnancy.[4]

Antacids can diminish the absorption of neuroleptic drugs from the gut. Neuroleptic drugs can decrease the blood levels of warfarin sodium. Neuroleptics and tricyclic antidepressants reduce the metabolism of each other, allowing for increased plasma concentrations of both drugs. Thioridazine can prevent the metabolism of phenytoin allowing toxic blood levels to occur. Smoking can decrease the blood levels of antipsychotic agents.[4] When neuroleptic drugs are used with tricyclic antidepressants or antiparkinsonian drugs, a powerful anticholinergic effect can result.

Malignant neuroleptic syndrome represents a rare but very serious side effect of antipsychotic drugs. This syndrome combines autonomic dysfunction, extrapyramidal dysfunction, and hyperthermia. The patient develops tachycardia, labile blood pressure, dyspnea, masked facies, tremors, muscle rigidity, catatonic behavior, dystonia, and marked elevation in temperature (106° F). The syndrome was first reported in 1960 and since that time about 200 cases have been described. It occurs after the use of neuroleptic drugs given in therapeutic doses. Malignant neuroleptic syndrome is most common in young male adults with mood disorders. The symptoms continue 5 to 10 days after the drug has been stopped. Mortality rate is 10% to 20%. Treatment consists of stopping all neuroleptic medication, body cooling, rehydration, and treatment with bromocriptine (a dopamine agonist).[21,39]

DENTAL MANAGEMENT
PATIENTS' ATTITUDE TOWARD THE DENTIST

Childhood experiences and learned social roles of the patient are important factors in the development of the patient's feelings and attitudes toward the dentist. Children learn role expectations through the teaching of physicians, dentists, parents, and peers. The patient may come to believe that the physician and dentist are powerful and dangerous and thus may feel awe, envy, and wonder in their presence.[1,5-7]

If the patient holds this belief, past behavior used to please parents may be transferred or displaced to the physician or dentist in an attempt to please. Other emotions, attitudes, and actions associated with a patient's relationship with his or her parents also may be transferred. Such behavior has nothing to do with who the physician really is but is displaced behavior toward a symbolic authority figure who represents the parent in the patient's mind. Transference of socially acceptable behavior such as respect and politeness usually is not destructive to the patient-dentist relationship. However, the transference of a need for unending love, a demand for unceasing attention, the need for protection, a fear of tyranny, and feelings of resentment and hate can be destructive to the relationship if not understood and dealt with. The patient may place the physician in a role that is impossible to fulfill—that is, the physician as a miracle worker, lordly, powerful, protective, fatherly, etc. However, when the patient begins to see who the physician really is, disappointment and anger may result.

The more that dentists reveal of themselves to the patient from the first contact, the less likely are these attitudes and feelings to be encouraged. Unrealistic expectations and inappropriate behavior should be open for discussion between the dentist and patient if a solid relationship is to be developed and maintained.

PSYCHOLOGIC SIGNIFICANCE OF THE ORAL CAVITY

The soft tissues of the mouth are an important and highly emotional part of the body. The mouth is the area of the body that early in life is involved with feelings of pleasure and satisfaction during feeding or with frustration and anger if the feeding is late or difficult. The mouth is an area of the body that may be involved with sexual sensations and is used to show the expression of an emotion that a person is feeling. The mouth is important for speech, appearance, and aesthetics. It is involved in our society with the images of health, sex, and youth[5] (Table 25-21).

Dental treatment and manipulation in the mouth may allow the patient to become aware of many of these feelings. For example, if as an infant the patient was frustrated and angry because of difficulty in feeding, these feelings may be "activated" during a dental visit and expressed as anger toward the dentist. Sexual feelings also may be activated by dental manipulations and, depending on the patient's feelings, a degree of satisfaction regarding sexual needs, affection, or anger may be misdirected to the dentist.

Teeth also have important psychologic significance. They may be symbolic of the expression of aggression because they were the first weapons of the child. A patient's body image may be reflected in his or her attitude toward teeth. To some people the loss of teeth means body destruction. Individuals who have a tendency toward self-destructive feelings may view the need to lose teeth as a means of gaining some degree of satisfaction for having these feelings. A person may view the loss of teeth as an indication of premature aging; or it may be seen as a loss of sexual potency and youthful optimism.

The dentist may not be aware of the source of a patient's strong feelings expressed in the dental setting, but the dentist should appreciate the fact that these feelings may have origins having nothing to do with the procedure being performed.

BEHAVIOR TOWARD ILLNESS

The dentist-patient relationship may be influenced by the way the dentist deals with a patient's reaction to illness. Because the emphasis of this book is the dental management of the medically compromised patient, the reaction of such a patient to medical disease as well as to dental problems must be considered when the patient is seen in the dental office. Ten major behavioral reactions to sickness are listed in Table 25-22.[5]

The patient may believe that it is bad to be sick, which leads to self-blame and self-rejection. The patient may also see the illness as representing a deserved punishment for being an imperfect person, or the illness may be viewed as a loss of personal power or personal control. These views may lead to feelings of worthlessness, hopelessness, and guilt.

One of the most intense reactions to illness is fear—fear that the illness will prevent the patient from achieving his or her immediate goals and desires; fear of pain, discomfort, and disability; fear of the unknown; or fear of death. It is unfortunate that Western culture tends to inhibit the expression of these natural fears.

The failure or inability to express fear leads to counterphobia in some patients. These individuals demonstrate actions directly opposite to

---

TABLE 25-21
Psychologic Significance of the Oral Cavity

Oral manipulation may activate old feelings associated with feeding as an infant
  If difficulties often occurred—anger and frustration
  If difficulties seldom occurred—pleasure and satisfaction
Oral manipulation may activate sexual sensations
Oral cavity and facial tissues may often be used to express emotions
Appearance of oral cavity important in our culture
Desire to present image of health, sex, and youth

TABLE 25-22
Major Behavioral Reactions to Sickness

Depression and self-rejection
Fear
Counterphobia
Anxiety
Frustration and anger
Withdrawal or apathy
Exaggeration of symptoms
Regression
Dependency
Self-centeredness

Based on Bloom SW: *The doctor and his patient: a sociological interpretation*, New York, 1963, Russell Sage.

the fear they feel to prove to themselves and others that they are not afraid. For example, this reaction may be seen in the cardiac patient who continues strenuous activities that may endanger his or her life.

Anxiety is a common response to illness that occurs in response to the patient's appraisal of what the illness may mean to his or her life-style and self-esteem at an unconscious level.

Patients may be frustrated by illness, possibly leading to feelings of aggression that are often expressed as irritability, crankiness, anger, and loud demands. Angry feelings may develop toward the dentist or physician, but there is often a reluctance to express the anger because the role of the patient demands politeness. Thus the anger may be expressed by other behaviors such as not following orders, not keeping appointments, or being late for appointments.

A sick person will often withdraw and become apathetic. Part of this reaction may be physiologically the direct result of the illness; however, the frustrated and angry patient who cannot express feelings because of fear of disapproval may retaliate by withdrawal and apathy. In addition, exaggerated conformance to the role of being a good patient may appear as withdrawal and apathy.

Patients may exaggerate symptoms to obtain care or to avoid doing things such as attending school or going to work. Often patients may be unaware of their actions. Persons who feel inadequate, who are shy, or who are crafty manipulators are those who most often demonstrate this reaction.

Another important patient response to illness is regressive, childish behavior. When a person is faced with a problem without a "solution," it is not unusual to regress, which may take the form of throwing things, crying, pouting, sorrowful looks, temper tantrums, or exaggerated helplessness and submission. Such regressive behavior in patients is usually an indication that the patient is having a difficult time coping with illness. It should be viewed by the dentist or physician in that light.

Severe and chronic illnesses foster a certain dependency by the patient on others. The more severe the disability, the greater the need for the patient to rely on others. Some individuals cannot accept this dependency and become anxious and try to deny their need for help.

Feelings of resentment, anger, and hostility can develop toward persons in contact with such a patient. Once again, an understanding of this process will allow individuals caring for such a patient to be empathetic and supportive.

Sick people tend to view the world around them as being small and develop a preoccupation with their sickness, needs, and fears. They may retreat to highly personal or magical notions about the cause of their illness. For example, cancer patients may believe that their illness is a punishment for swearing at their mother or for some "evil" thoughts they may have had.

MANAGEMENT OF THE ANXIOUS PATIENT

GENERALIZED ANXIETY

The dentist may detect anxiety in persons by their physical appearance, speech, dress, and the presence of certain signs and symptoms.

The anxious person looks overalert: sitting forward in a chair; moving fingers, arms, or legs; getting up and moving; pacing around the room; checking certain parts of clothing; and straightening ties or scarves, etc. On the other hand, sloppy dress habits and other signs, just the opposite of a concern with perfection, may be seen. Anxious persons may show signs of being watchful of possessions, always trying to keep them in sight.

The anxious person may speak mechanically and rapidly and at times may seem to block out or not connect thoughts together. The anxious person may respond to questions quickly; in fact, the dentist is often not even allowed to finish a question.

Signs of sweating, tension in muscles, increased breathing, and rapid heart rate may be seen. The patient may complain of an inability to sleep, may wake at an early hour, and may not be able to go back to sleep. There may be attacks of diarrhea and increased frequency of urination. In general, anxious persons are overalert and tense, feel apprehensive, and have a sense of impending disaster that has no apparent cause. Insomnia, tension, and apprehension lead to fatigue, which makes it even more difficult for the individual to deal with anxiety.

The dentist should talk with the patient and show personal interest. Verbal and nonverbal communication must be consistent. The dentist should confront the patient with the observation that he or she appears anxious and then ask if the individual would like to talk about how he or she feels, which may include the person's attitude toward the dentist. During these discussions, tension-free pauses should be allowed to develop between ideas, allowing a temporary state of regression to occur that will help the patient to restore a more anxiety-free state. Some patients may respond well to this approach without ever indicating why they were anxious.

If the patient remains anxious in the dental situation, the dentist may plan to use oral or parenteral sedation or nitrous oxide to better manage the dental treatment (Table 25-23).

POSTTRAUMATIC STRESS DISORDER

Many veterans with posttraumatic stress disorder (PTSD) may view the dentist as an authority figure who misled them and sent them to war. They may associate dental treatment with loss of control; hence the dentist must attempt to establish communication and trust with these patients. Those patients with IV drug habits may be carriers of the hepatitis B virus (HB$_s$Ag positive) and the AIDS virus. Those who are heavy drinkers may have liver and bone marrow involvement and be at an increased risk for infection, excessive bleeding, delayed healing, and altered drug metabolism. During the depressive stage of PTSD, patients often show a total disregard for oral hygiene procedures and are at an increased risk for dental caries, periodontal disease, and pericoronitis. They may complain of glossodynia, TMJ disorder, and bruxism.[18]

MANAGEMENT OF THE DEPRESSED PATIENT

During the depth of a depressive episode there may be significant impairment of all personal hygiene, including a total lack of oral hygiene. Salivary flow may be reduced, and patients may complain of dry mouth, increased rate of dental caries, and periodontal disease. In addition, complaints of glossodynia and various facial pain syndromes are common.[12]

Signs of low-grade chronic depression include tiredness even after enough sleep; difficulty getting up in the morning; restlessness; loss of interest in family, work, and sex; inability to

TABLE 25-23
Management of the Anxious Patient

Show interest
Carry on consistent verbal and nonverbal communication
Confront patient about appearing anxious
"You seem tense today."
"Would you like to talk about it?"
Administer sedation (oral or parenteral)
Administer nitrous oxide–oxygen

make decisions; anger and resentment; chronic complaining; self-criticism; feelings of inferiority; and excessive daydreaming.[10]

Signs of more severe depression in a patient include excessive crying, change in sleeping habits, thoughts of food making one sick, weight loss without dieting, strong feelings of guilt, nightmares, thoughts about suicide, feeling unreal or in a "fog," and an inability to concentrate.[10]

Individuals with severe depression should be encouraged to seek professional help; however, until that is sought and available, there are some things that can be done to help the person. Depressed individuals should be encouraged to try to stop feeling guilty about being depressed and should be assured that it is not their fault—they are not depressed because they want to be but because it seems to be the best way to keep themselves together. These persons should be told not to look on the depression as something that they will be able to recover from immediately because it will take time. They should be encouraged to remain active with physical activities such as jogging, tennis, or swimming. If it is too difficult for the patient to talk with people, notes can be used to communicate, and friends and family should be encouraged not to scold or criticize. The patient should be reminded that the depression will end and should be encouraged to eat properly and to find a person who is trustworthy so that the patient's feelings of anger can be expressed.[10]

It is important that patients with severe depression be referred for medical evaluation and treatment. If the patient is not responsive to this recommendation, the problem should be shared with a family member and every attempt made to get the individual in for medical attention. During severe depression, suicide is an ever-possible outcome; however, medical treatment is currently able to reduce this possibility.

MANAGEMENT OF THE PATIENT WITH A BIPOLAR DISORDER

From a dental standpoint lithium, used to manage bipolar disorders, can cause xerostomia and stomatitis. However, there are no adverse drug interactions between lithium and other agents used in dentistry.[13,31]

Patients who do not respond to lithium or those who can no longer take lithium are usually treated with a phenothiazine type of drug. Phenothiazines can cause bone marrow suppression and fluctuations in blood pressure. The dentist must be aware of these side effects and examine the patient for signs of thrombocytopenia and leukopenia (Chapter 23) because serious problems with infection and/or excessive bleeding can occur. The sedative action of sedative medications is potentiated by phenothiazine drugs, and serious respiratory depression could occur when using these agents in their normal dosage. Therefore, if these agents must be used, the dosage needs to be reduced. The dentist should consult with the patient's physician regarding this point. Epinephrine used in small amounts (three cartridges of 1:100,000 in local anesthetics) usually will produce no adverse effects when used in patients taking phenothiazine-type drugs[13] (Table 25-24).

MANAGEMENT OF THE COCAINE PATIENT

Patients who are "high" on cocaine should not receive any dental treatment for at least 6 hours following the last administration of cocaine.[16] Peak blood levels occur within 30 minutes and usually are gone by 2 hours. The danger of significant myocardial ischemia and cardiac arrhythmias is the main concern in patients who are "high" on the drug. Local anesthetics with epinephrine must not be used during the 6-hour waiting period following cocaine administration because cocaine potentiates the response of sympathetically innervated organs to epinephrine, which could result in a hypertensive crisis, cerebral vascular accident, or a myocardial infarction.[16]

TABLE 25-24
Dental Management of the Patient with a Bipolar Disorder

1. Consult with patient's physician
   a. Determine patient's current status
   b. Confirm drugs patient is being treated with
   c. Establish presence of side effects to these drugs
   d. Determine agents to be avoided or modified during dental treatment
2. Examine for and manage injuries to oral tissues
   a. Abrasion of teeth—excessive brushing
   b. Gingival ulceration or laceration—excessive flossing
3. Manage xerostomia and related problems
4. Patients receiving antidepressants or neuroleptic agents
   a. Local anesthetics with small amounts of epinephrine can be used (1:100,000); aspirate, inject slowly, limit to three cartridges
   b. Avoid use of all other forms of epinephrine (retraction cord, control of bleeding, etc.)
   c. Examine for possible side effects—thrombocytopenia, leukopenia, etc.
   d. Avoid or use in reduced dosage
      (1) Sedative agents
      (2) Narcotics for pain control
      (3) Hypnotic agents

Before treating a patient who is in a cocaine treatment program, the dentist should consult the patient's physician concerning the medications the patient may be taking and how to manage the patient in pain.

MANAGEMENT OF THE PATIENT WITH A PSYCHOPHYSIOLOGIC DISORDER

Oral diseases that are thought to be examples of psychophysiologic disorders include acute necrotizing ulcerative gingivitis, aphthous ulcers (PMNR), lichen planus, temporomandibular joint (TMJ) dysfunction, myofascial pain, and geographic tongue[8,26,28] (Figs. 25-1 to 25-3).

In these disorders there is an identifiable lesion with an emotional component to the cause. The pathologic process is potentially dangerous to the patient. The disorder does not reduce the level of anxiety or depression but rather increases it, and the increased anxiety aggravates the condition. Oral psychophysio-

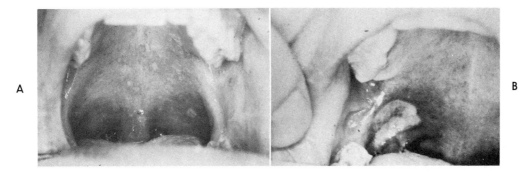

FIG. 25-1 Emotional factors appear to play important roles in some cases of aphthous stomatitis, **A,** and periadenitis mucosa necrotica recurrens (major aphthous), **B.**

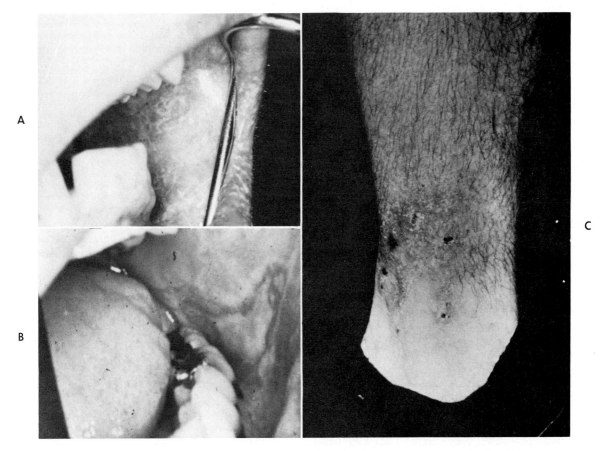

FIG. 25-2 **A,** Lichen planus involving the gingival and buccal mucosae. **B,** Erosive lichen planus involving the buccal mucosa. **C,** Skin lesions of lichen planus. Many patients with this disorder have a history of emotional crisis occurring just before the onset of oral and/or skin lesions.

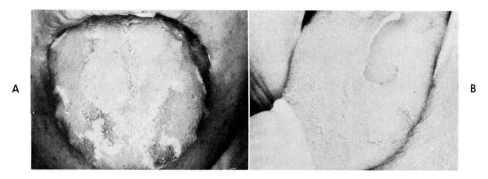

FIG. 25-3   Geographic tongue. This benign condition is thought to be related to emotional tension. It is an example of a psychophysiologic disorder.

logic disorders can be treated using the indicated regimen in Appendix B. The anxious patient can be sedated using one of the agents shown in Table 25-5.

MANAGEMENT OF THE PATIENT WITH A SOMATOFORM DISORDER (CONVERSION)

The characteristics of a somatoform disorder include the following: no identifiable lesion or pathologic condition can be found, the disorder or reaction has an emotional cause, it is not dangerous to the patient, and it is a defense for the patient in terms of reducing the level of anxiety. The reduction of anxiety by converting it into a symptom is called the *primary gain.* These patients may also have secondary gains resulting from their condition; for example, because of their symptom they may not be able to work or they may receive increased attention from their family.

The following are examples of oral symptoms that can be produced by somatoform disorders: burning tongue, painful tongue, numbness of soft tissue, tingling sensations of oral tissues, and pain in the facial region.[7,17] To the patient the symptom is real, and, if it is pain, it really hurts.

The diagnosis of a somatoform disorder should be made only under the following circumstances: (1) a thorough search from a clinical standpoint has failed to provide any evidence of a disease process that could explain the symptoms, (2) the symptoms have been

present long enough that if they were related to a disease process, it would be reasonable to expect that a lesion would have developed, (3) the symptoms have not followed known anatomic distribution of nerves, or (4) the underlying systemic conditions that could produce the symptoms have been ruled out by laboratory tests or by a referral to a physician. Systemic conditions that must be ruled out include anemia, diabetes, cancer, and a nutritional deficiency (vitamin B complex).[11]

The process of establishing the diagnosis of somatoform disorders is slow and time consuming. Dental treatment should not be performed on the basis of the patient's symptoms unless a dental cause can be found. Many patients have had needless extractions, root canals, etc. performed in an attempt to correct conversion symptoms. Complex dental care should not be attempted until the conversion problem has been managed. The diagnosis of a somatoform disorder should not be reached until a thorough search has been made over a period of time for pathologic findings that could explain the symptoms.

After a diagnosis of an oral somatoform disorder has been established, the patient can be managed as follows:

1. The findings should be discussed with the patient in the presence of a close relative, husband, wife, etc. During this discussion it should be pointed out that no organic source for the patient's problem could be found, that he or she does not have oral

cancer, and that the pain or symptom is real to the patient.

2. The possibility that feelings of unhappiness are the source of the symptoms should be pointed out, which will be difficult for the patient to understand and accept, but it is important to establish this "groundwork." Complex or unnecessary dental procedures should not be performed, even if the patient demands them in the belief that this will cause the symptoms to disappear.

The dentist should pay close attention to his or her feelings toward the patient. The symptoms may be viewed only as a device to gain attention and sympathy, and this may cause feelings of hostility and anger, which will not help in proper management of the patient. The dentist should try to feel empathy toward the patient, try to understand the cause of the problem, and react in a positive manner.

An attempt should be made by the dentist to manage the patient with a mild somatoform disorder (mild in the sense that the patient is able to function at a reasonable level even with the symptom, the patient's emotional status appears to be "stable," and he or she has shown or expressed no suicidal tendencies). Such patients should be assured that they do not have a life-threatening disease such as cancer. A series of regular short appointments should be scheduled to reexamine the patient for possible signs of disease, to discuss symptoms, and to reassure the individual that no tissue changes are present. The patient should be charged for this time and told what this fee will be before the appointments are set up (Table 25-25).

Patients with a severe somatoform disorder should be referred to a psychiatrist; however, once a patient has been referred, the dentist should still be willing to be involved. The patient may need to be reexamined and the psychiatrist consulted concerning the findings. If the patient feels that the dentist only wants to get rid of him or her, the suggestion of referral will not be helpful or effective.

MANAGEMENT OF THE SCHIZOPHRENIC PATIENT

Routine dental treatment of the schizophrenic patient should not be attempted unless the patient is under medical management. Even

TABLE 25-25

Management of the Patient with a Somatoform Disorder (Conversion Reaction)

Mild conversion reaction

Establish diagnosis
Talk with relative and patient
Suggest relation of feelings to problem
Examine patient to rule out serious disease such as oral cancer
Do not perform treatment that is not indicated
Do not become involved in complex treatment
Recall for support and reexamination

Severe conversion reaction

Refer to psychiatrist
Be available to continue to serve role as patient's dentist

---

then these patients may be difficult to deal with. It is advisable to have an attendant or family member accompany the patient to maximize comfort and familiarity. Patients should be scheduled for morning appointments. Confrontation and an authoritative attitude on the part of the dentist should be avoided.[12,35] If such an approach does not allow for proper dental management, the dentist should consider sedation or tranquilization, which should be done in consultation with the patient's physician. Chlorpromazine (Thorazine), chloral hydrate, haloperidol (Haldol), diazepam (Valium), or oxazepam can be considered.[12]

MANAGEMENT OF THE PATIENT WITH ALZHEIMER'S DISEASE

Alzheimer's patients are best managed by an understanding and empathetic approach. A patient's attention should be kept, and the dentist should explain what is going to happen before doing it. The dentist should communicate using short words and sentences and should repeat instructions and explanations. Nonverbal communication can be very helpful. Facial motion and body posture of the dentist should show support, cues that the patient is understood and that the dentist cares for the patient. Positive nonverbal communication includes direct eye contact, smiling, touching the patient on the arm, etc. Patients with Alzheimer's disease should be placed on an aggressive preventive dentistry program including 3-month recall, oral examination, prophylaxis, fluoride gel application, oral hygiene education, and adjustment of prosthesis.[17] Patients with advanced dementia may require sedation and short appointments. The choice of the sedative medication should be made in consultation with the patient's physician. Chloral hydrate or oxazepam have been used with some success.[24,28]

DRUG INTERACTIONS AND SIDE EFFECTS OF PARTICULAR CONCERN TO THE DENTIST IN PATIENTS WITH MENTAL DISORDERS

TRICYCLIC ANTIDEPRESSANTS

Many of the heterocyclic antidepressants can cause hypotension, orthostatic hypotension, tachycardia, and cardiac arrhythmias. When sedatives, hypnotics, barbiturates, and narcotics are used with the heterocyclic antidepressants, severe respiratory depression can result. If these agents must be used, the dosage needs to be reduced.[12] Atropine should be used with care in these patients because increased intraocular pressure can result.[12] Small amounts of epinephrine (1:100,000) can be used in patients taking heterocyclic antidepressants if the dentist aspirates before injecting and injects the anesthetic slowly. No more than three cartridges should be injected at any appointment (see Table 25-16). Other, more concentrated, forms of epinephrine must be avoided.

MONOAMINE OXIDASE INHIBITORS

Patients taking monoamine oxidase (MAO) inhibitors can receive small amounts of epinephrine in local anesthetics as described previously. Other forms of epinephrine (retraction cord, topical for control of bleeding) must be avoided. Phenylephrine must not be used in patients taking MAO inhibitors. MAO inhibitors may interact with sedatives, narcotics, nonnarcotic analgesics, antihistamines, and atropine to prolong and intensify their effect on the central nervous system (Table 25-15).

ANTIANXIETY DRUGS

Important drug interactions can occur between benzodiazepines and barbiturates, opioids, psychotropic agents, cimetidine, and erythromycin. In general, these agents will potentiate the central nervous system depressant effects of benzodiazepines. Two situations of concern to the dentist regarding the use of these agents exist: (1) barbiturates and opioids used for dental sedation or pain control must be administered with caution in patients taking a benzodiazepine for an anxiety disorder; (2) on the other hand, the dentist may prescribe a benzodiazepine for sedation to control dental-related anxiety, but care must be taken in dealing with the individual being treated with psychotropic agents for a psychiatric disorder. Usually the dosage of the medication can be reduced to avoid overdepression of the CNS. The dentist should consult with the patient's physician before using these drug combinations.[21,33,37,39]

ANTIPSYCHOTIC DRUGS

Several important drug interactions can occur in patients taking neuroleptic drugs. Extreme care must be taken if sedatives, hypnotics, antihistamines, and opioids are used in patients taking neuroleptic agents because the respiratory depressant effect of these agents is increased by neuroleptic drugs. This can be dangerous particularly in patients with compromised respiratory function. If these types of drugs must be used, the dosage needs to be reduced. The dentist must consult with the patient's physician before using these agents.

Epinephrine must be used with great care in patients receiving a neuroleptic drug because a severe hypertensive episode can result. Small amounts of epinephrine (1:100,000) can be used in patients taking neuroleptic drugs if the dentist aspirates before injecting, injects the anesthetic solution slowly, and uses no more than three cartridges. Epinephrine in retraction cords or for topical application for control of bleeding is contraindicated (Table 25-20).

Older patients taking antipsychotic drugs present several important problems concerning drug usage. These patients usually have decreased levels of serum albumin; hence many of them have a higher percentage of the drug in an unbound state. This increases the risk for toxic reaction. In addition, many of these patients have marginal liver function; hence drugs metabolized by the liver may remain in circulation for longer periods and in increased concentrations.

TREATMENT PLANNING CONSIDERATIONS

The goals of treatment planning for patients with psychiatric disorders are to maintain oral health, comfort, and function and to prevent and control oral diseases. Without an aggressive approach to prevention, many of these patients will be susceptible to dental caries and periodontal disease. Susceptibility to such diseases increases because of the side effect of xerostomia associated with most of the medications and the fact that some of the psychiatric conditions for which these patients are being treated reduce interest in or the ability to perform oral hygiene procedures. Also, many of these patients' diets contain foods or drinks that increase the risk for dental disease.[22,30]

The dental treatment plan should contain the following elements: The daily oral hygiene procedures must be identified. The treatment plan must be realistic for the patient's psychiatric disorder and physical status. The plan must be dynamic in order to take into account changes in the status of the psychiatric disorder and the patient's physical status. For example, a patient with Alzheimer's disease has progression to more severe symptoms that will make dental care very difficult in the later stages of the disorder. The patient with advanced dementia is often anxious, hostile, and uncooperative in the dental office. Complex dental procedures should be done in such a patient before the disease has reached the advanced stage. Another example of the need for a flexible, dynamic treatment plan is for patients with major depression or bipolar disorder. During affective episodes the emphasis should be on maintenance and prevention. Complex dental procedures should be performed only when the patient is in a stable condition regarding the mood disorder. The treatment plan should minimize any stress of the dental visit. This can best be accomplished by effective patient management efforts and the use of nonverbal communication.[30] The dental team should communicate to the patient and the family members a positive, hopeful attitude toward maintenance of the patient's oral health.

The last aspect of the treatment plan deals with the selection of medications to be used in the dental treatment of the patient. Certain agents may need to be avoided while others will require a reduction in their usual dosage. Medical consultation is suggested to establish the patient's current status, confirm the medications the patient is taking, identify any complications that may be present, and confirm dental medications and doses that will minimize possible drug interactions.[30]

Treatment planning for the patient with Alzheimer's disease demonstrates some of these principles. In a patient with mild dementia, good oral health should be quickly restored because of the progressive nature of the disease. Subsequent care should concentrate on preventing dental disease as the dementia progresses. A patient with moderate dementia may not be as amenable to dental treatment as the patient in earlier stages of the disease. For such patients treatment consists of maintaining the dental status and minimizing any deterioration.[30] A patient with advanced dementia often is very difficult to treat and will, most likely, require sedation, short appointments, and noncomplex procedures.[30]

ORAL COMPLICATIONS

Antipsychotic drugs can cause agranulocytosis, leukopenia, or thrombocytopenia. Oral lesions associated with this reaction may occur. If the dentist notes oral lesions, fever, or sore throat in patients taking antipsychotic drugs, the patient must be evaluated for possible agranulocytosis.

Patients who are taking antipsychotic agents may develop muscular problems in the oral and facial regions. If symptoms of dysfunction are first observed by the dentist, the patient should be referred to his or her physician for evaluation and management.[21] Patients with Tourette's syndrome often show oral tics, consisting of lip licking, lip smacking, cheek licking, tongue protrusion, and simultaneous contraction of the muscles of the lower face and blinking of the eyes. These involuntary orofacial movements have been misconstrued as obscene.[14]

Certain oral conditions—such as acute necrotizing ulcerative gingivitis, aphthous ulcers, lichen planus, temporomandibular joint (TMJ) dysfunction syndrome, myofascial pain, and geographic tongue[8,26,28] (Figs. 25-1 to 25-3)—may have psychologic factors that contribute to their etiology or affect the patient's physical condition.

Patients with psychiatric disorders may engage in painful self-destructive acts. Acts of orofacial mutilation such as eye gouging, pushing sharp objects into the ear canal, lip biting, cheek biting, tongue biting, burning of oral tissues with the tip of a cigarette, or mucosal injury with a sharp or blunt object have been reported.[14]

Patients with severe psychiatric disorders may not have the interest or the ability to care for themselves. Hence, oral hygiene is poor and increased dental problems develop. Prosthetic appliances are misplaced, lost, or improperly worn. In advanced cases, removable prosthetic devices may need to be taken from the patient because of the danger of self-injury.

Most of the medications used to treat psychiatric disorders contribute to increased dental problems in such patients because xerostomia is one of their main side effects. This may lead to an increased incidence of smooth surface caries. Stiefel et al.[36] reported on the oral health of persons with and without chronic mental illness in community settings. Patients with chronic mental illness were found to have a significantly higher incidence of dry mouth, mucosal lesions, coronal smooth surface caries, and severity of plaque and calculus build up.

Patients with dementia often have oral injuries from falls and ulcerations of the tongue, cheeks, and alveolar mucosa from accidents with forks, spoons, or mastication.[17] They may also have poor oral hygiene with an increased incidence of periodontal disease, root and crown caries, missing teeth, attrition and abrasion of teeth, and migration of teeth. It is not unusual for edentulous patients to misplace or lose their dentures and at times even attempt to wear the upper denture on the lower arch and vice versa. Xerostomia is common in patients on antipsychotic medications. It is important to establish good oral hygiene and dental repair early in the course of Alzheimer's disease because things only get progressively worse.[35]

REFERENCES

1. Adelson H: The psychodynamics of the doctor-patient relationship, *NY State Dent J* 36:95-103, 1970.
2. Alzheimer's Disease and Related Disorders Association: *Fact sheet on Alzheimer's disease,* Publ. no. ED2002-6, Chicago, 1988, The Association.
3. Beal MF, Richardson EP, Martin JB: Degenerative diseases of the nervous system. In Wilson JD, et al, editors: *Harrison's Principles of internal medicine,* ed 12, New York, 1991, McGraw-Hill, pp 2060-2076.
4. Black JL: Antipsychotic agents: a clinical update, *Mayo Clin Proc* 60:777-789, 1985.
5. Bloom SW: *The doctor and his patient: a sociological interpretation,* New York, 1963, Russell Sage.
6. Blum LH: Psychological aspects and the dentist-patient relationship, I, *NY State Dent J* 39:8-10, 1969.
7. Blum LH: Psychological aspects and the dentist-patient relationship, II, *NY State Dent J* 39:51-55, 1969.
8. Brightman VJ: Oral symptoms without apparent physical abnormality. In Lynch MA, editor: *Burket's Oral medicine, diagnosis and treatment,* ed 7, Philadelphia, 1977, JB Lippincott.
9. Brown MM, Hachinski VC: Acute confusional states, amnesia and dementia. In Wilson JD, et al, editors: *Harrison's Principles of internal medicine,* ed 12, New York, 1991, McGraw-Hill, pp 183-193.
10. DeRosin HA, Pellegrino VY: *The book of hope,* New York, 1976, Macmillan.
11. *Diagnostic and statistical manual of mental disorders,* ed 3, revised, Washington DC, 1987, American Psychiatric Association.
12. Friedlander AH, Brill NQ: Dental management of patients with schizophrenia, *Spec Care Dent* 6(5):217-219, 1986.
13. Friedlander AH, Brill NQ: The dental managment of patients with major depression, *Oral Surg* 71:573-578, 1991.
14. Friedlander AH, Cummings JL: Dental treatment of patients with Gilles de la Tourette's syndrome, *Oral Surg* 73:299-303, 1992.
15. Reference deleted in proofs.
16. Friedlander AH, Gorelick DA: Dental management of the cocaine addict, *Oral Surg* 65:45-48, 1988.
17. Friedlander AH, Jarvik LF: The dental management of the patient with dementia, *Oral Surg* 64:549-553, 1987.
18. Reference deleted in proofs.
19. Friedlander AH, Soloman DH: Dental management of the geriatric alcoholic patient, *Gerodontics* 4(1):23-27, 1988.
20. Hampf G, Aalberg V, Sunden B: Experiences from a facial pain unit, *J Craniomandib Disord* 4(4):267-272, 1990.
21. Judd LL: The therapeutic use of psychotropic medications. In Wilson JD, et al, editors: *Harrison's Principles of internal medicine,* ed 12, New York, 1991, McGraw-Hill, pp 2139-2154.
22. Judd LL, Braff DL, Britton KT, et al: Psychiatric disorders. In Wilson JD, et al, editors: *Harrison's Principles of internal medicine,* ed 12, New York, 1991, McGraw-Hill, pp 2123-2151.
23. Katzman R: The dementias. In Rowland LR, editor: *Merritt's Textbook of neurology,* ed 8, Philadelphia, 1989, Lea & Febiger, pp 637-644.

24. Magarian GJ, Middaugh DA, Linz DH: Hyperventilation syndrome: a diagnosis begging for recognition, *JAMA* 155:732-740, 1983.

25. McKhann G, Drachman D, Folstein M, et al: Clinical diagnosis of Alzheimer's disease: report of the NINCDS-ADRDA Work Group, *Neurology* 34:939-944, 1984.

26. Michels R, Schoenberg BB: Psychogenic disturbances. In Zegarelli EV, editor: *Diagnosis of diseases of the mouth and jaws,* ed 2, Philadelphia, 1978, Lea & Febiger.

27. Missri JC, Alexander S: Hyperventilation syndrome, *JAMA* 240:2093-2096, 1978.

28. Mitchell RJ: Etiology of temporomandibular disorders, *Curr Opin Dent* 1:471-475, 1991.

29. Morris JH: The nervous system. In Cotran RS, et al, editors: *Robbin's Pathologic basis of disease,* ed 4, Philadelphia, 1989, WB Saunders, pp 1385-1449.

30. Niessen LC, Jones JA: Professional dental care for patients with dementia, *Gerodontology* 6(2):67-71, 1987.

31. Roth JA: Drugs used in the treatment of mood disorders. In Smith CM, Reynard AM, editors: *Textbook of pharmacology,* Philadelphia, 1992, WB Saunders, pp 271-298.

32. Seltzer B: Dementia: its diagnosis and medical management, *Gerodontology* 6(2):47-52, 1987.

33. Smith CM: Antianxiety drugs. In Smith CM, Reynard AM, editors: *Textbook of pharmacology,* Philadelphia, 1992, WB Saunders, pp 271-298.

34. Somerman MJ: Dental implications of pharmacological management of the Alzheimer's patient, *Gerodontology* 6(2):59-66, 1987.

35. Steinberg BJ, Brown S: Dental treatment of the health compromised elderly: medical and psychological considerations, *Alpha Omegan* 79:34-41, 1986.

36. Stiefel DJ, Truelove EL, Menard TW, et al: A comparison of oral health of persons with and without chronic mental illness in community settings, *Spec Care Dent* 10(1):6-12, 1990.

37. VanDer Bijl P: Benzodiazepines in dentistry: a review, *Compendium* 13(1):46-49, 1992.

38. Winkler S: Psychological aspects of treating complete denture patients: their relation to prosthodontic success, *J Geriatr Psychiatry Neurol* 2(1):48-51, 1989.

39. Winter JC: Antipsychotic drugs (antipsychotics). In Smith CM, Reynard AM, editors: *Textbook of pharmacology,* Philadelphia, 1992, WB Saunders, pp 298-309.

26

Organ Transplantation

The first human heart transplantation was performed in 1967. During 1968, 102 heart transplants were done with a 1-year survival rate of only 22%.[12] The first orthotopic liver transplantation was performed in 1963 and the first extended survival, 13 months, was achieved in 1967.[25] The first successful kidney transplant occurred in 1954 involving identical twin brothers. The first successful kidney allograft transplant was done in 1959 using total body radiation, and the first successful human kidney cadaver transplant was performed in 1962, using azathioprine (Imuran).[14] The first pancreas transplant was performed in 1966, along with duodenum and kidney, for a patient with diabetic nephropathy.[15] Bone marrow transplantation (BMT) was initiated in 1957 when large quantities of marrow were infused intravenously into patients with leukemia. In 1958 BMT was performed in six victims of a radiation accident.[19]

These first attempts at organ transplantation in the 1950s and 1960s were all followed by increased activity in transplantation that resulted in very poor results. A period followed during which few transplants were attempted. Increased research activity in the 1960s led to techniques that dealt with the major limiting factor in organ transplantation—rejection of the organ by the host immune system. With the development of effective immunosuppressive agents, improved surgical techniques (including percutaneous biopsy of solid transplanted organs to monitor rejection), and the acceptance of the concept of "brain death" as a definition for determining the death of potential donors, the stage was set for major advances in organ transplantation.[12,25,30] Transplantation of the heart, liver, and kidney is now no longer considered an experimental procedure and is available as a treatment option for selected patients with end-organ disease. Transplantation of the pancreas is also considered a major treatment option for uremic diabetic patients who are receiving a kidney transplant.[26,27] BMT is an indicated treatment for patients with myelogenous leukemia as well as for other blood dyscrasias[19] (Table 26-1).

GENERAL DESCRIPTION

Various types of organ transplants can be performed, depending on the mix of recipients and donors. The ideal combination involves the transplantation of an organ from an identical twin to the other twin. The next best match for organ survival is transplantation of an organ from one living relative to another. This is followed by transplantation of an organ between living nonrelated individuals. Each of these combinations, however, is limited by the fact that unless two organs are present the donor could not survive. Thus these types of matches are basically limited to kidney and bone marrow donors. Nevertheless, recent studies have shown success with transplantation of a portion of a liver or pancreas from living donors. The largest organ pool for transplantation is cadaver organs, but the match is also poorest.

Matching of blood type and HLA antigens, along with tissue compatibility tests, usually results in longer graft and patient survival. The best matching, of course, occurs in identical twins; however, with appropriate screening tests, acceptable matches can be found for other potential organ recipients and living or cadaver donors.

TABLE 26-1
Patient or Graft Survival for Transplanted Organs*

Organ	Source	Period	Number	Survival	1-Year (%)	5-Year (%)
Heart	University of Minnesota	1983-1988	139	Patient	92	78
Heart	International registry	1980-1989	14,589	Patient	80	72
Liver	United Network for Organ Sharing— United States	1988-1989	3343	Patient	78.5	–
Kidney	University of Minnesota	1980-1990	1831	Patient	93	88
Kidney	International registry	1987-1990 (cadaver donors)	14,203	Graft	78	–
		1987-1990 (living donors)	2273	Graft	90	–
Pancreas	University of Minnesota	1987-1989	138	Patient	93	–
				Graft	56	–
Pancreas	International registry	1986-1989	1220	Patient	87	–
				Graft	40	–
Bone marrow	International registry	1984-1989	3458	Patient	–	–
	Aplastic anemia	1984-1989	573	Patient	–	32
	Acute myelogenous leukemia	1984-1989	964	Relapse free	–	77
	Acute lymphoblastic leukemia	1984-1989	422	Relapse free	–	75
	Chronic myelogenous	1984-1989	1499	Relapse free	–	71

Based on Belle SH, et al. In Terasaki P, editor: *Clinical transplants,* Los Angeles, 1990, UCLA Tissue Typing Laboratory, pp 11-19; Horowitz MM, Bortin MM. In Terasaki P, editor: *Clinical transplants*, Los Angeles, 1990, UCLA Tissue Typing Laboratory, pp 41-52; Kriett JM, et al. In Terasaki P, editor, *Clinical transplants*, Los Angeles, 1990, UCLA Tissue Typing Laboratory, pp 21, 27; Najarian JS, Sutherland DER: Pancreas transplantation (accepted for publication, *Transplantation Proc*, 1991); Seymour RA, et al: *J Clin Periodontol* 14(10):610-613. 1987; and Sutherland DER, Moudry-Munns KC: *Transplantation Proc* 22(2): 571-574, 1990.

PREVALENCE

Since 1987 all organ transplant procedures performed in the United States have been reported to the United Network For Organ Sharing (UNOS). In 1980 the Registry of the International Society For Heart Transplantation was established. Similar international registries have been established for other organ transplants.[1,6,11,27,32] By the end of 1991, 1342 pancreas transplants had been performed in the United States. This represented more than half of the 2144 transplants that were reported worldwide to the International Registry. Over half of all the pancreas transplants reported to the UNOS Registry (United States) were performed in 1990.[16,27]

As of October 1, 1990, data from over 14,500 heart transplant patients were collected by the Registry of the International Society for Heart Transplantation.[11] Before 1980, fewer than 100 heart transplantations were performed annually. In 1988 about 2450 heart transplants were reported worldwide. Over 85% of all heart transplantations that have been performed worldwide have been done since 1985. In the United States there are over 118 centers performing heart transplantations. Further growth in the annual number of heart transplant procedures is now limited by the supply of donor organs.[11]

During 1988 to 1989 some 3343 patients received their first orthotopic liver transplantation as reported to the UNOS. Most patients received a single liver graft; however, 419 patients received two livers, 51 received three livers, and 4 patients received four liver grafts. From 1988-1989 there was a 25% increase in the number of liver transplantations performed. Survival for patients transplanted in 1988 was 75.5% at 1 year and 68.6% at 2 years following the operation. One-year survival for patients transplanted in 1989 was 73.45%. There was insufficient follow-up to calculate 2-year survival for patients transplanted in 1989. The difference in 1-year survival between 1988 and 1989 was not statistically significant.[1]

The International Bone Marrow Transplant Registry reported that over 20,000 patients have received allogenic bone marrow transplants between 1955 and 1987. Over 50% of these were performed during the 3 years between 1985 and 1987. Bone marrow transplants are the treatment of choice for patients with aplastic anemia and chronic myelogenous leukemia, those who fail conventional therapy for acute leukemia, and patients with a variety of immune deficiency disorders.[9] Tables 26-2 to 26-7 show the number of all types of transplants reported through the end of 1991.

The Cincinnati Transplant Tumor Registry

TABLE 26-2
Total Heart Transplants

	Centers	1989	1990	1991	Total
United States	31	1594	2065	2100	11,353
Foreign	89	1497	1649	869	8,092
Total	222	3091	3714	2969	19,445

From Terasaki P, editor: *Clinical transplants*, Los Angeles, 1991, UCLA Tissue Typing Laboratory, p 513.

TABLE 26-3
Total Heart-Lung Transplants

	Centers	1989	1990	1991	Total
United States	39	121	127	51	625
Foreign	36	193	242	90	975
Total	75	314	369	141	1600

From Terasaki P, editor: *Clinical transplants*, Los Angeles, 1991, UCLA Tissue Typing Laboratory, p 521.

TABLE 26-4
Total Liver Transplants

	Centers	1989	1990	1991	Total
United States	72	2039	2624	2889	13,009
Foreign	83	1393	1697	1290	8315
Total	155	3432	4321	4179	21324

From Terasaki P, editor: *Clinical transplants*, Los Angeles, 1991, UCLA Tissue Typing Laboratory, p 540.

TABLE 26-5
Total Kidney Transplants

	Centers	1989	1990	1991	Total
United States	202	8760	9704	9577	120,832
Foreign	240	9955	10,717	6059	120,216
Total	442	18,715	20,421	15,636	241,048

From Terasaki P, editor: *Clinical transplants*, Los Angeles, 1991, UCLA Tissue Typing Laboratory, p 476.

TABLE 26-6
Total Pancreas Transplants

	Centers	1989	1990	1991	Total
United States	40	121	233	511	1342
Foreign	54	129	126	5	802
Total	94	250	359	516	2144

From Terasaki P, editor: *Clinical transplants*, Los Angeles, 1991, UCLA Tissue Typing Laboratory, p 548.

TABLE 26-7
Total Bone Marrow Transplants

	Centers	1989	1990	1991	Total
United States	79	2634	2744	2027	21,311
Foreign	183	3221	3148	1707	20,453
Total	262	5855	5892	3734	41,764

From Terasaki P, editor: *Clinical transplants*, Los Angeles, 1991, UCLA Tissue Typing Laboratory, p 495.

since 1968 has collected and analyzed data from transplant centers throughout the world. As of November 1990, 5435 post-transplant malignancies were reported, occurring in 5103 recipients. The incidence of cancer in patients with transplanted organs ranged from 1% to 18%, with a mean of 6%.[18]

ETIOLOGY

The most common indications for heart transplantation are cardiomyopathy and severe coronary artery disease. The most common diseases in adults for which liver transplantation is indicated are primary biliary cirrhosis, chronic hepatitis, sclerosing cholangitis, fulminant hepatic failure, and metabolic disorders. In children, most liver transplants are performed for extrahepatic biliary atresia or metabolic disorders. Common indications for kidney transplantation are bilateral chronic disease or end-stage renal disease. Glomerulonephritis, pyelonephritis, diabetic nephropathy, and congenital renal disorders are the most frequent conditions leading to end-stage renal disease. The most common indication for pancreas transplantation is severe diabetes leading to end-stage renal disease. Diabetic patients who are going to receive a kidney transplant are also good candidates for pancreas transplantation. The most common indications for bone marrow transplantation are acute and chronic myelogenous leukemia, acute lymphoblastic leukemia, aplastic anemia, and immune deficiency syndromes.[1,9,11,15-17]

PATHOPHYSIOLOGY AND COMPLICATIONS

All candidates for heart, liver, and bone marrow transplantation have severe end-stage organ disease and would die without transplantation. Patients with end-stage renal disease can be kept alive by hemodialysis. However, the quality of their life can be greatly improved by renal transplantation. Patients with severe diabetes can also be kept alive with daily insulin injections, but their life also will be greatly improved by pancreas transplantation.[16,26,27]

CLINICAL PRESENTATION
SIGNS AND SYMPTOMS

Signs and symptoms for the following are discussed in the chapters indicated:

Advanced cardiac disease, Chapters 6 to 9
Advanced liver disease, Chapter 12
End-stage renal disease, Chapter 11
Advanced diabetes mellitus, Chapter 17
Bone marrow transplantation, Chapters 22 to 24

LABORATORY FINDINGS

Laboratory findings of particular importance to the dentist who may be involved with patients before transplantation include

Bleeding time	Serum creatinine
Differential WBC	Specific gravity of urine
Prothrombin time	Platelet count
Hematocrit	White blood cell count
Partial thrombo-	Serum bilirubin
plastin time	Alkaline phosphatase
Blood urea nitrogen	Testing urine for pro-
Aspartate amino-	teins
transaminase	

Elevation of *aspartate aminotransaminase, alkaline phosphatase, prothrombin time,* and *serum bilirubin* would suggest advanced liver disease. Increased *bleeding time,* low *platelet count,* decreased *white blood cell count,* and decreased *hematocrit* are associated with many of the blood dyscrasiases. Elevation of *serum creatinine* and *blood urea nitrogen* and increased *specific gravity of urine* and *proteinuria* are associated with advanced renal disease. In addition, a low *hematocrit,* prolonged *partial thromboplastin time,* and decreased *WBC count* can be found in patients with advanced renal disease. These patients may be potential bleeders, prone to infection, and build up toxic levels of drugs that are metabolized by the liver or kidney, depending on the organ involved (Table 26-8).

MEDICAL AND SURGICAL MANAGEMENT
IMMUNOSUPPRESSION

The immunosuppressive agents now used for most heart, liver, kidney, and pancreas transplantations are cyclosporine, azathioprine, prednisone, and an antilymphocyte agent. Antilymphocyte agents include the Minnesota antilymphocyte globulin, equine antithymocyte globulin, rabbit antithymocyte globulin, or Orthoclone monoclonal antibody. The best clinical results are obtained with triple-drug immunosuppressive therapy—cyclosporine, azathio-

TABLE 26-8

Screening Laboratory Tests Used to Evaluate Status of Kidney, Liver, Pancreas and Bone Marrow Function*

Test	Normal Range	Abnormal Result	Organ
Alanine aminotransferase (ALT)to 45 U/L		Elevated	Liver
Alkaline phosphatase	1 to 4 Bodahsky units	Elevated	Liver
	3 to 13 King-Amstrong units		
	3 to 110 IV		
Aspartate aminotransferase (AST)	8 to 50 U/L	Elevated	Liver
Bleeding time (BT)	1 to 6 seconds (Ivy)	Prolonged	Kidney
			Bone marrow
Differential WBC			
Neutrophils	43% to 47%	Decreased	Bone marrow
Lymphocytes	17% to 47%		
Monocytes	0% to 9%		
Platelet count	140,000 to 400,000/mm³	Less than 80,000/mm³	Bone marrow, kidney, liver
Prothrombin time (PT)	11-15 seconds	Prolonged	Liver
Activated partial thrombo-plastin time (APTT)	21 to 30 seconds	Prolonged	Liver
			Kidney
Serum albumin	3.3 to 5 mg/dl	Elevated	Kidney
Serum amylase	60 to 180 U/L	Decreased	Pancreas
Serum bilirubin	0.1.5 mg/dl	Elevated	Liver
Serum chloride	95 to 103 mmol/L	Elevated	Kidney
Serum glucose	70 to 100 mg/dl (fasting), less than 120 mg/dl (2 hours postprandial)	Elevated	Pancreas
Serum creatinine	0.6 to 1.2 mg	Elevated	Kidney
Serum potassium	3.8 to 5 mmol/L	Elevated	Kidney
Serum sodium	136 to 142 mmol/L	Elevated	Kidney
Thrombin time (TT)	9 to 13 seconds	Prolonged	Liver
Urinalysis			
Specific gravity	1.003 to 1.03	Elevated	Kidney
pH	4.8 to 7.5	Decreased	Kidney
Protein	2 to 8 mg/dl	Elevated	Kidney
Glucose	Less than 180 mg %	Elevated	Pancreas
BUN	8 to 18 mg	Elevated	Kidney
Amylase	35 to 260 Somogyi units	Decreased	Pancreas
White blood cell count (WBC)	4000 to 10,000/mm³	Decreased	Bone marrow

*Normal values may vary depending on techniques used.

prine, and prednisone. Antilymphocyte agents are used at the time of induction of immuno-suppression and for acute rejection episodes. The immunosuppression regimens vary from center to center in terms of dosage, timing, and duration of use of the various agents. Following transplantation, doses of the immunosuppression agents are reduced as much as possible to a level that still prevents rejection of the graft.[9,15,16,20,26]

Total body irradiation (1000 rads) has been the most effective means of conditioning a bone marrow graft recipient. Cyclophosphamide is usually used in the immunosuppressive phase before (4 to 5 days) transplantation. Busulfan has also been used for conditioning the graft recipient. Cyclosporine, prednisone, and methotrexate are used after marrow transplantation to prevent or ameliorate graft-versus-host disease.[6,9,30]

SURGICAL PROCEDURE

HEART TRANSPLANTATION

Heart transplantation involves the surgical removal of the heart from the donor by one surgical team and then the removal of the recipient's diseased heart and the attachment of the donor's heart to the major vessels of the recipient's heart by a second surgical team (Fig. 26-1). In addition to the immunosuppressive agents given to the recipient, other medications are given at the time of transplantation. These include agents such as dipyridamole (platelet suppression), sulfa-methoxazole-trimethoprim (to prevent infection), and mycostatin (*Candida* prophylaxis). Surveillance right-ventricular endomyocardial biopsies are obtained following transplantation to check for signs of acute or chronic rejection. Starting 1 year after transplantation, coronary angiography is often performed to look for evidence of coronary artery disease.[17]

LIVER TRANSPLANTATION

Liver transplantation involves the excision of the diseased recipient's liver with reconstruction of the vena cava, portal vein, and biliary tree (Figs. 26-2 and 26-3). The transplant

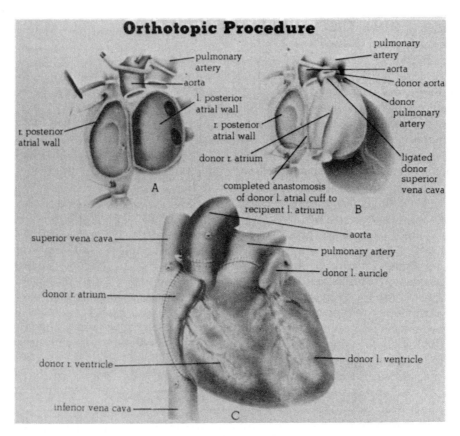

FIG. 26-1 Orthotopic heart transplant. By this procedure a patient's atria and ventricles are completely replaced. (From Herman M: *Am J Nurs* 80[10]:1786, 1980.)

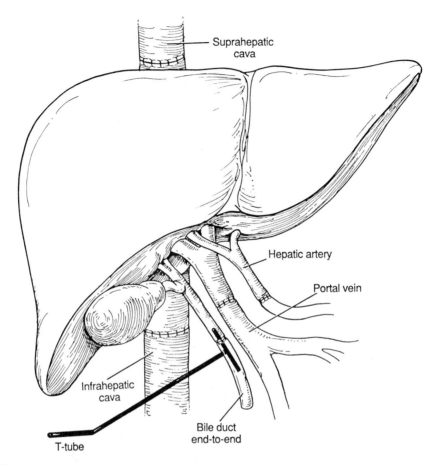

FIG. 26-2 Completed transplant. Vascular anastomoses include the suprahepatic vena cava, infrahepatic vena cava, portal vein, and hepatic artery. A choledochocholedochostomy biliary reconstruction is depicted. (From Howard TK, et al: In Kaplowitz N, editor: *Liver and biliary diseases,* Baltimore, 1992, Williams & Wilkins.)

procedure is commonly divided into three phases: (1) *dissection phase,* during which the recipient's liver is dissected free of surrounding structures; (2) *anhepatic phase,* when blood flow through the vena cava, portal vein, and hepatic artery is interrupted (during this time the recipient liver is resected and the donor liver revascularized); (3) and *reperfusion phase,* in which the implanted donor's liver is filled with blood. The final step is biliary anastomosis.[20]

KIDNEY TRANSPLANTATION

Patients who have a living related donor available for kidney transplantation are usually admitted to the hospital 2 days before transplantation. When a kidney recipient is to receive a cadaver kidney, the patient is admitted to the hospital on an urgent basis. Current preservation techniques allow kidney storage for up to 72 hours. In addition to being given immunosuppressive medications, the patient receives a bladder injection of antibiotic solution by means of a Foley catheter and a second-generation cephalosporin is given. The donor renal artery is usually anastomosed to the aorta and the renal vein to the vena cava in children. In adults, the renal artery is anastomosed to either the internal or the external iliac artery. After the

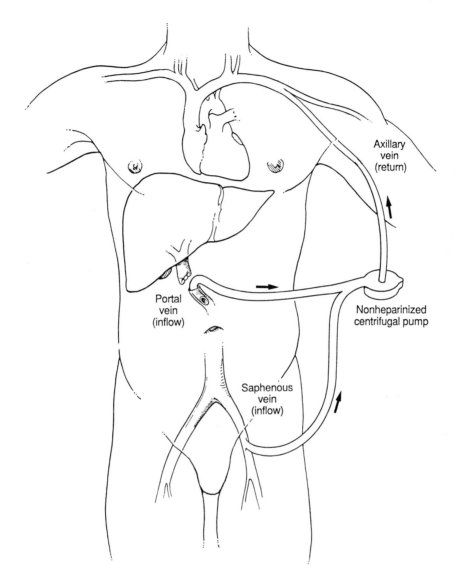

FIG. 26-3 Venovenous bypass. The portal vein is divided, and devascularization of the liver is completed. Then the portal vein is cannulated and a second cannula is placed in the iliac vein via the saphenous vein. The blood is pumped by a centrifugal pump through a nonheparinized system and returned to the patient via a cannula placed in the axillary vein. Flows of 2 to 5 L/min are commonly attained. Flow must be maintained above 700 to 1000 ml/min to prevent thrombosis. (From Howard TK, et al: In Kaplowitz N, editor: *Liver and biliary diseases,* Baltimore, 1992, Williams & Wilkins.)

kidneys are reperfused, urethral implantation is done. Three days after surgery the patient is taken off the antibiotics that were started just before surgery and is given trimethoprim-sulfamethoxazole (Bactrim) daily for as long as the graft is functioning. Acyclovir and nystatin are usually given for the first 3 months to prevent CMV and *Candida* infection.[15]

PANCREAS TRANSPLANTATION

Pancreas transplantation can be done (1) simultaneously with kidney transplantation (Fig. 26-4), (2) following kidney transplantation, or (3) as a separate procedure (Figs. 26-5 and 26-6). Living related donor grafts are usually used for recipients of pancreas transplants alone or a pancreas transplant after a previous kidney. However, cadaver grafts can be transplanted to all recipient categories. Cadaver donor pancreas grafts can be preserved by cold storage in a silica gel–filtered plasma solution for about 10 to 24 hours. In most grafts the pancreatic duct is drained into the bladder. Urine amylase levels (25% reduction) are used in bladder-drained patients to monitor for rejection. Decreased urinary amylase activity precedes hyperglycemia as a manifestation of rejection. In patients who have simultaneous kidney and pancreas transplants, an increase in serum creatinine indicates the possible onset of rejection before changes in urinary amylase are detected.[16,26]

BONE MARROW TRANSPLANTATION

Patients who are going to receive a bone marrow transplant are prepared using different preoperative regimens depending on the patient's disease. Cyclophosphamide and total body irradiation or busulfan may be used for patients with leukemia. Patients with a lymphoma may be given cyclophosphamide and total body irradiation, busulfan and cyclophosphamide, or busulfan alone. Patients with aplastic anemia may be given cyclophosphamide alone. The preoperative regimens start several days before transplantation. At transplantation, the donor's marrow is infused into the recipient. Most patients are given cyclosporine, methotrexate, or steroids following transplantation. Patients testing positive for HSV are given prophylactic IV acyclovir. Patients are usually given an antifungal medication such as IV miconazole to prevent *Candida* infection. These medications are continued following bone marrow transplantation throughout the critical period needed for the transplanted marrow to begin functioning. This critical period may last up to 20 days or more. Once the transplanted marrow starts to function, the risk of infection decreases. However, long-term therapy using broad spectrum antibiotics such as Bactrim is needed to reduce the risk of infection. Patients who develop evidence of graft-versus-host disease (GVHD) are treated with methotrexate.[7,9,19]

COMPLICATIONS

Complications associated with organ transplantation generally consist of technical problems involving the surgical procedure, problems related to immunosuppression, and special problems specific to the organ transplanted. A discussion of the surgical complications is beyond the scope of this text and would seldom apply to the dentist's management of such patients (Table 26-9).

IMMUNOSUPPRESSION

Excessive immunosuppression increases the risk for infection and must be avoided. Invasive (biopsy) and noninvasive techniques are used to evaluate patients for signs of excessive immunosuppression. Clinical evidence of such immunosuppression are opportunistic infections and tumors known to be related to these agents. When evidence of excessive immunosuppression is found, the dosage of the immunosuppressant drugs must be reduced.[11,15,16,20]

REJECTION

Rejection of the transplanted organ is evidenced when signs and symptoms of organ failure begin to occur. Organ biopsies are used to confirm the rejection reaction (Fig. 26-7). When evidence of acute rejection is found, the dosage of the immunosuppressive agents is usually increased.

Chronic rejection occurs insidiously and is progressive. It cannot be reversed with intensified therapy. Chronic rejection of the organ graft is associated with signs and symptoms of organ failure. Classical evidence of chronic rejection is found by biopsy.[11,15,16,20]

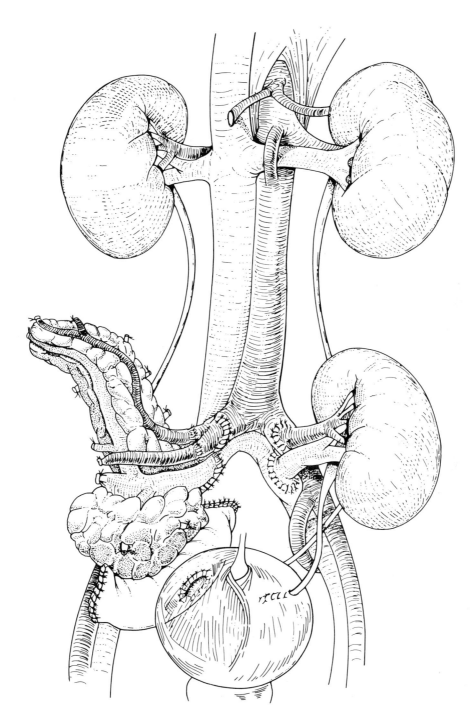

FIG. 26-4 Pancreaticoduodenocystostomy. Combined kidney and pancreas transplants. (From Groshek M, Smith VL: In Norris MK, House MA, editors: *Organ and tissue transplantation,* Philadelphia, 1991, FA Davis, p 159.)

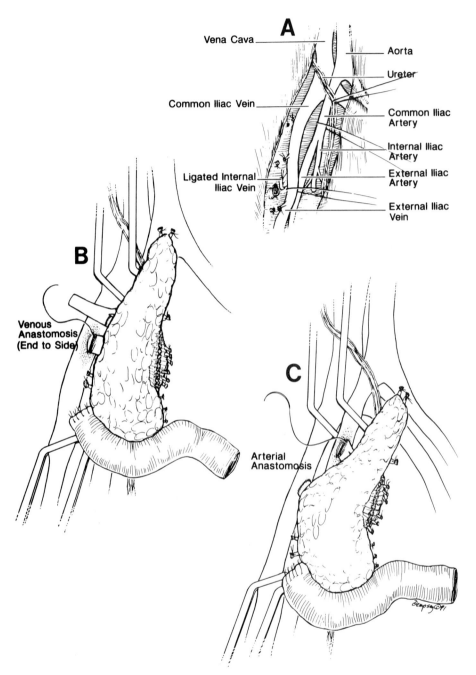

FIG. 26-5 Transplantation of the pancreaticoduodenal allografts. **A,** Preparation of the recipient vessels. Note that all deep branches of the common and external iliac veins are ligated and divided. The vein is brought lateral to the artery. The ureter is mobilized and brought medial to the artery. **B,** The venous anastomosis is performed end-to-side, with the portal vein of the pancreas graft anastomosed to the proximal external or distal common iliac vein. **C,** The arterial anastomosis is performed after the venous anastomosis and placed superior to the venous anastomosis. The common iliac artery of the recipient is used as the site for the arterial anastomosis. (From Brayman KL, et al: In Cameron JL, editor: *Current surgical therapy,* ed 4, St Louis, 1992, Mosby–Year Book, p 466.)

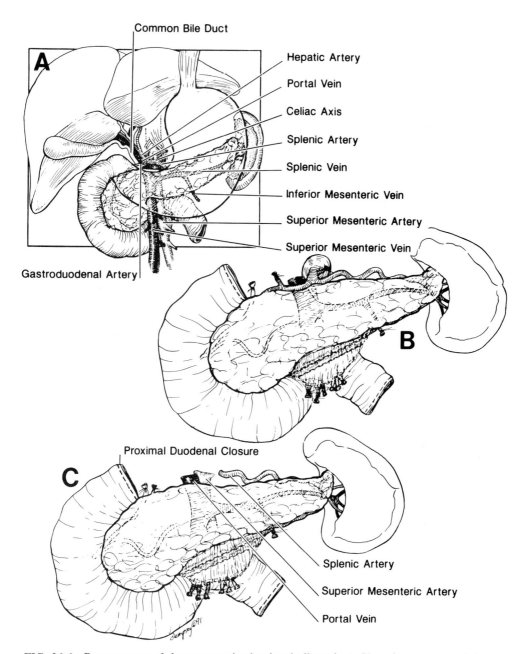

FIG. 26-6 Procurement of the pancreaticoduodenal allograft. **A,** Vascular anatomy of the liver and pancreas. Note the gastroduodenal artery, which is divided during simultaneous procurement of the liver and the pancreas but not during procurement of the pancreas alone. **B,** Pancreaticoduodenal allograft following procurement (nonliver donor). Note that the proximal duodenum has been divided with the GIA stapler. The mesentery of the small intestine inferior to the pancreas has also been ligated and divided following placement of two parallel rows of TA 90 staples. **C,** Pancreaticoduodenal allograft following procurement from a donor whose liver was also procured. Note the splenic and superior mesenteric arteries, which require ex vivo reconstruction. (From Brayman KL, et al: In Cameron JL, editor: *Current surgical therapy,* ed 4, St Louis, 1992, Mosby–Year Book, p. 461.)

DRUG SIDE EFFECTS

The agents used for immunosuppression have several important side effects. One of the major side effects of azathioprine is bone marrow suppression with resulting leukopenia, thrombocytopenia, and anemia. These changes place the patient at greater risk for infection and excessive bleeding. Cyclosporine has replaced azathioprine as the key agent for immunosuppression in transplant patients because it does not suppress the bone marrow. However, cyclosporine does have important side effects. It may cause severe kidney and liver changes, which can lead to hypertension, bleeding problems, and anemia; and it may potentiate renal injury caused by other agents. Cyclosporine is also related to an increased incidence of gingival hyperplasia, hirsutism, gynecomastia, and cancer of the skin and cervix. Antithymocyte globulin (ATG) and antilymphocyte globulin (ALG) both act as lymphocyte-selective immunosuppressants. Important side effects associated with these agents include fever, hemolysis,

TABLE 26-9

Major Medical Complications Associated with Transplantation

Complications	Specifics
Excessive immuno-suppression	Infection
	Tumors
	Delayed healing
Rejection of allograft	Graft failure—heart, kidney, liver, pancreas
	Increased risk for excessive bleeding—liver, kidney, bone marrow
	Overdosage—if drugs metabolized or excreted by kidney or liver are administered in normal amounts
	Death or retransplantation—heart, liver, bone marrow
	Insulin, hemodialysis or retransplantation—kidney, pancreas
Side effects caused by immunosuppressent agents	Hypertension
	Diabetes mellitus
	Infection
	Excessive bleeding
	Anemia
	Osteoporosis
	Adrenal crisis (significant stress from surgery, trauma)
Special organ complications	Accelerated coronary artery atherosclerosis—heart
	Graft versus host disease—bone marrow

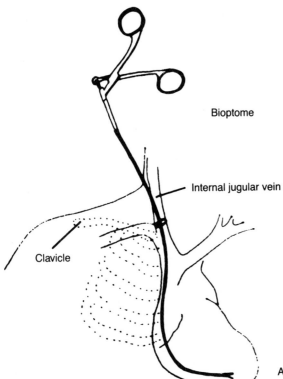

Bioptome

Internal jugular vein

Clavicle

Apex of right ventricle

FIG. 26-7 Endomyocardial biopsy technique showing the bioptome in place in the right ventricle. (From Copeland JG, Stinson EB: *Curr Probl Cardiol* 4(8):1-5, 1979.)

leukopenia, thrombocytopenia, tumor development, and increased risk for infection.[8,22,31]

Prednisone has important side effects, including hypertension, diabetes mellitus, osteoporosis, impaired healing, mental depression, psychoses, and increased risk for infection. In addition to these side effects, prednisone therapy may cause adrenal gland suppression. If adrenal suppression occurs, the patient is unable to produce and release increased amounts of steroids needed to deal with the stress of infection, trauma, surgery, or extreme anxiety.[14]

Immunosuppressed patients have an increased incidence of certain cancers. Overall, about 6% of these patients develop various forms of cancer. Cancers commonly seen in the general population (carcinomas of lung, breast, prostate, and colon) show no change in occurrence in immunosuppressed patients. However, two types of cancer found commonly in the general population are found with increased frequency in immunosuppressed patients: squamous cell carcinoma of the skin and in situ carcinomas of the uterine cervix.[18]

Cancers that are uncommon in the general population but that occur with increased frequency in immunosuppressed patients are lymphomas, lip carcinomas, Kaposi's sarcoma, carcinomas of the kidney, and carcinomas of the vulva and perineum (Table 26-10). It appears that cancer is a complication of intense immunosuppression per se, rather than being related to the use of any particular agent. However, certain agents may play a more direct role. Cyclosporine appears to be one of these agents,

as well as monoclonal antibodies. Both of these agents are associated with a higher incidence of lymphoma. Such lymphomas tend to occur earlier and show more nodal involvement.[18]

SPECIAL ORGAN COMPLICATIONS

The major specific organ complications of immunosuppression involve the heart and bone marrow. Recent improvements in immunosuppressant agents have not altered the development of *graft coronary artery disease.*[17] In a recent study the incidence of coronary artery disease in transplanted patients was 10% at 1 year, 25% at 3 years and 36% at 5 years. Coronary artery disease was responsible for 60% of late deaths.[17] One study showed a possible association between CMV infection and coronary atherosclerosis in transplanted hearts.[4]

Graft-versus-host disease (GVHD) is an important and often lethal complication of allogenic bone marrow transplantation. Acute GVHD occurs within the first 2 months after transplantation and is characterized by skin, liver, and gastrointestinal tract involvement. Chronic GVHD occurs later and is characterized by skin changes similar to scleroderma, sicca syndrome, malabsorption, and features of autoimmunity. Cyclosporine appears to be more effective than methotrexate in preventing GVHD in HLA-identical siblings who have received a bone marrow transplant for severe aplastic anemia. Methotrexate appears to be more effective for acute leukemia.[7,9,19]

DENTAL MANAGEMENT
PRETRANSPLANT MEDICAL CONSIDERATIONS

A number of significant medical problems must be considered during the dental management of patients being prepared for transplantation. The problems associated with congestive heart failure, advanced coronary artery disease, and significant cardiac arrhythmias are discussed in Chapters 7, 8, and 9. The medical considerations that impact on the dental treatment of patients with end-stage liver and renal failure are discussed in Chapters 11 and 12. The medical considerations impacting on dental treatment for severe diabetic patients being considered for pancreas and/or kidney transplantation are covered in Chapters 11 and 17. The patient who is a candidate for a bone

TABLE 26-10

Cancer Development in the General Population and in Transplant Patients

Tumor	General Population (%)	Transplant Patients (%)
Lymphomas	5	20
Lip carcinomas	0.3	8
Kaposi's sarcoma	<0.1	6
Carcinoma of kidney	2	5
Carcinoma of vulva and perineum	0.6	4

From Najarian JS, Sutherland DER: *Transplantation Proc* 24(4):1293-1296, 1992.

marrow transplant is generally very ill and is prone to infection, bleeding, and delayed healing because of thrombocytopenia and leukopenia (Chapter 23).

POSTTRANSPLANT MEDICAL CONSIDERATIONS

Medical considerations of importance to the dentist in the management of the transplanted patient fall into three stages: (1) *immediate posttransplant period,* (2) *stable transplant period,* and (3) *chronic rejection period.*

During the *immediate posttransplant period* the patient is at the greatest risk for technical complications, acute rejection, and infection. The length of this period will vary depending on a number of factors. The dentist needs to consult with the patient's physician to confirm that the patient has progressed beyond this critical stage.

The next stage is the period when the *graft is stable and functional.* The medical considerations during this stage relate to the effects of over-immunosuppression, which increase the risk for infection, and under-immunosuppression, which increase the risk for acute rejection. If rejection of the graft occurs, the organ begins to fail and the problems associated with end-stage heart, liver, kidney, and/or pancreas failure will have to be considered and managed when found.

The side effects of the immunosuppressive agents may present significant medical problems during any of the stages following transplantation. However, those occurring during the stable graft stage are of greatest concern to the dentist. These side effects may increase the risk for infection, excessive bleeding, bone fractures, circulatory collapse following significant emotional, physical, or surgical stress, hypertension, diabetes mellitus, and anemia.

Special organ complications found in heart and bone marrow transplantation recipients must be considered during the stable graft period. Symptomatic coronary artery disease develops in many of the heart transplantation patients. However, one important clinical feature of angina or myocardial infarction is missing in these patients. The transplanted heart has no nerve supply; thus, pain is not associated with angina or infarction.

Bone marrow transplantation patients may develop graft-versus-host disease (GVHD) following transplantation. Acute GVHD occurs during the *immediate post-transplant period* whereas the chronic form of the disease may appear in the *stable period.*

The *chronic rejection period* begins with signs and symptoms usually associated with organ failure along with histologic findings on biopsy indicating chronic rejection of the graft. This reaction is not reversible and will necessarily lead to retransplantation or death in heart and liver recipients. Kidney patients will require dialysis or retransplantation. Pancreas patients will require insulin or retransplantation.

TREATMENT PLANNING CONSIDERATIONS
PRETRANSPLANT PATIENTS

Patients being prepared for transplantation should be referred for an evaluation of their dental status. Whenever possible, patients found to have active dental disease should receive indicated dental care before the transplant operation. Patients with advanced periodontal disease may best be advised to have their teeth extracted and dentures constructed. The same consideration would be involved for patients who have extensive caries and have demonstrated little interest or ability to improve their level of oral hygiene or to modify their diet.

Patients who have a very good level of dental health should be encouraged to keep their teeth, but they must be advised of the risks and problems involved if significant dental disease were to develop following transplantation. The need for effective preventive dental procedures and more frequent recall visits to the dentist following transplantation must be pointed out to the patient.

Recommendations concerning retention of teeth for patients who have a dental status that falls between the extremes of poor and very good are more difficult to make. The risks involved regarding infection, the steps needed to prevent these complications, and the costs involved must be discussed with the patient and transplant surgeon. A patient with poor oral hygiene who has failed to become motivated to improve her or his level of home care should be encouraged to consider the extraction of teeth and the construction of dentures.

Before transplantation, all nonrestorable

teeth and teeth with advanced periodontal disease should be extracted in those patients deciding to retain their dentition. Nonvital teeth should be endodontically treated or extracted and all active carious lesions should be restored in these patients. Preventive dentistry techniques—including toothbrushing and flossing, diet modification, and the use of topical fluorides—should be initiated, reviewed, and implemented. The importance of using effective hygiene procedures, including antiseptic mouth rinses such as Peridex or Listerine, and the need for maintenance of good oral hygiene must be emphasized.

Before invasive dental procedures are performed on the patient, prior to transplantation, the dentist must consult with the patient's physician in order to establish the degree of organ dysfunction, need for prophylactic antibiotics to prevent local or distant infection, the ability of the patient to tolerate dental treatment, and the need to obtain other management suggestions.

There are no data to show that prophylactic antibiotics are indicated in the dental management of patients with advanced heart, liver, kidney, and/or pancreatic disease unless patients are subject to endocarditis or endarteritis (heart or kidney patients on hemodialysis). In patients with a depressed WBC count, a strong case can be made for using prophylactic antibiotics. The presence of infection in the operative field might be used as an additional indication for the use of antibiotics. Patients being prepared for bone marrow transplantation usually will require antibiotic prophylaxis. The need for prophylactic antibiotic treatment for invasive dental procedures in patients with advanced, heart, liver, kidney, or bone marrow disease should be discussed with the patient's physician before treatment.[5,28]

If the decision is made to use prophylactic antibiotics for certain patients, there is no general agreed-upon antibiotic, dosage, or duration of administration. The current American Heart Association's standard regimen used for prevention of endocarditis appears to be adequate for this need (Table 26-11). Patients facing bone marrow transplantation may require a more aggressive prophylactic regimen than those with advanced heart, liver, and kidney disease.

TABLE 26-11
Recommended Standard Prophylactic Regimen for Dental–Oral–Upper Respiratory Tract Procedures in the Patient at Risk for Bacterial Endocarditis*

Medication	Regimen
Amoxicilin	3 g orally 1 hour before procedure, then 1.5 g 6 hours after innitial dose
Amoxicillin-penicillin allergy	
Erythromycin ethyl-succinate	800 mg 2 hours before procedure, then half dose 6 hours after initial administration
Erythromycin stearate	1 g orally 2 hours before procedure, then half dose 6 hours after initial administration
Or: Clindamycin	300 mg 1 hour before procedure and 150 mg 6 hours after initial dose

NOTE: Initial pediatric doses are listed below. Follow-up doses should be half the initial dose. Total pediatric dose should not exceed total adult dose.
Amoxicillin: 50 mg/kg
Erythromycin ethylsuccinate or stearate: 20 mg/kg
Clindamycin: 10 mg/kg
*Including those with prosthetic heart valves and other high-risk patients.

Results of selective screening tests shown in Table 26-8 should be reviewed. If they are not available through medical consultation, they should be ordered before any invasive dental procedure is performed. If the screening tests reveal significant alterations in bleeding time and/or coagulation status (PT, TT, and APTT), the dentist should consider using antifibriolytic agents, fresh frozen plasma, vitamin K, and/or platelet replacement. The approach selected should be based on consultation with the patient's physician. The physician should also be consulted regarding drug selection and dosage modification. In patients with end-stage liver or kidney disease, the dentist should avoid drugs that are metabolized by these organs or reduce the dosage in order to prevent increased or unexpected effects (Table 26-12). Patients with severe diabetes mellitus must be managed as described in Chapter 11. If infection is present,

TABLE 26-12
Common Dental Drugs Metabolized Primarily by the Liver and Kidney

Drug	Route of Elimination and Metabolism	Normal Dosage OK	Method of Dose Adjustment	Requires Dosage Supplementation Following Hemodialysis
Lidocaine (Xylocaine)	Liver (kidney)	Yes		
Aspirin	Liver (kidney)	No	Increase interval between doses (avoid if possible)	Yes
Acetaminophen (Tylenol)	Liver	No	Increase interval between doses (avoid in severe failure)	Yes
Ibuprofen (Motrin)	Liver	Yes		No
Propoxyphene (Darvon)	Liver (kidney)	Yes		No
Codeine	Liver	Yes		No
Meperidine (Demerol)	Liver	Yes		No
Penicillin V	Kidney (liver)	No	Increase interval between doses	No
Erythromycin	Liver	Yes		
Cephalexin (Keflex)	Kidney	No	Increase interval between doses	Yes
Tetracycline (Doxycycline)	Kidney (liver)	No	Increase interval between doses (avoid if possible)	No
Diazepam (Valium)	Liver	Yes		No

Modified from Bennet WM, et al: *Am J Kidney Dis* 3:155-176, 1983.

an increase in insulin dosage may be required. Again, the dentist should consult with the patient's physician to confirm the patient's current status and specific management needs (Table 26-13).

POSTTRANSPLANT PATIENTS

The dental management of the patient following transplantation can be divided in three phases: (1) *immediate posttransplant period,* (2) *stable graft period,* (3) *chronic rejection period* (Table 26-14), or, in bone marrow transplants, the onset of *significant graft-versus-host disease.*

Immediate posttransplant period

During this phase, when operative complications and acute rejection of the graft are the major medical concerns, no routine dentistry is indicated. Only emergency dental care should be provided, following medical consultation, and it should be as noninvasive as possible.

Stable posttransplant period

Once the graft has healed and the acute rejection reaction has been controlled, the patient is considered to be in the stable phase. This period should be confirmed by medical

TABLE 26-13
Dental Management of the Patient Being Prepared for Transplantation

Complete dental evaluation

1. Poor dental status—consider extractions and dentures
2. Good dental status—maintain dentition
3. Other—decide on individual patient basis

Patients maintaining their dentition

1. Extract all nonrestorable teeth
2. Extract all teeth with advanced periodontal disease
3. Endodontic treatment or extraction of nonvital teeth
4. Initiate an active, effective, oral hygiene program
   a. Toothbrushing, flossing
   b. Diet modification if indicated
   c. Topical fluorides
   d. Plaque control, calculus removal
   e. Chlorhexidine or Listerine mouthwash

Patients receiving dental treatment including dental prophylaxis

1. Medical consultation
   a. Establish degree of organ failure
   b. Current status of patient
   c. Need for antibiotic prophylaxis (WBC count depressed)
   d. Need to modify drug selection or dosage (kidney or liver failure)
   e. Need to take special precautions to avoid excessive bleeding
   f. Other special management procedures that may be required
2. Laboratory tests (surgical procedures planned)
   a. Access to current PT, APTT, BT, platelet count
   b. Access to WBC count and differential

TABLE 26-14
Dental Management of the Patient with Transplanted Organs

Immediate posttransplant period (6 months)

1. Avoid routine dental treatment
2. Continue oral hygiene procedures
3. Emergency dental care as needed
   a. Medical consultation
   b. Conservative selection of treatment

Stable graft period

1. Maintain effective oral hygiene procedures
2. Active *recall* program every 3 to 6 months
3. *Medical consultation* regarding patient status and management
4. Treat all new *dental disease*
5. Infection control—use *universal precautions*
6. Staff *vaccinated* against HBV infection
7. Avoid *infection*
   a. Medical consultation—need for antibiotic prophylaxis
   b. Screening tests—WBC count, differential, CD_4 and CD_8 counts
   c. AHA standard regimen as option
8. Avoid excessive *bleeding*
   a. Screening tests—BT, PT, APTT, platelet count
   b. Special precautions
9. Need to alter *drug selection* or reduced dosage
   a. Liver or kidney failure
   b. Avoid drugs toxic to liver or kidney
10. Establish need for *steroid supplementation* and be able to identify and deal with acute adrenal crisis if it should occur
11. Examine for oral signs and symptoms of *over-immunosuppression or graft rejection*
12. Monitor blood pressure for patients taking cyclosporine or prednisone; if blood pressure increases above baseline established, refer for medical evaluation

Chronic rejection period

1. Render immediate or emergency dental treatment
2. Follow recommendations for patients with stable grafts if dental treatment is needed

consultation with the transplant surgeon. Usually any indicated dental treatment can be performed during this period if the procedures shown in Table 26-14 are adhered to completely. Many of the dental management problems with stable graft patients are similar regardless of the organ that was transplanted. However, some problems are unique to patients with specific transplanted organs.

RISK OF INFECTION

The increased risk for infection in the immunosuppressed transplant patient makes the case for use of prophylactic antibiotics stronger. In fact, many transplant centers recommend prophylactic coverage for all dental procedures that can produce transient bacteremias in these patients. The rationale for this practice is based on the increased risk for local and systemic infection resulting from suppression of the immune system. Again, there are no data to indicate if this practice is effective or necessary for all immunosuppressed transplant patients. To further complicate the situation, the oral flora in these patients appears to be altered by the immunosuppressive therapy, making the selection of the best antibiotic(s) for prophylaxis difficult. In addition, repeated antibiotic prophylaxis itself may alter the oral flora. Patients who have shown evidence of rejection and are receiving an increased dose of immunosuppressive agents are considered to be at greater risk for infection. A stronger case for the use of prophylactic antibiotics could be made for these patients.

Based on the lack of scientific information indicating whether or not antibiotic prophylaxis prevents local or systemic infection in organ transplant patients receiving invasive dental procedures, it is suggested that antibiotic use be decided on an individual patient basis. Thus the decision to use antibiotic prophylaxis and the regimen to follow should be made in consultation with the patient's transplant physician. Patients in excellent-to-good dental health and whose graft is stable may not require prophylaxis. By contrast, patients needing increased dosage of immunosuppressants or those with active dental infection (chronic periodontitis) may best be managed using antibiotic prophylaxis for invasive dental procedures.

The immunosuppressive agents used in the transplant patient may mask the early signs and symptoms of oral infection, making the diagnosis of the problem more difficult. When acute infection does occur, it is often more advanced and severe than that found in normal patients. The dentist should examine carefully for any evidence of acute infection in all transplant patients. The over-immunosuppressed patient can be more prone to oral infection as well as the patient with bone marrow suppression caused by the side effects of azathioprine, ALG, or ATG.

INFECTION CONTROL

Effective infection control procedures must be used when transplant patients receive dental treatment. Patients transplanted because of chronic hepatitis complications may still be infected with HBV or HCV. In addition, during transplant surgery additional blood is used, increasing the risk of infection with HBV or HCV. A few transplant patients also become HIV infected.[23,24] Excessively immunosuppressed patients may be infected with HSV, CMV, EBV, or other microorganisms that could be transmitted to dental staff or other patients. They are also at increased risk for infection transmitted to them in the dental operatory. The use of barrier techniques and the practice of universal precautions (recommended for all patients being treated in the dental office) are considered adequate to manage transplantation patients with stable grafts. In addition, hepatitis B vaccine should be administered to all dental staff to protect against infection from HBV.

EXCESSIVE BLEEDING

Liver transplant patients may be taking anticoagulants to prevent recurrence of hepatic vein thrombosis. Heart transplant patients may be taking anticoagulants to prevent thrombosis of the coronary vessels. Transplant patients on anticoagulants may need to have the dosage reduced by their physician before any dental surgical procedures. If the level of anticoagulation is greater than 2½ times the normal prothrombin time, the dosage of the medication may need to be reduced. It will take at least 3 to 4 days for the effect of the reduced dosage to lower the prothrombin time. When the patient's prothrombin time has been reduced to 2½ times normal or less, the surgery can be performed. If the prothrombin time is still above 2½ times normal, the surgery may need to be delayed. Following surgery, the dentist must be prepared to deal with excessive bleeding, if it should occur, by use of splints, thrombin, antifibrinolytic agents, etc.

Liver, kidney, and bone marrow transplant patients who are not taking anticoagulants could still be potential bleeders if there is rejection of the graft or graft-versus-host disease and significant organ dysfunction. Therefore, before any dental surgical procedure, the patient's physician should be consulted to determine the patient's current status. If necessary, selected screening tests should be ordered (partial thromboplastin time, prothrombin time, bleeding time, etc.).

ADVERSE REACTION TO STRESS

Transplant patients who are receiving steroids may not be able to adjust to the stress of various dental surgical procedures because of adrenal suppression and may require additional steroids before and after these surgical procedures to protect against an acute adrenal crisis. The need for supplemental steroids should be established by medical consultation. If steroid supplementation is recommended, the dosage and timing in relation to the dental procedure should be confirmed with the patient's physician. In general, patients taking more than 5 mg of prednisone/day should double or triple their normal maintenance dose on the morning of and 1 hour before the dental procedure. If postoperative pain or complications are anticipated, the maintenance dose also should be doubled the day following surgery. Patients taking a very large daily dose of prednisone usually will not require supplementation (Chapter 18).

Even though precautions are taken and patients are managed with increased steroid levels, the dentist should remain alert to the possibility of an acute adrenal crisis. Signs and symptoms of acute adrenal insufficiency include hypertension, weakness, nausea, vomiting, headache and, frequently, fever. Immediate treatment of this complication is required and consists of 100 mg of hydrocortisone (Solu-Cortef), IV or IM, and emergency transportation to a medical facility (Chapter 18).

HYPERTENSION

An important side effect of cyclosporine is renal damage and associated hypertension. Prednisone can also cause hypertension. It is important for the dentist to determine, by medical consultation once the graft is stable, what the "baseline" blood pressure is for each patient treated with cyclosporine or prednisone. As a part of each visit to the dentist, the patient's blood pressure should be measured

and, if it becomes elevated above the patient's "baseline" level, the patient's physician should be consulted immediately.[13]

Chronic rejection period

The third posttransplant period begins when significant signs and symptoms appear of chronic rejection of the graft or graft-versus-host disease. This phase should be established by medical consultation. In general, only emergency or immediate dental needs should be treated during this period.

ORAL COMPLICATIONS

Oral complications associated with advanced heart, liver, and kidney disease are discussed in Chapters 7, 8, 9, 11, and 12. Oral complications found in patients with blood dyscrasias are covered in Chapters 24 and 25. Oral complications found in patients with organ transplants are usually due to (1) *rejection,* (2) *over-immunosuppression,* (3) *side effects of the immunosuppressive agents,* (4) and, in bone marrow transplants, *graft-versus-host disease.*

Oral findings associated with *graft rejection* are the same as those found in patients with organ failure before transplantation. If lesions are found by the dentist that could be associated with organ failure, the patient should be immediately referred to the transplant physician for evaluation of possible organ rejection. Management of ulcerative or infectious lesions is described in Appendix B.

Oral findings that may indicate over-immunosuppression include herpes simplex infections, herpes zoster, candidiasis, large and slow-to-heal aphthous ulcers, and, on occasion, lymphoma, Kaposi's sarcoma, squamous cell carcinoma of the lip, and hairy leuko-plakia.[10,18,21] In addition, the potential is present for progressive gingival and periodontal disease. The presence of any of these lesions may indicate the transplant patient is over-immunosuppressed, and, after proper investigation, the transplant physician may need to reduce the dosage of the immunosuppressant agents. The dental management of these lesions is covered in Chapter 14 and Appendix B.

Oral complications associated with the *side effects of the immunosuppressive agents* include *infection, bleeding, poor healing,* and *tumor formation.* Azathioprine may cause bone marrow suppression, and, when it occurs, patients may develop oral ulceration, petechiae, and bleeding. ATG and ALG may cause bone marrow suppression, thus increasing the risk for bleeding and infection. Cyclosporine may cause poor healing, increase the risk for infection, and produce gingival hyperplasia.[3] The increased incidence of lymphoma in transplant patients is related to immunosuppression in general but is also related to the side effects of cyclosporine and antilymphocyte monoclonal antibodies.[18]

REFERENCES

1. Belle SH, Detre KM, Berringer KC, et al: Liver transplantation in the United States: 1988 to 1989. In Terasaki P, editor: *Clinical transplants,* Los Angeles, 1990, UCLA Tissue Typing Laboratory, pp 11-19.

2. First MR: Annual review of transplantation. In Terasaki P, editor: *Clinical transplants,* Los Angeles, 1990, UCLA Tissue Typing Laboratory, pp 357-373.

3. Friskopp J, Klintmalm G: Gingival enlargement: a comparison between cyclosporine and azathioprine-treated renal allograft recipients, *Swed Dent J* 10(3): 85-92, 1986.

4. Grattan MT, Moreno-Cabral CE, Starnes VA, et al: Cytomegalovirus infection is associated with cardiac allograft rejection and atherosclerosis, *JAMA,* 261:3561-3566, 1989.

5. Harms KA, Bronny AT: Cardiac transplantation: dental considerations. *J Am Dent Assoc* 112(5):677-781, 1986.

6. Heck CF, Shumway SJ, Kaye MP: The registry of the International Society for Heart Transplantation: sixth official report—1989, *J Heart Trans* 8(4):271-276, 1989.

7. Heimdahl A, Mattsson T, Dahllöf G, et al: The oral cavity as a port of entry for early infections in patients treated with bone marrow transplantation, *Oral Surg* 68:711-716, 1989.

8. Henderson RG: Complications of immunosuppression. In Hunter AR, et al, editors: *Transplant surgery: anesthesia and perioperative care,* New York, 1988, Elsevier Science Publishing, pp 73-111.

9. Horowitz MM, Bortin MM: Current status of allogenic bone marrow transplantation. In Terasaki P, editor: *Clinical transplants,* UCLA Tissue Typing Laboratory, Los Angeles, 1990, pp 41-52.

10. Itin P, Rufli T, Rüdlinger R, et al: Oral hairy leukoplakia in a HIV-negative renal transplant patient: a marker for immunosuppression? *Dermatologica* 177:126-128, 1988.

11. Kriett JM, Tarazi RY, Kaye MP: The registry of the international society for heart transplants. In Terasaki P, editor: *Clinical transplants,* Los Angeles, 1990, UCLA Tissue Typing Laboratory, pp 21-27.

12. Lansman SL, Ergin MA, Grieff RB: History of cardiac transplantation. In Wallwork J, editor: *Heart and heart-lung transplantation,* Philadelphia, 1989, WB Saunders, pp 3-21.

13. Little JW, Rhodus NL: Dental management of the heart transplant patient. *Gen Dent* 40(2):126-131, 1992.

14. Little JW, Rhodus NL: Dental management of the liver transplant patient. *Oral Surg* 73:419-426, 1992.

15. Matas AJ, Najarian JS: Therapeutic approaches to renal transplantation. In *Current therapy in allergy, immunology, and rheumatology,* ed 4, St Louis, 1992, Mosby–Year Book, pp 106-113.

16. Najarian JS, Sutherland DER: Pancreas transplantation—1991, *Transplantation Proc* 24(4):1293-1296, 1992.

17. Olivari MT, Kubo SH, Braunlin EA, et al: Five-year experience with triple-drug immunosuppressive therapy in cardiac transplantation, *Circulation* 82(Suppl 5):276-280, 1990.

18. Penn I: Occurrence of cancers in immunosuppressed organ transplant recipients. In Terasaki P, editor: *Clinical transplants,* Los Angeles, 1990, UCLA Tissue Typing Laboratory, pp 53-62.

19. Rhodus NL, Little JW: Dental management of the bone marrow transplantation (BMT) patient. (Submitted for publication, 1992.)

20. Roberts JP, Ascher NL, Payne WD: Clinical and surgical considerations in hepatic transplantation. In Letourneau JG, et al, editors: *Radiology of organ transplantation,* St Louis, 1991, Mosby–Year Book, pp 161-169.

21. Schiodt M, Greenspan D, Greenspan JS: Can you recognize the oral manifestations of AIDS? *J Resp Dis* 10(4):91-108, 1989.

22. Seymour RA, Smith DG, Rogers SR: The comparative effects of azathioprine and cyclosporin on some gingival health parameters of renal transplant patients: a longitudinal study, *J Clin Periodontol* 14(10):610-613, 1987.

23. Starzl TE, Demetris AJ, Van Thiel D: Liver transplantation: I, *N Engl J Med* 321:1014-1021, 1989.

24. Starzl TE, Demetris AJ, Van Thiel D: Liver transplantation: II, *N Engl J Med* 321:1092-1099, 1989.

25. Starzl TE, Iwatsuki S, Van Thiel DH, et al: Evolution of liver transplantation, *Hepatology* 2:614-636, 1982.

26. Sutherland DER, Dunn DL, Goetz FC, et al: A 10-year experience with 290 pancreas transplants at a single institution, *Ann Surg* 210:274-288, 1989.

27. Sutherland DER, Moudry-Munns KC: International Pancreas Transplantation Registry analysis, *Transplantation Proc* 22(2):571-574, 1990.

28. Svirsky JA, Saravia ME: Dental management of patients after liver transplantation, *Oral Surg* 67:541-546, 1989.

29. Thomas ED, Lochte HL Jr, Lu WC, et al: Intravenous infusion of bone marrow in patients receiving radiation and chemotherapy, *N Engl J Med* 257:491-496, 1957.

30. Thomas ED, Storb R: Technique for human marrow grafting, *Blood* 36:507-515, 1970.

31. White DG: Immunosuppression for cardiac transplantation. In Wallwork J, editor: *Heart and heart-lung transplantation,* Philadelphia, 1989, WB Saunders, pp 155-173.

32. Worldwide transplantation: reports of various registries. In Terasaki P, editor: *Clinical transplants,* Los Angeles, 1991, UCLA Tissue Typing Laboratory, pp 476-548.

27

Prosthetic Implants

Many patients with implanted prosthetic devices seek dental treatment. An issue of considerable importance to both the patient and the dentist is whether or not there is an increased risk for infection at the site of the prosthesis secondary to transient bacteremias that can occur with invasive dental procedures. National guidelines provided by the American Heart Association concern the increased risk for infection in patients with prosthetic heart valves and the steps to be taken to minimize this risk.[5] However, no such guidelines or recommendations from other national medical organizations are available to dentists regarding the level of risk or the need for prophylaxis in patients with other types of implanted prosthetic devices, such as knees, hips, intraocular lenses, vascular grafts, breast implants, penile implants, or intravascular access devices. The purpose of this chapter is to review data concerning the risk of infection at the site of the prosthetic device from dental procedures and to provide recommendations regarding the dental management of patients with such devices.

Discussion of the dental management of patients with prosthetic devices does not lend itself to the chapter organization used elsewhere in this textbook. Therefore this chapter will deviate from the usual format. In this chapter each of the prosthetic devices covered will be presented as separate headings, with the medical and dental considerations discussed as they relate to the need to use prophylactic antibiotics for invasive dental procedures. At the end of the chapter, a summary statement will compare the need for antibiotic prophylaxis for patients with various devices.

THE PROBLEM

A major problem in attempting to decide on the need for prophylactic antibiotics to prevent infection at the site of prosthetic devices is the method by which postoperative infection rates are reported. The current system results in under-reporting of late prosthetic device infection. Most accurately reported are acute infections that occur while patients are still in the hospital. Such infections are usually caused by wound contamination at the time of surgery. These infections usually have no relationship to transient dental bacteremias resulting from invasive dental procedures. However, in rare cases, acute oral infections can cause hematogenous seeding of bacteria that could infect the prosthetic device in the early postoperative period.[12]

Reporting of late prosthetic device infections is much less complete than for the cases occurring within the first 2 months following surgery.[12] However, some infections do not occur until several months or years after the surgery. Coagulase-negative *Staphylococcus* organisms can be present in the wound area for long periods before causing clinical infection. Thus even some cases of very late infections of prosthetic devices can be the result of wound contamination.[12] Nevertheless, the longer the period from surgery to the onset of infection, the more likely is hematogenous seeding of bacteria from distant sites of acute or chronic infection to occur. In some types of prosthetic devices, transient dental bacteremias may increase the risk for infection.

Under-reporting of prosthetic device infections can also occur because of the referral patterns involved. Many of the patients receiving prosthetic devices are referred to larger centers for surgery. Unless the infection occurs early in the postoperative period, it may go unreported. Once patients return home and infection occurs, they are often treated at the local area hospital, with no report occurring to the larger initial center.[12]

To initiate more accurate reporting of early and late prosthetic device infections, improvements must be made in the surveillance system. Hopkins[12] suggests that improved communication is needed between infection control workers in hospitals where patients with prosthetic device infections are treated and specialty physicians in the centers where the devices were implanted. This networking could lead to improved data concerning the frequency and types of infections involving prosthetic devices.

Based on current reporting methods, prosthetic devices implanted into a clean field have an overall acute wound infection rate of less than 5%.[12] The overall infection rate for most of these devices is 0.5% to 3% for the first year.[12] Acute infections are defined as early infections occurring during the first 2 months following insertion of the prosthetic device. Late infections are usually defined as those occurring 2 months following device implantation.[12]

SPECIFIC PROSTHETIC DEVICES
PROSTHETIC HEART VALVES

Mechanical and tissue prosthetic heart valves are used to replace damaged natural cardiac valves (Fig. 27-1). Over 120,000 prosthetic heart valves are implanted each year worldwide, with the majority being placed in the United States.[26] These prosthetic valve replacements are susceptible to infective endocarditis or prosthetic valve endocarditis (PVE).[11,24,26] The incidence of PVE is about the same for both mechanical and tissue valves.[17,26] Table 27-1 shows data reported from four studies involving more than 10,000 prosthetic heart valve patients, showing an incidence of PVE ranging from 0.98% to 4.4%.[11] PVE is described as early or late depending on the time from surgical placement of the valve to the onset of PVE. Early PVE occurs within 2 months, and most cases are considered to be the result of wound contamination at the time of surgery. Coagulase-negative staphylococci are responsible for about 43% of the early infec-

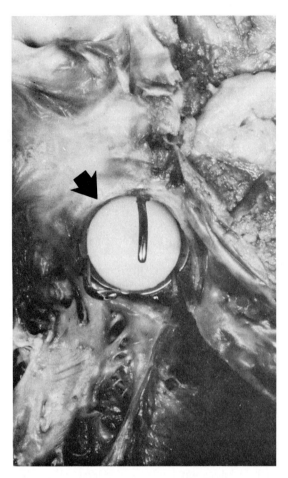

FIG. 27-1 Mechanical prosthetic heart valve *(arrow)*. (Courtesy Jesse E. Edwards, M.D., St Paul Minn.)

tions whereas streptococci are the cause of roughly only 3% of such early infections.[11,17,24,26] Late PVE occurs 2 months or longer following the surgical placement of the prosthetic heart valve. Staphylococci account for about 27% of the cases of late PVE, and streptococci are responsible for about 27% of the cases.[11]

Wound contamination accounts for some of the late PVE cases but does not explain all of them. Hematogenous spread of bacteria from distant sites of acute and chronic infection accounts for some cases of late PVE, and bacteremias resulting from surgical procedures performed elsewhere in the body appear to be

TABLE 27-1
Prosthetic Valve Endocarditis—Four Studies Totaling 260 Cases (1962-1982)

		Incidence of PVE			
Location	Number of Patients with Valves	Early	Late	Total	Overall (%)
Cornell Medical Center	1282	16	32	48	3.7
Mayo Clinic	4586	16	29	45	0.98
Stanford University Hospital	2184	9	42	51	2.3
Massachusetts General Hospital	2608	38	78	116	4.4
Totals	10,660	79	181	260	2.44

From Heimberger TS: *Infect Dis Clin North Am* 3:2:221-245, 1989.

responsible for the remaining cases.[5,11,17,24,26] Any invasive dental procedure has the potential to release oral bacteria into the bloodstream.[17] The frequency and magnitude of the bacteremia increase with the amount of gingival and periodontal inflammation present.[17] The bacteremias produced by invasive dental procedures last only 5 to 30 minutes and are termed *transient bacteremias*.[17] However, they appear capable of causing PVE in patients with prosthetic heart valves.

The American Heart Association[5] issues guidelines to dental health professionals for the prevention of endocarditis and PVE. The most current AHA guidelines (1990) published appear in Table 27-2. The American Heart Association recommendations have become the "standard of care" for the prevention of PVE, although there are no controlled studies on humans demonstrating that the recommended antibiotic regimens are effective in preventing PVE.[5]

VASCULAR GRAFTS

Synthetic vascular grafts are used to replace segments of major arteries, such as the aorta, that have developed an aneurysm secondary to atherosclerotic disease (Fig. 27-2). The material most commonly used is dacron. Infections of arterial grafts are not common, but, when they occur, wound contamination at the time of surgery is the major source for infection. In the United States, about 60,000 vascular grafts are implanted each year.[26] The rate of vascular graft infection is approximately 2%.[26] At the present time, the American Heart Association does not

TABLE 27-2
American Heart Association Recommended Standard Prophylactic Regimen for Prevention of Prosthetic Valve Endocarditis in Patients at Risk (1990)

Medication	Regimen
Amoxicillin	3 g orally 1 hour before procedure, then 1.5 g 6 hours after initial dose
Amoxicillin/penicillin allergy	
Erythromycin ethylsuccinate	800 mg 2 hours before procedure, then half dose 6 hours after initial administration
Erythromycin stearate	1 g orally 2 hours before procedure, then half dose 6 hours after initial administration
or	
Clindamycin	300 mg 1 hour before procedure and 150 mg 6 hours after initial dose

NOTE: Initial pediatric doses are listed below. Follow-up doses should be half the initial dose. Total pediatric dose should not exceed total adult dose.
  Amoxicillin: 50 mg/kg
  Erythromycin ethylsuccinate or stearate: 20 mg/kg
  Clindamycin: 10 mg/kg

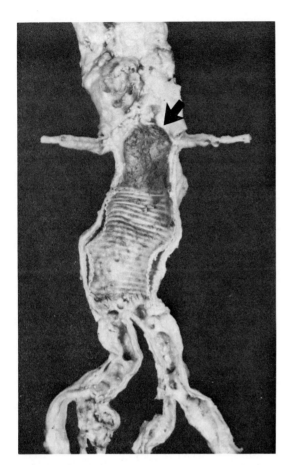

FIG. 27-2   Dacron arterial graft sutured into place (*arrow* points to the beginning of the graft). (Courtesy Jesse E. Edwards, M.D., St Paul Minn.)

feel there are sufficient data linking the risk of dental bacteremias with vascular graft infection to recommend antibiotic prophylaxis for patients undergoing invasive dental procedures.[5] It is suggested that the dentist consult with the patient's physician on an individual basis to determine the need for antibiotic prophylaxis. If it is determined that prophylaxis is needed, the standard American Heart Association regimen is recommended (Table 27-2).

IMPLANTED TRANSVENOUS PACEMAKERS

Transvenous pacemakers usually consist of a bipolar catheter that is inserted through the external jugular vein into the right ventricle[17]

(Fig. 27-3). The lead is connected to a generator that is usually implanted in the subcutaneous tissues in the chest.[17] In the United States about 90,000 pacemakers are surgically implanted each year.[26] Most infections associated with pacemakers occur in the tissues around the generator and are caused by wound contamination. The infection rate ranges from 1% to 5%.[11,13,24,26] Infection of the electrode catheter can lead to endocarditis, but this is an uncommon event. The current American Heart Association guidelines do not recommend antibiotic prophylaxis for patients with permanent transvenous cardiac pacemakers.[5]

CEREBROSPINAL FLUID SHUNTS

The condition that most often requires shunting to reduce increased cerebrospinal fluid pressure is hydrocephalus. Several types of shunts are used to decrease fluid pressure. Ventriculoperitoneal, ventriculoatrial, and lumboperitoneal are the most common types of shunts.[7-9] In the United States around 75,000 cerebrospinal fluid shunts are placed each year.[26] The infection rate ranges from about 5% to 15%, with most infections resulting from wound contamination.[6] Almost 70% of the infections are caused by skin flora staphylococcal organisms.[6] Cerebrospinal fluid shunt infections usually occur within 2 months following implantation.[1] The infection rate is higher for ventriculoperitoneal shunts than for ventriculoatrial shunts.[9] However, other types of complications include thromboemboli, severe complications of infection, and shunt malfunctions that make ventriculoatrial shunts more risky.[7,9]

Ventriculoperitoneal and lumboperitoneal shunts do not appear to cause increased risk for infection from hematogenous seeding of bacteria.[7-9, 24,26] However, ventriculoatrial shunts can become infected by transient bacteremias resulting from distant acute infection or invasive dental procedures.[5] The need for antibiotic prophylaxis should be established by medical consultation. If prophylaxis is indicated, the standard regimen of the current American Heart Association's guidelines should be used (see Table 27-2).

PROSTHETIC JOINTS

Severe arthritis, avascular necrosis of the femoral head, nonunion of a fracture, and acute trauma may require surgical replacement of a

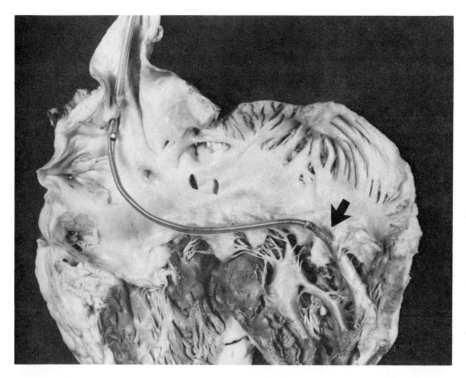

FIG. 27-3 Transvenous pacemaker (*arrow* points to the lead). (Courtesy Jesse E. Edwards, M.D., St Paul Minn.)

joint with a prosthesis (Fig. 27-4). Most experience, to date, has been with total hip replacement and knee replacement; however, other joints have been replaced, including shoulder, elbow, wrist, and metacarpophalangeal joints.[18] During the last 10 years, the number of prosthetic joints inserted has doubled.[26] In the United States some 400,000 joints a year are now being replaced with prosthetic devices. These include about 140,000 total hip prostheses and 115,000 knee prostheses annually.[26] The postoperative infection rate for total hip replacements is 1% to 2%[18,26] (Fig. 27-5). Most infections occur because of wound contamination at the time of surgery.[24] Various types of staphylococci *(S. aureus, S. epidermidis)* are the organisms most commonly implicated in these patients.[18,24,26]

In rare cases, hematogenous seeding from distant sites of acute infection has caused prosthetic joint infection.[13,19] However, there is no documentation of transient bacteremias from invasive dental procedures infecting prosthetic joint replacements.[13,18,19] In fact, the American Dental Association's Council on Dental Therapeutics and the American Academy of Oral Medicine have published statements indicating the lack of scientific information associating transient dental bacteremias with increased risk of joint prosthesis infection.[4,20,25] These groups do not recommend antibiotic prophylaxis for prosthetic joint patients but do suggest that the dentist consult with the patient's orthopedic surgeon on an individual basis to determine the need for prophylaxis. In 1992 a British medical organization, the Working Party of the Society for Antimicrobial Chemotherapy, reported that it did not support the practice of administering prophylaxis to prosthetic joint patients receiving dental treatment.[24a] Some factors that would favor prophylaxis for a given patient include previous history of joint infection, a loose prosthesis, severe rheumatoid arthritis, hemophilia, altered immune function, diabetes mellitus, or steroid therapy.

In a recent nationwide survey of 1666 orthopedic surgeons,[13] 57% of the respondents

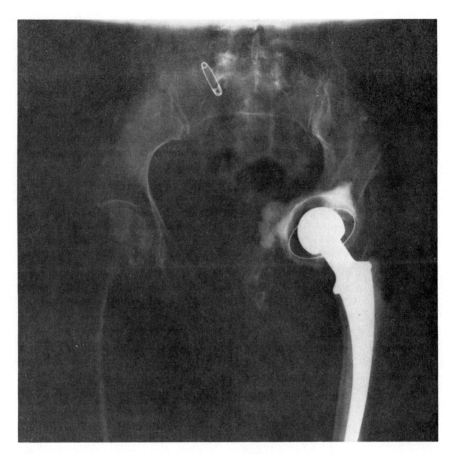

FIG. 27-4   Radiograph of a prosthetic hip joint. (The safety pin was on the patient's clothing.)

indicated that they believed a relationship between transient dental bacteremias and secondary infections of prosthetic joints had not been established or was of minor significance. Paradoxically, however, 93% of the same respondents indicated they considered antibiotic prophylaxis necessary before dental treatment that might cause a bacteremia, while 70% of these respondents recommended a cephalosporin antibiotic be given in lieu of other antibiotics.[13]

PENILE IMPLANTS

Two types of penile implants are now being placed: semirigid or rigid rod and inflatable. Six models of noninflatable and six models of inflatable devices are on the market. The inflatable devices still have a rather high intrinsic and surgically related mechanical failure rate.[2,10,15,22] The infection rate for all penile implants is 2% to 4%.[26] Kabalin and Kessler[14] reported their experience at Stanford University Medical Center over a 10-year period during which they found nine cases of infection among 417 total penile implants. Two of these followed dental treatment (infection appearing in one patient a week after and in the second 4 weeks after treatment). The authors concluded by suggesting that patients with penile implants should receive prophylactic antibiotics for invasive dental procedures.

A review of the literature found the postoperative infection rate to be higher for semirigid penile implants than for the inflatable prosthe-

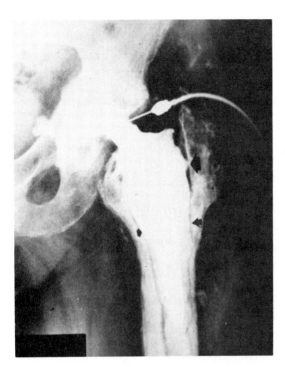

FIG. 27-5 Infected hip prosthesis. (Courtesy H.J. Robinson, M.D., Minneapolis Minn.)

sis.[2,10,15,22,26] Most infections occur within several months following implantation, and over 67% of the infections are caused by *Staphylococcus epidermidis*.[14,22] Gram-negative enteric bacteria also are found with some frequency in infected prostheses.[14] With the exception of the Kabalin and Kessler study,[14] however, no other studies have been done associating transient dental bacteremias with infections of penile implants. Therefore the suggestion is that the vast majority of postoperative infections of penile implants result from wound contamination at the time of the surgical insertion of the prosthesis.

In a recent survey of 1756 urologists in the United States,[21] 14% reported that they felt transient dental bacteremias did not pose a risk of infecting a healed penile implant whereas 58% felt dental bacteremias presented only a slight risk of infection. Fifty-seven percent of the urologists did not recommend antibiotic prophylaxis for penile implant patients who under-

went invasive dental procedures[21]; however, of those who did recommend prophylaxis, 56% selected a cephalosporin. None of the responding urologists reported infection occurring in a penile implant patient following dental treatment.[21]

INTRAOCULAR LENSES

About 90% of the operations for removal of cataracts are accompanied by the insertion of a prosthetic intraocular lens.[26] In the United States, about 900,000 intraocular lenses are inserted each year.[26] The postoperative infection rate is 0.3% to 1%.[16,27,26] Bacterial endophthalmitis usually will occur within 7 days of initial cataract surgery and is rare after 32 days.[16] The most common bacterial agents causing infection are coagulase-negative staphylococci and *Staphylococcus aureus*.[16] Most cases of intraocular lens implant infections appear to be from wound contamination.[3,16,27,26] A review of the literature failed to find any reports associating an increased risk for infection of prosthetic intraocular lenses from transient dental bacteremias. There is no evidence that patients with prosthetic intraocular lenses need prophylactic antibiotics for invasive dental procedures.

BREAST IMPLANTS

In the United States about 90,000 bilateral breast implants are placed each year for aesthetic reasons.[26] In addition, about 50,000 breast implants are performed for reconstructive needs following cancer treatment.[26] The postoperative infection rate is 1% to 4%.[26,28] No reports were found associating breast implant infection with transient dental bacteremias. Prophylactic antibiotics are not indicated for these patients when receiving dental treatment.

INTRAVASCULAR ACCESS DEVICES

Table 27-3 shows various types of intravascular access devices and the rate of postoperative infection associated with them. Uldall catheters, used for hemodialysis and plasmapheresis, have the highest postoperative infection rate—37%. Other devices have infection rates of less than 1% to as high as 15%.[26] Few data are available regarding the association of transient dental bacteremias and infection of intravascular access devices. When

TABLE 27-3
Intravascular Access Devices and Infection

Device	Use	Complication	Rate
Peripheral intravenous lines	Fluids, medications	Thrombophlebitis, bacteremia	74/1,000,000 2.5 to 5/1000
Central intravenous lines	Fluids, medications, monitoring	Bacteremia	2% to 8%
Central intravenous (tunnelled) Broviac/ Hickman devices	Chemotherapy	Catheter-related infections	1 to 2/1000 days of use
Central intravenous lines	Hyperalimentation	Catheter-related infections	15%
Uldall catheters	Hemodialysis, plasmapheresis	Catheter-related infections	37%

From Sugarman B, Young EJ: *Infect Dis Clin North Am* 3(2):187-198, 1989.

TABLE 27-4
Type, Frequency, and Infection Rate for Prosthetic Devices

Prosthetic Device	Number Inserted (Approximate %)	Infection Rate (Approximate %)
Joints	400,000/year (USA)	
Total hips	140,000/year	1 to 2
Knees	115,000 per year	
Intraocular lenses	900,000/year (USA)	0.3 to 1
Pacemakers	90,000/year (USA)	1 to 5
Cardiac valves	120,000/year (worldwide)	1 to 4
Vascular grafts	60,000/year (USA)	2
Cerebrospinal fluid shunts	75,000/year (USA)	10 to 15
Breast implants		
Aesthetic	90,000/year (USA)	1 to 4
Reconstruction	50,000/year (USA)	
Penile implants	35,000	2 to 4

Modified from Sugarman B, Young EJ: *Infect Dis Clin North Am* 3(2): 187-198, 1989.

invasive dental treatment must be provided to a patient with an intravascular access device, the dentist should consult with the patient's physician regarding the need for antibiotic prophylaxis.

SUMMARY

The frequency of insertion and the usual postoperative infection rate for prosthetic devices described in this chapter are shown in Tables 27-3 and 27-4. Intraocular lenses are the most common devices implanted. Intravascular access devices were found to have the highest rate of infection and intraocular lens implants the lowest rate of infection. The most common cause of infection with all devices was found to be from wound contamination at the time of surgical insertion. However, hematogenous spread of organisms from distant sites of acute infection, in rare cases, can infect prosthetic devices, such as prosthetic heart valves, joints, synthetic vascular grafts, ventriculoatrial cerebrospinal fluid shunts, cardiac pacemakers, and intravascular access devices.

Infection of prosthetic devices by transient bacteremias produced by invasive dental procedures appears to be very rare. Only prosthetic heart valves are considered to be at increased risk for such an infection. By contrast, no evidence has been found indicating increased risk for infection associated with intraocular lenses or breast implants. Also, little evidence has been found to indicate an increased risk of infection from transient dental bacteremias for prosthetic joints or penile implants.

Based on recommendations from the American Heart Association (AHA), patients with prosthetic heart valves should receive antibiotic coverage for invasive dental procedures. Patients with cardiac pacemakers do not require antibiotic prophylaxis. The AHA made no recommendation for patients with synthetic vascular grafts because evidence has been inconclusive. The need for prophylaxis in patients with vascular grafts should be determined on an individual patient basis by medical consultation.

There is some evidence suggesting the need for antibiotic prophylaxis for patients with certain intravascular access devices and ventriculoatrial cerebrospinal fluid shunts. Again, medical consultation regarding the need for prophylaxis on an individual basis should be obtained for patients with these devices. Although there is little evidence indicating increased risk for infection from transient dental bacteremias in patients with joint and penile implants, medical consultation should be obtained on an individual basis to determine the need for prophylaxis.

REFERENCES

1. Aoki N: Lumboperitoneal shunt: clinical applications, complications and comparison with ventriculoperitoneal shunt, *Neurosurgery* 26(6):998-1003, 1990.
2. Benson GS, Boileau MA: The penis: sexual function and dysfunction. In Gillenwater JY, editor: *Adult and pediatric urology*, St Louis, 1990, Mosby–Year Book, pp 1599-1642.
3. Carslon AM, Tetz MR, Apple DJ: Infectious complications of modern cataract surgery and intraocular lens implantation, *Infect Dis Clin North Am* 3(2):339-345, 1989.
4. Council on Dental Therapeutics: Management of dental patients with prosthetic joints, *J Am Dent Assoc* 121:1, October 1990.
5. Dajani AS, Bisno AL, Chung KJ, et al: Prevention of bacterial endocarditis: recommendations of the American Heart Association, *JAMA* 264:2919-2922, 1990.
6. Drucker MH, Vanek VW, Franco AA, et al: Thromboembolic complications of ventriculoatrial shunts, *Surg Neurol* 22(5):444-448, 1984.
7. Fan-Havard P, Nahata MC: Treatment and prevention of infections of cerebrospinal fluid shunts, *Clin Pharm* 6(11):866-880, 1987.
8. Fernell E, VonWendt L, Serlo W, et al: Ventriculoatrial or ventriculoperitoneal shunts in the treatment of

hydrocephalus in children, *Z Kinderchir* 40(suppl 1): 12-14, 1985.
9. Gardner P, Leipzig TJ, Sadigh M: Infections of mechanical cerebrospinal fluid shunts, *Curr Clin Top Infect Dis* 9:185-214, 1989.
10. Goldstein I, Krane RJ, Greenfield AJ, Padima-Nathan H: Vascular disease of the penis—impotence and priapism. In Pollack HM, editor: *Clinical urology*, Philadelphia, 1990, WB Saunders.
11. Heimberger TS, Duma RJ: Infections of prosthetic heart valves and cardiac pacemakers, *Infect Dis Clin North Am* 3(2):221-245, 1989.
12. Hopkins CC: Recognition of endemic and epidemic prosthetic device infections: the role of surveillance, the hospital infection control practitioner, and the hospital epidemiologist, *Infect Dis Clin North Am* 3(2):211-219, 1989.
13. Jaspers MT, Little JW: Prophylactic antibiotic coverage in patients with total arthroplasty: current practice, *J Am Dent Assoc* 111(6):943-948, 1985.
14. Kabalin JW, Kessler R: Infectious complications of penile prosthesis surgery, *J Urol* 139:953-955, 1988.
15. Kirkemo A: Complications of penile surgery. In Smith RB, Ehrlich RM, editors: *Complications of urologic surgery*, ed 2, Philadelphia, 1990, WB Saunders, pp 534-548.
16. Klimek JJ, Ajemian E, Andrews L, et al: Outbreak of bacterial endophthalmitis after cataract surgery and lens implantation: lack of direct evidence for exogenous contributing factors, *Am J Infect Control* 14(4):184-187, 1986.
17. Little JW: The need for antibiotic coverage for dental treatment of patients with joint replacements, *Oral Surg* 55:20-23, 1983.
18. Little JW: Is there a need for antibiotic prophylaxis in dental patients with prosthetic joints? [Editorial.] *Oral Surg* 66:430-431, 1988.
19. Little JW, Falace DA: *Dental management of the medically compromised patient*, ed 3, St Louis, 1988, CV Mosby, pp 83-100, 120-136.
20. Little JW, Falace DA: *Dental management of the medically compromised patient*, ed 3, St Louis, 1988, CV Mosby, pp 269-279.
21. Little JW, Rhodus NL: The need for antibiotic prophylaxis of patients with penile implants during invasive dental procedures: a national survey of urologists, *J Urol* 148(6):1801-1804, 1992.
22. Mallory TR, Wein AJ: Surgery of the penis. In Walsh PC, editor: *Campbell's Urology*, ed 5, Philadelphia, 1986, WB Saunders, pp 2896-2899.
23. Mueller X, Sadeghi H, Kappenberger L: Complications after single versus dual chamber pacemaker implantation, *Pace* 13(6):711-714, 1990.
24. Segreti J, Levin S: The role of prophylactic antibiotics in the prevention of prosthetic device infections, *Infect Dis Clin North Am* 3(2):357-371, 1989.
24a. Simmons NA, Ball AP, Cawson RA, et al: Case against

antibiotic prophylaxis for dental treatment of patients with joint prostheses. [Letter.] *Lancet* 339:301, 1992.

25. Strom T: Prosthetic joint patients: is premedication a must? *Pharmacy Times,* 48-53, July 1990.

26. Sugarman B, Young EJ: Infections associated with prosthetic devices: magnitude of the problem, *Infect Dis Clin North Am* 3(2):187-198, 1989.

27. Weber DJ, Hoffman KL, Thoft RA, Baker AS: Endophthalmitis following intraocular lens implantation, *Rev Infect Dis* 8(1):12-20, 1986.

28. Weber J Jr, Hentz RV: Salvage of the exposed breast implant, *Ann Plast Surg* 16(2):106-110, 1986.

A

Infection Control

The American Dental Association (ADA) and the Centers for Disease Control (CDC) have recommended that all dental patients be considered as potentially infectious and that universal precautions be used. These guidelines have been available since 1985.

The Federal Government, through the Occupational Safety and Health Administration (OSHA), has now expanded these guidelines to include how to prevent blood-borne pathogen transmission in the workplace. The standards, which apply to dental offices with one or more employees, went into effect on March 6, 1992, with all provisions being enforced after July 6, 1992. OSHA requires a written exposure control plan for the dental office as well as information and training programs on infection control offered to all employees. Other aspects of the regulations deal with personal protective equipment, housekeeping, engineering and work controls, hepatitis vaccination, post-exposure follow-up, medical records on all employees, and the posting of the OSHA poster in the dental office.[4,11,12]

Dentists should check with their OSHA office in the state in which they practice to obtain a copy of the regulations. In many states, a state plan will be responsible for the program, and they may have slightly different regulations than the Federal program. By law, the state plan must be as effective as the Federal program. Dentists need to check with their state health department to gain access to the state regulations as well as with OSHA.[1] The ADA published an excellent question and answer paper on the new OSHA standards. This paper is available on request from the ADA.[12]

OSHA, by law, cannot give advanced notice of an inspection. Most of the dental office inspections OSHA has conducted, during the time temporary regulations were being enforced, were based on employee complaints. However, random spot check inspections were conducted. Seventy-five percent of the inspections conducted resulted in citations. Violations fell into the following categories: willful, repeated, serious, other than serious, and no OSHA poster.[1,11] Fines for willful or repeated violations are up to $70,000.00. The fine for no OSHA poster is $1000.00. The dentist has 15 days to either pay the fine and correct the problem, call the regional office for a conference, or contest the citation. Most of the citations issued to date (66%) were related to serious violations that carried a fine of up to $7000.[1,11]

A new Federal Clinical Laboratory Regulation is in the final stages of development. Once enforced, this regulation will impact on dental offices performing clinical laboratory tests on blood, urine, and saliva. Facilities that collect specimens for forwarding to a laboratory for analysis will not be effected by this new regulation.[3]

PROCEDURES

The following steps for sterilization, disinfection, barrier protection, universal precautions, and office management meet the Federal OSHA Standards.

STERILIZATION

Ultrasonic cleaning is an effective method for cleaning instruments before sterilization. After ultrasonic cleaning, the instruments are rinsed and, if still visibly dirty, they are hand scrubbed. If ultrasonic cleaning is not used, all instruments

TABLE A-1
Suitable Methods for Sterilizing Common Dental Instruments and Items*

Materials	Steam autoclave†	Dry heat oven	Chemical vapor	Ethylene oxide
General hand instruments				
Stainless steel	1	1	1	2
Carbon steel	3	1	1	2
Mirrors	2	1	1	2
Burrs‡				
Steel	2	1	1	2
Carbon steel	3	1	1	2
Tungsten-carbide	2	1	2	2
Stones				
Diamond	2	1	1	2
Polishing	1	2	1	2
Sharpening	2	1	2	2
Polishing wheels and disks				
Rubber	2	4	3	2
Garnet and cuttle	4	3	3	2
Rag	1	2	2	2
Rubber dam equipment				
Carbon or carbide steel clamps	3	1	1	2
Stainless steel clamps	1	1	1	2
Punches	3	1	1	2
Plastic frames	3	4	4	2
Metal frames	1	1	1	2
Impression trays				
Aluminum metal, chrome plated	1	1	1	2
Custom acrylic resin	4	4	4	2
Plastic (discarding is preferred)	4	4	4	2
Fluoride gel trays				
Heat-resistant plastic	1	4	3	2
Non-heat-resistant plastic	4	4	4	2
Orthodontic pliers				
High quality stainless	1	1	1	2
Low quality stainless	4	1	1	2
With plastic parts	4	4	3	1
Endodontic instruments				
Reamers and files, broaches, stainless metal handles	1	1	1	1
Nonstainless metal handles	4	1	1	1
Stainless with plastic handles	3	3	3	1
Pluggers and condensers	1	1	1	2
Glass slabs	1	2	1	2
Dappen dishes	1	2	1	2

TABLE A-1
Suitable Methods for Sterilizing Common Dental Instruments and Items*—cont'd

Materials	Steam autoclave†	Dry heat oven	Chemical vapor	Ethylene oxide
Handpieces§				
High speed	3	3	3	2
Low-speed straight	3	3	3	2
Prophy angles	2	2	2	2
Contra-angles	4	4	4	2
Radiographic equipment				
Plastic film holders, columating devices	3	4	4	2
Stainless steel surgical instruments	1	1	2	2
Ultrasonic scaling tips	2	4	4	2
Electrosurgical tips and handles	4	4	4	4
Needles				
Disposable (do not reuse)	4	4	4	4
Reusable	2	2	4	4

*1, Indicates preferred method with minimum risk of damage; 2, indicates that materials should withstand treatment with minimum risk of damage; 3, indicates that treatment is usually not suitable and may damage materials, manufacturer should be consulted; 4, indicates that materials are likely to be damaged or process may be ineffective.
†Chemical protection of certain nonstainless instruments may permit steam autoclaving. A rust-preventive dip (1% sodium nitrate) is recommended before sterilization.
‡Steel burrs may be sterilized in hot endodontic sterilizer for 15 to 20 seconds at 475° F (246° C), but the process may not be suitable for carbide burrs.
§Some common latch-type contra-angles cannot withstand repeated heat sterilization; short, heat-sterilizable contra-angle handpieces are now available.

should be hand scrubbed. If ultrasonic cleaning is used, the ultrasonic machine needs to be tested on a regular basis to ensure that energy is being delivered throughout the tank and power is not being lost. These procedures should be performed while dental personnel are wearing nitrile utility gloves to reduce the possibility of puncture wounds. Clean instruments are placed into sterilization bags. Heat sterilization bags that meet ADA acceptance standards should be used. Packaging of instruments protects them from being contaminated after sterilization.[5] Studies have demonstrated that these sterile packs can be stored up to 12 months without the loss of sterile integrity.[2]

Heat sterilization is required for all instruments and items that can withstand repeated exposure to high temperatures. Steam under pressure, prolonged dry heat, and unsaturated chemical vapor sterilization are the preferred methods for sterilization (Table A-1). The efficiency of office sterilization procedures should be monitored by the dentist. Chemically treated indicator tapes and biologic monitors are used to check for proper functioning of an office sterilizer. Indicator tapes should be used for every cycle. Color change in the tape indicates sterilizing conditions occurred. Calibrated biologic monitors guarantee sterilization. Proof of spore destruction by culturing after exposure to the sterilization cycle infers that all microorganisms exposed to the same conditions have been destroyed. Biologic monitors should be used once a week with dental office sterilizers (Table A-2). A record of all tests results must be kept for at least 3 years.[5]

A number of products are on the market for immersion sterilization and surface disinfection.

TABLE A-2
Sterilization Method, Biologic Indicator Spore
Type, and Incubation Temperature

Sterilization method	Spore type*	Incubation temperature (C)
Autoclave Chemical vapor	*Bacillus stearother-mophilus*	56°
Dry heat Ethylene oxide	*Bacillus subtilis*	37°

*For most dental practices, weekly verification should be adequate. Contact Council on Dental Materials, Instruments, and Equipment of the ADA for information regarding monitoring services.
Based on Merchant VA: *Dent Teamwork*, pp 13-15, 1990.

Those for immersion sterilization use glutaraldehyde as the active agent. The general directions for disinfection are not designed for dental use. The glutaraldehyde products used for sterilization can be compared by reviewing the tuberculocidal directions. The newer Quantitative Logarithmic Reduction Test method for determining tuberculocidal action is preferred to the Association of Official Analytical Chemists' Test. However, only a few of the current products have been reevaluated using the Quantitative Logarithmic Reduction test. Product labels do not provide directions for the test used to determine tuberculocidal action. The reuse days mentioned on product labels also do not relate well to dentistry. Glutaraldehyde products found to be ineffective are those that are highly diluted or used to the end of their reuse time. Tables A-3 and A-4 list the products available for immersion sterilization and surface disinfection.[4,12]

DISINFECTION

Environmental surfaces should be cleaned before they are disinfected. Diluted iodophors, chlorines, or synthetic phenolics are good cleaners in addition to being effective disinfectants (Table A-3). Products with high alcohol content are generally poorer cleaners. Alcohol will precipitate proteins in saliva and blood, making it more difficult to clean the surface. A recommended method for surface cleaning and disinfection is the "spray-wipe-spray" technique.

The first spray and wipe is for cleaning; the second spray is for disinfection. If the product is a good cleaner it can be used for both steps. An ADA-accepted surface disinfectant should provide documented evidence of bactericidal, tuberculocidal, and virucidal activity. Disposal barriers should be used, whenever possible, to reduce the need for surface disinfection. Aluminum foil, plastic wrap, plastic bags, or plastic-lined paper can be used as disposable barriers for equipment and surfaces.[4,12]

Hand washing and gloves Hand washing should be done throughout the day with antimicrobial soaps that have residual action. Disposable latex gloves should be used, *one pair for each patient, unless tears occur that would require new gloves immediately*. Individuals allergic to latex can try cotton liners or hyoallergenic gloves. Not all hypoallergenic gloves are free of latex so allergy may still occur. Utility gloves should be worn when using chemical disinfectants or cleaning the operatory.[4,12]

Face mask and eye wear A disposable face mask that can filter 95% of particles 3 to 5 μm in size or a full face mask should be used for each patient. Protective eye wear should be worn for all procedures except for examination procedures. A side shield should be used with corrective glasses.[4,12]

Gowns A clinic gown should be worn and changed, at least once per day, or anytime it becomes soiled. Impervious gowns are not required by OSHA. Long sleeves are recommended. Work clothes (gowns, etc.) should not be worn away from the workplace and must not be laundered at home.[4,12]

Sharps disposal A sharps disposal system is needed. The sharps container must be rigid, puncture proof, leak resistant, sterilizable or burnable, and labeled. Needles, sutures, scalpel blades, burrs, glass, pointed instruments, anesthetic capsules, and orthodontic wire should be discarded in it. A one-handed scoop technique or a specific resheathing device should be used to resheath needles.[4,12]

Handpieces Disinfection of handpieces is still acceptable, but sterilizable handpieces are recommended. (This may soon be changed to

TABLE A-3
Office Sterilization and Asepsis Procedures Research Foundation (OSAP) Guide to Chemical Agents for Disinfection and/or Sterilization

Products	EPA Reg. No.	TB directons (Test timer temp)*	ADA accepted	Sterilization	Sterilant reuse (days)
Immersion only					
Multicide Plus	1043-36	1 : 32, 20 min, 20°C† (AOAC)	No	No	None
CoeSteril, ColdSpor	55195-2	1 : 20, 10 min, 20°C (AOAC)	Yes	1 : 5, 6 hr, 20°C 1 : 20, 12 hr, 20°C	30
Sporicidin	8383-5	1 : 16, 10 min, 20°C (AOAC)	Yes	FS*, 6¾ hr, 20°C	1 to 14 (1 : 8, 8 hr);15 to 30 (1 : 8, 10 hr)
Glutarex	7182-4	FS, 10 min, 20°C (AOAC)	Yes	FS, 10 hr, 20°C	Not estab-lished
Banicide					
Sterall	15136-1	1 : 4 or FS* 30 min (AOAC)	Yes	FS, 10 hr, 21°C	30
Wavicide 01	"	"			
Cidex Plus (3.2%)	7078-14	FS, 20 min, 25°C† (Quant)	Yes	FS, 10 hr, 20°C	28
Cidex 7	7078-1	FS, 90 min, 20°C (AOAC)	Yes	FS, 10 hr, 25°C	28
Germ-X	10352-29	FS, 10 min, 20°C (AOAC)	Yes	FS, 10 hr, 20°C	Not estab-lished
Baxter/Omnicide	46851-2	FS, 45 min, 20°C (AOAC)	Yes	FS, 10 hr, 20°C	28
Glutall	"	"			
K-Cide	"	"			
Omnicide	"	"			
Procide	"	"			

Continued.

TABLE A-3
Office Sterilization and Asepsis Procedures Research Foundation (OSAP) Guide to Chemical Agents for Disinfection and/or Sterilization—cont'd

Products	EPA Reg. No.	TB directons (Test timer temp)*	ADA accepted	Sterilization	Sterilant reuse (days)
CoeCide XL	46781-2	FS, 20 min, 20°C (AOAC)	Yes	FS, 6 hr, 20°C	30
Maxicide	"				
Metricide	"	FS, 20 min, 25°C† (AOAC)			
Protect-Top	"	"			
Vitacide	"	"			
Surface Only					
Alcide LD	45631-15	10 : 1 : 1, 3 min, 20°C	Yes	No	None
Exspor	45631-03	4 : 1 : 1, 3 min, 20°C		4 : 1 : 1, 6 hr, 20°C	None
Bleach (5.25%)	–	1 : 10, 10 min, 20°C	No	No	None
Sporicidin Spray	8383-3	10 min, 20°C (AOAC)	Yes	No	None
Lysol Spray	777-53	10 min, 20°C (AOAC)	Yes	No	None
Coe Spray—The Pump	334-417	10 min, 20°C (AOAC)	Yes	No	None
Procide Spray	46851-5	10 min, 20°C (AOAC)	Yes	No	None

*Test used for TB label claim: *FS*, full strength; *AOAC*, Association of Official Analytical Chemists; *Quant*, Quantitative TB Test.
†20°C = 68°F; 25°C = 77°F.
From Cottone JA, Molinari JA: *J Am Dent Assoc* 122(9):33-41, 1991.

TABLE A-4
2% Alkaline Glutaraldehydes, EPA-approved for Sterilant Reuse* (1991)

Product	EPA Reg. No.	TB directions (test, time, temp)†	Sterilization
Cidex 7	7078-1	(Quant) 90 min, 25°C	10 hr 20°C
Cidex Plus (3.2%)	7078-14	(Quant) 20 min, 25°C	10 hr 20°C
Asepti-Steryl 28	46851-2	(AOAC) 45 min, 20°C	10 hr 20°C
Baxter/Omnicide	46851-2	(AOAC) 45 min, 20°C	10 hr 20°C
Glutall	"	(AOAC) 45 min, 20°C	10 hr 20°C
K-Cide	"	(AOAC) 45 min, 20°C	10 hr 20°C
Omnicide	"	(AOAC) 45 min, 20°C	10 hr 20°C
Procide	"	(AOAC) 45 min, 20°C	10 hr 20°C
CoeCide XL	46781-2	(AOAC) 20 min, 20°C†	6 hr 20°C
Maxicide	"	(AOAC) 20 min, 20°C‡	6 hr 20°C
Metricide	"	(AOAC) 20 min, 20°C‡	6 hr 20°C
Protec-Top	"	(AOAC) 20 min, 20°C‡	6 hr 20°C
Vitacide	"	(AOAC) 20 min, 20°C‡	6 hr 20°C

*All products are to be used undiluted on precleaned instruments. All products are ADA accepted. Other products are available. Listing does not imply endorsement, recommendation, or warranty. Purchasers are legally required to consult the package insert for changes in formulation and recommended product uses. Updated tables are available from the OSAP Research Foundation, (800) 243-1233.
†Test used for TB label claim: *AOAC*, Association of Official Analytical Chemists, *Quant*, Quantitative TB Test.
‡20 min at 25°C; 20°C = 68°F; 25°C = 77°F.

"are required.") Antiretraction valves should be used to prevent water and saliva from being drawn into the fluid line.

Impressions Dental impressions should be rinsed with water and then disinfected. Diluted sodium hypochlorite is effective for all impression materials except zinc oxide–eugenol (ZOE) impression paste. Glutaraldehydes are suggested for ZOE. The manufacturer's directions for disinfection should be followed. The impression can be immersed in the disinfectant. An optional method of disinfection is to spray the disinfectant onto the impression and then place it in a plastic bag. Stone models can be sprayed with an iodophor solution. The impression should be rinsed with water before and following disinfection. A suggested disinfectant for dental prostheses being sent to a dental laboratory is an iodophore. Prostheses, following disinfection, should be rinsed with water before being

---

**DENTAL LABORATORY INFECTION
CONTROL PRECAUTIONS**

Clean and disinfect all impressions and other
impressions and other appliances as soon
as they are removed from patient's mouth.
Advise dental laboratory of disinfection so
that they will not have to repeat it.
Require laboratory personnel to wear gloves,
mask, and protective eyewear when working with infected materials.
Use sterile wheel and small dish of pumice
for each case and dispose or sterilize between uses.
Clean laboratory work surfaces with diluted
household bleach after each case.
Disinfect or sterilize all laboratory burrs and
stones after each use.
Wash hands with iodine soap at lunch time
and at end of day.
Require laboratory personnel to wear fresh
uniforms or gowns daily; do not wear
home.

**MANAGEMENT OF BIOPSY
SPECIMENS**

Place usual specimen container with fixative
into rigid container for transport.
Require laboratory personnel to wear gloves
and mask when processing specimen.
Remind laboratory personnel to be
extremely careful to avoid accidental injury.

---

placed into the patient's mouth.[6-9,13] The
boxes above summarize precautions that the
dental laboratory and clinical laboratory personnel should take in dealing with impressions, dental prostheses, or biopsy specimens.

EFFICACY CONFLICTS

Clinical Research Associates has been evaluating the effectiveness of the various products
for use in the dental office for infection control
for over 5 years. They are involved with continuous evaluations and issue monthly updates

concerning their findings. An important consideration to take into account when selecting a
glutaraldehyde-based disinfectant is the fact
that the agencies that approve the use of these
agents do not actually test disinfectants to
confirm efficacy. These agencies (EPA, FDA,
CDC, and ADA) use reports submitted by the
companies to establish efficacy, and these reports may not always be accurate. For example
testing of 12 brand names of glutaraldehyde-
based disinfectants by Clinical Research Associates found that (1) disinfectants with similar
active ingredients had equivalent performance
despite diverse label claims; (2) contact time
needed to be increased beyond the conventional
10 minutes; (3) contact time increased as the
active agent(s) was diluted; and (4) all solutions
tested were effective if the clinician was willing
to tolerate the increased contact time needed
for products with diluted active agents. The
infection control products recommended as of
May 1992 by Clinical Research Associates are
shown in Table A-5.

TABLE A-5
State-of-the-Art Infection Control Products*

Product	Source	Approximate Cost

Eye coverings

(Criteria: Tolerate routine disinfection, comfortable and economical)

Tuff-Spec	Local dental dealers and EFOS Inc., (800) 826-8701 and (716) 634-5601	$5.95/pr
OP-D-OP Shield	OP-D-OP, Inc., (916) 783-5741	$39.95/kit (3 shields and accessories)

Face masks

(Criteria: Fit face well, have high filtration of very small particles [$\geq 95\%$ filtration of 3.0 to 3.5 μm particles], comfortable, and economical)

Magic Arch	Alpha ProTech, (800) 527-7689 and (801) 298-3240	38¢/mask
Surgical Comfort Cup	Healthco, (800) 225-2360 and (617) 423-6045	31¢/mask
Triple Layer	Local dental dealers and 3M, (800) 634-2249 and (612) 733-8524	54¢/mask
Laser Face Masks		
Laser Plume Face Mask	Local dental dealers and J&J Medical	44¢/mask
Sub-Micron Molded Surgical Mask	Local dental dealers and 3M	$1.20/mask
Technol Laser Mask, regular and fog-free	Local medical dealers and Baxter Hospital Supply Division	$1.25 and $1.28/mask

Hand protection (antiseptics)

(Criteria: For protection under operating gloves—rapid antimicrobial activity, plus residual and cumulative activity)

Bactoshield	Amsco, (800) 444-9009 and (919) 362-0842	Price/gal—25¢/oz
CHG	Dexide, (800) 645-3378 and (817) 589-1454	Price/qt—43¢/oz
Excelle	Local dealers	Price/gal—29¢/oz
Hibiciens	GC America, Schein, and local medical dealers	Price/gal—39¢/oz
Luroscrub	The Dial Corporation, (800) 528-0849 and (602) 207-4000	Price/gal—20¢/oz
Novoclens	Septodont/Deproco, (800) 872-8305 and (302) 328-1102	Price/gal—35¢/oz
(Criteria: For particular attention to virucidal activity)		
Alcare	Calgon-Vestal, (800) 325-8005 & (314) 535-1810)	78¢/oz
TLC	Amadent, (800) 289-6367 & (609) 429-8297)	68¢/oz

*Recommendations for infection control (May 1992) based on evaluations performed over a 5-year period by Clinical Research Associates, 3707 North Canyon Road, Provo, Utah 84604. Reproduced with permission from Dr. Rella P. Christensen.

Continued.

TABLE A-5
State-of-the-Art Infection Control Products*—cont'd

Product	Source	Approximate Cost

Hand protection (gloves)

(Criteria: Nonsterile latex or vinyl operating gloves—combination of low number of manufacturing-defects [pinholes below 4%], economical, good clinical characteristics [i.e., fit, tactile sensitivity, amount and texture of powder, taste, tackiness after wetting, resistance to tearing])

Product	Source	Approximate Cost
APO Health "White" by Shield Gloves (latex)	APO Health, (800) 365-2839 and (516) 485-6700	7¢/glove
Bio-flex by Aliga Ind. (latex)	Premium Latex, (800) 755-4588 and (213) 287-0380	6¢/glove
C. Rubber by C. Rubber Co. (latex)	Columbia World, (800) 225-3881 and (509) 946-3993	6¢/glove
Micro-Touch by J&J Medical (latex)	Local dental and medical dealers	10¢/glove
Triflex Vinyl Exam Glove by Baxter Healthcare (vinyl)	Baxter, (800) 423-2311 and (708) 940-1990	14¢/glove

(Criteria: Utility gloves—resist punctures and tears during cleanup procedures)

Product	Source	Approximate Cost
Asep Gluv (nitrile rubber)	Local dealers or Health Sonics, (800) 342-3096 and (510) 462-4610	$2.66/glove

Uniforms

(Criteria: Long sleeves, high neck, moisture resistant, can be discarded or sent to commercial laundry)

Product	Source	Approximate Cost
Scrubs by Doc (lab coat or jacket)	Healthco and Scrubs by Doc, (314) 846-8300	$38-49/uniform
Compel jacket	Pro-Safe Professional Linens, (800) 354-2084	$29/uniform
Overgarment	American Linen, (503) 283-2233 (leased)	$1.50/laundering

Hepatitis vaccine

(Criteria: Render most humans immune to infection by hepatitis B virus)

Product	Source	Approximate Cost
Engerix-B (3 innoculations)	SmithKline Beecham, (800) 366-8900 and (215) 751-5644	$156.75
Recombivax HB (3 innoculations)	Merck, Sharp, & Dohme, (800) 637-2579 and (215) 661-5000	$128.49

Ultrasonic cleaners

(Criteria: Remove debris rapidly with minimal adverse effects to instruments)

Product	Source	Approximate Cost
Biosonic	Coltene/Whaledent, (800) 221-3046 and (212) 696-8000	$485.00
T3.3C	Health Sonics, (800) 342-3096 and (510) 462-4610	$444.50
Colster 3 (provides ultrasonic clean and rinse with blow dry)	Esma Chemicals, (708) 433-6116	$2300.00

TABLE A-5
State-of-the-Art Infection Control Products*—cont'd

Product	Source	Approximate Cost

Heat sterilization
(Criteria: Does not corrode or rust carbide burrs and high carbon steel instruments; has relatively short cycle time)
Heat Sterilizers that meet above criteria

Product	Source	Approximate Cost
Cox Sterilizer (rapid dry heat)	Cox Sterile Products, (800) 247-6493 and (214) 528-8900	$3550.00
Guardian 2000 (rapid dry heat)	Dentronix, Inc., (800) 523-5944 and (215) 322-4220	$2750.00
Harvey Chemi-Clave (chemical vapor)	MDT, (800) 347-4638 and (213) 608-2290	$2300 to $6235 (depending on chamber size)

Monitors for the four types of sterilizers used in dentistry (use weekly)

Product	Source	Approximate Cost
Rapid dry heat	SporView Culturing Set (SPS Medical), (800) 722-1529 and (716) 328-2150	$3.00/monitor $190 incubator NDB-037
Chemical vapor	SporTest (MDT), (800) 347-4638 and (213) 608-2290	Media $91/box of 100 77¢/monitor $250 incubator
Steam heat	Attest (3M), (800) 634-2249 and (612) 733-8524	$4.28/monitor $155 incubator
Dry heat oven	SporView Culturing Set (SPS Medical), (800) 722-1529 and (716) 328-2150	$3.00/monitor $190 incubator NDB-037

Handpiece sterilization
(Criteria: All surfaces of handpiece rendered sterile rapidly, without harming or shortening life of handpiece; presently no products meet the criteria; current handpiece components and design are eventually affected adversely by routine heat sterilization causing need for servicing or part replacement; new handpiece designs, new sterilization methods, and new clinician expectations are all needed to solve problem)
Products that are usable but will eventually affect handpiece performance
Sterilization

Product	Source	Approximate Cost
Statim	SciCan, (800) 572-1211 and (412) 281-6789	$3595.00
KavoKlave	Kavo America, (800) 323-8029 and (708) 885-3855	$895.00 ($39 @ additional cassette)

Disinfection of external surfaces only

Product	Source	Approximate Cost
Decident	Nevin Laboratories, (800) 544-5337 and (312) 624-4330	§70¢/bag
Disposable disinfectant sleeve	Lares Research, (800) 347-3289 and (916) 345-1767	§70¢/bag

Continued.

TABLE A-5
State-of-the-Art Infection Control Products*—cont'd

Product	Source	Approximate Cost

Instrument disinfection

(Criteria: Relatively rapid broad spectrum kill of organisms; heat sterilizaton is best final step in treatment of *all* instruments; chemicals are useful for predisinfection of instruments before cleaning and disinfection of items that do not tolerate heat)

3.2% glutaraldehyde products—for predisinfection of all instruments prior to ultrasonic and hand cleaning

Product	Source	Approximate Cost
Cidex Plus	J & J Medical, (800) 433-5170 and (817) 465-3141	Price/gal—18¢/oz
Metricide Plus 30	Metrex, (800) 841-1428 and (303) 841-5842	Price/gal—19¢/oz
Maxicide Plus	Schein, (800) 772-4346 and (516) 621-4300	Price/gal—15¢/oz

2% glutaraldehyde products—alkaline pH, for disinfection of items that will not tolerate heat

Product	Source	Approximate Cost
Cidex 7	J & J Medical, (800) 433-5170 and (817) 465-3141	Price/gal—18¢/oz
Metricide 28	Metrex, (800) 841-1428 and (303) 841-5842	Price/gal—18¢/oz
Maxicide	Schein, (800) 772-4346 and (516) 621-4300	Price/gal—15¢/oz

Glutaraldehyde monitors

Product	Source	Approximate Cost
Cidex solution test strip	J & J Medical, (800) 433-5170 and (817) 465-3141	93¢/strip

Environmental surface disinfection

(Criteria: Fast-acting, broad-spectrum kill that includes the tuberculosis organism and a resistant nonenveloped virus in presence of heavy protein challenge)

Product	Source	Approximate Cost
Amphyl	National Laboratories, (800) 753-4855 and (201) 573-5280	26¢/oz
Citrace and Citrex	Caltech Industries, (800) 234-770 and (517) 496-3110	36¢/oz
Coespray—The Pump	GC America, (800) 323-7063 and (708) 597-0900	73¢/oz
Lysol Spray (any fragrance)	Healthco, drug, and grocery stores	29¢/oz
Lysol Spray with Accusol sprayer	Healthco, Patterson, or Schein	29¢/oz (if buy case of 12)

Aerosol and odor control

Product	Source	Approximate Cost
Ultraviolet Air Sterilight	Allseasons, (416) 475-9795	$549.00

Pretreatment mouth rinse with chlorhexidine

Product	Source	Approximate Cost
Peridex (0.12% CHG)	Local drug stores, prescription item in US	$1.19/oz

TABLE A-5
State-of-the-Art Infection Control Products*—cont'd

Product	Source	Approximate Cost
Rubber dam		
Dental dam—green or gray, 6 × 6 heavyweight		29¢/dam
Punch #01251	Hygienic Corp., (800) 321-2135 and (216) 633-8460	@ $66.95/punch
Clamp forceps # 01252		@ $38.95/forceps
Clamps (NW or PW for molars; A for partially erupted molars; L or E for premolars; C for Class 5)	Ash/Dentsply, (800) 877-9929 and (717) 845-7511	@ $7.60/clamp
Needle recapping and sharps disposal		
(Criteria: Safely recaps anesthetic needle, plus provides safe disposal after recapping)		
DisposiNeedle	Septodont/Deproco, (800) 872-8305 and (302) 328-1102	$59/kit

REFERENCES

1. Be ready for inspections: OSHA official stresses planning. An ADA official stresses planning, *ADA News,* Jan 6, 1992.
2. Butt WE, Bradley DV, Mayhew RB, Schwartz RS: Evaluation of the shelf life of sterile instrument packs, *Oral Surg* 72:650-654, 1991.
3. Clinical lab regulations prompt federal survey: dentists flood ADA with questions, *ADA News,* Jan 6, 1992.
4. Cottone JA, Molinari JA: State-of-the-art infection control in dentistry, *J Am Dent Assoc* 122(9):33-41, 1991.
5. Council on Dental Materials, Instruments, and Equipment; Council on Dental Practice; and Council on Dental Therapeutics: Infection control recommendations for the dental office and dental laboratory, *J Am Dent Assoc* 116(2):341-343, 1988.
6. Merchant VA: Infection control and prosthodontics, *J Calif Dent Assoc* 17(2):49-53, 1989.
7. Merchant VA: Disinfection of dental impressions, *Dent Teamwork,* pp 13-15, 1990.
8. Merchant VA, Molinari JA: Infection control in prosthodontics: a choice no longer, *Gen Dent* 37(1):29-32, 1989.
9. Miller CH: Barrier techniques for infection control, *CDA J* 13(10):54-59, 1985.
10. Mitchell EW: Chemical disinfecting/sterilizing agents, *CDA J* 13(10):64-67, 1985.
11. OSHA issues regulations: ADA foresees unnecessary costs, *ADA News,* Dec. 16, 1991.
12. OSHA's bloodborne pathogens standard: questions and answers, *J Am Dent Assoc* (Suppl) 123:1, February 1992.
13. Schaefer ME: Infection control in dental laboratory procedures, *CDA J* 13(10):81-84, 1985.

B

Therapeutic Management of Common Oral Lesions

This appendix is designed to serve as a quick reference to currently accepted therapeutic management for many oral conditions the dentist may be involved with. Its emphasis, of course, is on the medical conditions with oral manifestations or complications covered in this text. For many of these there is no "cure," but the treatment regimens listed here are designed to (1) relieve discomfort, (2) shorten the clinical duration, and (3) in some cases delay recurrences. The treatment protocols were taken from the third edition of *Clinician's Guide to Treatment of Common Oral Conditions,* developed by a committee of the American Academy of Oral Medicine in 1992 (William K. Bottomley and Simon W. Rosenberg, editors).

Clinicians are reminded that therapeutic success is predicated on an accurate diagnosis. Every effort must be made to establish a diagnosis of the oral condition and any associated systemic cause before initiating treatment. When signs, symptoms, screening laboratory tests, and/or referral have failed to establish a definitive diagnosis, treatment can be started and evaluated on a therapeutic trial basis. Further treatment can be based on the patient's response. Patient management should be directed by the philosophy that there is a palliative, supportive, or curative treatment for every oral condition.

HERPES SIMPLEX

Infection with the herpes simplex virus produces a disease that has a primary, or acute, phase and a secondary, or recurrent, phase.

A. PRIMARY HERPETIC GINGIVOSTOMATITIS

ETIOLOGY

A transmissible infection with herpes simplex virus (HVS), usually type I or, less commonly, type II

CLINICAL DESCRIPTION

Clear, then yellowish, vesicles develop intra- and extraorally. These rupture within hours and form shallow, painful ulcers. The gingival tissues are erythematous, enlarged, and painful. The patient may have systemic signs and symptoms—including regional lymphadenitis, fever, and malaise. Usually the disease is self-limiting with healing in 7 to 14 days.

RATIONALE FOR TREATMENT

Treatment should relieve symptoms, prevent secondary infection, and support general health. Supportive therapy includes forced fluids, protein, vitamin and mineral food supplements, and rest.*

Acyclovir and vidarabine are effective in treating herpes in immunocompromised patients. Topical steroids should be avoided as they tend to permit spread of the viral infection on mucous membranes, particularly ocular. Patients should be cautioned to avoid touching the herpetic lesions and then touching the eyes, genitals, or other body areas because of the possibility of self-inoculation.

---

* References 16, 30, 33, 34, 36, 40.

556

1. Topical Anesthetics and Coating Agents*

Rx

Diphenhydramine HCl (Benadryl) [OTC] elixir 12.5 mg/5 ml mixed with Kaopectate [OTC], 50% mixture by volume

Disp: 8 oz
Sig: Rinse with 1 teaspoonful q2h and spit out.

Maalox [OTC] can be used in place of Kaopectate.

Rx

Diphenhydramine HCl (Benadryl [OTC], Benylin [OTC]) elixir 12.5 mg/5 ml

Disp: 4 oz bottle
Sig: Rinse with 1 teaspoonful for 2 minutes every 2 hours and before each meal, then spit out.

Rx

Lidocaine HCl (Xylocaine) viscous 2%†

Disp: 450 ml bottle
Sig: Swish with 1 tablespoonful, hold for 1 minute, then spit out.

Rx

Dyclonine HCl (Dyclone) 0.5% or 1%†

Disp: 1 oz bottle
Sig: Rinse with 1 teaspoonful for 2 minutes before each meal and spit out.

2. Systemic Antiviral Therapy

Acyclovir oral capsules may relieve and decrease the duration of symptoms.

Rx

Acyclovir (Zovirax) capsules 200 mg‡

Disp: 25 capsules
Sig: Take 1 capsule 5 times a day for 5 days, or 2 capsules 3 times per day for 5 days.

3. Systemic Antibiotics*

Rx

Penicillin V tablets 500 mg

Disp: 40 tablets
Sig: Take 1 tablet qid.

For patients allergic to penicillin:

Rx

Erythromycin tablets 250 mg†

Disp: 40 tablets
Sig: Take 1 tablet qid.

4. Nutritional Supplements

Rx

Meritene (protein-vitamin-mineral supplement) [OTC]

Disp: 1 lb can (plain vanilla, chocolate, and eggnog flavors)
Sig: Take 3 servings qd. Prepare as indicated on the label. Serve cold.

Rx

Ensure Plus (protein-vitamin-mineral food supplement) [OTC]

Disp: Twenty cans
Sig: Drink 3-5 cans in divided doses throughout the day as tolerated. Serve cold.

5. Analgesic and Antipyretic

Rx

Acetaminophen tablets 325 mg [OTC]

Sig: Take 2 tablets q4h prn for pain and fever (Limit 4 g per 24 hours).

Tylenol #3 for more severe pain

Disp: 24 tablets
Sig: Take 1-2 tablets q4h for pain (requires narcotic number).

B. RECURRENT (OROFACIAL) HERPES SIMPLEX

ETIOLOGY

Reactivation of the latent virus that resides in the sensory ganglion of the trigeminal nerve. Precipitating factors include fever, stress, exposure to sunlight, trauma, and hormonal alterations.

---

*Dyclonine (Dyclone) HCl 0.5% 1 oz may be added for greater anesthetic efficacy.

†When topical anesthetics are used, patients should be cautioned concerning reduced gag reflex and the need for care while eating and drinking to avoid possible airway compromise. Allergies are rare but may occur.

‡Current FDA recommendation is that systemic acyclovir be used to treat oral herpes only in immunocompromised patients.

---

*For secondary bacterial infection in susceptible individuals. Do not use routinely.

†If nausea or stomach cramps occur, prescribe enteric-coated preparations (E-Mycin, ERYC, Ery-Tab, etc.)

CLINICAL DESCRIPTION

Intraoral — single or small clusters of vesicles that quickly rupture forming painful ulcers. The lesions usually occur on the keratinized tissue of the hard palate and gingiva. In immunocompromised patients, HSV lesions occur on any mucosal surface and may have atypical appearance. They can resemble major aphthae or allergic responses.

Labialis — clusters of vesicles on the lips that rupture within hours and then crust.*

RATIONALE FOR TREATMENT

Treatment should be initiated as early as possible in the *prodromal stage* with the objective of reducing the duration and symptoms of the lesion.[27] Prophylactically as well as therapeutically, oral acyclovir may be considered where frequent recurrent herpetic episodes interfere with daily function and nutrition. (Current FDA recommendation is that systemic acyclovir be used to treat oral herpes only in immunocompromised patients.)

1. Prevention

Rx

PreSun 15 sunscreen lotion [OTC]

Disp: 4 fl oz
Sig: Apply to susceptible area 1 hour before sun exposure and every hour thereafter.

Rx

PreSun 15 lip gel [OTC]

Disp: 4 oz
Sig: Apply to lips 1 hour before sun exposure and every hour thereafter.

If a recurrence on the lips is usually precipitated by exposure to sunlight, the lesion *may be prevented* by the application to the area of a sunscreen with a higher skin protection factor.[1,13]

2. Topical Antiviral Agents

Antiviral creams and ointments are minimally effective for recurrent herpes simplex (RHS). Their value may be attributed to coating of the lesion by the petrolatum vehicle, which reduces the possibility of self-inoculation. Constant or intermittent application of ice to the area for 90 minutes during the prodromal phase may result in aborting the lesion.

Cocoa butter ointment, lanolin-based lip preparations, or petrolatum (Vaseline) as an emollient may be palliative.

Rx

Acyclovir (Zovirax) topical ointment 5%

Disp: 15 g tube
Sig: Apply to area q2h during waking hours, beginning when symptoms first occur.

VARICELLA ZOSTER (SHINGLES)

ETIOLOGY

Reactivation of a latent herpes-varicella virus present since the occurrence of an original varicella infection (chickenpox). Precipitating factors include thermal, inflammatory, radiologic, or mechanical trauma.

CLINICAL DESCRIPTION

Usually painful segmental eruption of small vesicles that rupture to form punctate or confluent ulcers. Acute zoster follows a portion of the trigeminal nerve distribution in about 20% cases. It is rare in the young, very common in the elderly.

RATIONALE FOR TREATMENT

Initiate antiviral therapy promptly on diagnosis to reduce duration and symptoms of the lesions. Patients over 60 years of age are particularly prone to post-herpetic neuralgia (PHN). In the absence of specific contraindications, consideration should be given to prescribing short-term, high-dose corticosteroid prophylaxis for PHN in conjunction with oral acyclovir.[3,31,35]

Rx

Acyclovir (Zovirax) capsules 200 mg

Disp: 200 capsules
Sig: Take 4 capsules five times daily for 10 days.

RECURRENT APHTHOUS STOMATITIS (RAS)

ETIOLOGY

Exact etiology is unknown. An altered local immune response is postulated as the predisposing factor. Patients with frequent recurrences should be screened for conditions such as

---

* References 1, 16, 27, 30, 33, 34, 36, 40.

anemia, inflammatory bowel disease, and immunosuppression.

Precipitating factors include stress, trauma, allergies, and endocrine alterations, as well as dietary components such as acidic foods and juices, and foods that contain gluten. Inspect the oral cavity closely for sources of trauma.

CLINICAL DESCRIPTION

Minor aphthae (canker sores), less than 0.6 cm — small, shallow, painful ulcerations covered by a gray membrane and surrounded by a narrow erythematous halo — usually occur on nonkeratinized (movable) oral mucosa.

Major aphthae, greater than 0.6 cm — large, painful ulcers — are more severe and can last weeks or months. May mimic other conditions such as granulomatous and malignant lesions.

Herpetiform ulcers — crops of small, shallow, painful ulcers — can occur anywhere on the oral mucosa and resemble recurrent intraoral herpes simplex clinically but are not of viral etiology.*

RATIONALE FOR TREATMENT

Since RAS is a T-lymphocytic disease, effective treatment involves topical and/or systemic corticosteroids and immunosuppressants when indicated.

1. Topical Steroids
Rx

Triamcinolone acetonide (Kenalog) in Orabase 0.1%

Disp: 5 g tube
Sig: Coat the lesion with a thin film pc and hs.

Other topical steroid preparations include:
- Betamethasone valerate (Valisone) ointment 0.1%
- Fluocinonide (Lidex) gel 0.05%
- Fluocinonide (Lidex) ointment 0.5%
- Clobetasol propionate (Temovate) ointment 0.05% (mixing of above agents with equal part of Orabase promotes adhesion to oral mucosa)

Rx

Dexamethasone (Decadron) elixir 0.5 mg/5 ml

Disp: 100 ml
Sig: Rinse with 1 teaspoonful for 2 minutes qid and spit out.

Oral candidiasis may result from topical steroid therapy. The oral cavity should be monitored for emergence of fungal infection in patients who are placed on therapy. Prophylactic antifungal therapy should be initiated in patients with a history of fungal infections with prior steroid administration (see Candidiasis).

Nutritional supplements may be indicated (see Primary Herpetic Gingivostomatitis).

2. Systemic Steroids and Immunosuppressants*

For severe cases:

Rx

Dexamethasone (Decadron) elixir 0.5 mg/5 ml

Disp: 237 ml
Sig: (1) For 3 days, rinse with 1 tablespoonful (15 ml) qid and swallow. Then, (2) for 3 days, rinse with 1 teaspoonful (5 ml) qid and swallow. Then, (3) for 3 days, rinse with 1 teaspoonful (5 ml) qid and swallow every other time. Then, (4) rinse with 1 teaspoonful qid and spit out. Discontinue medication when mouth becomes comfortable.

If mouth discomfort recurs, begin treatment at step #3. Rinsing should be done after meals and at bedtime. Refill × 1.

For very severe cases:

Rx

Prednisone tablets 5 mg

Disp: 100 tablets
Sig: Take 9 tablets in the morning until lesions recede. Then decrease by 1 tablet qd.

Azathioprine may be prescribed concomitantly with prednisone and topical steroid rinses for managing very severe conditions of minor or major aphthae. This addition gives the clinical effects of a higher dosage of prednisone without the side effects. Azathioprine should not be taken during pregnancy.

---

* References 2, 4, 6, 8, 15, 18, 32.

* Therapy with systemic steroids and immunosuppressants is presented to inform the clinician that such modalities are available. Because of the potential for side effects, close collaboration with the patient's physician is recommended when these medications are prescribed.[4,6,26]

Rx

Azathioprine (Imuran) tablets 50 mg

> *Disp:* 30 tablets
> *Sig:* Take 1 tablet bid.

Concomitant systemic therapy with ketoconazole for candidiasis should be considered (see Candidiasis).

CANDIDIASIS
ETIOLOGY

Candida albicans, a yeastlike fungus, is an opportunistic organism that tends to proliferate with the use of broad-spectrum antibiotics, corticosteroids, medicines that reduce salivary output, and cytotoxic agents. Conditions that contribute to candidiasis include xerostomia, diabetes mellitus, poor oral hygiene, prosthetic appliances, and suppression of the immune system (i.e., AIDS or the side effects of some medications). It is important to determine the predisposing factors.

CLINICAL DESCRIPTION

Soft, white, slightly elevated plaques that usually can be wiped away, leaving an erythematous area (pseudomembranous type). Candidiasis also may appear as generalized erythematous, sensitive areas (atrophic or erythematous type) or as confluent white areas (hypertrophic form). When the clinical diagnosis is questionable, it is advisable to culture for *Candida albicans* concurrent with starting medication.

RATIONALE FOR TREATMENT

To reestablish a normal balance of oral flora and improve oral hygiene. Medication should be continued for 48 hours after disappearance of clinical signs to prevent immediate recurrence.[19,20,29,41]

1. Topical Antifungal Agents
Rx

Nystatin (Mycostatin, Nilstat) oral suspension 100,000 units/ml

> *Disp:* 60 ml
> *Sig:* Take 2-5 ml qid. Rinse for 2 minutes and swallow. Nystatin suspension has a high sugar content; therefore, good oral hygiene should be reinforced.

A few drops of nystatin oral suspension can be added to the water used for soaking acrylic prostheses.

Rx

Nystatin ointment

> *Disp:* 15 g tube
> *Sig:* Apply a thin coat to inner surface of denture and to the affected area pc.

Rx

Nystatin topical powder

> *Disp:* 15 g
> *Sig:* Apply a thin layer under the prosthesis pc.

Rx

Nystatin pastilles 200,000 u

> *Disp:* 50 pastilles
> *Sig:* Let 1 pastille dissolve in mouth five times a day.

Rx

Clotrimazole (Mycelex) troches 10 mg

> *Disp:* 70 troches
> *Sig:* Let 1 troche dissolve in mouth five times a day.

Rx

Clotrimazole (Gyne-Lotrimin, Mycelex-G) vaginal cream 1%*

> *Disp:* One tube
> *Sig:* Apply small dab to tissue side of denture or to the infected oral mucosa qid.

Rx

Miconazole nitrate (Monistat 7) vaginal cream 2%*

> *Disp:* One tube
> *Sig:* Apply small dab to tissue side of denture or to the infected oral mucosa qid.

2. Systemic Antifungal Agents

When topical therapy is not practical or is ineffective, ketoconazole (Nizoral) and fluconazole (Difuican) are effective, well tolerated, systemic drugs for mucocutaneous candidiasis. They should be used with caution in patients with impaired liver function (i.e., with a history of alcoholism or hepatitis). Liver function tests should be performed initially and conducted monthly when ketoconazole and fluconazole are prescribed for an extended period. Several drug interactions have been reported.

---

*Whereas some consultants might disagree with the use of vaginal creams intraorally, their efficacy has been observed clinically in selected cases when other topical antifungal agents have failed.

Rx

Ketoconazole (Nizoral) tablets 200 mg

Disp: 20 tablets
Sig: Take 1 tablet qd with a meal.

Rx

Fluconazole (Diflucan) tablets 100 mg

Disp: 20 tablets
Sig: Take 1 tablet qd with a meal.

CHEILITIS AND CHEILOSIS

A. ANGULAR CHEILITIS AND CHEILOSIS

ETIOLOGY

Fissured lesions in the corners of the mouth are caused by a mixed infection of the microorganisms—*Candida albicans,* staphylococci, and streptococci. Predisposing factors include local habits, drooling, a decrease in intermaxillary space, anemia, and an extension of oral infections.

CLINICAL DESCRIPTION

The commissures may appear wrinkled, red, fissured, cracked, or crusted.

RATIONALE FOR TREATMENT

Identification and correction of predisposing factors and elimination of the secondary infection. Since this is usually a mixed infection, an effective therapeutic agent is a preparation of multiple agents (e.g., Mycolog II [nystatin–triamcinolone acetonide]).*

Rx

Mycolog II (nystatin–triamcinolone acetonide) ointment

Disp: 15 g tube
Sig: Apply to affected area pc and hs. Concomitant intraoral antifungal treatment may be indicated.

B. ACTINIC CHEILITIS AND SOLAR CHEILOSIS

ETIOLOGY

Prolonged exposure to sunlight results in irreversible degenerative changes in the vermilion of the lips, especially the everted lower lip.

CLINICAL DESCRIPTION

The normal red translucent vermilion with regular vertical fissuring of a smooth surface is replaced by a white flat surface that may exhibit periodic ulceration.

RATIONALE FOR TREATMENT

If exposure to the UV light in the sun's rays is allowed to continue, the degenerative changes may progress to a malignancy. Sunscreens with a high skin protection factor (SPF 15) should be used constantly.[1,13,27]

Rx

Several over-the-counter preparations with PABA are available (e.g., PreSun 15 lotion and lip gel). For those patients allergic to PABA, Vaseline sunscreens may be prescribed.

DENTURE SORE MOUTH

ETIOLOGY

Discomfort under prosthetic appliances may result from combinations of candidal infections, poor denture hygiene, an occlusive syndrome, or overextension or excessive movement of the denture. In rare cases allergy to the denture may occur, usually caused by an uncured monomer.

CLINICAL DESCRIPTION

The tissue covered by the denture, especially one made of acrylic, is erythematous and smooth or granular. If the erythema is caused solely by candidiasis, it may be asymptomatic.

RATIONALE FOR TREATMENT

Therapy is directed toward all possible etiologies (i.e., antifungal therapy [see Candidiasis]), improvement of oral hygiene and denture hygiene, construction of a new denture, or rebasing the existing denture and leaving it unworn for extended periods. The denture should be soaked in a cleanser (e.g., 1% sodium hypochlorite for 15 minutes). Systemic conditions such as diabetes and poor nutrition should be ruled out.[19,20,29,41]

XEROSTOMIA

ETIOLOGY

Acute or chronic reduced salivary flow may result from drug therapy, mechanical blockage, dehydration, emotional stress, infection of the salivary glands, local surgery, avitaminosis, diabetes, anemia, connective tissue diseases,

---

* References 8, 15, 19, 20, 29, 41.

Sjögren's syndrome, radiation therapy, and congenital factors (e.g., ectodermal dysplasia).

CLINICAL DESCRIPTION

The tissues may be dry, pale, or red and atrophic. The tongue may be devoid of papillae, atrophic, fissured, and inflamed. Multiple carious lesions may be present, especially at the gingival margin and on exposed root surfaces.

RATIONALE FOR TREATMENT

Salivary stimulation or replacement therapy to keep mouth moist, prevention of caries and candidal infection, and palliative relief.*

1. Saliva Substitutes
Rx

Sodium carboxymethyl cellulose 0.5% aqueous solution [OTC]†

Disp: 8 fl oz
Sig: Use as a rinse prn.

Commerical saliva substitutes:
- Xero-Lube
- Salivart
- Moi-Stir
- Orex [and others]

Relief from oral dryness and accompanying discomfort can be achieved conservatively by
- Sipping water *frequently* all day long
- Letting ice melt in the mouth
- Restricting caffeine intake
- Avoiding mouth rinses that contain alcohol
- Humidifying sleeping area
- Coating lips with Vaseline

2. Saliva Stimulants

Chewing sugarless gum and/or sucking sugarless mints are conservative methods to temporarily stimulate salivary flow in patients with medication xerostomia or with salivary gland dysfunction. Patients should be cautioned against using products that contain sugar.

Rx

Pilocarpine HCl solution 1 mg per 1 ml

Disp: 100 ml
Sig: Take 1 teaspoon tid. Swish and swallow.

---

* References 10, 11, 19-21, 23, 29, 39, 41, 43.
† Generic carboxymethyl cellulose solutions may be prepared by a pharmacist.

Rx

Bethanechol chloride (Urecholine) 25 mg

Disp: 100 tablets
Sig: Take 1 tablet tid.

These cholinergic agents should be prescribed in consultation with the patient's physician.

3. Caries Prevention[22]
Rx

Stannous fluoride gel 0.4%

Disp: 24 ml bottles
Sig: Apply to teeth daily for 5 minutes—5-10 drops in a plastic carrier. The manufacturer advises not swallowing this solution.

SnF_2 gels available include:

Flo Gel	Omni-Gel	Perfect Choice
True Gel	Control	Basic Gel
Nova Gel	Gel-Pro	Gel-Tin
IDP Gel-Oh	Stan-Gard	Thera-Flur
Gel-Kam	Easy-Gel	

When the taste of acidulated SnF_2 gels is poorly tolerated or where there is etching of ceramic restorations, neutral pH sodium fluoride gel 1% (Thera-Flur-N) should be considered.

Rx

Neutral NaF gel (Thera-Flur-N) 1.0%

Disp: 24 ml
Sig: Place 1 drop/tooth in the custom tray. Apply for 5 minutes qd. Avoid rinsing or eating for 30 minutes following treatment.

FDA regulations have limited the size of bottles of fluoride because of toxicity if ingested by infants. Since most preparations do not come in child-proof bottles, the sizes of topical fluoride preparations vary; 24 ml is approximately a 2-week supply for application to a full dentition in custom carriers. Xerostomia provides an excellent environment for the overgrowth of *Candida albicans*. The patient is likely to require treatment for candidiasis along with, possibly, a prescription for the treatment of dry mouth.

In a dry oral environment, plaque control becomes more difficult. Scrupulous oral hygiene is a must for these patients.

EROSIVE LICHEN PLANUS
ETIOLOGY

Unknown. It is postulated to be an autoimmune disorder with a genetic predisposition, possibly initiated by a variety of factors including emotional stress, general debilitation, hypersensitivity to drugs, or bacterial or viral infections.

CLINICAL DESCRIPTION

Painful, eroded areas ranging in size from a few millimeters to several centimeters surrounded by characteristic radiating white striae. The lesions are commonly found on the buccal mucosa, gingiva, and tongue. They occur less frequently on the lips and palate.

Any chronic lesion should be biopsied to establish a diagnosis and to rule out a malignancy.

RATIONALE FOR TREATMENT

Systemic and local relief with anti-inflammatory and immunosuppressant agents, and treatment or prevention of a secondary fungal infection with a systemic antifungal agent.*

1. Topical Steroids
Rx

Fluocinonide (Lidex) gel 0.05%

Disp: 15 g tube
Sig: Apply to affected areas pc and hs.

Rx

Betamethasone valerate (Valisone) ointment 0.1%

Disp: 15 g tube
Sig: Apply to affected areas pc and hs.

Rx

Triamcinolone acetonide (Kenalog) in Orabase 0.1%

Disp: 5 g tube
Sig: Apply to affected areas pc and hs.

Rx

Dexamethasone (Decadron) elixir 0.5 mg/5 ml

Disp: 100 ml bottle
Sig: Rinse with 1 teaspoonful for 2 minutes qid and spit out

2. Systemic Steroids and Immunosuppressants*

For severe cases:

Rx

Dexamethasone (Decadron) elixir 0.5 mg/5 ml

Disp: 237 ml
Sig: (1) For 3 days, rinse with 1 tablespoonful (15 ml) qid and swallow. Then, (2) for 3 days, rinse with 1 teaspoonful (5 ml) qid and swallow. Then, (3) for 3 days, rinse with 1 teaspoonful (5 ml) qid and swallow every other time. Then, (4) rinse with 1 teaspoonful qid and spit out. Discontinue medication when mouth becomes comfortable.

If mouth discomfort recurs, begin treatment at step #3. Rinsing should be done after meals and at bedtime. Refill × 1.

For very severe cases:

Rx

Prednisone tablets 5 mg

Disp: 100 tablets
Sig: Take 9 tablets in the morning.

Alternate day therapy tends to reduce side effects. Concomitantly administer azathioprine.

Rx

Azathioprine (Imuran) tablets 50 mg

Disp: 30 tablets
Sig: Take 1 tablet bid.

Monitor the patient weekly and taper medications as indicated by clinical response. Discontinue if severe nausea occurs. Treatment should be in collaboration with the patient's physician.

3. Injectable Steroids

Dexamethasone phosphate injectable, one ampule (4 mg/ml), may be used in the following manner. After anesthetizing the area with lidocaine, inject 0.5 to 1 ml around margins of ulcer with a 25-gauge needle twice a week until ulcer heals.

PEMPHIGUS AND PEMPHIGOID

These are relatively uncommon oral lesions. They should be suspected when there is chronic

---

* References 1, 8, 14, 15, 24, 38.

* See comment under Recurrent Aphthous Stomatitis (p. 558) on the use of systemic steroids and immunosuppressants.

oral ulceration and a history of oral and skin blisters. Diagnosis is based on history and on the histologic and immunofluorescent characteristics of a primary lesion biopsy.[7,24,38]

TREATMENT

Either refer to a dermatologist or treat as indicated in the section on very severe lichen planus.*

BURNING MOUTH SYNDROME
ETIOLOGY

Xerostomia, candidiasis, referred pain from the tongue musculature, other chronic infections, reflux of gastric acid, medications, habits, blood dyscrasias, nutritional deficiencies, hormonal imbalances, allergic and inflammatory disorders, psychogenic factors, or idiopathic.

TREATMENT

On the basis of history, physical evaluation, and specific laboratory studies, rule out all possible organic etiologies. Minimal blood studies should include CBC and differential, glucose, iron, ferritin, folic acid, and B_{12}. For symptomatic relief, elixir of diphenhydramine (Benadryl) is a useful antihistaminic, and it also has a mild topical anesthetic effect.†

Rx

Diphenhydramine (Benadryl) elixir 12.5 mg/5 ml

Disp: 4 oz bottle
Sig: Rinse with 1 teaspoonful for 2 minutes before each meal and swallow.

If the burning mouth is considered psychogenic or idiopathic, tricyclics or benzodiazepines in low doses exhibit the properties of analgesia and sedation and are frequently successful in reducing or eliminating the symptoms after several weeks or months. Dosage is adjusted according to patient reaction and clinical symptomatology.

Rx

Amitriptyline (Elavil) tablets 25 mg

Disp: 100 tablets
Sig: Take 1 tablet hs for 1 week, then 2 tablets hs.

---

* See comment under Recurrent Aphthous Stomatitis (p. 558) on the use of systemic steroids and immunosuppressants.
† References 5, 12, 17, 22, 36, 37.

Increase to three tablets hs after 2 weeks and maintain at that dosage for several months or until symptoms clear.

Rx

Alprazolam (Xanax) tablets 0.25 mg

Disp: 100 tablets
Sig: Take 1 tablet tid.

Rx

Chlordiazepoxide (Librium) 5 mg

Disp: 30 tablets
Sig: Take 1 tablet tid.

Rx

Diazepam (Valium) 5 mg

Disp: 30 tablets
Sig: Take 1 tablet tid.

The dosage should be adjusted according to the individual response of the patient. Anticipated side effects are dry mouth and morning drowsiness. The rationale for using tricyclic antidepressant medications and other psychotropic drugs should be thoroughly explained to the patient, and the physician should also be made aware of the therapy. These medications have a potential for addiction and dependency.

CHAPPED OR CRACKED LIPS
ETIOLOGY

Alternate wetting and drying, resulting in inflammation and possible secondary infection

CLINICAL DESCRIPTION

The surface of the vermilion is rough and peeling and may be ulcerated with crusting. The normal vertical fissuring may be lost.

RATIONALE FOR TREATMENT

An interrupted and chronically inflamed surface invites secondary infection. An antiinflammatory agent in a petrolatum or adhesive base will block the irritating factors and allow healing.[8,15,36]

Rx

Betamethasone valerate (Valisone) ointment 0.1%

Disp: 15 g tube
Sig: Apply to lips pc and hs.

Prolonged use of corticosteroids can result in

thinning of the tissue and should be closely monitored.

For maintenance, the frequent application of petrolatum-based products (e.g., Chapstick, Vaseline, or cocoa butter) should be suggested.

GINGIVAL ENLARGEMENT
ETIOLOGY

Phenytoin sodium (Dilantin), calcium channel blocking agents (nifedipine and others), and cyclosporine medications may predispose some patients to gingival enlargement. Blood dyscrasias and hereditary gingival fibromatosis should be ruled out by history and laboratory tests as indicated.

CLINICAL DESCRIPTION

Gingival tissues, especially in the anterior region, are dense, resilient, insensitive, and enlarged but essentially of normal color.

RATIONALE FOR TREATMENT

Local factors, such as plaque and calculus accumulation, contribute to secondary inflammation and the hyperplastic process. This, in turn, further interferes with plaque control. Specific drugs tend to deplete serum folic acid levels, which results in compromised tissue integrity. Folic acid and drug serum levels should be determined every 6 months. This should be coordinated with the patient's physician.[9,28]

TREATMENT

Treatment consists of (1) meticulous plaque control, (2) gingivoplasty when indicated, and (3) folic acid supplement only when the serum folic acid level is low.*

Rx

Folic acid oral rinse 1 mg/ml

> *Disp:* 1 liter
> *Sig:* Rinse with 1 teaspoonful for 2 minutes bid and spit out.

---

* When testing for serum folate level, it is judicious to also check for vitamin B_{12} level since a B_{12} deficiency can be masked by the patient's use of a folic acid supplement. The phenytoin level also should be assessed for future reference.[9]

Rx

Chlorhexidine gluconate (Peridex) 0.12%

> *Disp:* 16 oz
> *Sig:* Rinse with ½ oz bid for 30 seconds and spit out. Avoid rinsing or eating for 30 minutes following treatment.

TASTE DISORDERS
ETIOLOGY

Taste acuity may be affected by both neurologic and physiologic changes and drugs. Diagnostic procedures should first rule out a neurologic deficiency, an olfactory deficit, or systemic influences such as malnutrition, metabolic disturbances, drugs, chemical and physical trauma, or radiation sequelae. Blood tests for trace elements should be conducted to identify any deficiencies.

RATIONALE FOR TREATMENT

A reduction in salivary flow may concentrate the electrolytes in the saliva, resulting in a salty or metallic taste (see treatment for xerostomia). A deficiency of zinc has been associated with a loss of taste (and smell) sensation.[35]

1. For Zinc Replacement (in Patients with Proven Zinc Deficiency)
Rx

Orazinc capsules 220 mg [OTC]

> *Disp:* 100 capsules
> *Sig:* Take 1 capsule with milk tid for at least 1 month.

Rx

Z-BEC tablets [OTC]

> *Disp:* 60 tablets
> *Sig:* Take 1 tablet qd with food or pc.

MANAGEMENT OF PATIENTS RECEIVING ANTINEOPLASTIC AGENTS AND RADIOTHERAPY
ETIOLOGY

Cancer chemotherapy and radiation to the head and neck tend to reduce the volume and alter the character of the saliva. The balance of the oral flora is disrupted allowing overgrowth of opportunistic organisms (e.g., *Candida albicans*). Also anticancer therapy damages fast-growing tissues, especially the oral mucosa.

CLINICAL APPEARANCES

The oral mucosa become red and inflamed. With radiation therapy, xerostomia develops and saliva may become viscous.

RATIONALE FOR TREATMENT

Treatment of these patients is symptomatic and supportive. Patient education, frequent monitoring, and close cooperation with the patient's physician are important.

The oral discomfort may be relieved with topical anesthetics, such as lidocaine HCl (Xylocaine) viscous, diphenhydramine elixir (Benadryl), and dyclonine (Dyclone). Artificial salivas (i.e., Moi-Stir, Salivart, Xero-Lube) will reduce oral dryness. Nystatin and clotrimazole preparations will control fungal overgrowth. Chlorhexidine rinses help control plaque and candidiasis. Fluorides can be applied for caries control. A patient information sheet that discusses this topic can be reproduced and given to the patient.*

1. Mouth Rinses
Rx

Alkaline saline (salt and bicarbonate) mouth rinse. Mix ½ teaspoonful each of salt and baking soda in a glass of water.

Sig: Rinse with copious amounts qid.

2. Gingivitis Control
Rx

Chlorhexidine gluconate mouth rinse (Peridex) 0.12%

Disp: 32 oz
Sig: Rinse with ½ oz bid for 30 seconds and spit out. Avoid rinsing or eating for 30 minutes following treatment.

In xerostomic patients, chlorhexidine (Peridex) should be used concurrently with an artificial saliva to provide the needed protein-binding agent for efficacy and substantiveness.

3. Caries Control
Rx

Neutral NaF gel (Thera-Flur-N) 1.0%

Disp: 24 ml
Sig: Place 1 drop/tooth in the custom tray; apply for

---

* References 10, 11, 19-21, 23, 29, 36, 39, 41, 43.

5 minutes qd. Avoid rinsing or eating for 30 minutes following treatment.

4. Topical Anesthetics for Pain Control
Rx

Diphenhydramine HCl (Benadryl) [OTC] elixir 12.5% mg/5 ml mixed with Kaopectate [OTC]. 50% mixture by volume.

Disp: 8 oz
Sig: Rinse with 1 teaspoonful q2h and spit out.

Maalox [OTC] can be used in place of Kaopectate. Dyclonine (Dyclone) HCl 0.5% 1 oz may be added to the above for greater anesthetic efficacy.

Rx

Lidocaine HCl (Xylocaine) viscous 2%*

Disp: 450 ml bottle
Sig: Swish with 1 teaspoonful qid and spit out.

Rx

Diphenhydramine HCl (Benadryl) [OTC] elixir 12.5 mg/5 ml

Disp: 4 oz bottle
Sig: Rinse with 1 teaspoonful for 2 minutes ac and spit out.

Rx

Dyclonine HCl (Dyclone) 0.5% or 1%†

Disp: 1 oz bottle
Sig: Rinse with 1 teaspoonful for 2 minutes ac and spit out.

5. Antifungals: Treatment for Candidiasis Control
Rx

Nystatine pastilles 200,000 u

Disp: 50 pastilles
Sig: Let 1 pastille dissolve in the mouth five times a day.

Rx

Clotrimazole (Mycelex) troches 10 mg

Disp: 70 troches
Sig: Let 1 troche dissolve in the mouth five times a day.

---

* When topical anesthetics are used, patients should be cautioned concerning reduced gag reflex and the need for care while eating and drinking to avoid possible airway compromise.

PATIENT INFORMATION SHEET

The oral regimen for patients receiving chemotherapy and radiotherapy[23] is outlined starting on p. 565. The following are general guidelines to be individualized by your doctor. Follow your doctor's advice or discuss any questions with your doctor if these guidelines differ from what you've been told or have heard.

A. Rinses
1. Rinse with warm, dilute solution of sodium bicarbonate (baking soda) or salt and bicarbonate every 2 hours to bathe the tissues and control oral acidity. Two teaspoonfuls of bicarbonate (or 1 teaspoonful of table salt plus one teaspoonful of bicarbonate) per quart of water is recommended.
2. If you are experiencing pain, rinse with 1 teaspoonful of elixir of Benadryl before each meal. Be careful when eating while your mouth is numb to avoid choking.
3. If your mouth is dry, sip cool water frequently (every 10 minutes) all day long. Allowing ice chips to melt in the mouth is comforting. Artificial salivas (e.g., Moi-Stir, Salivart, Xero-Lube, Orex) can be used as frequently as needed to make the mouth moist and "slick." Keep the lips lubricated with petrolatum or a lanolin-containing lip preparation. Commercial mouthrinses with alcohol or coffee, tea, and colas should be avoided as they tend to dry the mouth.
4. If an oral yeast infection develops, antifungal medications can be prescribed.
   a. Nystatin pastille*, let one dissolve in mouth 5 times a day or
   b. Let a 10 mg clotrimazole (Mycelex)* troche dissolve in the mouth five times a day.

B. Care of Teeth and Gums
1. Floss your teeth after each meal. Be careful not to cut the gums.
2. Brush your teeth after each meal. Use a soft even-bristle brush and a bland toothpaste containing fluoride (e.g., Aim, Crest, Colgate). Brushing with a sodium bicarbonate–water paste is also helpful. Arm & Hammer Dental Care toothpaste and tooth powder are bicarbonate based. If a toothbrush is too irritating, cotton-tip swabs (Q-Tips) or foam sticks (Toothettes) can provide some mechanical cleaning.
3. A pulsating water device (e.g., Water-Pik) will remove loose debris. Use warm water with a half teaspoonful of salt and baking soda and low pressure to prevent damage to tissue.
4. Have custom, flexible vinyl trays made by your dentist to self-apply fluoride gel to the teeth for 5 minutes once a day after brushing.
5. Rinse with an antiplaque solution (Peridex) (if prescribed by your dentist) two or three times a day when you cannot follow other oral hygiene procedures.
6. Follow any alternative oral hygiene instructions prescribed by your dentist.

C. Nutrition
Adequate nutrition and fluid intake are very important for oral and general health. Use diet supplements (e.g., Carnation Instant Breakfast, Meritene, Ensure). If your mouth is sore, a blender may be used to soften food.

D. Maintenance
Have your oral health status reevaluated at regularly scheduled intervals by your dentist.

E. Supportive
A humidifier in the sleeping area will alleviate or reduce nighttime oral dryness.

*Drugs that must be prescribed by your dentist or physician.

The above regimen is also applicable to patients with AIDS.

REFERENCES

1. Boger J, Araujo O, Flowers F: Sunscreens: efficacy, use and misuse, *South Med J* 77:1421-1427, 1984.
2. Brooke RI, Sapp JP: Herpetiform ulceration, *Oral Surg* 42:182-188, 1976.
3. Brown GR: Herpes zoster: correlation of age, sex, distribution and associated disorders, *South Med J* 69:576-587, 1976.
4. Brown RS, Bottomley WK: Combination immunosuppressant and topical steroid therapy for treatment of recurrent major aphthae, *Oral Surg* 69:42-44, 1990.
5. Browning S, Hislop S, Scully C, Shirlaw P: The association between burning mouth syndrome and psychosocial disorders, *Oral Surg* 64:171-174, 1987.
6. Burns RA, Davis WJ: Recurrent aphthous stomatitis, *Am Fam Physician* 32:99-104, 1988.
7. Bystryn JC: Adjuvant therapy of pemphigus, *Arch Dermatol* 120:941-951, 1984.
8. Dilley D, Blozis G: Common oral lesions and oral manifestations of systemic illnesses and therapies, *Pediatr Clin North Am* 29:585-611, 1982.
9. Drew HJ, Vogel RI, Molofsky W, et al: Effect of folate on phenytoin hyperplasia, *J Clin Periodontol* 14:350-356, 1987.
10. Duxbury AJ, Hayes NF, Thakkar NS, et al: Clinical trial of a mucin-containing artificial saliva, *IRCS Med Sci* 13:1197-1198, 1985.
11. Fardal O, Turnbull RS: A review of the literature on use of chlorhexidine in dentistry, *J Am Dent Assoc* 112(6):863-869, 1986.
12. Feinmann C: Pain relief by antidepressants: possible modes of action, *Pain* 23:1-8, 1985.
13. Fenske NA, Greenberg SS: Solar-induced skin changes, *Am Fam Physician* 25:109-117, 1982.
14. Gabriel SA, Jenson AB, Hartmann D, Bottomley WK: Lichen planus: possible mechanisms of pathogenesis, *J Oral Med* 40:56-59, 1985.
15. Gorsline J, Bradlow HL, Sherman MR: Triamcinolone acetonide 21-oic acid methyl ester: a potent local anti-inflammatory steroid without detectable systemic effects, *Endocrinology* 116:263-273, 1985.
16. Greenberg MS: Oral herpes simplex infections in immunosuppressed patients, *Compendium* 9(suppl):289-291, 1988.
17. Grushka M: Clinical features of burning mouth syndrome, *Oral Surg* 63:30-36, 1987.
18. Hay KD, Reade PC: The use of an elimination diet in the treatment of recurrent aphthous ulceration of the oral cavity, *Oral Surg* 57:504-507, 1984.
19. Holst E: Natamycin and nystatin for treatment of oral candidiasis during and after radiotherapy, *J Prosthet Dent* 51:226-231, 1984.
20. Hughes WT, Bartley DL, Patterson GG, Tufenkeji H: Ketoconazole and candidiasis: a controlled study, *J Infect Dis* 147:1060-1063, 1983.
21. Katz S: The use of fluoride and chlorhexidine for the prevention of radiation caries, *J Am Dent Assoc* 104(2):164-169, 1982.
22. Lamey PJ, Hammond A, Allam BF, McIntosh WB: Vitamin status of patients with burning mouth syndrome and the response to replacement therapy, *Br Dent J* 160:81-84, 1986.
23. Lang NP, Brecx MC: Chlorhexidine digluconate—an agent for chemical plaque control and prevention of gingival inflammation, *J Periodont Res* (suppl):74-89, 1986.
24. Lever WF, Schaumburg-Lever G: Treatment of pemphigus vulgaris: results obtained in 84 patients between 1961 and 1982, *Arch Dermatol* 120:44-47, 1984.
25. Loeser JD: Herpes zoster and post-herpetic neuralgia, *Pain* 25:149-164, 1986.
26. Lozada F, Silverman S Jr, Migliorati C: Adverse side effects associated with prednisone in the treatment of patients with oral inflammatory ulcerative diseases, *J Am Dent Assoc* 109(2):269-270, 1984.
27. Lundeen RC, Langlais RP, Terezhalmy GT: Sunscreen protection for lip mucosa: a review and update, *J Am Dent Assoc* 111(4):617-621, 1985.
28. O'Neil T, Figures K: The effects of chlorhexidine and mechanical methods of plaque control on the recurrence of gingival hyperplasia in young patients taking phenytoin, *Br Dent J* 152:130-133, 1982.
29. Owens NJ, Nightingdale CH, Schweizer RT, et al: Prophylaxis of oral candidiasis with clotrimmazole troches, *Arch Intern Med* 144:290-293, 1984.
30. Poland JM: The spectrum of HSV-1 infections in non-immunosuppressed patients, *Compendium* 9(suppl):320-312, 1988.
31. Portenoy RK, Duma C, Foley KM: Acute herpetic and post-herpetic neuralgia: clinical review and current management, *Ann Neurol* 20:651-664, 1986.
32. Porter SR, Scully C, Flint S: Hematologic status in recurrent aphthous stomatitis compared with other oral disease, *Oral Surg* 66:41-44, 1988.
33. Raborn GW, McGaw WT, Grace M, et al: Oral acyclovir and herpes labialis: a randomized, double-blind, placebo-controlled study, *J Am Dent Assoc* 11(1):38-42, 1987.
34. Rowe NH: Diagnosis and treatment of herpes simplex virus disease, *Compendium* 9(suppl):292-295, 1988.
35. Schiffman SS: Taste and smell in disease, *N Engl J Med* 308:1275-1279, 1337-1343, 1983.
36. Scully C, Mason DK: Therapeutic measures in oral medicine. In Jones JH, Mason DK, editors: *Oral manifestations of systemic disease*, Philadelphia, 1980, WB Saunders, pp 530-542.
37. Sharav Y, Singer E, Schmidt E, et al: The analgesic effect of amitriptyline on chronic facial pain, *Pain* 31:199-209, 1987.
38. Silverman S Jr, Gorsky M, Lozada-Nur F, Liu A: Oral mucous membrane pemphigoid, *Oral Surg* 61:233-237, 1986.
39. Sonis ST, Sonis AL, Lieberman A: Oral complications in patients receiving treatment for malignancies other than of the head and neck, *J Am Dent Assoc* 97(3):468-472, 1978.

40. Straus SE (moderator): Herpes simplex virus infection: biology, treatment and prevention, *Ann Intern Med* 103:404-419, 1988.

41. Thompson PJ, Wingfield HJ, Cosgrove RF, et al: Assessment of oral candidiasis in patients with respiratory disease and efficacy of a new nystatin formulation, *Br Med J* 292:1699-1700, 1986.

42. Wood MJ, Ogan PH, McKendrick MW, et al: Efficacy of oral acyclovir treatment of acute herpes zoster, *Am J Med* 85:79-83, 1988.

43. Wright WE, Haller JM, Harlow S, Pizzo PA: An oral disease prevention program for patients receiving radiation and chemotherapy, *J Am Dent Assoc* 110(1):43-47, 1985.

Index

A

Abuse, substance, 491-493
  dental management in, 42-45*t*
Acebutolol for hypertension, dosage ranges for, 166*t*
Acetaminophen for primary herpetic gingivostomatitis, 557
Acetone, urinary, determination of, in diabetes detection, 349
Acidosis, metabolic, in diabetes, 345
Acquired immune deficiency syndrome (AIDS), 289-315
  clinical presentation of, 295-296
  complications of, 293-295
  definition of, 289
  dental management in, 16-19*t*, 297-299
  etiology of, 293
  general description of, 291-295
  incidence of, 291-293
  laboratory findings in, 296
  medical complications of, prevention of, 299-300
  medical management of, 296-297
  oral complications of, 302, *303-305*, 305-306, 306*t*, 307*t*, 308, 308*t*, 309*t*, 310-313
  pathophysiology of, 293-295
  patient evaluation in, 300-301
  prevalence of, 291-293
  risk of, in chronic hemodialysis patient, 253
  signs and symptoms of, 295-296
  transmission of, 293-294
  treatment planning considerations in, 301-302
Actinic cheilitis, therapeutic management of, 561
Activated partial thromboplastin time (APTT) in evaluation of hemostasis, 94
Acyclovir (Zovirax)
  for genital herpes, 285
  for primary herpetic gingivostomatitis, 557
  for recurrent herpes simplex, 558
  for varicella zoster, 558
Addiction, drug, in health history, 85
Addison's disease, 363
  medical management of, 366
  pathophysiology of, 263
  signs and symptoms of, 365
Adrenal insufficiency, 361-369

Adrenal insufficiency—cont'd
  clinical presentation of, 365-366
  dental management in, 60-61*t*, 367-368
  general description of, 361-365
  incidence of, 361-363
  laboratory findings in, 365-366
  medical management of, 366-367
  pathophysiology of, 363-365
  prevalence of, 361-363
  signs and symptoms of, 365
Adrenergic inhibitors for hypertension
  considerations on, 169*t*
  dosage ranges for, 166-167*t*
Agonal rhythm, 210
Agoraphobia, 488
Agranulocytosis, dental management in, 34-35*t*, 444
AIDS related complex (ARC), dental management in, 16-17*t*
AIDS-related virus (ARV), 293
Albuterol for COPD and asthma, 240*t*
Alcohol
  abuse of, in health history, 85
  dependence on, 492-493
    incidence/prevalence of, 485
Alcoholic liver disease, 269-275
  clinical presentation of, 272
  complications of, 271
  dental management in, 52-55*t*, 272-274
  ental management in, 52-55*t*
  etiology of, 269
  general description of, 269-271
  incidence of, 269
  medical management of, 272
  pathophysiology of, 269-271
  sequelae of, 271
Aldosterone, secretion and function of, 363
Allergens, 391
Allergic reactions, infectious-type, 396
Allergy(ies), 390-411
  complications of, 392-398
  contact, 396-398
  dental management in, 399-411
    treatment planning modifications in, 406
  etiology of, 391-392
  general description of, 390-398
  in health history, 83, 86

The letter *t* after a page denotes table.

The letter *t* after a page denotes table.

The letter *t* after a page denotes table.

The letter *t* after a page denotes table.

The letter *t* after a page denotes table.

The letter *t* after a page denotes table.

The letter *t* after a page denotes table.

The letter *t* after a page denotes table.